Refractory Status Epilepticus

Xuefeng Wang • Shichuo Li
Editors

Refractory Status Epilepticus

Diagnosis and Treatment

Springer

Editors
Xuefeng Wang
Department of Neurology
The First Affiliated Hospital of Chongqing Medical University
Chongqing
China

Shichuo Li
Institute on Global Health (IGH)
Peking University & UN Consultative Committee on Life Science and Human Health (CCLH)
Beijing
China

ISBN 978-981-10-5124-1 ISBN 978-981-10-5125-8 (eBook)
DOI 10.1007/978-981-10-5125-8

Library of Congress Control Number: 2017951928

Printed on acid-free paper

This Springer imprint is published by Springer Nature
The registered company is Springer Nature Singapore Pte Ltd.
The registered company address is: 152 Beach Road, #21-01/04 Gateway East, Singapore 189721, Singapore

Abbreviations

2-DG	2-deoxy-D-glucose
5-HT	5-hydroxytryptamine
AA	Arachidonic acid
AC	Arm circumference
ADF	Acid detergent fiber
ADK	Adenosine kinase
AE	Autoimmune encephalitis
AED	Antiepileptic drug
aEEG	Amplitude integrated electroencephalogram
AERRPS	Acute encephalitis with refractory repetitive partial seizures
AMC	Arm muscle circumference
AMPA	α-amino-3-hydroxy-5-methyl-4-isoxazole-propionic acid
AMPAR	α-amino-3-hydroxy-5-methyl-4-isoxazole-propionic acid receptor
AMRF	Action myoclonus-renal failure
ANP	Atrial natriuretic peptide
AP	Action potential
ASIC	Acid sensitive ion channel
ASID	After-SE ictal discharge
ATL	Anterior temporal lobectomy
AWS	Alcohol withdrawal syndrome
BBB	Blood-brain barrier
BDNF	Brain-derived neurotrophic factor
BECTS	Benign childhood epilepsy with central temporal spikes
BHB	Beta-hydroxybutyrate
BiPED	Bilateral independent periodic epileptiform discharge
BMEI	Benign myoclonic epilepsy in infancy
BMI	Body mass index
BNP	Brain natriuretic peptide
BUN	Blood urea nitrogen
CAE	Childhood absence epilepsy
CASPR2	Contactin-associated protein-like 2
CBF	Cerebral blood flow
CBZ	Carbamazepine
C/D	Concentration/dose
cEEG	Continuous electroencephalogram
CHI	Creatinine height index
cIV-MDZ	Continuous intravenous MDZ

CK	Creatine kinase
CMV	Cytomegalovirus
CNS	Central nervous system
CO_2	Carbon dioxide
CPK	Creatine phosphokinase
CPR	Cardiopulmonary resuscitation
CPS	Complex partial seizures
CPSE	Complex partial SE
CPTII	Carnitine palmitoyltransferase type II
CRE	Creatinine
CRMP5	Collapsing response mediator protein 5
CRS	Cortical responsive stimulation
CSE	Convulsive status epilepticus
CSF	Cerebrospinal fluid
CSWS	Cerebral salt wasting syndrome
CSWS	Continuous spikes and waves during slow wave sleep
CZi	Caudal zona incerta
CZP	Clonazepam
DBS	Deep brain stimulation
DDD	Defined daily dose
DESC	Devastating epilepsy in school age children
DHA	Docosahexaenoic acid
DIC	Disseminated intravascular coagulation
DNET	Dysembryoplastic neuroepithelial tumor
DRE	Drug-resistant epilepsy
DRPLA	Dento-Rubro-Pallido-Luysian atrophy
DS	Dravet syndrome
DT	Delirium tremen
DZ/DPH	Combination diazepam and phenytoin
DZP	Diazepam
EAA	Excitatory amino acid
EBV	Epstein-Barr virus
ECG	Electrocardiography
ECS	Electroconvulsive shock
ECT	Electroconvulsive therapy
EEG	Electroencephalogram
EFNS	European Federation of Neurological Societies
eGFR	Estimated glomerular filtration rate
EGTCS	Epilepsy with generalized tonic-clonic seizures
EIMFS	Epilepsy in infancy with migrating focal seizures
EMA	Epilepsy with myoclonic absences
EMAS	Epilepsy with myoclonic-atonic seizures
EMG	Electromyogram
EPA	Eicosapentaenoic acid
EPC	Epilepsia partialis continua
EPSEP	Ege Pediatric SE Protocol
ER	Endoplasmic reticulum
ER	Epilepsy resolve

ESES	Electrical status epilepticus in sleep
FDA	Food and Drug Administration
FIRES	Fever-induced refractory epileptic encephalopathy syndrome
FLAIR	Fluid attenuated inversion recovery
GABA	γ-aminobutyric acid
GABAAR	γ-aminobutyric acid A receptor
GABAR	γ-aminobutyric acid receptor
GAD	Glutamic acid decarboxylase
GAD65	Glutamate decarboxylase 65kDa
GAD-Ab	Glutamic acid decarboxylase antibody
GalR1	Galanin receptor 1
GalR2	Galanin receptor 2
GCSE	Generalized convulsive status epilepticus
GED	Generalized epileptiform discharge
GHB	γ-hydroxybutyrate
GluR	Glutamate receptor
GPED	Generalized periodic epileptiform discharge
GRAW	Generalized periodic discharges related to anesthetic withdrawal
GTCS	Generalized tonic-clonic seizures
HDL	High-density lipoprotein
HE	Hashimoto encephalopathy
HE	Hypertensive encephalopathy
HFS	High-frequency stimulation
HIE	Hypoxic ischemic encephalopathy
HIV	Human immunodeficiency virus
hMPV	Human metapneumovirus
hPVB19	Human parvovirus B19
HS	Hypertonic saline
HSE	Herpes simplex encephalitis
HSV	Herpes simplex virus
HVPT	Hyperventilation provocation test
HVS	Hyperventilation syndrome
IAP	Intracisternal A-particle retrotransposon
ICP	Intracranial pressure
ICU	Intensive care unit
IF	Interferon
IGE	Idiopathic generalized epilepsy
IL	Interleukin
ILAE	International League Against Epilepsy
IOP	Intraocular pressure
IPG	Implantable pulse generator
IVIG	Intravenous immunoglobulin
JAE	Juvenile absence epilepsy
JME	Juvenile myoclonic epilepsy
KA	Kainic acid
KD	Ketogenic diet
KE	Ketamine
LDL	Low-density lipoprotein

LEV	Levetiracetam
LGI1	Leucine-rich glioma inactivating factor-1
LGIT	Low glycemic index treatment
LGS	Lennox-Gastaut syndrome
LKS	Landau-Kleffner syndrome
LTP	Long-term potentiation
LZP	Lorazepam
MAD	Modified Atkins diet
MAE	Myoclonic-atonic epilepsy
MAP	Mean arterial pressure
MCT	Medium chain triglyceride
MDPB	Mega-dose of phenobarbital
MDZ	Midazolam
mEPSC	Miniature excitatory postsynaptic current
MERRF	Myoclonic epilepsy with ragged red fiber
MFS	Mossy fiber sprouting
MGSE	Myoclonus-generalized status epilepticus
mIPSC	Miniature inhibitory postsynaptic current
MN	Metanephrine
MNA	Mini nutritional assessment
MNA-SF	The short form of the mini nutritional assessment
MPSI	Migrating partial seizures in infancy
MRI	Magnetic resonance imaging
MUST	Malnutrition universal screening tool
NAC	Nucleus accumbens
NCL	Neuronal ceroid lipofuscinosis
NCS	Neurocritical Care Society
NCSE	Nonconvulsive status epilepticus
NGF	Nerve growth factor
NICU	Neonatal intensive care unit
NICU	Neurology intensive care unit
NMDA	N-methyl-D-aspartic acid
NMDAR	N-methyl-D-aspartic acid receptor
NMN	Normetanephrine
NORSE	New-onset refractory status epilepticus
NPE	Neurogenic pulmonary edema
NPSLE	Neuropsychiatric systemic lupus erythematosus
NPY	Neuropeptide Y
NREM	Non-rapid eye movement
NRS	Nutritional risk screening
NSE	Neuron-specific enolase
OXC	Oxcarbazepine
PAWSS	Prediction of alcohol withdrawal severity scale
PB	Phenobarbital
PCS	Prolonged convulsive seizure
PE	Plasma exchange
PEBT	Partial exchange of blood therapy
PED	Periodic epileptiform discharge

PERSE	Refractory status epilepticus in patients with pre-existing epilepsy
PGES	Postictal generalized electroencephalography suppression
PG-SGA	Patient-generated subjective global assessment
pHyp	Posterior hypothalamus
PIKK	Phosphatidylinositol kinase-related kinase
PKC	Protein kinase C
PLED	Periodic lateral epileptiform discharge
PME	Progressive myoclonic epilepsy
PNES	Psychogenic nonepileptic seizures
PRIS	Propofol infusion syndrome
PRL	Prolactin
PSE	Pseudostatus epilepticus
PSE	Psychiatric side effect
PTZ	Pentylenetetrazole
PUFA	Polyunsaturated fatty acid
RAAS	Renin-angiotensin-aldosterone system
RAS	Renin angiotensin system
RCT	Randomized controlled trial
RE	Refractory epilepsy
RGCSE	Refractory generalized convulsive status epilepticus
rhEPO	Recombinant human erythropoietin
RNS	Responsive neurostimulator system
ROS	Reactive oxygen species
RPE	Reversible posterior encephalopathy
RSE	Refractory status epilepticus
SAGE	Serial analysis of gene expression
SBP	Systolic blood pressure
SE	Status epilepticus
SEP	Somatosensory evoked potential
SIADH	Syndrome of inappropriate antidiuretic hormone
SLE	Systemic lupus erythematosus
SMEI	Severe myoclonic epilepsy in infancy
SNR	Substantia nigra pars reticulata
SOD	Superoxide dismutase
SREAT	Steroid-responsive encephalopathy associated with autoimmune thyroiditis
SRSE	Super-refractory status epilepticus
SRS	Spontaneous recurrent seizure
SSRI	Selective serotonin reuptake inhibitor
SSTR	Somatostatin receptor
STESS	Status Epilepticus Severity Score
STN	Subthalamic nucleus
SUDEP	Sudden unexpected death in epilepsy
SV2A	Synaptic vesicle protein 2A
SWI	Spike-wave index
TBM	Tuberculous meningitis
TDM	Therapeutic drug monitoring

T1DM	Type 1 diabetes mellitus
TG-Ab	Thyroglobulin antibody
TLE	Temporal lobe epilepsy
TNF	Tumor necrosis factor
TPO-Ab	Thyroid peroxidase antibody
TSF	Triceps skinfold thickness
TSWA	Typical spike-and-wave activity
ULD	Unverricht-Lundborg disease
VEGF	Vascular endothelial growth factor
VEM	Video-EEG monitoring
VGCC	Voltage-gated calcium channel
VGKC	Voltage-gated potassium channel
VNS	Vagus nerve stimulation
VPA	Valproic acid
VTA	Ventral tegmental area
VZV	Varicella-zoster virus
WHO	World Health Organization
WNV	West Nile virus

Contents

Contributor List

We would like to thank the following authors for their participation in the preparation of this book:
Baobing Gao, Fei Xiao, Feng Li, Fangshuo Zheng, Guibo Feng, Hong Tang, Jing Jin, Kaiyan Tao, Peijia Lin, Qingxia Lin, Ruijiao Zhou, Tao Xu, Wei Jiang, Weixiang Liu, Xiaoyan Yang, Xin Xu, Xi Lu, Xinyuan Yu, Xin Tian, Yujiao Zhang, Yixue Gu, Yafei Shangguan, Yong Yang, Yanke Zhang, Yao Fang, Yi Yang, Yun Li, Yaxi Luo, Yuting Jiang, Ying Chen, Zijun Lin.

1 Epilepsy, Status Epilepticus, and Refractory Status Epilepticus

Yangmei Chen and Shichuo Li

Abstract

Epilepsy is a common nervous system disease that affects approximately 65 million people worldwide. Because it has diverse clinical manifestations, epilepsy is difficult to diagnose and treat. In contrast to epilepsy, status epilepticus (SE) is not self-terminating. The International League Against Epilepsy (ILAE) classifies SE into two types, SE with prominent motor symptoms and SE without prominent motor symptoms, which primarily include convulsive status epilepticus (CSE) and nonconvulsive status epilepticus (NCSE), respectively. Additionally, complex partial seizures, which are the main presentation in NCSE, have complex clinical manifestations. Refractory status epilepticus (RSE) is resistant to anti-SE drugs and requires special treatment to induce termination. It is currently thought that if the seizure does not terminate or reoccurs after 2–3 types of anti-SE drugs have been administered, it should be classified as RSE. In this chapter, we introduce the definitions, classifications, and clinical features of and evaluations used in epilepsy, SE, and RSE. Moreover, we describe what is currently known regarding epilepsy and SE with a focus on new opinions regarding RSE. Throughout this discussion, we present our own views, and we hope to provide a solid foundation for the studies described in the other chapters presented in this book.

1.1 Epilepsy

Epilepsy is a common and frequently occurring disease, with a morbidity of 7% according to epidemiological investigations. The World Health Organization (WHO) estimates that approximately 65 million patients suffer from epilepsy worldwide, and the disease can occur at any age, but it is especially prevalent among teenagers and the elderly.

Y. Chen (✉)
Department of Neurology, The Second Affiliated Hospital of Chongqing Medical University, 76 Linjiang Road, Yuzhong District, Chongqing 400010, China
e-mail: chenym1997@sina.com

S. Li
China Association Against Epilepsy (CAAE), Rm. 5102, Building 2, Beijing Exhibition Center Hotel, 135 Xizhimenwai Avenue, Xicheng District, Beijing 100044, People's Republic of China

X. Wang, S. Li (eds.), *Refractory Status Epilepticus*, DOI 10.1007/978-981-10-5125-8_1

1.1.1 Definition of Epilepsy

Epilepsy originates from the Greek word "epilepsia," which refers to recurrent seizures with different characteristics and levels. The definition of epilepsy summarizes the intrinsic characteristics of epilepsy in the pithiest and most concise scientific language. This definition is not only the guideline for clinical and research studies of epilepsy but also of vital importance for governments and institutions to establish social activities related to disability, pensions, driving vehicles, education, and employment. Therefore, experts from different eras of epileptology use different terminology to express the perception of epilepsy, giving it new definitions by adding new connotations to this old term based on a new understanding of the disease [1].

Written records related to epilepsy can date back to over 4000 years ago, and over this time, the definition of epilepsy has developed due to an increased understanding of the disease. In the Middle Ages, epilepsy was considered a result of possession; in the early eighteenth century, epilepsy was viewed as a phenomenon that occurred due to an unpredictable sudden excessive release of energy accumulated in a localized part of the brain. In the nineteenth century, Jackson proposed that epilepsy was an occasional, sudden, excessive, rapid, and self-limited discharge of gray matter. With the constant development of human bioscience, recognition of epilepsy has rapidly increased in the past 30 years, and its definition has been updated more frequently.

In 2001, the ILAE defined epilepsy as "a clinical manifestation with brain dysfunction resulting from sudden, paroxysmal, transient and abnormal discharge of cortical and deep nuclei, part of the thalamus and gray matter neurons in upper brain stem" [1].

In 2005, the ILAE defined epileptic seizures and epilepsy [2], and the condition of epileptic seizures was defined as "a transient occurrence of signs and/or symptoms due to abnormal excessive or synchronous neuronal activity in the brain." Meanwhile, the conceptual definition of epilepsy was established as follows: "Epilepsy is a disorder of the brain characterized by an enduring predisposition to generate epileptic seizures, and by the neurobiological, cognitive, psychological and social consequences of this condition. The definition of epilepsy requires the occurrence of at least one epileptic seizure." The core element of this definition is "enduring epileptogenic tendency or recurrent predisposition," which summarizes the essential features of epilepsy in an abstract and theoretical manner. However, this definition, to a certain extent, lacks operability and practicability in clinical practice.

In 2008, French et al. [3] proposed the practical definition of epilepsy, which requires at least two epileptic seizures without other diseases or situational inducements before seizures. This definition gives specific parameters to quantify the essential characteristics of epilepsy and provides good clinical operability. Verified by long-term clinical and epidemiological studies, the practicability of this definition is widely recognized, but it still has some deficiencies; for example, it requires at least two epileptic seizures. However, in clinical practice, patients with a high risk of recurrence should be given antiepileptic treatment after the first epileptic seizure, and these patients cannot be diagnosed as epileptics according to the old definition; moreover, this definition does not cover reflex epilepsy, nor does it define the resolution time of epilepsy.

To meet the requirements of clinical practice, the ILAE released a new practical definition of epilepsy in 2014 [4], which considers epilepsy as a brain disease, and its diagnosis must meet the following criteria: (a) at least two unprovoked (or reflex) epileptic seizures occurring more than 24 h apart; (b) one unprovoked (or reflex) seizure and a probability of further seizures similar to the general recurrence risk (at least 60%) after two unprovoked seizures, occurring over the next 10 years; and (c) diagnosis of an epilepsy syndrome. This definition added the diagnosis of reflex epilepsy based on the old definition. The risk of recurrence (at least 60%) in the definition is subjective and difficult to determine; nevertheless, it has positive effects on seizure control with the purpose of establishing an early diagnosis and initiating treatment measures. In clinical practice, epileptic seizures after stroke, infection, and trauma are conditions that result in a more than 60% risk of recurrence. The ILAE suggests that if a doctor cannot determine the risk of the recurrence accurately, the first criterion should be adopted, namely, a diagnosis should be made after the second seizure.

Epilepsy syndrome is an epileptic phenomenon consisting of a group of signs and symptoms. In general, once an epilepsy syndrome is diagnosed, epilepsy is diagnosed; however, in rare cases, sparse epileptic activity occurs in some types of epilepsy, such as benign epilepsy of childhood with centrotemporal spikes, epilepsy with continuous spike-and-waves during slow-wave sleep, and Landau–Kleffner syndrome. Therefore, the third criterion in the new definition highlights that the diagnosis of epilepsy and epilepsy syndrome can be made under certain circumstances even without seizures. In the new practical definition of epilepsy, a new terminology was specifically proposed, epilepsy resolve (ER), which includes epileptic individuals who had an age-dependent epilepsy syndrome but are now past the applicable age or those who have remained seizure-free for the past 10 years, with no seizure medications for the past 5 years [4]. It is different from "relieved" and "cure"; ER is a condition of individuals without epilepsy at present, but the condition may recur in the future. Compared to the old definition, the new definition is more applicable to clinical diagnosis and more accepted by current experts of epileptology, which improves the management and prognosis of epileptics.

1.1.2 Classification of Epilepsy

In 1960, the ILAE first released the classification of epileptic seizures, but it has constantly changed due to various types of epileptic seizures and complex clinical manifestations. Currently, common classifications are based on the types of epileptic seizures or epilepsy syndrome.

In 1981, the ILAE proposed the international classification of epileptic seizures (Table 1.1) [5]. This classification is based on two criteria: (a) seizures originating from unilateral or bilateral hemispheres and (b) whether a loss of consciousness occurs during seizures. The classification mainly depends on the clinical manifestations and characteristics of electroencephalogram (EEG) when seizures occur. Partial seizures constitute a condition in which the EEG and initial manifestations of seizures indicate that they are generated from a unilateral hemisphere without loss of consciousness, while generalized seizures are generated from the bilateral hemispheres with a loss of consciousness.

Table 1.1 International classification of epileptic seizures (ILAE 1981)

I. Partial seizures (originating from one side of the cerebral hemisphere)	Simple partial seizures (consciousness not impaired)	With motor signs With somatosensory or special sensory symptoms With autonomic symptoms or signs With psychic symptoms
	Complex partial seizures (with impairment of consciousness)	Simple partial onset, followed by impairment of consciousness With impairment of consciousness at onset
	Partial seizures evolving into secondarily generalized seizures	Simple partial seizures evolving into generalized seizures Complex partial seizures evolving into generalized seizures Simple partial seizures evolving into complex partial seizures then evolving into generalized seizures
II. Generalized seizures	Absence seizures and atypical absence seizures Myoclonic seizures Clonic seizures Tonic seizures Tonic–clonic seizures Atonic seizures	
III. Unclassified epileptic seizures	Epileptic seizures that cannot be classified due to inadequate or incomplete data and some that defy classification in the described categories	

Reproduced with permission from ILAE [5]

In 1989, the ILAE proposed the revised classification of epilepsies and epileptic syndromes (Table 1.2) [6]. This classification integrated the etiology, pathogenesis, clinical manifestations, evolution, and therapeutic effects of epilepsy, which provided a good basis for clinical and research studies at that time and promoted the study of epileptology.

However, due to the constantly increasing understanding of epilepsy, the old classification gradually became limited. In 2001, the ILAE proposed the international classification of epileptic seizures and epilepsy syndrome (Table 1.3) [1]. This classification continued "the dichotomy" proposed in 1981 but classified SE as a unique type of seizure because the treatment and prognosis are different from self-limited epileptic seizures. Therefore, it is more practical for clinical application.

In 2010, the ILAE again revised the classification of epileptic seizures (Table 1.4) [7]. This classification retained "the dichotomy" of

Table 1.2 International classification of epilepsy syndrome (1989)

I. Localization related (focal, local, partial)	Idiopathic (with age-related onset)	Benign childhood epilepsy with centrotemporal spikes Childhood epilepsy with occipital paroxysms Primary reading epilepsy
	Symptomatic	Temporal lobe epilepsy Frontal lobe epilepsy Occipital lobe epilepsy Partial lobe epilepsy Persistent focal epilepsy Syndromes characterized by seizures with specific modes of precipitation
	Cryptogenic	Types of seizures, clinical features, etiology, and anatomic structures should be confirmed
II. Generalized epilepsy	Idiopathic (with age-related onset)	Benign neonatal familial convulsions Benign neonatal convulsions Benign myoclonic epilepsy in infancy Childhood absence epilepsy (pyknolepsy) Juvenile absence epilepsy Juvenile myoclonic epilepsy (impulsive petit mal) Epilepsy with generalized tonic–clonic seizures on awakening Other generalized idiopathic epilepsy Epilepsies with seizures precipitated by specific modes of activation
	Cryptogenic or symptomatic	Infantile spasms (West syndrome) Lennox–Gastaut syndrome Epilepsy with myoclonic–astatic seizures Epilepsy with myoclonic absences
	Symptomatic	Nonspecific etiology Early myoclonic encephalopathy Early infantile epileptic encephalopathy with suppression bursts Other symptomatic generalized epilepsies not defined above
	Specific syndrome	Epileptic seizures with other diseases
III. Epilepsy and syndrome undetermined whether focal or generalized	With both generalized and focal seizures	Neonatal seizures Severe myoclonic epilepsy in infancy Epilepsy with continuous spike-and-waves during slow-wave sleep Acquired epileptic aphasia (Landau–Kleffner syndrome) Other undetermined epilepsies not defined above
	Without unequivocal generalized or focal features	
IV. Special syndromes	Febrile convulsions	
	Isolated seizures or isolated status epilepticus	
	Seizures occurring only when in the presence of an acute metabolic or toxic event (alcohol, drugs, eclampsia, nonketotic hyperglycemia)	

Reproduced with permission from ILAE [6]

Table 1.3 International classification of epileptic seizures and epilepsy syndrome (ILAE 2001)

ILAE International Classification of epileptic seizures and epileptic syndrome		
I. Self-limited seizures	Generalized epilepsy	Tonic–clonic seizures Tonic seizures Clonic seizures Typical absence seizures Atypical absence seizures Myoclonic absence seizures Myoclonic seizures Myoclonic–atonic seizures Atonic seizures Eyelid myoclonia Negative myoclonic seizures Spasm (mainly infantile spasms) Reflex seizures in generalized epilepsy syndromes
	Focal seizures	Focal sensory seizures Focal motor seizures (including epileptic automatism) Gelastic seizures Hemiclonic seizures Secondarily generalized seizures Reflex seizures in focal epilepsy syndromes
II. Continuous seizures	Generalized status epilepticus	Generalized tonic–clonic status epilepticus Tonic status epilepticus Clonic status epilepticus Myoclonic status epilepticus Absence status epilepticus
	Focal status epilepticus	Epilepsia partialis continua of Kojevnikov Aura continua Limbic status epilepticus Hemiconvulsive status with hemiparesis

International classification of epileptic syndrome (ILAE)	
Benign familial neonatal seizures	Idiopathic photosensitive occipital lobe epilepsy
Early myoclonic encephalopathy	Other visual-sensitive epilepsies
Ohtahara syndrome	Primary reading epilepsy
Migrating partial seizures of infancy	Startle epilepsy
West syndrome	Autosomal dominant nocturnal frontal lobe epilepsy
Benign myoclonic epilepsy in infancy	Familial temporal lobe epilepsies
Benign familial infantile seizures	Generalized epilepsy with febrile seizures plus
Benign infantile seizures (nonfamilial)	Familial focal epilepsy with variable foci
Dravet syndrome (DS)	Symptomatic (or likely symptomatic) focal epilepsies
Hemiconvulsion–hemiplegia (HH) syndrome	Limbic epilepsies
Myoclonic status in nonprogressive encephalopathies	Medial temporal lobe epilepsy with hippocampal sclerosis
Benign childhood epilepsy with centrotemporal spikes	Medial temporal lobe epilepsy defined by specific etiologies
Early-onset benign childhood occipital epilepsy Late-onset childhood occipital epilepsy (Gastaut type) Epilepsy with myoclonic absences	Other types defined by location and etiology Neocortical epilepsies Rasmussen syndrome
Epilepsy with myoclonic–astatic seizures	Other types defined by location and etiology

(continued)

Table 1.3 (continued)

ILAE International Classification of epileptic seizures and epileptic syndrome	
Lennox–Gastaut syndrome Landau–Kleffner syndrome (LKS) Epilepsy with continuous spike-and-waves during slow-wave sleep (other than LKS) Childhood absence epilepsy	Conditions with epileptic seizures that do not require a diagnosis of epilepsy Benign neonatal convulsions Febrile convulsion Reflex seizures
Progressive myoclonic epilepsy	Alcohol-withdrawal seizures
Idiopathic generalized epilepsies with variable phenotypes Juvenile absence epilepsy Juvenile myoclonic epilepsy Epilepsy with generalized tonic–clonic seizures only	Drug or other chemically induced seizures Immediate and early posttraumatic seizures Single seizures or isolated clusters of seizures Rarely repeated seizures (oligoepilepsy)
Reflex epilepsy	

Reproduced with permission from Parra et al. [1]

Table 1.4 International classification of epileptic seizures and transitional classification of epilepsy and epilepsy syndrome (ILAE 2010)

International classification of epileptic seizures (IALE)		
I. Generalized seizures	Tonic–clonic seizures	
	Absence seizures	Typical absence seizures
		Atypical absence seizures
		Absence with special manifestations (myoclonic absence seizures, eyelid myoclonic seizures)
	Myoclonic	Myoclonic seizures
		Myoclonic atonic seizures
		Myoclonic tonic seizures
	Clonic seizures	
	Tonic seizures	
	Atonic seizures	
II. Focal seizures	Specifically explained by a particular situation	
III. Unclassified seizures	Epileptic spasms	
Transitional classification of epilepsy and epileptic syndrome (ILAE): electroclinical syndromes and other epilepsies		
Electroclinical syndrome classified by age at onset[a]	Neonatal period (0–30 days)	Benign familial neonatal epilepsy (BFNE) Early myoclonic encephalopathy (EME) Ohtahara syndrome
	Infancy (1 month–2 years old)	Epilepsy of infancy with migrating focal seizures West syndrome Myoclonic epilepsy in infancy (MEI) Benign infantile epilepsy Benign familial infantile epilepsy Dravet syndrome Myoclonic encephalopathy in nonprogressive disorders

Table 1.4 (continued)

International classification of epileptic seizures (IALE)		
	Childhood (2–12 years old)	Febrile seizures plus (FS+, can start in infancy) Panayiotopoulos syndrome Epilepsy with myoclonic atonic (previously astatic) seizures Benign epilepsy with centrotemporal spikes (BECTS) Autosomal dominant nocturnal frontal lobe epilepsy (ADNFLE) Late-onset childhood occipital epilepsy (Gastaut type) Epilepsy with myoclonic absence Lennox–Gastaut syndrome Epileptic encephalopathy with continuous spike-and-wave during sleep (CSWS)[b] Landau–Kleffner syndrome (LKS) Childhood absence epilepsy (CAE)
	Adolescence-adult (≥12 years old)	Juvenile absence epilepsy (JAE) Juvenile myoclonic epilepsy (JME) Epilepsy with generalized tonic–clonic seizures alone Progressive myoclonic epilepsies (PME) Autosomal dominant epilepsy with auditory features (ADEAF) Other familial temporal lobe epilepsies
	Variable onset age	Familial focal epilepsy with variable foci (childhood to adult) Progressive myoclonie epilepsy (PME) Reflex epilepsy
Other epilepsies/ surgical syndrome	Medial temporal lobe epilepsy with hippocampal sclerosis (MTLE with HS)	
	Rasmussen syndrome	
	Gelastic seizures with hypothalamic hamartoma	
	Hemiconvulsion–hemiplegia epilepsy	
Other epilepsies not defined above	Epilepsies that do not fit into any of these diagnostic categories can be distinguished first based on the presence or absence of a known structural or metabolic condition (presumed cause) and then according to the primary mode of seizure onset (generalized vs. focal)	
Non-syndrome epilepsy	Epilepsy attributed to and organized by structural-metabolic causes	Malformations of cortical development (hemimegalencephaly, heterotopias, etc.) Neurocutaneous syndromes (tuberous sclerosis complex, Sturge–Weber, etc.) Tumor, infection, trauma, angioma, perinatal insults, stroke, etc.
	Epilepsy with unknown causes	
Conditions with epileptic seizures that are traditionally not diagnosed as a form of epilepsy	Febrile seizures (FS) Benign neonatal syndrome (BNS)	

Reproduced with permission from Berg et al. [7]
[a]The order of electroclinical syndrome does not reflect the etiology
[b]Sometimes indicates electrical status epilepticus in slow-wave sleep (ESES)

seizures and suggested calling partial seizures as focal seizures; it also suggested eliminating the further classification of seizures (simple and complex seizures). However, it proposed that focal seizures could be described in detail if needed. Meanwhile, the ILAE revised the definition of focal epileptic seizures and generalized epileptic seizures. Focal epileptic seizures are seizures that constantly originate from a unilateral hemisphere, with a localized or more widely distributed epileptogenic network. These seizures have a benign discharge pathway and can subsequently involve the other hemisphere. Focal seizures may originate from subcortical structures. Although some patients have more than one epileptogenic network and various seizure types, the onset site is constant for each seizure type. Generalized epileptic seizures are seizures that originate from one point in the bilateral cerebral cortices or epileptogenic networks composed of cortices and subcortical structures and quickly spread to the entire network. The onset site is variable for each seizure, and the entire cortex may not be involved when generalized seizures, which can be asymmetric, occur. In 2010, the ILAE proposed the transitional classification of epilepsy and epilepsy syndrome, using age as the main factor (Table 1.4) [7]. However, during practical application, the type of disease constantly changes with increasing age, and therefore the clinical practicability of this classification is much lower than the classifications proposed in 1981 and 2001. Currently, various classifications include only a summary of the disease to facilitate drug development and clinical and basic research of drugs, without describing the characteristics of epileptic seizures or epilepsy syndrome.

1.1.3 Refractory Epilepsy (RE)

Epilepsy is a curable disease, and approximately 80% of epileptic seizures can be controlled with current therapies; however, it is still difficult for the other 20% of epileptics to obtain satisfactory relief with available treatments, and this type of epilepsy is called RE. The basis of RE is that epilepsies and epilepsy syndrome have been proven to be refractory or cannot be terminated by current antiepileptic treatments during the effective treatment period. RE, in a broad sense, is epilepsy that cannot be terminated or undergo a significant reduction in seizures using current therapies, including drugs, operations, and vagus nerve stimulations. In narrow sense, RE is limited to drug-resistant epilepsy (DRE). DRE, in a broad sense, is epilepsy that cannot be completely controlled by current antiepileptic drugs (AEDs). With the introduction of new AEDs, epilepsy that can be treated is no longer called DRE. DRE, in narrow sense, is limited to epilepsy that cannot be completely controlled by first-line AEDs, such as carbamazepine, phenytoin sodium, valproic acid, phenobarbital, and ethosuximide [8, 9].

In 2010, the ILAE released a definition of DRE, namely, "failure of adequate trials of two tolerated and appropriately chosen and used AED schedules (whether as monotherapies or in combination) to achieve sustained seizure freedom" [10]. In this definition, "two AEDs" refer to monotherapy or combined therapy; "appropriately" refers to drug selection based on seizure types; "tolerated" refers to tolerable side effects or no significant side effects; "properly used AED" refers to a sufficient course of treatment and defined daily dose (DDD), which is consistent with the average daily dose of AEDs defined by the WHO (Table 1.5) [11]. For the practical application of this definition, the ILAE gave detailed methods to measure the treatment outcome of patients through the treatment outcome of drugs, thus determining whether to diagnose epilepsy as DRE (Tables 1.6 and 1.7). The current definition of DRE released by the ILAE in 2010 is the most practicable definition, which is widely used by clinicians.

Table 1.5 Defined daily doses (DDD) of AEDs (WHO)

Name of drug	DDD (mg)	50% DDD (mg)
Carbamazepine	1000	500
Clonazepam	8	4
Gabapentin	1800	900
Lacosamide	300	150
Levetiracetam	1500	750
Oxcarbazepine	1000	500
Lamotrigine	300	150
Phenobarbital	100	50
Valproic acid	1500	750
Phenytoin	300	150
Pregabalin	300	150
Tiagabine	30	15

Reproduced with permission from the WHO [11]

Table 1.6 Scheme for categorizing outcome of an intervention for epilepsy

Outcome	Definition	Side effect	Classification
I. Successful	Remission period reaches 12 months or 3 times the seizure interval before treatment	A: Yes B: No C: Undetermined	1A 1B 1C
II. Failed	Treatment is not effective	A: Yes B: No C: Undetermined	2A 2B 2C
III. Undetermined	Information is insufficient to evaluate therapeutic effects and/or the evaluation is interrupted by side effects	A: Yes B: No C: Undetermined	3A 3B 3C

Reproduced with permission from Kwan et al. [10]

Table 1.7 Outcomes of AED treatments in epileptics

Therapeutic review	Definition
Effectiveness	After treatment with the current AED, the remission period of epileptics reaches 12 months or 3 times the seizure interval before treatment
Drug resistance	Failure of effective seizure control after administrating two types of appropriate and tolerated drugs with proper use of AED schedules (reasonable dose and regimen)
Undetermined conditions	Failing to meet the diagnosed standard of effectiveness or ineffectiveness

Reproduced with permission from Kwan et al. [10]

1.2 Status Epilepticus

The "transient" type of epileptic seizures emphasizes the duration, indicating that a seizure starts suddenly and ends quickly, while SE involves epileptic seizures with a long duration of seizure or recurrent seizure without complete recovery of consciousness during seizure intervals. The duration of an epileptic seizure is the key to distinguishing an ordinary seizure and SE. Due to a lack of substantial epidemiological, clinical, and animal experimental evidence, the definition of SE was obscure and inaccurate until the 1990s—SE was regarded as a seizure with a long duration or a fixed and enduring condition that resulted from repeated epileptic seizures. No concise definition exists for the time standard of SE, and no corresponding classification of SE is described in previous definitions [12].

1.2.1 Definition of SE

In 1993, the ILAE defined SE as "a single epileptic seizure of >30 min in duration or a series of epileptic seizures during which function is not regained between ictal events in a >30-min period" [13]. This definition listed specific time limits for the diagnosis of SE, facilitating the clinical application. However, subsequent research showed that a longer duration results in a poorer prognosis. Thus, SE should be terminated as soon as possible. Subsequently, Lowenstein et al. defined SE among adults and children over 5 years old as (a) one generalized convulsive seizure that lasts for more than 5 min or (b) recurrent generalized convulsive seizures without recovery (returning to baseline) between seizures [14]. This definition increased the standard of SE to 5 min mainly due to two reasons. On one hand, both video-EEG and clinical research found that most single clinical or EEG-suggested epileptic seizure could self-terminate within 5 min, but epileptic seizures that lasted for more than 5 min rarely self-terminated and could easily evolve into SE. On the other hand, animal experiments indicated that 30 min of epileptic seizures could lead to permanent injury of the central nervous system (CNS) and RSE. Therefore, most clinicians recognized "≥5 min" as the standard to diagnose SE, advocating early and timely treatments of SE to reduce CNS injury and RSE. In 2010, the European Federation of Neurological Societies (EFNS) released the EFNS guideline on the management of SE, which did not give an explicit standard for SE diagnosis (5 min, 10 min, or 30 min) due to the tremendous controversy

Table 1.8 Historical evolution of the definition of SE

Time	Definition of SE
1904	A status of frequent epileptic seizures; with consciousness impairment during the epileptic seizure intervals [21]
1940	The most serious epileptic seizures; convalescence becoming shorter for relapses of epileptic seizures [22]
1964	One seizure with a long duration (no explicit time) or a fixed and enduring condition resulting from repeated epileptic seizures [23]
1981	One seizure with a long duration (no explicit time), or recurrent epilepsy, without recovery of consciousness during seizure intervals [5]
1993	ILAE considered: (a) a single seizure lasting for more than 30 min; (b) a series of epileptic seizures of more than 30 min, during which function is not regained between ictal events in a >30-min period. Although this definition is disputed, it is well accepted by the majority of epilepsy societies and clinicians and is widely used [13]
1998	Treiman et al. first defined 10 min as the shortest time of SE and regarded this as an inclusive criterion for subjects. The research results suggest that early SE termination can significantly decrease mortality and disability [24]
1999	Lowenstein et al. proposed one generalized convulsive seizure lasting for more than 5 min or recurrent generalized convulsive seizures with incomplete recovery of consciousness during seizure intervals [14]
2015	ILAE: Status epilepticus is a condition caused either by the failure of the mechanisms responsible for seizure termination or by the initiation of mechanisms that lead to abnormally prolonged seizures (after time point t1) or a condition that can have long-term consequences (after time point t2), consisting of neuronal death, neural injury, and alteration of neural networks, which depends on the type and duration of seizures [17]

among neurologists in European countries [15]. In 2012, "≥5 min" was suggested as the time standard for SE diagnosis in the guidelines published by the Neurocritical Care Society (NCS) (Table 1.8) [16].

In 2015, the ILAE proposed a definition and classification of SE [17]. The revised definition of SE is more detailed and improves clinical practice. The definition is as follows: status epilepticus is a condition caused either by the failure of the mechanisms responsible for seizure termination or by the initiation of mechanisms that lead to abnormally prolonged seizures (after time point t1) or a condition that can have long-term consequences (after time point t2), consisting of neuronal death, neural injury, and alteration of neural networks, which depends on the type and duration of seizures. To facilitate clinical use, the definition includes two time points (t1 and t2). In the case of generalized convulsive (tonic–clonic) SE, t1 and t2 are defined as 5 min and 30 min, respectively. In the case of focal SE with impairment of consciousness, t1 is defined as 10 min, and t2 is 60 min. In cases of other types of SE, evidence is not sufficient to define the two time points. The clinical significance and indications vary between t1 and t2. The seizures should be regarded as "continuous epileptic activity" when the period of seizures exceeds time point t1, indicating the initiation of SE treatment in clinical practice. When the duration of seizures exceeds t2, a risk of long-term consequences caused by SE is present, and a more active treatment should be adopted in clinical practice to prevent long-term consequences [17].

1.2.2 Classification of SE

The classification of SE is mainly based on the semiology of epileptic seizures (types of seizures), EEG findings during the period, interval of seizures, anatomical structures, etiology, and age of the patient. In 1981, the ILAE suggested that SE should be classified as focal SE (such as Jacksonian seizures) and generalized SE (including absence seizures and tonic–clonic seizures), which is primarily consistent with the types of seizures and EEG results [5]. In 2001, the ILAE proposed a more detailed classification of SE based on the types of seizures and EEG results (Table 1.9) [18].

Table 1.9 Classifications of SE (ILAE 2001; America NCS 2012)

ILAE Classification (2001)
I. Generalized SE
Tonic–clonic SE
Clonic SE
Absence SE
Tonic SE
Myoclonic SE
II. Focal SE
Kojevnikov partial SE
Persistent aura
Limbic systematic SE (psycho-motorial)
Hemiconvulsive status epilepticus with hemiparesis (reproduced with permission from Engel et al. [18])
American NCS Classification (2012)
I. Convulsive status epilepticus
Definition: Convulsive status epilepticus (CSE) presents with a rhythmic movement of the arms and legs
Clinical characteristics of generalized convulsive SE:
1.1 Generalized tonic–clonic movement of arms and legs
1.2 Consciousness impairment (coma, somnolence, and confusion)
1.3 Focal neurologic deficits in the postictal period (such as Todd's paralysis)
There are no explanations of focal motor SE and partial SE in this definition
II. NCSE
Definition: Abnormal epileptiform discharges can be observed on EEG, without clear motor symptoms
Two types of NCSE:
2.1 Mild consciousness impairment, confusion, with good prognosis
2.2 Severe consciousness impairment often occurs in the late period of CSE, with or without subtle motor symptoms (such as limb or facial muscle abstraction or tonic eyeball heterotropia), which is called subtle SE (reproduced with permission from Brophy et al. [16])

In 2012, the American NCS guidelines categorized SE as convulsive status epilepticus and nonconvulsive status epilepticus according to the semiology (with or without motor symptoms) and EEG results (Table 1.9) [16].

In 2015, the ILAE published a further detailed classification of SE. This classification contained four main factors: (a) semiology, (b) etiology, (c) EEG-related manifestations, and (d) ages. It provides a clinical framework for the diagnosis and treatment available to every patient. At the onset of SE, this method can be used to classify cases by ages and types of seizures without delay. Compared to this method, the etiological classification would take a longer period to further analyze and confirm the findings. Because its results could influence the choice of treatment protocols and suggest the prognosis of SE, EEG is of vital importance for the classification of SE. Therefore, the fact that EEG classification should be initiated as early as possible is suggested in the definition. The diagnosis and treatment for some types of SE (particularly NCSE) rely on EEG. In addition, the performance of semiology and EEG might be dynamic during the period of SE; hence, the classification of SE would also be dynamic. For example, in the initial stage, SE could exhibit focal motor secondarily generalized CSE and then exhibit NCSE with coma and subtle motor seizures. At the early stage of SE, EEG results could also show unilateral periodic discharges that evolve into bilateral synchronous epileptiform discharges [17].

The evidence of semiology involves the clinical manifestations of SE, namely, the types of seizures, which is crucial for SE classification. Currently, it is suggested that SE should be

Table 1.10 Semiology classification of SE (ILAE 2015)

I. Obviously generalized or focal motor symptoms during seizures
1.1 Tonic–clonic SE, namely, CSE
Generalized motor SE
Focal SE secondary to generalized SE
Occurrence of obvious motor symptoms, failing to differentiate generalized SE and focal SE
1.2 Myoclonic SE, showing obvious epileptic myoclonic twitch
Consciousness impairment
Without consciousness impairment
1.3 Focal motor seizures
Recurrent focal motor seizures
Partial SE
Adversive status
Oculoclonic status
Ictal paresis (focal inhibitory SE)
1.4 Tonic SE
1.5 Hyper-motor SE
II. Without obvious motor component, namely, NCSE
2.1 Coma, including subtle SE
2.2 Without coma
2.2.1 Generalized
Typical absence
Atypical absence
Myoclonic absence
2.2.2 Focal
Without consciousness impairment (aura persistent status, with symptoms of autonomic nerves, sensation, sense of vision, sense of smell, affection/spirit/experience, or auditory perception)
Aphasia status
With consciousness impairment
2.2.3 Failure of classification as generalized status or focal status, such as autonomic nerve SE
III. Undetermined status ("marginal syndrome")
3.1 Epileptic encephalopathy
3.2 Coma with non-variable EEG epileptiform discharges
3.3 Behavior disorders
3.4 Acute mental disorders (such as delirium and fugue) with EEG epileptiform discharge

Reproduced with permission from Trinka et al. [17]

further classified based on whether motor symptoms are apparent and the degree of consciousness impairment (Table 1.10) [17].

The etiological classification of SE is consistent with previous proposals released by the ILAE, and it adopts some terminology often used by professionals in various areas [16, 17]. SE is mainly divided into known and unknown causes. The known causes include acute causes (such as stroke, trauma, and encephalitis), remote causes (including post-trauma, postencephalitis, and post-stroke), and progressive causes (including brain neoplasm, Creutzfeldt–Jakob disease, Alzheimer's disease, and other progressive myoclonic epilepsies).

EEG does not show specificity during seizure intervals for all types of SE. Currently, no EEG classification standard exists based on evidence-based medicine. A description of EEG findings is recommended according to Table 1.11 [12, 17].

The definition in 2015 [17] also lists representative SE characteristics of different age stages,

Table 1.11 EEG of SE (ILAE 2015)

Site	Generalized, including bilateral synchronous discharge; bilateral; independently bilateral; multifocal
Name of discharge pattern	Periodic discharge; rhythmic motor; spike slow-wave/sharp slow-wave syndrome
Morphology	Sharp wave; phase (triphasic wave); absolute and relative amplitude; polarity
Characteristics related to time	Occurrence; frequency; time limit; duration and index of daily discharge pattern; onset pattern of discharge (sudden or gradual); variation (change, fluctuation, or no change)
Modulation	Stimulus provoked or spontaneous
Drugs	Effect of intervention on EEG

Reproduced with permission from Trinka et al. [17]

Table 1.12 Representative characteristics of SE in different age stages

SE in infantile (1 month–2 years old) epileptic syndrome	SE in childhood (2–12 years old) and adolescent period	SE in adolescence and adulthood (12–59 years old)	SE in the elderly (at least 60 years old)
a. Myoclonic status in Dravet syndrome b. Focal status c. Febrile status d. Tonic status	a. Self-limited SE in early benign childhood occipital epilepsy b. NCSE in exceptional childhood epileptic syndrome (such as epilepsy with myoclonic–atonic seizures and other childhood myoclonic encephalopathy) c. Myoclonic status in progressive myoclonic epilepsy d. Tonic status in Lennox–Gastaut syndrome e. Discharge SE in slow-wave sleep f. Aphasia status in Landau–Kleffner syndrome	a. Myoclonic status in juvenile myoclonic epilepsy b. Absence status in juvenile myoclonic epilepsy c. Myoclonic status in Down syndrome	a. Myoclonic status in Alzheimer's disease b. NCSE in Creutzfeldt–Jakob disease c. Occurrence or recurrent absence in the elderly, such as SE after stoke

Reproduced with permission from Trinka et al. [17]

which facilitates learning and mastering the relevant semiology, etiology, and EEG manifestations that are caused by SE (Table 1.12).

1.3 Definition and Classification of RSE

RSE is defined as a condition that when treated with standard protocols, convulsive seizures and epileptic discharges on EEG cannot be terminated when sufficient first-line drugs are used for the treatment of SE (benzodiazepines and one subsequent AED). This definition was proposed in the guidelines published by the American NCS in 2012 [16].

Currently, controversy exists regarding the definition of RSE, and no universal definition has been proposed. The two main controversial aspects are as follows. One issue is the number of AEDs used. One view holds that RSE can be diagnosed when two sufficient AEDs (one type of benzodiazepine and one subsequent AED) are used, but convulsive seizures and epileptic discharges on EEG are not terminated. However, others have proposed that RSE can be diagnosed when convulsive seizures and epileptic discharges on EEG are still not terminated after using three sufficient AEDs (a type of benzodiazepine and two subsequent other AEDs). The other issue is the duration of seizures after treatment, particularly, of the length of epileptic seizures after using two or three types of AEDs and when the disease can be diagnosed as RSE. The opinion in the guidelines published by the NCS (America) in 2012 is that the diagnosis of RSE can be made without considering the duration of epileptic seizures after using two types of AEDs. If seizures cannot be terminated after two types of drugs are used, RSE can be diagnosed. The guideline, published by the EFNS in 2010, mentions that the duration of epileptic seizures after using two or three types of AEDs is not standardized (1 h, 2 h, or irrespective of the time) [15]. Currently, the main opinion is that RSE can be diagnosed after the failure of two types of AEDs without considering the duration of epileptic seizures. At present, no specific report related to RSE classification exists. Therefore, the classification of RSE is also consistent with the semiology, EEG findings, and etiology of seizures as well as the patient age, which is similar to the classification of SE.

In 2011, Shorvon et al. [19] noted that super-RSE could be defined when the period of anesthetic pharmacotherapy for SE exceeds 24 h but the clinical convulsive seizures or epileptic discharges on EEG are still not terminated or when the condition relapses. Super-RSE is well known by clinicians and mainly found in following two conditions: patients with severe brain trauma and patients with no history of epilepsy who have SE without obvious causes.

Not all SE is epilepsy. Some patients without a history of seizure or epilepsy may demonstrate SE; however, after an episode of SE, even without the use of AEDs, most of these patients do not have a recurrent seizure. However, in many patients, RSE is caused by delayed diagnosis or inappropriate treatment during the initial stage of the disease. Some patients with epileptic syndrome are also prone to SE. When that occurs, treatments vary from those for other types of SE. Therefore, some experts suggested that according to the prognosis of SE, SE should be classified as new-onset SE, SE refractory to treatment, and special types of SE, for the purpose of SE treatment [20].

The above is the brief description of the definitions and classifications of epilepsy, SE, and RSE. Currently, the definitions and classifications of epilepsy and SE are accepted by the majority of clinicians due to their increasing clinical operability and wide application. However, controversy still exists regarding the definition of epilepsy, which requires clinicians to judge actual situations. With the development of clinical research and animal experiments, definitions of epilepsy, SE, and RSE will be further revised.

1.4 Diagnosis of Convulsive Epilepsy and Status Epilepticus

SE is one of the most common critical illnesses of the nervous system; it has a high mortality rate and requires emergency treatment, but the diagnosis of SE is very difficult [25–27]. Studies have reported that more than half of the patients admitted to neurological intensive care units with SE do not have actual seizures, as the onset of epilepsy lacks specificity. Clinically, convulsive epilepsy must be differentiated from ten other types of convulsive disorders. Moreover, the clinical manifestations of epilepsy are also very complex. For complex partial seizures, which belong to the category of NCSE, more than 18 types of academically reported clinical manifestations have been described. Due to its comorbidity, some patients with epilepsy may simultaneously experience both epileptic and nonepileptic attacks, which increases the difficulty of diagnosis and treatment in clinical settings and thus requires caution in the differentiation from other diseases [25–33].

1.4.1 Convulsive Epilepsy Versus Nonepileptic Convulsion

Convulsion is the sudden, involuntary, and uninhibited tonic and/or clonic contraction of systemic or local muscle group(s), often accompanied by disturbance of consciousness. Although the ILAE does not recommend the term convulsion for the classification of epilepsy, the term convulsive epilepsy, which mainly encompasses generalized tonic–clonic seizures, tonic seizures, clonic seizures, and partial seizures with prominent motor symptoms, is still widely adopted and reported in the literature. Convulsion is not specific to epilepsy; it is one of the clinical manifestations of more than ten types of nonepileptic seizures. Nonepileptic seizure is not a separate identity but a general term for many nonepileptic diseases with similar clinical manifestations. Although nonepileptic convulsions are similar to epilepsy in clinical manifestations, they are not epilepsy and cannot be treated as epilepsy, especially SE. No susceptibility to repeated epileptic seizures exists in the brains of these patients, and abnormal electrical discharges of brain neurons are not found during clinical monitoring. The clinical importance of nonepileptic convulsion lies in its extremely easy misdiagnosis as convulsive epilepsy, and inappropriate antiepileptic treatment may lead to serious consequences. Therefore, clinicians, especially those specializing in critic neurological disorders, should pay serious attention to this issue [29–32].

1.4.2 Characteristics of Convulsive Epilepsy

Human epilepsy includes two main features: epileptiform discharges on EEG in patients and clinical attacks. In theory, epileptiform discharges are present on the EEG of every patient with epilepsy; however, in clinical practice, they are not detectable in a considerable number of epilepsy patients due to technical limitations or differences in the location of lesions. Therefore, the diagnosis of epilepsy still relies on clinical attacks. Because convulsive epilepsy is a type of epileptic disorder, it exhibits the common characteristics of epilepsy, that is, it is paroxysmal, transient, stereotyped, and repetitive. "Paroxysmal" means epileptic attacks often begin abruptly and end shortly afterward, with clear start and end points. In the interictal period, most patients appear normal. "Transient" means that epileptic attacks usually last for a very short time, no longer than 5 min, except for those with SE. Although the clinical manifestations of epilepsy are very complex, almost all attacks in an individual patient are similar. This is known as the stereotype of epilepsy. "Repetitive" refers to repeated attacks of epilepsy in most patients, and it is necessary to be particularly careful with the diagnosis of epilepsy when only one attack has occurred. However, not all disorders with the common characteristics of epilepsy can be diagnosed as epilepsy, including trigeminal neuropathy, a clinically common disorder that displays paroxysmal, transient, stereotyped, and repetitive clinical manifestations but is not epilepsy because its clinical manifestations are not consistent with the "individuality" of seizures. This "individuality" distinguishes epilepsy from other seizure-like attacks. The "individuality" of convulsive epilepsy is loss of consciousness and generalized tonic events followed by a series of clonic activities [20].

A typical course of convulsive epilepsy can be divided into three phases: (a) pre-convulsion, (b) convulsion, and (c) post-convulsion phases. The pre-convulsion phase mainly manifests as loss of consciousness, often accompanied by falls. The convulsion phase mainly manifests as the sequential emergence of tonic activities and clonic activities. During the tonic phase, the skeletal muscles of the entire body contract continuously, with eyes turning upward, gazing, locked jaws, screaming, upper limb adduction and pronation, and lower limb straightening. These manifestations continue for 10–20 s before the patient enters the clonic phase, which is mainly characterized by tonus developing into episodes of clonus, each succeeded by a brief interval. The frequency of clonus gradually decreases, the intervals are extended, and then the patient enters the post-convulsion phase. The tonic and clonic phases are both accompanied by respiratory arrest, increased blood pressure, pupil dilation, increased secretion, and other symptoms. In the post-convulsion phase, transient clonus is still present, but breathing, blood pressure, and heart rate gradually return to normal. At this point, the patient appears easily irritated, confused, and agitated. A small number of patients exhibit focal seizures.

1.4.3 Characteristics of CSE

Recurrent convulsive seizures without recovery of interictal neurological function or a single attack longer than 5 min with continuous epileptiform discharges on EEG is known as CSE. In view of clinical diagnosis and treatment, it is also advocated that convulsive seizures with frequent recurrence during a short time should be termed CSE, but the specific frequency of recurrence is not unified; it has been stated to be as low as once per hour or as high as four times per hour. Recently, a new classification system for epilepsy has been proposed by the ILAE, in which CSE is classified as SE with prominent motor symptoms.

Childhood CSE is the most common febrile seizure in children. Hayakawa et al. [34] analyzed 381 cases of CSE accompanied by fever and found that 81.6% developed from febrile seizures, 6.6% were due to encephalitis, 0.8% were due to meningitis, and 7.6% developed from epilepsy. Other studies of refractory SE have found that 60.3% of cases originated from infection of the central nervous system [35]. Clinically, childhood CSE primarily manifests as systemic myoclonus, which is repeated, paroxysmal, and bilateral, and it may be asymmetric and arrhythmic. EEG shows synchronized bilateral spikes, while outbreaks of sharp waves or spike-and-waves may occur. In some children, generalized tonic SE, mainly demonstrated by paroxysmal, transient, and frequent tonic contraction of limbs, is the primary manifestation, often accompanied by gazing and muscle contraction of the face, neck, and throat, which occur once over several minutes. EEG shows desynchronization, but more typically low-voltage fast activities of 20–30 Hz that gradually slow to 10–20 Hz with an increase in amplitude are observed. Polyspike-and-waves can also be seen [20, 35].

Before the onset of CSE, a prodromal period lasting for several hours often occurs, manifested as more epileptic activity than usual, gradually increased frequency and increased intensity of attacks. Progressive myoclonus, mental changes, or consciousness disorders due to subclinical epileptic activities may also be present in some patients. In patients without a history of seizures, it is possible that SE can occur suddenly.

The frequency of seizure attacks is variable, ranging from 4 to 6 times to thousands of times per hour according to reports. As CSE proceeds, the duration of each attack is shortened, the tonic phase is prolonged, and the clonus is relieved; finally, these manifestations disappear completely.

1.4.4 Evaluation of Convulsive Epilepsy

Firstly, it is necessary to determine whether a patient's seizures have the common and individual qualities of epileptic seizures, especially the details of the attack, which usually serve as an important basis for correct diagnosis.

Secondly, although not every patient's EEG is abnormal, abnormalities on EEG are still important evidence of the diagnosis of epilepsy. Video-EEG monitoring (VEM), in particular, is highly valuable for the differentiation of epileptic and nonepileptic seizures. Serological tests, especially the detection of prolactin (PRL) levels, and neuroimaging are also helpful for diagnosis.

Thirdly, it is very important to exclude other nonepileptic paroxysmal disorders. Antiepileptic treatment has almost no curative effect on disorders misdiagnosed as epileptic seizures, and the iatrogenic harm caused by medical workers in pursuit of successful disease control needs to be strongly emphasized as it often poses great threat to the health of patients.

In addition, there are some notes on the evaluation of convulsive epilepsy. The diagnosis of epilepsy depends on the patient's medical history; however, history taking is the most difficult part of the diagnostic process. Since loss of consciousness is common in CSE, patients are unable to provide critical details of attacks. The transient nature of seizure attacks also makes it difficult for the medical staff to have the opportunity to observe seizures. Therefore, the history of seizures is often provided by nurses who are deficient in the essential knowledge of epilepsy and attention to details of attacks. However, these details are particularly important for diagnosis. For example, it should be noted whether respiratory arrest occurs during the attack. Its existence supports the diagnosis of epilepsy, while deep respiration should lead to the consideration of hyperventilation syndrome. In addition, family members of the patient or nurses with Munchausen syndrome may provide a false history, which increases the uncertainty of the diagnosis of epilepsy. Therefore, effective measures, such as videotaping or recording using mobile phones and educating patients' families and the nursing staff on epilepsy, are fundamental for obtaining the medical history of a patient suspected of having epilepsy.

Meanwhile, attention should be paid to the state of consciousness. Disturbance of consciousness is one of the most important manifestations of convulsive epilepsy. When a seizure event is witnessed, all efforts should be made to ascertain whether disturbance of consciousness occurs. Commonly used methods include the menace reflex (when an object rapidly approaches the patient's eyes from the front, observe whether blinking occurs; blinking indicates the presence of consciousness and, therefore, does not support the diagnosis of convulsive epilepsy) and the "man in the mirror" (move a mirror in front of the patient; if the patient reacts to follow the mirror, it suggests that his or her consciousness is not lost). It is also useful to repeat some words used in everyday conversations, such as "banana," "car," or "house" during the attack and to ask the patient to recite what they heard during the attack after its termination. The ability to do so does not support the previous existence of consciousness disorders [20].

Attention should also be paid to the details of the attack. Tonic events during the course of convulsive epilepsy tend to be characterized by manifestations such as gazing and upward turning of both eyes, locked jaws, screaming, and foaming (saliva) at the mouth. These manifestations serve as important evidence for the consideration of convulsive epilepsy. Convulsive epilepsy is often accompanied by changes in vital signs essential for the diagnosis of epilepsy. During attacks of convulsive epilepsy, patients tend to have facial cyanosis, while the possibility of psychogenic seizures should be considered in case of pallor.

In laboratory examinations, elevated PRL and neuron-specific enolase (NSE) are very common after a convulsive event. The diagnosis of epilepsy is supported by serum PRL reaching 2–3 times the interictal level within the first hour of the postictal period and an increased level of NSE 24–28 h after an event. Postictal serum creatine phosphokinase (CPK) tends to be elevated and provides an important reference for the clinical diagnosis, although it lacks specificity [35, 36].

1.4.5 Distinguish Nonepileptic Convulsion from Convulsive Epilepsy

Nonepileptic seizure is not an independent identity but a general term for nonepileptic disorders similar to epileptic seizures in clinical manifestations. It is often misdiagnosed as refractory epilepsy, and the coexistence of both disorders makes the diagnosis even more difficult [37–39].

1.4.5.1 Convulsive Syncope

Syncope is a transient loss of consciousness caused by transient global cerebral hypoperfusion, or ability to maintain postural tone due to lack of perfusion to the brain. When syncope is accompanied by tonic or clonic movements, it can be diagnosed as convulsive syncope. The manifestations of convulsive syncope were first reported by Cooper [40]. Santy et al. [41] found that syncope in children was accompanied by convulsions, which attracted attention to convulsive syncope. In 1957, Gastaut et al. [42] experimentally induced syncope in humans for the first time and studied its clinical and EEG features. After observing that patients in syncope had tonus and myoclonus in the absence of epileptiform discharges on EEG, they proposed the concept of convulsive syncope.

Convulsive syncope is easily misdiagnosed. Some patients have been initially misdiagnosed with epilepsy and have undergone inappropriate treatment, only to be correctly diagnosed when they were ultimately found to have convulsive syncope induced by tilt table testing. Some patients under long-term antiepileptic treatment have been found to have cardiogenic convulsive syncope only after occasional electrocardiographic examinations revealed severe cardiac arrhythmia. Grubb et al. [43] found that 1/3 of cases evaluated for epilepsy were actually cases of nonepileptic convulsions.

Convulsive syncope is often induced by significant factors, such as pain, fear, emotional stress, blood loss, and carotid artery stimulation. The onset of syncope is preceded by prodromal symptoms, such as fatigue, unclear vision, tinnitus, pale countenance, and excessive sweating. Convulsion usually occurs 10 s after loss of consciousness and manifests as limb rigidity, clonic events, or tonic–clonic events with a short duration and mild intensity. Additionally, apnea, decreased heart rate, or even cardiac arrest, at which time the pulses of the radial artery and the carotid artery are unlikely to be palpable, may be present. These symptoms generally last for 20–30 s, after which full recovery can be expected. After the attack, patients may experience retrograde amnesia, somnolence, or confusion, while psychiatric symptoms such as excitement, euphoria, fear, and visual or auditory hallucinations may also appear. Simultaneously, the patient may also have manifestations of the primary disease. Bădilă et al. [44] analyzed 217 cases of syncopal patients and found that the most common causes of syncope were orthostatic hypotension and cardiac and vasovagal causes; some patients had multiple factors.

Convulsive syncope and epileptic seizures are very similar clinically; therefore, it is very difficult to differentiate them. Many patients with convulsive syncope may receive long-term antiepileptic treatment because they were misdiagnosed with epilepsy at their first clinical visit, and many patients undergo operations due to drug resistance. Therefore, careful identification is necessary [45].

Often, significant inducements of the onset of convulsive syncope exist, such as bleeding, pain, and rapid postural changes, especially when suddenly standing from the sitting position. In general, convulsive syncope does not occur during sleep. Epileptic seizures often are not significantly associated with these factors, and occurrence during sleep is very common.

Preceding warning symptoms, such as blurred vision, palpitation, dizziness, excessive sweating, and tinnitus, usually appear before syncope. The recovery is slow. The auras of epileptic seizures mainly include central nervous symptoms, such as hallucinations, or paresthesia, such as limb numbness.

The most important part of identification is finding the cause. Cardiogenic syncope patients often have a variety of arrhythmias and cardiomyopathy. Cerebral syncope patients may show manifestations such as subclavian steal syndrome. Primary orthostatic hypotension, levodopa, and chlorpromazine can lead to orthostatic syncope. Hypoglycemia or severe anemia may also lead to syncope.

Auxiliary examinations are necessary. Blood glucose and hemoglobin should be examined routinely. Electrocardiography, especially 24-h dynamic electrocardiography plus echocardiography, is important for the exclusion of cardiogenic shock. For suspected cerebral syncope, examinations should include EEG, cranial CT or MRI, transcranial Doppler sonography, and, if necessary, cerebral angiography. If carotid sinus massage induces sinus arrest longer than 3 s and/or a systolic blood pressure decrease of more than 30 mmHg, hypersensitive carotid sinus syndrome can be diagnosed. Additionally, the upright tilt table test is relatively sensitive for the identification of unexplained recurrent syncope. In patients with abnormalities found upon examination of the nervous system, considerations should include peripheral neuropathies, such as diabetes, nutritional disorders, and amyloidosis, and lesions of the central nervous system, such as multiple system atrophy. Sometimes, autonomic function tests such as the Ewing's batteries may contribute toward the investigation of a patient with syncope by diagnosing autonomic dysfunctions.

1.4.5.2 Pheochromocytoma-Induced Convulsion

Pheochromocytoma is a type of tumor that is derived from pheochromocytes of the adrenal medulla or extra-adrenal paraganglia and secretes large amounts of catecholamines. Pheochromocytoma may occur at any age, most commonly between 20 and 50 years, and the incidence is slightly higher in males than in females. Approximately 10% of pheochromocytomas are malignant. The first report of convulsions induced by pheochromocytoma was from Becker [46]. Later, Leiba et al. [47] reported a case with only a slight increase in blood pressure (170/100 mmHg) but with loss of consciousness and limb convulsions as the primary manifestations. During convulsions, the patient's blood pressure was only mildly elevated, while CT and MRI showed no abnormalities; in the absence of antihypertensive treatment, the attack was terminated by active anticonvulsant therapy. The possibility of cerebral tumors had been excluded by cranial MRI. Thus, the authors believed that the convulsions were induced by the pheochromocytoma. Anderson et al. [48] retrospectively analyzed 93 patients with confirmed pheochromocytoma, five of whom showed convulsions as manifestations. Manger [49] summarized the clinical features of nonepileptic convulsions induced by pheochromocytoma based on the literature, noting the great danger of this condition, the extreme difficulty of diagnosis, and the near certainty of fatal cardiovascular complications or metastasis without timely treatment. In 2016, the first human genetic screen for pheochromocytoma was performed [50, 51].

Patients with pheochromocytoma often have headache, palpitations, tachycardia, pallor, chest and abdominal pain, nausea, and vomiting; however, the most typical clinical symptom is paroxysmal hypertension. Anderson et al. [48] analyzed the clinical manifestations of 93 patients and found that 68 (73%) had paroxysmal neurological symptoms, of whom 47 had headaches, 24 had anxiety, 12 had nausea, and five had convulsions. Manger [49] found that patients with paroxysmal hypertension accounted for 50% of patients with this disease. Paroxysmal hypertension may, through hypertensive encephalopathy, lead to convulsions that manifest as generalized tonic–clonic events. These events last for 1–2 min before self-alleviation but may be as brief as several seconds or as long as several hours, as reported in some studies. Recurrence is common, and the frequency of paroxysm varies from once per several months to a few times per week. The patients are easily misdiagnosed with epilepsy and thus receive antiepileptic therapy or even suffer serious consequences from surgical treatment. Therefore, the issue of misdiagnosis should be adequately addressed [46–51].

The main cause of convulsions is a large amount of norepinephrine secreted by the pheochromocytoma. The sudden release of norepinephrine not only elevates blood pressure but also promotes the occurrence of convulsions.

Auxiliary examinations available for pheochromocytoma can be divided into two categories. The first is biochemical testing. Because metanephrine (MN) and normetanephrine (NMN), metabolites of catecholamines, are not associated with the stimulated secretion of catecholamines, blood and urine screens for MN and NMN have become the first choice for the biochemical diagnosis of pheochromocytoma. The second category is imaging methods. Adrenal tumors greater than 1 cm and extra-adrenal tumors greater than 2 cm can be discovered by CT scans, which serve as an important means of noninvasive imaging. More than 90% of adrenal tumors can be precisely located. MRI does not require the injection of contrast agents and is highly valuable for the diagnosis of extra-adrenal tumors. Ultrasound examinations are convenient, simple, cheap, and noninvasive but are less sensitive than CT and MRI and less likely to find small tumors. A functional metaiodobenzylguanidine (MIBG) scan, which has high specificity, helps distinguish pheochromocytoma from other space-occupying lesions and can be used to identify multifocal tumors and metastatic tumors [49] and to perform further screening on patients with otherwise negative findings.

The early diagnosis of pheochromocytoma-induced convulsions is extremely important. However, the diagnosis is quite difficult as it is easily confused with epilepsy. Misdiagnosis and mistreatment may endanger patients' lives. Therefore, patients with abrupt onset of generalized tonic–clonic seizures should be highly suspected of pheochromocytoma, especially those with high blood pressure or tachycardia. In senior patients and individuals with a history of hypertension, if acute brain dysfunction arises with significantly increased blood pressure, it is imperative to determine the cause of hypertension. In young individuals with sudden convulsions, inadequate blood pressure monitoring may result in missed diagnosis of pheochromocytoma. For patients with positive findings in further biochemical tests, such as blood and urine MN, NMN, and others, imaging should be performed to locate the tumors and confirm the diagnosis.

Pheochromocytoma-induced convulsions are easily misdiagnosed as epilepsy; they should be carefully differentiated from the latter. Although similar to epilepsy in some respects, they are not actual epileptic seizures and can be identified with caution. First of all, pheochromocytoma-induced convulsions are usually preceded by severe headache, nausea, vomiting, palpitations, tachycardia, anxiety, pallor, chest pain, abdominal pain, and other symptoms. The existence of pheochromocytoma can be confirmed by biochemical tests and imaging. Secondly, in pheochromocytoma-induced convulsions, EEG findings are normal between attacks, while interictal epileptic discharges on EEG are an important diagnostic indication of epilepsy. Thirdly, the most common clinical manifestation of pheochromocytoma is persistent or paroxysmal hypertension, which tends to prompt the occurrence of convulsions, leading to paroxysmal confusion, rigidity, or twitching. Finally, regarding other manifestations, despite the paroxysm of symptoms, signs of pheochromocytoma, such as hypertension, headache, and palpitation, are still present between convulsive attacks. In this regard, pheochromocytoma differs from the interictal period of epilepsy, which shows almost no abnormalities.

1.4.5.3 Insulinoma-Induced Convulsion

Insulinoma is a rare type of pancreatic endocrine tumor. It was first reported by Thorling [52] in 1948. In 1954, Smyth et al. [53] noted that this disease could induce convulsions with peculiar EEG changes. Subsequently, Ding et al. [54] analyzed 42 patients with insulinoma, 12 of whom were misdiagnosed with epilepsy because the main clinical manifestations were convulsions. Current studies have recognized that coma followed by recurrent involuntary convulsions is an outstanding manifestation of fatal hypoglycemia, and a delay in diagnosis may lead to death of the patient [55, 56].

Insulinoma-induced convulsions have a variety of forms. Although patients with manifestations similar to complex seizures are not uncommon, convulsion is still the main manifestation in the majority of patients. Ding et al. [54] analyzed 42 cases of insulinoma, of whom 25 were misdiagnosed as neurological or psychiatric disorders and 12 were initially misdiagnosed as epilepsy; of these 12 cases, three showed epileptic discharges on EEG. Similar to epilepsy, insulinoma-induced convulsion starts suddenly; then, generalized or focal twitching or limb rigidity accompanied by loss of consciousness occurs. The convulsion lasts from a few seconds to several hours and can be immediately terminated by the ingestion of carbohydrates or an intravenous glucose drip [54–56].

Insulinoma-induced convulsions are similar to epileptic seizures and are not responsive to antiepileptic drugs; therefore, they are likely to be confused with refractory epilepsy and misdiagnosed. Many reports have described the misdiagnosis of insulinoma as refractory epilepsy. Sympathetic excitatory symptoms and neuropsychiatric symptoms associated with insulinoma-induced convulsions, in particular, should not be regarded as an aura or a postictal reaction of epileptic seizures [54].

The first issue in differential diagnosis is the chronological pattern of convulsion. Hyperinsulinemic hypoglycemia is the underlying cause of insulinoma-induced convulsions. Almost all of the energy used in brain cells is supplied by glucose. Hypoglycemia and the lack of carbohydrate supplementation may result in acute cerebral lesions. Paroxysmal hypoglycemia secondary to insulinoma mostly occurs at night or before meals. Correspondingly, insulinoma-induced convulsions mostly occur at dawn or during fasting at night. These convulsions can be induced by hunger, fatigue, mental stimulation, menstruation, fever, and other factors. If timely treatment is not received, the frequency of attacks may gradually increase to several times per week. Intake of carbohydrates or an intravenous glucose drip can immediately terminate an attack [57]. In comparison, epileptic events are more frequent at night and are not associated with eating.

The second issue in differential diagnosis is concomitant symptoms. In patients with insulinoma, a rapid decline in the blood glucose level is generally followed by sympathetic activation syndrome and later cerebral dysfunction. Therefore, before the onset of convulsions, patients often experience symptoms of sympathetic hyperfunction, such as sweating, trembling of the extremities, hunger, palpitation, anxiety, pallor, and emotional agitation. Symptoms of hypoglycemic brain dysfunction may also be present, such as loss of concentration, dizziness, blurred vision, and gait instability. Between convulsive attacks, patients may also have other neurological symptoms, such as confusion, coma, hemiplegia, paraparesis, monoparesis, visual disturbances, headache, dysarthria, ataxia, strabismus, and hypothermia [54–57]. In contrast, epilepsy mostly exhibits preictal manifestations, such as visual hallucinations and numbness, as well as normal interictal manifestations. This difference is helpful for the differentiation of these two types of disorders.

The third issue is the stereotype of attacks. Unlike epileptic events, insulinoma-induced convulsions are not stereotyped, and their clinical manifestations, which evolve as the blood glucose level changes, are often diverse and dramatic. Detailed investigations and close observation regarding whether a stereotype can be found for attacks can facilitate the clinical diagnosis.

The fourth issue is auxiliary examinations. The main purpose of auxiliary examinations is to confirm the presence of epilepsy and hypoglycemia.

- EEG: The differentiation between epilepsy and convulsions induced by pancreatic islet cell tumors relies heavily on EEG. Interictal epileptic discharges on EEG are critical evidence of epilepsy.
- Blood glucose level: Because the clinical manifestations of patients are associated with hypoglycemia, it is necessary to determine the blood glucose level. Particularly, patients with onset during fasting or unexplained resistance to antiepileptic drugs should be examined promptly to determine whether hyperinsulinemia-induced hypoglycemia is a possibility. Nevertheless, random blood glucose levels can be normal as hypoglycemia secondary to insulinoma may be paroxysmal; therefore, frequent and dynamic blood glucose monitoring is necessary, especially for detecting blood glucose levels during attacks, which may help clarify the diagnosis [53, 57].
- Insulin release index and corrected insulin release index: The insulin release index (the ratio of fasting insulin to blood glucose) has more significance in the determination of inappropriate insulin secretion. An insulin release index higher than 0.3 is a reliable indication of insulinoma [55].
- Fasting and exercise tests: When fasting hypoglycemia is strongly suspected in a patient whose blood glucose level is normal or above the cutoff value, fasting and exercise tests can be used to confirm the diagnosis. After 24–36 h of fasting, hypoglycemic symptoms will appear in almost all patients with insulinoma, accompanied by inappropriate insulin secretion, which increases plasma insulin to 100–220 U/mL.
- Imaging: Imaging techniques such as abdominal ultrasound and CT examination still play an important role in locating insulinomas, but positive findings are unlikely to be obtained when the tumor has a diameter less than 2 cm or a signal intensity close to that of normal tissue. Therefore, in the case of negative imaging findings, an exploratory laparotomy should be promptly performed for the histopathological diagnosis of patients highly suspected of insulinoma based on the results of laboratory examinations.

1.4.5.4 Hypertensive Encephalopathy-Induced Convulsion

Hypertensive encephalopathy (HE) is global cerebral dysfunction caused by a sharp increase in blood pressure, with convulsions, disturbance of consciousness to varying degrees, and severe headache as primary manifestations, in addition to transient hemiplegia, hemianopia, and hemidysesthesia. HE may be induced by nephritis, eclampsia, hypertensive crisis, pheochromocytoma, Cushing's syndrome, renal artery thrombosis, or the sudden withdrawal of antihypertensive drugs. As one of the common neurological manifestations of HE, convulsion is caused by ischemia and hypoxia of the cerebral hemispheres, which is usually considered a consequence of cerebral arteriovenous spasm and collapse of the mechanism of cerebral vascular autoregulation.

The incidence of HE-induced convulsions is not clear. Batouche et al. [58] found that 33.3% of 66 children with severe hypertension had hypertension-induced convulsions. In a retrospective study, McEnery et al. [59] discovered that 31% of 48 children who had received renal transplantation experienced convulsive seizures, and 60% of them had convulsions as the only manifestation.

As reported, HE can be observed in all age groups, from children to the elderly, but it is most common in youth or middle age. The typical symptoms are severe headache, nausea, vomiting, disturbance of consciousness, and convulsions, along with sudden elevation of blood pressure [58–62].

Convulsions induced by HE are mainly manifested as generalized tonic–clonic events with loss of consciousness, falling, upward turning of the eyes, gazing, and limb rigidity followed by clonus. During an episode, respiratory arrest, pupil dilation, and sometimes tongue biting and incontinence can occur. The convulsions, which last for 1–2 min, are often recurrent. In some cases, they may evolve into status convulsivus, which easily induces heart failure. Between episodes, patients show other common symptoms of HE, such as irritability, nausea, vomiting, disorientation, delirium, stupor, and coma. After the blood pressure is controlled, the symptoms often disappear completely within 1–2 h.

Because the clinical manifestations of HE-induced convulsions and epilepsy are very similar, the main purpose of identification is to exclude the possibility of HE. The following conditions should prompt a suspicion of HE: (a) sharply increased blood pressure in patients with a history of primary or secondary hypertension plus exacerbating factors, such as fatigue, nervousness, and excitement, especially if the diastolic blood pressure is >120 mmHg; (b) the clinical emergence of neurological abnormalities mainly manifesting as increased intracranial pressure and focal lesions of brain tissue, particularly the following three types of global cerebral manifestations: sudden onset of severe headache, nausea, and vomiting, varying degrees of disturbance of consciousness, and convulsions; and (c) the rapid disappearance of global cerebral manifestations following a decrease in blood pressure with no sequelae. There is an overlap between hypertensive encephalopathy and posterior reversible leukoencephalopathy syndrome, both of which may contribute to seizures, but the latter is associated with hypertension, the use of immunosuppressive agents, preeclampsia, and chronic renal failure.

1.4.5.5 Convulsive Psychogenic Nonepileptic Seizures

Psychogenic nonepileptic seizures (PNES) are defined as changes in behavior or consciousness resembling epileptic seizures but which have a psychological origin and are not clinically characterized by epileptic seizures or epileptiform discharges on EEG [63]. By 1800, psychiatrists had recognized the existence of this entity and regarded it as a form of hysteria. In 1996, Schachter et al. [64] surveyed the American epilepsy specialists regarding the terminology for this disorder, and most experts believed that nonepileptic seizures were a better summarization of the characteristics of the attacks because this term more accurately described the clinical manifestations and the pathophysiological process. Therefore, nonepileptic seizures have been adopted as the new diagnostic terms for such disorders.

Nonepileptic seizures can be classified as either physiological or psychogenic. The former include panic attacks, paroxysmal dystonia, and nonepileptic myoclonus; the latter are mainly associated with psychological factors and are more likely to be confused with epileptic seizures.

The prevalence of PNES varies in different reports. In the general population, the incidence of PNES confirmed by EEG or VEM is approximately 1.4–3 per ten million [65, 66]. However, the actual incidence is much higher. Szaflarski et al. [66] conducted a retrospective survey of the population of Hamilton County, Ohio, USA, in which the mean incidence of PNES was 3.03/100,000.

Silva et al. [67] classified PNES into five different types: (a) tonic–clonic mimicking movements, such as generalized tonic, clonic, or tonic–clonic movements and myoclonus activities; (b) falling/syncope, characterized by gradual slipping to the floor or the bed, with unresponsiveness or decreased responsiveness sustained for a certain period; (c) unresponsiveness/complex partial mimicking events, characterized by apparent unresponsiveness or decreased responsiveness with or without partial seizures; (d) other event types; and (e) more than one event type.

Of the clinical features of PNES, three main aspects are noteworthy. First, PNES may occur at any age, with typical onset generally between 10 and 40 years of age and a peak incidence between 25 and 40 years. PNES is more common in females than males, and the ratio of male to female cases is 1:3. Cases are rare among the elderly and children under 3 years old. Childhood onset is mostly due to the conversion of an unconscious psychological conflict into somatic symptoms, which acts as a method of self-protection from stressful emotions. The symptoms are relatively simple, mostly involving motor symptoms, primitive reactions, or significant autonomic dysfunction. Chinta et al. [68] studied PNES in children (mean age of 10 years) and found that most patients showed prolonged gazing and unresponsiveness, with less than one-third of patients presenting with pelvic thrusting, upper and lower limb movements, head movements, vocalization, and other symptoms. Clinical manifestations of PNES in adolescents are not significantly different from those in adults and include seizure-like motor, sensory, autonomic, or behavioral abnormalities, with one or more of these as the primary manifestation. Second, various forms of motor symptoms occur, such as trembling, clonus, intermittent rigidity, and dyssynchrony of limb movements. Using a cluster analysis, Groppel et al. [69] classified PNES into three clusters. Cluster 1, called "psychogenic motor seizures," consists of clonic and hyper-motor movements of the extremities, pelvic thrusting, head movements, and tonic posturing of the head. Cluster 2 comprises trembling of the extremities and was termed "psychogenic minor motor or trembling seizures." Cluster 3 is characterized by falling to the floor and was termed "psychogenic atonic seizures." Third, PNES may manifest as one or several types of sensory abnormalities, such as symptoms of irritation, including numbness, pain, foreign body sensation, or electric shock sensation, or symptoms of sensory deficit, such as hypesthesia or anesthesia. Other manifestations can occur, such as emotional outbreaks, rage, chest thumping, feet stamping, rolling on the ground, tearing clothes, and hair pulling. Typically, ictal crying is thought to be one of the characteristic symptoms of PNES and can be evidence favoring the diagnosis of PNES [70]. Autonomic symptoms, such as urinary incontinence, fecal incontinence, shortness of breath, breath holding, and coughing, may also be present.

The differentiation between nonepileptic seizures and epilepsy is very difficult, and the difficulty is particularly increased by the possible coexistence of both disorders [71]. Long duration of seizures, closed eyes, asymmetric movement, frequent recurrence, the presence of consciousness during and after attacks, and the lack of a postictal state are all useful indications in the differentiation of nonepileptic seizures from epilepsy. Mental complications, drug abuse, cognitive impairment, and multiple nonspecific somatic symptoms facilitate the identification of nonepileptic seizures. However, confirmation of the diagnosis relies on the capture of the seizure event by VEM [72].

The following conditions support the diagnosis of PNES: (a) risk factors including anxiety, depression, posttraumatic stress, somatization, anxiety sensitivity, life adversities, suggestibility, attention deficit, family/relationship problems, defense mechanisms, disorders of emotional regulation, alexithymia, and affective disorders; female gender, young age, significant previous traumatic experiences, and attacks induced or aggravated by memories or suggestion of previous traumatic events are all indications of nonepileptic seizures [73]; (b) all types of strange feelings, unilateral or bilateral limb numbness, tonic or clonic seizures, and other clinical manifestations that cannot be explained by neuroanatomy, physiology, or other medical knowledge, in addition to clear purposefulness of displaying symptoms; (c) diverse symptoms and violent, dramatic behavior often accompanied by groaning or weeping without emotional elements; paroxysmal weeping, in particular, is strongly supportive of PNES; and (d) evidence against the presence of epilepsy: nonepileptic seizures rarely occur at night, and they do not have the stereotyped or transient nature of epileptic seizures. The onset and termination of PNES are relatively slow. Once the seizures are terminated, the patient's response is immediately resumed, and no postictal state occurs. Although PNES may be similar to SE, no lip cyanosis, mydriasis, or loss of light reflex occurs, and patients have clear consciousness. The motor symptoms are neither synchronous nor symmetrical, such as nonsynchronous and nonsymmetrical limb swinging or head twisting from side to side, pelvic thrusting, and biped pedal-like movements, which differ significantly from the regular motor symptoms of epilepsy. During PNES, patients keep their eyes closed and are resistant to opening them. Additionally, paroxysmal stuttering and whispering can occur after the attacks, which is evidently different from epileptic seizures. Tongue biting, urinary incontinence, self-mutilation, and bodily injury are common in epileptic seizures but are rare in nonepileptic seizures.

VEM is the most important method used to distinguish epilepsy from nonepileptic seizures. Hupalo et al. [74] monitored 202 patients with paroxysmal disorders and found that the diagnoses of 36% of patients were changed based on the results of VEM. However, the duration of EEG monitoring should be taken into consideration because epilepsy and nonepileptic seizures are both paroxysmal disorders without patterns of onset. Hupalo et al. [74] also conducted EEG monitoring on 117 females and 85 males for 3–9 days and found that 62% of patients with nonepileptic seizures had clinical onset during the first 24 h of monitoring, while the rate for patients with epilepsy was only 15%; thus, they believed that patients with a probable diagnosis of epilepsy should be monitored for at least 72 h; for nonepileptic seizures, the duration of monitoring could be shortened to 49 h. Shen et al. [75] summarized the VEM evidence supporting the diagnosis of nonepileptic seizures as follows: (a) observation through VEM of onset similar to previous attacks in the same patient without epileptiform discharges; (b) nonepileptic seizures are indicated when alteration of consciousness or bilateral limb movement and sensory symptoms appear during onset in the absence of EEG changes; (c) significant alpha rhythm on EEG simultaneous with consciousness alteration; and (d) normal background activity on continuous electroencephalogram (cEEG) records in different physiological states. However, EEG findings may be normal for some types of epileptic seizures, such as simple partial seizures, complex partial seizures, and especially frontal lobe epilepsy, in which it is difficult to detect epileptiform discharges deep within the brain. In these cases, the medical history, clinical manifestations, and results of other auxiliary examinations should be integrated into the process of diagnosis [76, 77]. Studies have found that 5–10% of patients with nonepileptic seizures also have epilepsy, and epileptiform discharges may appear on EEG during psychogenic seizure events. Therefore, an abnormal EEG cannot exclude the possibility of epileptic seizures combined with psychogenic seizures.

In addition to VEM, studies have shown that serum PRL, serum CPK, NSE, and other biochemical markers play an important role in the differential diagnosis between nonepileptic seizures and certain types of epilepsy. First of all, serum PRL is generally thought to peak within 1 h after generalized tonic–clonic seizures (GTCS) and complex partial seizures (CPS) but soon returns to normal. The sensitivity values for the diagnosis of GTCS and CPS are 60% and 46%, respectively, but the specificity is not high. The serum PRL level does not significantly change after frontal lobe seizures, myoclonic seizures, CPS without motor symptoms, or other simple partial seizures. Therefore, the postictal serum PRL level has some significance only in the differential diagnosis between nonepileptic seizures and some types of epilepsy, such as GTCS and CPS. Secondly, serum CPK has also been found to significantly increase after GTCS in most patients, but not after the absence seizures, tonic seizures, CPS, or nonepileptic seizures. Serum CPK usually begins to increase 12 h after seizures, peaks at the 40th hour after seizures, and persists for 3–8 days. Its sensitivity and specificity for the diagnosis of epileptic seizures are 75% and 86%, respectively, making serum CPK a useful index in the differential diagnosis. Petramfar et al. [78] found that postictal serum CPK helped distinguish nonepileptic seizures from GTCS.

1.4.5.6 Hyperventilation Syndrome and Its Differentiation from Epilepsy

Hyperventilation syndrome (HVS) is the most common type of disordered respiratory syndrome. HVS is a complex of symptoms induced by dysfunctional hyperventilation, featuring various physical and psychological manifestations. Increases in the respiratory rate and tidal volume can both result in hyperventilation. The clinical manifestations include dyspnea, chest tightness, sighing, chest pain, and changes in respiratory patterns and rate. Despite the diversity of clinical manifestations, its related symptoms are all associated with respiratory alkalosis and hypocapnia. Rigidity, clonus, and limb convulsion are considered primary manifestations. The most important features of HVS are hyperventilation, decrease in the carbon dioxide level to the lower limit of the normal range, and patterns of symptoms that can be partially or completely reproduced during hyperventilation [79]. Acute HVS accompanied by significantly accelerated breathing accounts for only a very small number of cases, while 99% of patients have chronic HVS that is accompanied by increased tidal volume but not accelerated respiration.

The incidence of HVS in the general population is 6–11%; it occurs more often in females than in males, with a male-to-female ratio of 1:(2–7) [80]. In HVS with neurological symptoms, 50–87% of patients are females. Cases of HVS have also been seen in children and adolescents, many of which are accompanied by chronic anxiety [81].

The exact cause of hyperventilation is not yet clear, and multiple causes may exist. Five percent of cases are caused by organic factors, 60% of cases are associated with psychological factors, and the remaining cases result from the interaction of multiple factors. The main pathogenic process involves hyperventilation leading to a reduction in the carbon dioxide level, which triggers a series of acid-base and/or ion imbalance disorders [82].

Due to its diversity and instability, the clinical manifestations of HVS are very complex. During a single episode, manifestations may involve multiple systems; additionally, each attack may differ. A comprehensive understanding of the manifestations, both systemic and neurological, is beneficial for the diagnosis of this disease.

Systemic manifestations include fatigue, nausea, palpitations, precordial pain, shortness of breath, inspiratory difficulties, suffocation, anxiety, neuroticism, a sense of non-reality, and disorientation. In addition, cognitive and memory disorders, shouting, confusion, panic, and nervousness can be observed. Williamson et al. [83] analyzed 207 cases, 55% of whom had spontaneous hyperventilation, and found that common non-neurological manifestations included pneumonia, neurogenic myocardial injury, systemic inflammatory response syndrome, and radiographic vasospasm. Perkin examined 78 patients who were diagnosed with HVS without any neurological disorder according to a complete neurological examination. The distribution of various neurological symptoms was as follows: dizziness in 36 cases (59%), paresthesia in 28 cases (36%), loss of consciousness in 24 cases (31%), visual impairment in 22 cases (28%), ataxia (including tremor and tinnitus) in 14 cases (18%), and headache in 17 cases (22%) [84]; vertigo was also among the most common manifestations [85]. Generalized convulsions of the extremities are not common clinically. Loss of consciousness is not frequent in HVS; it is generally not associated with posture, but patients with frequent attacks may suffer from head injury due to falling. If the patient simultaneously shows loss of consciousness, convulsion of the limbs, or generalized tonus, HVS should not be considered.

As HVS often manifests as a paroxysmal mental disorder, paresthesia, transient loss of consciousness, or limb twitching, HVS is easily misdiagnosed as epilepsy or another disorder. HVS can also induce CPS, convulsive seizures and NCSE, which increases the difficulty of differentiation from epilepsy [86]. However, HVS can be distinguished from epilepsy based on the factors of age, sleep, stereotype, disturbance of consciousness, paresthesia, twitching, paroxysmal psychiatric symptoms, EEG, and so on. Firstly, HVS is common between the age of 15 and 55 years, while epilepsy onset occurs before 20 years of age in 60% of cases. The incidence of HVS is significantly higher in women than in men, while the incidence of epilepsy shows no significant gender difference. Secondly, over half of epileptic seizures are associated with the sleep–wake cycle, including onset at awakening in the morning. Generalized tonic–clonic seizures mostly occur after awakening or before sleep, while infantile spasms arise during sleep. The onset of HVS occurs during a sober and calm state but rarely occurs during sleep. Thirdly, the manifestations of HVS are complex and highly variable. In a single episode, the symptoms often appear in various forms that involve multiple organs and systems, and they seldom completely coincide with those of other episodes. Epileptic seizures are stereotyped, and the manifestations of each attack are consistent in most cases. Fourthly, the disturbance of consciousness in HVS is shorter and milder. It often manifests as reticence, meditation, and a lack of response when called. Patients have a better understanding of their surroundings than those with epilepsy, while most patients who have epileptic seizures with disturbance of consciousness do not remember events that occur during the seizure attack. After the attack, some patients experience apnea and hypoxemia, which can also lead to disturbance of consciousness [87]. Fifthly, paresthesia in HVS, especially unilateral asymmetric paresthesia, may be mistaken for frontal lobe epilepsy. Paresthesia may be associated with increased axon excitability of peripheral neurons resulting from hyperventilation-induced acid-base imbalance and ion disorders. It may appear alone or be combined with other symptoms. When paresthesia emerges as the only symptom, careful identification is required. Epileptic paresthesia is brief and is mostly lateralized with consistent symptoms; this is a key point in the differentiation of paresthesia from HVS. Sixthly, generalized convulsions of the upper and lower extremities are uncommon in HVS. Twitching often manifests as trembling of the limbs, and the patient simultaneously has clear consciousness. The trembling exhibits a low amplitude and a high frequency, which is significantly different from epileptic convulsions of the limbs, which are accompanied by loss of consciousness. With careful observation, it is not difficult to differentiate these symptoms from epilepsy [86]. Seventhly, paroxysmal psychiatric symptoms include anxiety, neuroticism, a sense of non-reality, and orientation disorders. The psychiatric symptoms are more diverse in epilepsy and include various types of amnesia, emotional abnormalities, illusions, and complex hallucinations. Eighthly, although some patients of HVS exhibit global slow waves, occasional cases of abnormal focal or global delta waves during awakening have been observed on EEG. However, no obvious epileptiform discharge is seen on EEG either during or after attacks, while the EEGs of patients with epilepsy often show epileptic discharges (such as typical spikes, spike-and-wave complexes, or sharp-and-wave complexes). Hyperventilation is a technique often used by neurologists to induce epileptiform discharges. If epileptiform discharges occur during hyperventilation, it should be determined whether they are induced by the latter. Finally, the hyperventilation provocation test (HVPT) is a routine examination for HVS. In the HVPT, hypocapnia should be sustained for 3 min, and it should be ensured that the end tidal partial pressure of carbon dioxide is lower than 1.9 kPa or 50% of the baseline. Partial or complete replication of onset in daily life is key evidence in the differentiation of HVS from epilepsy; low partial pressure of carbon dioxide in blood gas analysis is another key point of identification.

1.4.5.7 Eclampsia

Convulsive epileptic seizures during pregnancy mainly involve epileptic convulsions intensified during pregnancy or existing specifically during pregnancy. The former is caused by a reduced seizure threshold and aggravation of epileptic seizures due to poor compliance of medication during pregnancy or specific physiological conditions, such as nausea, vomiting, sleep disorders, and others; the latter involve a particular pathophysiological condition that occurs during pregnancy. Although eclampsia and epileptic seizures have similar manifestations, they are two separate disorders.

Globally, eclampsia is a public health issue and a major cause of pregnancy-related maternal mortality. It occurs in approximately 6–8% of pregnancies, and it is the direct cause of 12.3% of maternal mortality. In low-income and middle-income countries, eclamptic convulsions are directly associated with 10–15% of maternal deaths. The cause of convulsions in eclampsia is not clear. The general view is that cerebral edema, hypertension, and cerebral ischemia in eclampsia trigger the massive release of neurokinin B, inflammatory cytokines, endothelin, tissue plasminogen activator, and other bioactive molecules. These molecules stimulate excitatory neuronal receptors and alter synaptic transmission, leading to the occurrence of eclamptic convulsions [60, 88].

Eclampsia involves convulsions that cannot be explained by any other reason than the existence of preeclampsia. Primiparas are more susceptible to eclampsia, which often occurs in the middle or late stage of pregnancy. In approximately 10% of patients, eclampsia occurs before the 28th week of pregnancy, with a few cases of onset before the 20th week. Eclampsia arises with acute onset. Some patients may have auras, such as severe forehead pain, nausea, vomiting, blurred vision, photophobia, or epigastric pain, which are followed by convulsions. The convulsions manifest as a sudden loss of consciousness, falling, upward turning of the eyes, locked jaws, and tonus–clonus of the limbs. After a few minutes, the patient recovers but cannot recall the attack. The seizures may be recurrent.

Eclamptic encephalopathy is acute global cerebral dysfunction induced by the onset of eclampsia. Posterior reversible encephalopathy syndrome is a type of eclamptic encephalopathy that is reported to have an extremely high incidence in patients with eclampsia [89]. The clinical manifestations of eclamptic encephalopathy include severe headache, blurred vision, epileptic seizures, nausea, vomiting, and disturbance of consciousness or coma in severe cases. Elevated blood pressure (≥170/100 mmHg) can be found on physical examination. Laboratory findings may include proteinuria and thrombocytopenia. With timely treatment, full recovery can be expected; otherwise, patients may suffer from irreversible damage or even death.

For sudden convulsions accompanied by high blood pressure or proteinuria during the middle or late stage of pregnancy, the first consideration should be eclampsia, but other causes of convulsions should be excluded. For an atypical course of onset, such as onset before the 20th week of pregnancy or late onset of postpartum eclampsia without hypertension or proteinuria, the diagnosis should be made with caution; relevant examinations should be completed to reveal evidence of preeclampsia.

Misdiagnosis is not uncommon due to the similar clinical manifestations of eclampsia and epileptic seizures as well as the abnormal EEG findings in both. However, eclampsia is different from epileptic convulsions in that the convulsions are accompanied by hypertension and proteinuria, which occur during pregnancy and can be terminated with magnesium sulfate.

1.5 Diagnosis of NCSE

NCSE is SE without generalized convulsion. Due to its complex etiology, diverse clinical manifestations, and frequent complication with other diseases, NCSE is easily masked by the primary disease or misdiagnosed as other disorders (such as hysteria, encephalitis, metabolic disease, or postictal state). NCSE may cause irreversible damage to the nervous system with delayed treatment.

1.5.1 Definition of NCSE

Controversy remains over the definition of NCSE. It is currently considered a series of nonconvulsive epileptic events that result from continuous epileptiform electroencephalographic activities [16, 17]. NCSE describes a continuous nonconvulsive clinical condition associated with continuous epileptiform discharges on EEG, and it may involve changes in behavioral and/or mental–psychological processes, disorders of consciousness, or visceral dysfunction. Clinically, NCSE is mainly characterized as an episodic disorder of sensation, thinking, consciousness, behavior, or visceral function or a decline in arousal level. To understand the definition of NCSE, three aspects should be considered. The first aspect is symptoms, especially changes in the psycho-behavioral state and/or the state of consciousness. Niedermeyer et al. [90] described the two stereotypes of NCSE: the walking wounded and the ictally comatose. The walking wounded refers to patients with absence status or focal SE, with only a slight disturbance of consciousness or behavioral abnormalities. The ictally comatose mainly includes patients with subtle SE who are often left with slight motor symptoms after convulsive seizures and comatose patients with epileptiform discharges. The second aspect is EEG changes as a prerequisite for establishing the diagnosis of NCSE (please refer to Chap. 5). The third aspect is the duration of clinical manifestations or EEG changes, which should be sufficiently long, although the specific length remains to be defined. Traditionally, an episode of NCSE is defined as longer than 30 min or recurrent without complete interictal recovery of consciousness, but some studies support the thought that treatment should be initiated as early as 5–10 min after onset [91]. Therefore, if a patient shows more than 10 min of continuous clinical and EEG changes that suggest NCSE, the presence of NCSE should be considered.

1.5.2 Incidence of NCSE

The incidence of NCSE is high, but a specific value is difficult to estimate. According to epidemiologic surveys and other clinical studies, the estimated incidence is approximately 18.3–85 per ten million person-years [92–95], and Towne et al. [96] suggested in a prospective study that 8% of all patients treated in an ICU had NCSE. Although these data suggest a relatively high incidence of NCSE, some researchers still believe that the incidence of NCSE is underestimated because the absence of timely diagnosis results in numerous missed cases [97]. NCSE accounts for 25–50% of SE cases [98] and of patients who had tonic–clonic seizures, more than 14% experienced postictal NCSE [99].

1.5.3 Etiology of NCSE

The etiology of NCSE is complex. NCSE may originate from primary dysfunction of the central nervous system or may be an aggravation of preexisting seizure events. Other common causes include metabolic disorders, systemic disorders, and drugs.

NCSE often occurs in patients with a history of convulsions or epilepsy. It has been reported that before the occurrence of NCSE, approximately 1/3 to 2/3 of patients have a history of convulsions or epilepsy [96, 100–102]. Improper withdrawal and improper use of antiepileptic drugs are important factors in the incidence of NCSE in these patients [16, 101, 103]. Compared to adults with epilepsy, patients under 18 years of age are more prone to NCSE [100–102, 104]. In addition, Shorvon et al. [105] summarized the characteristics of NCSE, finding that NCSE is associated not only with age and brain maturity but also with epileptic encephalopathy and epilepsy syndrome.

Hypoxic–ischemic encephalopathy [106, 107], intracranial infection [108–112], ischemic stroke [113, 114], intracranial hemorrhage [115–117], cerebral sinovenous thrombosis [112], brain tumors [118, 119], traumatic brain injury [120], and autoimmune encephalitis [121] are all common causes of NCSE. Alroughani et al. [122] found that before the onset of NCSE, 38.1% of patients had a history of hypoxic–ischemic brain injury, which indicates that this type of acute brain injury is a common cause of NCSE. Little et al. [117] found that after subarachnoid hemorrhage, 2.8% of patients had NCSE, while the incidence was even higher in other studies [115, 123]. Greiner et al. [124] analyzed data from an 11-year follow-up of 73 patients with traumatic brain injury and found that 27.4% of patients had nonconvulsive seizures and 4.1% had NCSE.

Disorders of metabolism and the internal environment may induce NCSE. For example, NCSE may occur in patients with dysglycemia and electrolyte imbalance [125, 126]. There are also reports of NCSE during the terminal stages of systemic disorders, such as hepatic failure [127, 128]. NCSE may also occur in patients with reversible posterior leukoencephalopathy syndrome and HE [129].

Drugs are also important factors that induce SE [130]. Antibiotics (e.g., cephalosporins or quinolones) often induce NCSE [131, 132]. In an analysis of 117 patients, Misra et al. [133] found that approximately 3.4% of the cases were associated with the use of antibiotics. Antipsychotics, such as lithium, olanzapine, and tricyclic antidepressants, are also common causes of convulsion and NCSE [134–137]; some complications of antipsychotic therapy, such as serotonin syndrome and neuroleptic malignant syndrome, may also lead to the occurrence of NCSE [138]. Reports have also described NCSE associated with chemotherapeutic drugs for malignant tumors, immunosuppressive agents, and alcoholism [139–143].

1.5.4 Clinical Manifestations of NCSE

The clinical manifestations of NCSE are sometimes atypical. Jirsch et al. [144] summarized the common positive and negative symptoms of NCSE and noted that manifestations such as anorexia, catatonia, nystagmus, amnesia, lethargy, blinking, crying, and laughter are all indications of NCSE. These symptoms are very common in the NICU but are easily overlooked by healthcare providers.

1.5.4.1 Generalized Typical Absence in NCSE Without Coma

Typical absence status is a type of epileptic activity with specific clinical manifestations. It is common in patients with idiopathic generalized seizures, especially absence seizures or juvenile myoclonic absence seizures. Typical absence status is often induced by inappropriate antiepileptic therapy, fever, hyperventilation, sadness, excitement, or fatigue. The primary manifestation is disturbance of consciousness of varying degrees, which is sometimes accompanied by slight eyelid twitching. It lasts a few seconds, several days, or several weeks and is often followed by secondary generalized convulsive SE. The overall prognosis is good.

1.5.4.2 Generalized Atypical Absence in NCSE Without Coma

From a clinical point of view, it is difficult to distinguish between typical and atypical absence status in the absence of a reliable medical history, clinical features, aura, and other information. In atypical absence status, the level of disturbance of consciousness is deeper, and blinking, grimacing, and other manifestations are present.

The prognosis is poor, and a tendency toward recurrence and drug resistance has been observed.

The EEG changes of atypical absence SE are similar to the ictal EEG changes of typical absence status, but the interictal background EEG activity is often slowed.

1.5.4.3 Myoclonic Absence in NCSE Without Coma

Myoclonic absence status is common in children with idiopathic generalized epilepsy. It manifests as frequent rhythmic limb myoclonus with disturbance of consciousness during absence events; the elements of myoclonus are more obvious than the elements of absence.

1.5.4.4 Focal NCSE Without Impairment of Consciousness

This type of NCSE primarily involves the neocortex and is similar to the previous notion of simple partial NCSE. The main manifestations are aphasia and disorders of hearing, speech, gustation, olfaction, vision, autonomic nerve function, sensation, mental state, and behavior. Focal NCSE without impairment of consciousness is different from complex partial SE in that the patient's consciousness is not impaired. As the attacks originate from focal discharges, they are easily overlooked because the lack of characteristics of generalized convulsions can be misleading. If the patient has only subjective experiences that have not been witnessed, it is called aura continua.

1.5.4.5 Focal NCSE with Aphasic Status

Aphasic status is a rare type of SE characterized by speech disorders. This concept was first proposed by Bender [145] in 1966. In addition to continuous or fluctuating sensory, motor, or mixed aphasia, most patients experience mild myoclonus, hemianopia, or hemiplegia. The lesions are often in the dominant hemisphere, especially the temporal and frontal regions. cEEG monitoring is very helpful for the diagnosis and treatment of aphasic status [146]. Imaging studies suggest that in SE with aphasic manifestations, the temporoparietal cortex and thalamic nuclei, including areas far from the epileptic foci or speech areas, show high signal intensity on DWI after onset [147].

1.5.4.6 Focal NCSE with Impairment of Consciousness

The main clinical manifestations of this type of NCSE include varying degrees of disturbance of consciousness and mental–behavioral abnormalities. Disturbance of consciousness includes confusion, indifference, somnolence, or stupor; its main characteristic is the inability to recall the attack. Mental–behavioral abnormalities include silence, dullness, loss of concentration, fear, impulsiveness, delusion, and automatism of the mouth or hands. During an attack, patients are often unable to take care of themselves, recognize their family, or understand speech. After the attack, patients have no memory of the event and often feel tired. An attack may last several hours, several days, or even over a month but can be alleviated spontaneously. In some patients, focal NCSE may be complicated by other types of seizures.

1.5.4.7 NCSE Failure of Classification as Generalized or Focal Status

Among the most common subtypes of this category of NCSE is autonomic SE, which is common in Panayiotopoulos syndrome [148, 149] but rare in other epilepsy syndromes. Patients often have autonomic symptoms, such as nausea, vomiting, hiccups, tachycardia, bradycardia, pallor, flushing, increased or decreased blood pressure, fever, and frequent micturition.

1.5.5 Diagnosis of NCSE

The diagnosis of NCSE requires comprehensive consideration of clinical manifestations and EEG changes. Repeated clinical events are important clues. If EEG shows typical epileptic discharges, the diagnosis is easy. However, considering that EEG changes of NCSE are often confounded with those of other encephalopathies, verification of the effectiveness of antiepileptic drugs (AEDs) on clinical presentation and EEG are needed [150]. The diagnosis can be divided into three steps as follows.

Step 1: Identify patients with suspected NCSE.
Step 2: Perform EEG monitoring with a definite duration.
Step 3: Assess whether the diagnosis of NCSE is supported by the medical history and EEG; if the diagnosis is difficult, tests with intravenous AEDs may be performed.

Since the clinical symptoms of NCSE are nontypical, theoretically, patients with continued alterations of mental state, behavior, or state of consciousness and those with similar previous manifestations should be suspected of NCSE. In the NICU, sustained disorder of consciousness after a generalized tonic–clonic event, especially those lasting over 10 min after the attack, is a warning of the possible development of NCSE [151–153]. In patients with severe neurological disorders, NCSE should be considered in cases of coma or aggravated disturbance of consciousness [96, 103, 116].

The European Society of Intensive Care Medicine and the Neurocritical Care Society of the US recommend cEEG monitoring as a routine procedure for patients with critical neurological disorders [16, 123]. Regarding the duration of monitoring, Claassen [102] and colleagues performed cEEG monitoring on 570 patients and observed epileptic attacks in 110 of them, of whom 88% had their first attacks observed within the first 24 h of cEEG monitoring and 93% were found to have epileptic attacks when the monitoring was prolonged to 48 h. However, Shafi et al. [154] monitored 242 patients without prior generalized convulsive seizures or active seizures and discovered that in the majority of patients with observed seizure attacks, the attacks occurred during the first 30 min of monitoring (52 cases in 70 patients; 74.3%). If no epileptiform discharges were detected within the first 4 h of monitoring, the likelihood of a subsequent seizure was very low. This evidence suggests the necessity of cEEG monitoring in NICU patients, and we advocate cEEG monitoring within 48 h after admission if possible. If the patient experiences generalized convulsive SE or an aggravated disturbance of consciousness during this period, monitoring can be extended to 72 h.

To read about the evaluation of the diagnosis of NCSE based on patient history and EEG as well as the intravenous AED test, please refer to Chap. 5.

1.5.6 Treatment of NCSE

Identification of the primary disorder should be actively sought to treat NCSE based on etiology. Meanwhile, the stability of vital signs should be maintained. For specific solutions, please refer to Chaps. 6, 7, and 8.

The goal of SE treatment is the clinical termination of attacks and epileptiform discharges on EEG. As a type of SE, NCSE is not fundamentally different from other types in terms of methods of termination. However, due to the insignificant clinical manifestations of NCSE, much of the diagnosis relies on EEG, and the treatment is also dependent on EEG guidance.

1.6 Diagnosis of RSE

A principle characteristic of epilepsy is that it self-terminates. Epileptic seizures terminate as a result of the refractory period that occurs following seizure activity. If the refractory period is disrupted, the seizure will continue, resulting in status epilepticus. Although RSE has not been uniformly defined, one of its major characteristics is that it is resistant to first-line antiepileptic drugs, especially benzodiazepines, and therefore requires special treatment. Despite the effort to define RSE, no international agreement has been reached regarding how many types of drugs a patient must be resistant to for their seizures to be defines as "resistant." The current view is that if an epileptic seizure does not stop or begins again after 2–3 types of antiepileptic drugs have been used, it is considered RSE [155–174].

The first person to propose the concept of refractory status epilepticus was Lebedev

[175]. Then, Vajda et al. [176] reported the use of valproate to treat refractory status epilepticus in patients who were resistant to diazepam. When valproate was administered at a dose of 200–800 mg every 6 h, it produced satisfactory results. In 1980, Young et al. [177] explored the use of barbiturates to treat refractory status epilepticus. In 1984, Orlowski [178] began to use low temperature therapy to treat refractory status epilepticus in children, and three such patients showed improvements. In recent years, treatments using electro-convulsion and a ketogenic diet have received increased attention, and these results have enriched the study of this condition [179, 180].

1.6.1 Epidemiological Investigation of RSE

The incidence rate is the frequency at which new cases of a disease appear in a population during a specified period of time. The prevalence is the proportion of the total population that has a certain disease during a given period of time. Because the definition of persistent refractory status epilepticus is not clear, and because medical level and social factors are different in each study area, an accurate incidence of the disease has not been obtained. Epidemiological investigations have shown that the status epilepticus incidence rate is between 100/1 million and 160/1 million [99]. Retrospective studies showed that in adults, the rate of refractory status epilepticus in patients with status epilepticus was 14–46% [155, 181–183]. Rossetti et al. [184] evaluated 127 instances of refractory status epilepticus in 107 patients and found that the rate of refractory status epilepticus was 39% in patients with status epilepticus. Barzegar et al. [185] investigated 132 children with status epilepticus and found that the incidence of refractory status epilepticus was 40.15%. Because of the aging of society and ongoing increases in a variety of diseases, the incidence of refractory status epilepticus may be higher.

The mortality rate is the proportion of total deaths resulting from a specific disease among all patients or animals suffering from that disease during a certain period of time. If refractory status epilepticus is not controlled, a patient can die from a severe fever, internal disturbances, respiratory depression, or cardiac arrest. Rohracher et al. [186] found that the mortality rate in patients with refractory status epilepticus who were hospitalized in an intensive care unit was 38%, similar to the 39%~65% mortality rate reported in other studies. Sinha et al. [187] found that mortality in older patients with refractory status epilepticus was 34%. The highest reported mortality rate reached 60% in patients with high blood pressure, hypoxia, and intracranial infections [181, 183]. In a retrospective cohort study, Juhasz et al. [188] found that the mortality rate in patients with refractory status epilepticus was 30–50% and was influenced by the presence of different etiologies. Tumors, hypoxia, infection, and onset age were the main risk factors for death, and the mortality was two–three times higher in patients with these risk factors than in other patients. Delaj et al. [181] found that 25% of patients with refractory status epilepticus died and 44% experienced subsequent serious neurological disease. Lai et al. [189] studied 78 patients with refractory status epilepticus, of whom 41 died, resulting in a mortality rate of 52.5%. Twenty-six of the patients died of infection and multiple organ failure (33.2%), two died of cardiac arrest (2.5%), and one died of malignant intracranial hypertension (1.3%). Liberalesso et al. [190] conducted electroencephalography monitoring in 15 patients with refractory epilepsy. Nine of these patients (60%) died, including all of the patients over 80 years old and 50% of the patients over 50 years old. One patient (6.6%) had a sequelae, and five patients (33.3%) had a good prognosis. Therefore, the mortality rate in patients with refractory status epilepticus is generally between 30 and 60%. Because there is currently no accurate definition for refractory status epilepticus, it is difficult to make comparisons between data in different studies.

1.6.2 Relative Factors of RSE

1.6.2.1 Age

The incidence rate of refractory status epilepticus has a bimodal distribution and peaks in patients less than 1 year old and over 60 years old. Additionally, 49.1% of patients are older than 50 years old, and 24.2% of affected patients are older than 80 years old, indicating that its incidence increases with age [99]. Studies have also suggested that the bimodal distribution has peaks at less than 5 years old and more than 60 years old [191]. In addition, other studies have shown that the distribution of the incidence of this condition exhibits a "J" type, with a smaller peak in patients less than 5 years old (incidence, 10.2/100,000) and a lager peak in those more than 60 years old (incidence, 13.9/100,000) [191].

1.6.2.2 Type of Onset of Status Epilepticus

Nonconvulsive status epilepticus is more likely to develop into refractory status epilepticus than convulsive status epilepticus. Previous studies have shown that approximately 8% of critically ill patients in hospitals have nonconvulsive status epilepticus. In patients with nonconvulsive status epilepticus without a history of epilepsy, the mortality rate is as high as 80% [97]. Liberalesso et al. [190] conducted cEEG monitoring in 15 male patients with refractory status epilepticus and found that in 14 of these cases (93.3%), it developed from CPS. A multivariate analysis showed that nonconvulsive status epilepticus and partial motor status epilepticus were independent risk factors for refractory status epilepticus. Cardoso et al. [192] conducted a retrospective study of 15 hospitalized patients, including children and adolescents, with refractory status epilepticus (11 with convulsive status epilepticus and four with nonconvulsive status epilepticus). Six of these 11 patients developed nonconvulsive status epilepticus, and the average status epilepticus duration was 10.2 days. After treatment, one patient became drug resistant, one died, and 13 developed new neurological symptoms and epilepsy that became difficult to control.

1.6.2.3 Etiology

Etiology plays an important role in the formation of refractory status epilepticus. Epidemiological surveys have shown that common causes of refractory status epilepticus include anti-epilepsy drug withdrawal, central nervous system infections, stroke, hypoxia, and metabolic disorders [186, 187]. Other causes include acute craniocerebral injury, brain malformations, encephalitis, autoimmune diseases (e.g., systemic lupus erythematosus), Kufs disease, mitochondrial myopathy, acute drug poisoning, periodic stroke, cancer, and paraneoplastic syndrome, in addition to genes and genetic factors, such as mutations in mitochondrial DNA [193–195]. A multivariate analysis showed that central nervous system infections, metabolic encephalopathy, and hypoxia are the most common risk factors for refractory status epilepticus. Encephalitis and meningitis are the most common causes of refractory status epilepticus in children [185]. Glaser et al. [196] studied 1151 patients with encephalitis at the California Encephalitis Research Center and found that the incidence rate of refractory status epilepticus was 4% in patients with encephalitis. Fever caused by respiratory or digestive system disease is typically observed prior to status epilepticus. Sutter et al. [197] found that in 260 patients with refractory status epilepticus, the condition was caused by hypoxia, intracranial tumors, and stroke in 54%, 32%, and 18% of the cases, respectively, and in more than 40% of the patients, it had an additional cause, such as metabolic disease, hypertension, diabetes mellitus, or chronic congestive heart failure. Lingappa et al. [35] conducted a retrospective study of 73 children who were 2–12 years old and suffered from status epilepticus in developing countries. They found that 45.2% of the included children with convulsive status epilepticus developed refractory status epilepticus. In all, 60.3% of the cases were caused by intracranial infection, and affected patients had a poor prognosis over a short period of time.

1.6.3 Clinical Features of RSE

Refractory status epilepticus is different from epilepsy. Epilepsy is a chronic disease that requires long-term treatment, while refractory status epilepticus is a critical and severe condition. Drugs are not needed to prevent the recurrence of epilepsy if status epilepticus is stopped. However, status epilepticus will inevitably develop into epilepsy. Many cases of status epilepticus do not recur or develop into epilepsy if status epilepticus is stopped and the cause is eliminated. Therefore, the classification of refractory status epilepticus is not consistent with that of epilepsy. Although there is currently no consensus regarding the classification of refractory status epilepticus, the literature divides it into new-onset, preexisting epilepsy with initial treatment failure and special types of refractory status epilepticus.

1.6.3.1 New-Onset Refractory Status Epilepticus

Refractory status epilepticus can occur in patients who have no history of epilepsy but are resistant to first-line anti-status epileptic drugs. This is called new-onset refractory status epilepticus. Its exact cause is unknown, but most affected patients have an elevated temperature, suggesting that it may be associated with an infection in the central nervous system or an immune response.

1.6.3.2 Refractory Status Epilepticus in Patients with Preexisting Epilepsy with Initial Treatment Failure

Most of these patients have a history of epilepsy, and acute withdrawal is an important cause of its occurrence. If treatment is not administered quickly, alterations to the internal environment may occur, including changes in synaptic membrane receptors and neurotransmitter release. These changes result in drug resistance in these patients and lead to refractory status epilepticus. An epidemiological survey that examined refractory status epilepticus found that only 3.4–6% of patients with refractory status epilepticus have a history of epilepsy. This type of refractory status epilepticus can be prevented by treatment prior to hospital admission.

1.6.3.3 Special Types of RSE

This type of RSE is symptomatic of a primary disease, and improvement in the primary disease should lead to improvement in RSE without additional treatment. If the primary disease continues to develop but the epilepsy is controlled, its prognosis will not change. Overemphasis on controlling its onset can result in iatrogenic injury. Therefore, a reasonable strategy should be applied that targets both RSE and the primary disease.

1.6.4 Treatment for RSE

The management principles for treating RSE include controlling its clinical symptoms, eliminating epileptic discharges on EEG, avoiding or reducing iatrogenic injury, and effectively controlling complications.

The major characteristic of RSE is resistance to benzodiazepine drugs, such as diazepam and lorazepam, which are commonly used as a treatment option. It therefore requires anesthesia, hypothermia, or electroconvulsive therapy. The risk of iatrogenic injury is substantially increased in affected patients. The use of anesthetics can cause rhabdomyolysis, and the risk of drug-induced heart pulmonary dysfunction is also significantly increased. Additionally, the patient's internal environment is disrupted. Electrolyte disorders, coma-associated malnutrition, and combined infections that result from refractory status epilepticus can endanger the lives of affected patients. Correcting disorders in the internal environment should therefore be an important component of strategies to manage refractory status epilepticus.

1.6.5 Prognosis of RSE

Elderly patients have a higher mortality rate. Even when survivors are treated with endotracheal intubation and managed in an intensive care unit, their functional status will be significantly reduced [196]. A study by Sutter et al. [197] found that affected patients (60%) with periodic lateralized epileptiform discharges all died, and 2/3 of these deaths occurred in patients who were over 50 years old. Therefore, age and the type of epilepsy are closely associated with the prognosis.

In addition to its association with increased age, prognoses are worse in patients with a complex partial type of refractory status epilepticus than in patients with other epilepsy types [190].

Patients with a disturbance of consciousness before refractory status epilepticus have poor prognoses. Approximately 1/3 of these patients experienced symptoms of epilepsy 6 months after refractory status epilepticus [186]. A prospective study of 83 patients with status epilepticus in Italy found that the mortality rate in refractory status epilepticus was 54%, and only 19% of the included patients showed improvement and returned to normal baseline levels. Prolonged unconsciousness during the early stages of the disease suggested a poor prognosis [198, 199].

Lingappa et al. [35] found that the risk of refractory status epilepticus-induced sepsis is six times higher than the corresponding status epilepticus-induced risk. The risk of acidosis was 15 times higher in refractory than non-refractory status epilepticus patients. The mortality rate in refractory status epilepticus was 21.2%, and 1 year later, the disability rate was seven times higher than that observed in young patients with status epilepticus. The prognosis of patients with pulmonary infection is poor [200, 201].

The rate of reduction of the K-M survival curve is 3.1 times lower in patients with refractory status epilepticus caused by hypoxic encephalopathy than in patients without hypoxic encephalopathy. A study of 132 patients with status epilepticus in the children's hospital of Iran found that 40.15% of these children developed refractory status epilepticus. Encephalitis and meningitis were the most common causes of deterioration, and the mortality rate in affected patients was 8.3%. None of the encephalitis survivors returned to normal baseline levels [184]. Some studies also found that the etiology and duration of status epilepticus during the first 2 h have predictive value. For example, the mortality rate was 2.7% if the duration of refractory status epilepticus was less than 1 h, whereas it was 32% if the duration of refractory status epilepticus was more than 1 h. The duration loses its prognostic value when it is longer than a few hours [200]. Webster et al. [201] studied two patients with refractory status epilepticus that was induced by partial lung virus infection. In these patients, the disease was controlled by antiviral drug treatment for 2 weeks.

References

1. Parra J, Augustijn PB, Geerts Y, van Emde Boas W. Classification of epileptic seizures: a comparison of two systems. Epilepsia. 2001;42:476–82.
2. Fisher RS, van Emde BW, Blume W, Elger C, Genton P, Lee P, Engel J Jr. Epileptic seizures and epilepsy: definitions proposed by the International League Against Epilepsy (ILAE) and the International Bureau for Epilepsy (IBE). Epilepsia. 2005;46:470–2.
3. French JA, Pedley TA. Clinical practice. Initial management of epilepsy. N Engl J Med. 2008;359:166–76.
4. Fisher RS, Acevedo C, Arzimanoglou A, Bogacz A, Cross JH, Elger CE, Engel J Jr, Forsgren L, French JA, Glynn M, Hesdorffer DC, Lee BI, Mathern GW, Moshe SL, Perucca E, Scheffer IE, Tomson T, Watanabe M, Wiebe S. ILAE official report: a practical clinical definition of epilepsy. Epilepsia. 2014;55:475–82.
5. Commission on Classification and Terminology of the International League Against Epilepsy. Proposal for revised clinical and electroencephalographic classification of epileptic seizures. Epilepsia. 1981;22:489–501.
6. Commission on Classification and Terminology of the International League Against Epilepsy. Proposal for revised classification of epilepsies and epileptic syndromes. Epilepsia. 1989;30:389–99.
7. Berg AT, Berkovic SF, Brodie MJ, Buchhalter J, Cross JH, van Emde BW, Engel J, French J, Glauser TA, Mathern GW, Moshe SL, Nordli D, Plouin P, Scheffer IE. Revised terminology and concepts for organization of seizures and epilepsies: report of the ILAE Commission on Classification and Terminology, 2005-2009. Epilepsia. 2010;51:676–85.
8. Bwala SA, Gardner-Thorpe C. Intractable epilepsy. Br J Clin Pract. 1990;44:106–10.
9. Livingston JH. Management of intractable epilepsy. Arch Dis Child. 1991;66:1454–6.
10. Kwan P, Arzimanoglou A, Berg AT, Brodie MJ, Allen Hauser W, Mathern G, Moshe SL, Perucca E, Wiebe S, French J. Definition of drug resistant epilepsy: consensus proposal by the ad hoc Task Force of the ILAE Commission on Therapeutic Strategies. Epilepsia. 2010;51:1069–77.
11. World Health Organization. WHO defined daily doses of antiepileptic drugs. 2010. www.WHOCC.no/atc_ddd_index/?code=NO3A0. Accessed 10 Oct 2011.
12. Morimoto K, Fahnestock M, Racine RJ. Kindling and status epilepticus models of epilepsy: rewiring the brain. Prog Neurobiol. 2004;73:1–60.

13. Guidelines for Epidemiologic Studies on Epilepsy. Commission on Epidemiology and Prognosis, International League against Epilepsy. Epilpsia. 1993;34:592–6.
14. Lowenstein DH, Bleck T, Macdonald RL. It's time to revise the definition of status epilepticus. Epilepsia. 1999;40:120–2.
15. Meierkord H, Boon P, Engelsen B, Gocke K, Shorvon S, Tinuper P, Holtkamp M. EFNS guideline on the management of status epilepticus in adults. Eur J Neurol. 2010;17:348–55.
16. Brophy GM, Bell R, Claassen J, Alldredge B, Bleck TP, Glauser T, Laroche SM, Riviello JJ Jr, Shutter L, Sperling MR, Treiman DM, Vespa PM. Guidelines for the evaluation and management of status epilepticus. Neurocrit Care. 2012;17:3–23.
17. Trinka E, Cock H, Hesdorffer D, Rossetti AO, Scheffer IE, Shinnar S, Shorvon S, Lowenstein DH. A definition and classification of status epilepticus—report of the ILAE Task Force on Classification of Status Epilepticus. Epilepsia. 2015;56:1515–23.
18. Engel J Jr. A proposed diagnostic scheme for people with epileptic seizures and with epilepsy: report of the ILAE Task Force on Classification and Terminology. Epilepsia. 2001;42:796–803.
19. Shorvon S. Super-refractory status epilepticus: an approach to therapy in this difficult clinical situation. Epilepsia. 2011;52(Suppl 8):53–6.
20. Wang X. Diagnosis and treatment of status epilepticus. Beijing: People's Medical Publishing House; 2010.
21. Hunter RA. Status epilepticus; history, incidence and problems. Epilepsia. 1959;1:162–88.
22. Arnautova EN, Nesmeianova TN. A proposed international classifiaction of epileptic seizures. Epilepsia. 1964;5:297–306.
23. Bleck TP. Convulsive disorders: status epilepticus. Clin Neuropharmacol. 1991;14:191–8.
24. Treiman DM, Meyers PD, Walton NY, Collins JF, Colling C, Rowan AJ, Handforth A, Faught E, Calabrese VP, Uthman BM, Ramsay RE, Mamdani MB. A comparison of four treatments for generalized convulsive status epilepticus. Veterans Affairs Status Epilepticus Cooperative Study Group. N Engl J Med. 1998;339:792–8.
25. Malek AM, Wilson DA, Martz GU, et al. Mortality following status epilepticus in persons with and without epilepsy. Seizure. 2016;42:7–13.
26. Rohracher A, Reiter DP, Brigo F, et al. Status epilepticus in the elderly—a retrospective study on 120 patients. Epilepsy Res. 2016;127:317–23.
27. Mirsattari SM, Gofton TE, Chong DJ. Misdiagnosis of epileptic seizures as manifestations of psychiatric illnesses. Can J Neurol Sci. 2011;38(3):487–93.
28. Power KN, Gramstad A, Gilhus NE, et al. Prognostic factors of status epilepticus in adults. Epileptic Disord. 2016;18(3):297–304.
29. Rutka R, Denis A, Vercueil L, Hot P. Psychogenic nonepileptic seizures: current knowledge and contributions of the study of emotions. Sante Ment Que. 2016;41(1):123–39. French.
30. Wiseman H, Mousa S, Howlett S, et al. A multicenter evaluation of a brief manualized psychoeducation intervention for psychogenic nonepileptic seizures delivered by health professionals with limited experience in psychological treatment. Epilepsy Behav. 2016;63:50–6.
31. Asadi-Pooya AA, Asadollahi M, Tinker J, et al. Post-epilepsy surgery psychogenic nonepileptic seizures. Epilepsia. 2016;57(10):1691–6.
32. Russell LA, Abbass AA, Allder SJ, et al. A pilot study of reduction in healthcare costs following the application of intensive short-term dynamic psychotherapy for psychogenic nonepileptic seizures. Epilepsy Behav. 2016;63:17–9.
33. Rawlings GH, Reuber M. What patients say about living with psychogenic nonepileptic seizures: a systematic synthesis of qualitative studies. Seizure. 2016;41:100–11.
34. Hayakawa I, Miyama S, Inoue N, et al. Epidemiology of pediatric convulsive status epilepticus with fever in the emergency department: a cohort study of 381 consecutive cases. J Child Neurol. 2016;31(10):1257–64.
35. Lingappa L, Konanki R, Patel R, et al. Clinical profile and outcome of refractory convulsive status epilepticus in older children from a developing country. Seizure. 2016;36:31–5.
36. Chentli F, Akkache L, Daffeur K, et al. General seizures revealing macro-adenomas secreting prolactin or prolactin and growth hormone in men. Indian J Endocrinol Metab. 2014;18(3):361–3.
37. Sorge ST, Hesdorffer DC, Phelan JC, et al. Depression and genetic causal attribution of epilepsy in multiplex epilepsy families. Epilepsia. 2016;57:1643–50.
38. Camara-Lemarroy CR, Escobedo-Zúñiga N, Ortiz-Zacarias D, et al. Prevalence and impact of irritable bowel syndrome in people with epilepsy. Epilepsy Behav. 2016;63:29–33.
39. Mameniškienė R, Karmonaitė I, Zagorskis R. The burden of headache in people with epilepsy. Seizure. 2016;41:120–6.
40. Cooper BB. Alarming syncope, from the admission of air into a vein during an amputation at the shoulder-joint. Med Chir Trans. 1844;27:41–51.
41. Santy P, Bret J, Marion P. Convulsive and syncopal form of Fallot's tetralogy in a 7-month-old child; Pott's operation; disappearance of functional symptoms. Lyon Chir. 1950;45(4):456–7.
42. Gastaut H, Fischer-Williams M. Electro-encephalographic study of syncope; its differentiation from epilepsy. Lancet. 1957;273(7004):1018–25.
43. Grubb BP, Gerard G, Wolfe DA, et al. Syncope and seizures of psychogenic origin: identification with head-upright tilt table testing. Clin Cardiol. 1992;15(11):839–42.
44. Bădilă E, Negrea C, Rîpă A, et al. The etiology of syncope in an emergency hospital. Rom J Intern Med. 2016;54(3):173–8.
45. Sabu J, Regeti K, Mallappallil M, et al. Convulsive syncope induced by ventricular arrhythmia masquerading as epileptic seizures: case report and literature review. J Clin Med Res. 2016;8(8):610–5.

46. Becker MC, Bass RD, Robbins CM. Pheochromocytoma; a cause of post-partum convulsions. J Med Soc N J. 1949;46(7):339–42.
47. Leiba A, Bar-Dayan Y, Leker RR, et al. Seizures as a presenting symptom of phaeochromocytoma in a young soldier. J Hum Hypertens. 2003;17(1):73–5.
48. Anderson NE, Chung K, Willoughby E, et al. Neurological manifestations of phaeochromocytomas and secretory paragangliomas: a reappraisal. J Neurol Neurosurg Psychiatry. 2013;84(4):452–7.
49. Manger WM. The protean manifestations of pheochromocytoma. Horm Metab Res. 2009;41(9):658–63.
50. Liu P, Zu X, Liu L. Genetic screening in pheochromocytoma/paraganglioma. Pathol Oncol Res. 2017;23(1):217.
51. Zou HJ, Li YS, Shan ZY. Genetic analysis and clinical investigation of a pedigree with multiple endocrine neoplasia type 2A: a case report. Oncol Lett. 2016;12(4):2657–9.
52. Thorling L. Spontanhypoglykämi, insulom. Nord Med. 1948;37(5):217.
53. Smyth GA, Shields TW, Carroll WW. Functioning insulinoma superimposed on idiopathic epilepsy. Q Bull Northwest Univ Med Sch. 1954;28(2):129–33.
54. Ding Y, Wang S, Liu J, et al. Neuropsychiatric profiles of patients with insulinomas. Eur Neurol. 2010;63(1):48–51.
55. Wei J, Liu X, Wu J, et al. Diagnosis and surgical management of insulinomas in 33 consecutive patients at a single institution. Langenbecks Arch Surg. 2016;401(7):1019–25.
56. Sánchez-Bueno F, Rodríguez González JM, Torres Salmerón G, et al. Prognostic factors in resected pancreatic neuroendocrine tumours: experience in 95 patients. Cir Esp. 2016;94(8):473–80.
57. Gupta M, Batra A, Hirve M, et al. Paroxysmal dystonic choreoathetosis with symptomatic seizures secondary to hypoglycemia caused by insulinoma. Ann Indian Acad Neurol. 2011;14(4):313–5.
58. Batouche DD, Kerboua KE, Sadaoui L, et al. Clinical and etiological profile malignant hypertension in children in pediatric intensive care. Ann Cardiol Angeiol. 2016;65(3):165–70.
59. McEnery PT, Nathan J, Bates SR, et al. Convulsions in children undergoing renal transplantation. J Pediatr. 1989;115(4):532–6.
60. Wasseff S. Mechanisms of convulsions in eclampsia. Med Hypotheses. 2009;72(1):49–51.
61. Brown CM, Garovic VD. Drug treatment of hypertension in pregnancy. Drugs. 2014;74(3):283–96.
62. Moraes KR, Tavares LC, Machado RH, et al. HELLP syndrome: challenges for establishing diagnostic criteria. Pregnancy Hypertens. 2012;2(3):329.
63. Hingray C, Biberon J, El-Hage W, et al. Psychogenic non-epileptic seizures (PNES). Rev Neurol (Paris). 2016;172(4–5):263–9.
64. Schachter SC, Brown F, Rowan AJ. Provacative testing for nonepileptic seizures:attitudes and practices in the United States among American Epilepsy Society members. J Epilepsy. 1996;9:249–52.
65. Sigurdardottir KR, Olafsson E. Incidence of psychogenic seizures in adults: a population-based study in Iceland. Epilepsia. 1998;39(7):749–52.
66. Szaflarski JP, Ficker DM, Cahill WT, Privitera MD. Four-year incidence of psychogenic nonepileptic seizures in adults in Hamilton County, OH. Neurology. 2000;55(10):1561–3.
67. Silva W, Giagante B, Saizar R, et al. Clinical features and prognosis of nonepileptic seizures in a developing country. Epilepsia. 2001;42(3):398–401.
68. Chinta SS, Malhi P, Singhi P, Prabhakar S. Clinical and psychosocial characteristics of children with nonepileptic seizures. Ann Indian Acad Neurol. 2008;11(3):159–63.
69. Groppel G, Kapitany T, Baumgartner C. Cluster analysis of clinical seizure semiology of psychogenic nonepileptic seizures. Epilepsia. 2000;41(5):610–4.
70. Elzawahry H, Do CS, Lin K, Benbadis SR. The diagnostic utility of the ictal cry. Epilepsy Behav. 2010;18(3):306–7.
71. Nikolaev EL, Serli T, Rezvyi G. Psychogenic nonepileptic seizures: issues of comorbidity in the diagnosis and treatment. Zh Nevrol Psikhiatr Im S S Korsakova. 2016;116(4):58–61.
72. Takasaki K, Diaz Stransky A, Miller G. Psychogenic nonepileptic seizures: diagnosis, management, and bioethics. Pediatr Neurol. 2016;62:3–8.
73. Plioplys S, Doss J, Siddarth P. Risk factors for comorbid psychopathology in youth with psychogenic nonepileptic seizures. Seizure. 2016;38:32–7.
74. Hupalo M, Smigielski JW, Jaskolski DJ. Optimal time of duration of a long-term video-EEG monitoring in paroxysmal events—a retrospective analysis of 282 sessions in 202 patients. Neurol Neurochir Pol. 2016;50(5):331–5.
75. Shen W, Bowman ES, Markand ON. Presenting the diagnosis of pseudoseizure. Neurology. 1990;40(5):756–9.
76. Rathakrishnan R, et al. BOLD signal changes preceding negative responses in EEG-fMRI in patients with focal epilepsy. Epilepsia. 2010;51(9):1837–45.
77. Thornton R, Moeller F, Levan P, Dubeau F, Gotman J. EEG correlated functional MRI and postoperative outcome in focal epilepsy. J Neurol Neurosurg Psychiatry. 2010;81(8):922–7.
78. Petramfar P, Yaghoobi E, Nemati R, Asadi-Pooya A. Serum creatine phosphokinase is helpful in distinguishing generalized tonic-clonic seizures from psychogenic nonepileptic seizures and vasovagal syncope. Epilepsy Behav. 2009;15(3):330–2.
79. Boulding R, Stacey R, Niven R, Fowler SJ. Dysfunctional breathing: a review of the literature and proposal for classification. Eur Respir Rev. 2016;25(141):287–94.
80. Garssen B, Rijken H. Hyperventilation syndrome. In: Kaptein AA, van der Ploog HM, PJG S, Beunderman R, editors. Behavioural medicine. New York: Wiley; 1990. p. 159–72.
81. Herman SP, Stickler GB, Lucas AR. Hyperventilation syndrome in children and adolescents: long-term follow up. Pediatrics. 1981;67(2):183–7.

82. Brashear RE. Hyperventilation syndrome: managing elderly patients. Geriatrics. 1984;39(7):114–5.
83. Williamson CA, Sheehan KM, Tipirneni R, et al. The association between spontaneous hyperventilation, delayed cerebral ischemia, and poor neurological outcome in patients with subarachnoid hemorrhage. Neurocrit Care. 2015;23(3):330–8.
84. Perkin GD, Joseph R. Neurological manifestations of the hyperventilation syndrome. J R Soc Med. 1986;79(8):448–50.
85. Kim CH, Jeong KH, Ahn SH. Vibration- and hyperventilation-induced nystagmus in patients with Ramsay Hunt syndrome with vertigo. Otolaryngol Head Neck Surg. 2015;152(5):912.
86. Kang BS. A case of hyperventilation syndrome mimicking complex partial seizure: usefulness of EEG monitoring in emergency department. J Epilepsy Res. 2015;5(1):20–2.
87. Kobayashi M, Kurata S, Sanuki T, Okayasu I, Ayuse T. Management of post-hyperventilation apnea during dental treatment under monitored anesthesia care with propofol. Biopsychosoc Med. 2014;8(1):26.
88. Zeeman GG, Fleckenstein JL, Twickler DM, Cunningham FG. Cerebral infarction in eclampsia. Am J Obstet Gynecol. 2004;190(3):714–20.
89. Brewer J, Owens MY, Wallace K, et al. Posterior reversible encephalopathy syndrome in 46 of 47 patients with eclampsia. Am J Obstet Gynecol. 2013;208(6):468.e1–6.
90. Niedermeyer E, Ribeiro M. Considerations of nonconvulsive status epilepticus. Clin Electroencephalogr. 2000;31:192–5.
91. Capovilla G, Beccaria F, Beghi E, Minicucci F, Sartori S, Vecchi M. Treatment of convulsive status epilepticus in childhood: recommendations of the Italian League Against Epilepsy. Epilepsia. 2013;54(Suppl 7):23–34.
92. Bearden S, Eisenschenk S, Uthman B. Diagnosis of nonconvulsive status epilepticus (NCSE) in adults with altered mental status: clinico-electroencephalographic considerations. Am J Electroneurodiagnostic Technol. 2008;48:11–37.
93. Shorvon S. The definition, classification and frequency of NCSE. Epileptic Disord. 2005;7(13):255–8.
94. Walker M, Cross H, Smith S, et al. Nonconvulsive status epilepticus: Epilepsy Research Foundation workshop reports. Epileptic Disord. 2005;7:253–96.
95. Shorvon S, Walker M. Status epilepticus in idiopathic generalized epilepsy. Epilepsia. 2005;46(Suppl 9):73–9.
96. Towne AR, Waterhouse EJ, Boggs JG, et al. Prevalence of nonconvulsive status epilepticus in comatose patients. Neurology. 2000;54:340–5.
97. Jordan KG. Nonconvulsive status epilepticus in acute brain injury. J Clin Neurophysiol. 1999;16:332–40. discussion 53.
98. Knake S, Rosenow F, Vescovi M, et al. Incidence of status epilepticus in adults in Germany: a prospective, population-based study. Epilepsia. 2001;42:714–8.
99. DeLorenzo RJ, Waterhouse EJ, Towne AR, et al. Persistent nonconvulsive status epilepticus after the control of convulsive status epilepticus. Epilepsia. 1998;39:833–40.
100. Kennedy JD, Gerard EE. Continuous EEG monitoring in the intensive care unit. Curr Neurol Neurosci Rep. 2012;12:419–28.
101. Abend NS, Gutierrez-Colina AM, Topjian AA, et al. Nonconvulsive seizures are common in critically ill children. Neurology. 2011;76:1071–7.
102. Claassen J, Mayer SA, Kowalski RG, Emerson RG, Hirsch LJ. Detection of electrographic seizures with continuous EEG monitoring in critically ill patients. Neurology. 2004;62:1743–8.
103. Meierkord H, Holtkamp M. Nonconvulsive status epilepticus in adults: clinical forms and treatment. Lancet Neurol. 2007;6:329–39.
104. Jette N, Claassen J, Emerson RG, Hirsch LJ. Frequency and predictors of nonconvulsive seizures during continuous electroencephalographic monitoring in critically ill children. Arch Neurol. 2006;63:1750–5.
105. Shorvon S. What is nonconvulsive status epilepticus, and what are its subtypes? Epilepsia. 2007;48(Suppl 8):35–8.
106. Poothrikovil RP, Gujjar AR, Al-Asmi A, Nandhagopal R, Jacob PC. Predictive value of short-term EEG recording in critically ill adult patients. Neurodiagn J. 2015;55:157–68.
107. Wusthoff CJ, Dlugos DJ, Gutierrez-Colina A, et al. Electrographic seizures during therapeutic hypothermia for neonatal hypoxic-ischemic encephalopathy. J Child Neurol. 2011;26:724–8.
108. Carrera E, Claassen J, Oddo M, Emerson RG, Mayer SA, Hirsch LJ. Continuous electroencephalographic monitoring in critically ill patients with central nervous system infections. Arch Neurol. 2008;65:1612–8.
109. Greco F, Cocuzza MD, Smilari P, Sorge G, Pavone L. Nonconvulsive status epilepticus complicating Epstein-Barr virus encephalitis in a child. Case Rep Pediatr. 2014;2014:547396.
110. Misra UK, Kalita J, Nair PP. Status epilepticus in central nervous system infections: an experience from a developing country. Am J Med. 2008;121:618–23.
111. Kramer AH, Bleck TP. Neurocritical care of patients with central nervous system infections. Curr Treat Options Neurol. 2008;10:201–11.
112. Narayanan JT, Murthy JM. Nonconvulsive status epilepticus in a neurological intensive care unit: profile in a developing country. Epilepsia. 2007;48:900–6.
113. Fernandez-Torre JL, Burgueno P, Ballesteros MA, Hernandez-Hernandez MA, Villagra-Teran N, de Lucas EM. Super-refractory nonconvulsive status epilepticus secondary to fat embolism: a clinical, electrophysiological, and pathological study. Epilepsy Behav. 2015;49:184–8.
114. Kanazawa Y, Morioka T, Arakawa S, Furuta Y, Nakanishi A, Kitazono T. Nonconvulsive partial

status epilepticus mimicking recurrent infarction revealed by diffusion-weighted and arterial spin labeling perfusion magnetic resonance images. J Stroke Cerebrovasc Dis. 2015;24:731–8.
115. Crepeau AZ, Kerrigan JF, Gerber P, et al. Rhythmical and periodic EEG patterns do not predict short-term outcome in critically ill patients with subarachnoid hemorrhage. J Clin Neurophysiol. 2013;30: 247–54.
116. Fernandez-Torre JL, Hernandez-Hernandez MA. Utility of bilateral Bispectral index (BIS) monitoring in a comatose patient with focal nonconvulsive status epilepticus. Seizure. 2012;21:61–4.
117. Little AS, Kerrigan JF, McDougall CG, et al. Nonconvulsive status epilepticus in patients suffering spontaneous subarachnoid hemorrhage. J Neurosurg. 2007;106:805–11.
118. Punia V, Garcia CG, Hantus S. Incidence of recurrent seizures following hospital discharge in patients with LPDs (PLEDs) and nonconvulsive seizures recorded on continuous EEG in the critical care setting. Epilepsy Behav. 2015;49:250–4.
119. Fujioka H, Urasaki E, Izumihara A, Yamashita K. Nonconvulsive status epilepticus following implantation of subdural grid electrodes in a brain tumor patient. Clin Neurophysiol. 2016;127:975–6.
120. Vespa PM, Miller C, McArthur D, et al. Nonconvulsive electrographic seizures after traumatic brain injury result in a delayed, prolonged increase in intracranial pressure and metabolic crisis. Crit Care Med. 2007;35:2830–6.
121. Kadoya M, Onoue H, Kadoya A, Ikewaki K, Kaida K. Refractory status epilepticus caused by anti-NMDA receptor encephalitis that markedly improved following combination therapy with rituximab and cyclophosphamide. Intern Med. 2015;54:209–13.
122. Alroughani R, Javidan M, Qasem A, Alotaibi N. Nonconvulsive status epilepticus; the rate of occurrence in a general hospital. Seizure. 2009;18:38–42.
123. Claassen J, Taccone FS, Horn P, Holtkamp M, Stocchetti N, Oddo M. Recommendations on the use of EEG monitoring in critically ill patients: consensus statement from the neurointensive care section of the ESICM. Intensive Care Med. 2013;39: 1337–51.
124. Greiner MV, Greiner HM, Care MM, Owens D, Shapiro R, Holland K. Adding insult to injury: nonconvulsive seizures in abusive head trauma. J Child Neurol. 2015;30:1778–84.
125. Azuma H, Akechi T, Furukawa TA. Absence status associated with focal activity and polydipsia-induced hyponatremia. Neuropsychiatr Dis Treat. 2008;4:495–8.
126. Pro S, Randi F, Pulitano P, Vicenzini E, Mecarelli O. Nonconvulsive status epilepticus characterised exclusively by a language disorder induced by non-ketotic hyperglycaemia. Epileptic Disord. 2011;13:193–6.
127. Jo YM, Lee SW, Han SY, et al. Nonconvulsive status epilepticus disguising as hepatic encephalopathy. World J Gastroenterol. 2015;21:5105–9.
128. Jhun P, Kim H. Nonconvulsive status epilepticus in hepatic encephalopathy. West J Emerg Med. 2011;12:372–4.
129. Bhatt A, Farooq MU, Bhatt S, Majid A, Kassab MY. Periodic lateralized epileptiform discharges: an initial electrographic pattern in reversible posterior leukoencephalopathy syndrome. Neurol Neurochir Pol. 2008;42:55–9.
130. Cock HR. Drug-induced status epilepticus. Epilepsy Behav. 2015;49:76–82.
131. Anzellotti F, Ricciardi L, Monaco D, et al. Cefixime-induced nonconvulsive status epilepticus. Neurol Sci. 2012;33:325–9.
132. Mazzei D, Accardo J, Ferrari A, Primavera A. Levofloxacin neurotoxicity and nonconvulsive status epilepticus (NCSE): a case report. Clin Neurol Neurosurg. 2012;114:1371–3.
133. Misra UK, Kalita J, Chandra S, Nair PP. Association of antibiotics with status epilepticus. Neurol Sci. 2013;34:327–31.
134. Anzellotti F, Capasso M, Frazzini V, Onofrj M. Olanzapine-related repetitive focal seizures with lingual dystonia. Epileptic Disord. 2016;18:83–6.
135. Camacho A, Garcia-Navarro M, Martinez B, Villarejo A, Pomares E. Olanzapine-induced myoclonic status. Clin Neuropharmacol. 2005;28: 145–7.
136. Taniguchi G, Miyajima M, Watanabe M, et al. Nonconvulsive status epilepticus in the elderly associated with newer antidepressants used at therapeutic doses: a report of three cases. Epilepsy Behav Case Rep. 2015;3:8–11.
137. Schindler BA, Ramchandani D. Partial complex status epilepticus in a lithium-toxic patient. Psychosomatics. 1993;34:521–4.
138. Maganti R, Gerber P, Drees C, Chung S. Nonconvulsive status epilepticus. Epilepsy Behav. 2008;12:572–86.
139. Steeghs N, de Jongh FE, Sillevis Smitt PA, van den Bent MJ. Cisplatin-induced encephalopathy and seizures. Anticancer Drugs. 2003;14:443–6.
140. Patterson DM, Aries J, Hyare H, Holder D, Rees J, Lee SM. Nonconvulsive status epilepticus and leucoencephalopathy after high-dose methotrexate. J Clin Oncol. 2011;29:e459–61.
141. Bhatt A, Farooq MU, Majid A, Kassab M. Chemotherapy-related posterior reversible leukoencephalopathy syndrome. Nat Clin Pract Neurol. 2009;5:163–9.
142. Kim TK, Jung ES, Park JM, Kang K, Lee WW, Lee JJ. An atypical presentation of subacute encephalopathy with seizures in chronic alcoholism syndrome. J Epilepsy Res. 2016;6:28–30.
143. Fernandez-Torre JL, Kaplan PW. Subacute encephalopathy with seizures in alcoholics (SESA syndrome) revisited. Seizure. 2014;23:393–6.

144. Jirsch J, Hirsch LJ. Nonconvulsive seizures: developing a rational approach to the diagnosis and management in the critically ill population. Clin Neurophysiol. 2007;118:1660–70.
145. Bender MB. Diagnostic aids in the mental and aphasic status. J Mt Sinai Hosp N Y. 1966;33:208–12.
146. Ericson EJ, Gerard EE, Macken MP, Schuele SU. Aphasic status epilepticus: electroclinical correlation. Epilepsia. 2011;52:1452–8.
147. Toledo M, Munuera J, Sueiras M, Rovira R, Alvarez-Sabin J, Rovira A. MRI findings in aphasic status epilepticus. Epilepsia. 2008;49:1465–9.
148. Michael M, Tsatsou K, Ferrie CD. Panayiotopoulos syndrome: an important childhood autonomic epilepsy to be differentiated from occipital epilepsy and acute non-epileptic disorders. Brain Dev. 2010;32:4–9.
149. Ferrie CD, Caraballo R, Covanis A, et al. Autonomic status epilepticus in Panayiotopoulos syndrome and other childhood and adult epilepsies: a consensus view. Epilepsia. 2007;48:1165–72.
150. Mizobuchi M. Nonconvulsive status epilepticus. Brain Nerve. 2016;68:451–62.
151. Marchi NA, Novy J, Faouzi M, Stahli C, Burnand B, Rossetti AO. Status epilepticus: impact of therapeutic coma on outcome. Crit Care Med. 2015;43: 1003–9.
152. Rossetti AO, Trinka E, Stahli C, Novy J. New ILAE versus previous clinical status epilepticus semiologic classification: analysis of a hospital-based cohort. Epilepsia. 2016;57:1036–41.
153. Sutter R, Kaplan PW. Electroencephalographic criteria for nonconvulsive status epilepticus: synopsis and comprehensive survey. Epilepsia. 2012;53(Suppl 3):1–51.
154. Shafi MM, Westover MB, Cole AJ, Kilbride RD, Hoch DB, Cash SS. Absence of early epileptiform abnormalities predicts lack of seizures on continuous EEG. Neurology. 2012;79:1796–801.
155. Yazdi JS, Schumaker JA. Treatment of refractory status epilepticus with vagus nerve stimulator in an elderly patient. World Neurosurg. 2016;5:620.e1–7.
156. Vyas DD, Dash GK. Supra-recommendation treatment of super-refractory status epilepticus. J Epilepsy Res. 2016;6(1):39–41.
157. Sheikh Z, Wang W, Hillen M. A young man with recurrent coma and refractory status epilepticus. JAMA Neurol. 2016;73(10):1243–4.
158. Prasanth S, et al. Refractory status epilepticus due to pneumococcal meningitis in an infant with congenital immunodeficiency. J Pediatr Neurosci. 2016;11(2):125–7.
159. Niquet J, et al. Benzodiazepine-refractory status epilepticus: pathophysiology and principles of treatment. Ann N Y Acad Sci. 2016;1378(1):166–73.
160. Newey CR, et al. Observed medical and surgical complications of prolonged barbiturate coma for refractory status epilepticus. Ther Adv Drug Saf. 2016;7(5):195–203.
161. Legriel S, Oddo M, Brophy GM. What's new in refractory status epilepticus? Intensive Care Med. 2017;43(4):543–6.
162. KK K. Super refractory status epilepticus. J Assoc Physicians India. 2016;64(1):131.
163. Johnson EL, Martinez NC, Ritzl EK. EEG characteristics of successful burst suppression for refractory status epilepticus. Neurocrit Care. 2016;25(3):407–14.
164. Hofler J, et al. (S)-Ketamine in refractory and super-refractory status epilepticus: a retrospective study. CNS Drugs. 2016;30(9):869–76.
165. Hocker S, et al. Progressive brain atrophy in super-refractory status epilepticus. JAMA Neurol. 2016;73(10):1201–7.
166. Farias-Moeller R, et al. A practical approach to ketogenic diet in the pediatric intensive care unit for super-refractory status epilepticus. Neurocrit Care. 2017;26(2):267–72.
167. Dillien P, et al. New-onset refractory status epilepticus: more investigations, more questions. Case Rep Neurol. 2016;8(2):127–33.
168. Chiusolo F, et al. From intravenous to enteral ketogenic diet in PICU: a potential treatment strategy for refractory status epilepticus. Eur J Paediatr Neurol. 2016;20(6):843–7.
169. Bick SK, et al. Anterior temporal lobectomy for refractory status epilepticus in herpes simplex encephalitis. Neurocrit Care. 2016;25(3):458–63.
170. Bennett KS. Treatment of refractory status epilepticus in children: current practice and opportunities to improve care. Pediatr Crit Care Med. 2016;17(10):1006–7.
171. Beg JM, et al. Burden of illness for super-refractory status epilepticus patients. J Med Econ. 2017;20(1):45–53.
172. Appavu B, et al. Ketogenic diet treatment for pediatric super-refractory status epilepticus. Seizure. 2016;41:62–5.
173. Kramer U, et al. Severe refractory status epilepticus owing to presumed encephalitis. J Child Neurol. 2005;20(3):184–7.
174. Madzar D, et al. Effects of clobazam for treatment of refractory status epilepticus. BMC Neurol. 2016;16(1):202.
175. Lebedev VV, Ioffe IuS. Cooling of the brain in refractory status epilepticus. Vopr Neirokhir. 1972;36(2):32–6.
176. Vajda FJ, et al. Rectal administration of sodium valproate in status epilepticus. Neurology. 1978;28(9 Pt 1):897–9.
177. Young GB, et al. Anesthetic barbiturates in refractory status epilepticus. Can J Neurol Sci. 1980;7(4):291–2.
178. Orlowski JP, et al. Hypothermia and barbiturate coma for refractory status epilepticus. Crit Care Med. 1984;12(4):367–72.
179. Rosati A, et al. Efficacy of ketamine in refractory convulsive status epilepticus in children:

a protocol for a sequential design, multicentre, randomised, controlled, open-label, non-profit trial (KETASER01). BMJ Open. 2016;6(6):e011565.
180. Miras VA, et al. Effectiveness of electroconvulsive therapy for refractory status epilepticus in febrile infection-related epilepsy syndrome. Neuropediatrics. 2017;48(1):45–8.
181. Delaj L, et al. Refractory and super-refractory status epilepticus in adults: a 9-year cohort study. Acta Neurol Scand. 2017;135(1):92–9.
182. Sahin M, et al. Outcome of severe refractory status epilepticus in children. Epilepsia. 2001;42(11):1461–7.
183. Mayer SA, et al. Refractory status epilepticus: frequency, risk factors, and impact on outcome. Arch Neurol. 2002;59(2):205–10.
184. Rossetti AO, Logroscino G, Bromfield EB. Refractory status epilepticus: effect of treatment aggressiveness on prognosis. Arch Neurol. 2005;62(11):1698–702.
185. Barzegar M, et al. Refractory convulsive status epilepticus in children: etiology, associated risk factors and outcome. Iran J Child Neurol. 2015;9(4):24–31.
186. Rohracher A, et al. Perampanel in patients with refractory and super-refractory status epilepticus in a neurological intensive care unit. Epilepsy Behav. 2015;49:354–8.
187. Sinha S, et al. Refractory status epilepticus: a developing country perspective. J Neurol Sci. 2010;290(1–2):60–5.
188. Juhasz C, et al. Successful surgical treatment of an inflammatory lesion associated with new-onset refractory status epilepticus. Neurosurg Focus. 2013;34(6):E5.
189. Lai A, et al. Functional outcome of prolonged refractory status epilepticus. Crit Care. 2015;19:199.
190. Liberalesso PB, et al. Higher mortality rate is associated with advanced age and periodic lateralized epileptiform discharges in patients with refractory status epilepticus. Arq Neuropsiquiatr. 2013;71(3):153–8.
191. Ong CT, et al. Age-dependent sex difference of the incidence and mortality of status epilepticus: a twelve year nationwide population-based cohort study in Taiwan. PLoS One. 2015;10(3):e0122350.
192. Cardoso I, et al. Refractory status epilepticus in children: characterisation of epilepsies, continuous electroencephalographic monitoring and response to treatment. Rev Neurol. 2013;56(8):401–8.
193. Lowenstein DH, Alldredge BK. Status epilepticus at an urban public hospital in the 1980s. Neurology. 1993;43(3 Pt 1):483–8.
194. Lowenstein DH. The management of refractory status epilepticus: an update. Epilepsia. 2006;47(Suppl 1):35–40.
195. Scholtes FB, Renier WO, Meinardi H. Generalized convulsive status epilepticus: causes, therapy, and outcome in 346 patients. Epilepsia. 1994;35(5):1104–12.
196. Glaser CA, et al. Refractory status epilepticus in suspect encephalitis. Neurocrit Care. 2008;9(1):74–82.
197. Sutter R, et al. Mortality and recovery from refractory status epilepticus in the intensive care unit: a 7-year observational study. Epilepsia. 2013;54(3):502–11.
198. Murthy JM. Refractory status epilepticus. Neurol India. 2006;54(4):354–8.
199. Giovannini G, et al. A one-year prospective study of refractory status epilepticus in Modena, Italy. Epilepsy Behav. 2015;49:141–5.
200. Sivakumar S, et al. Clobazam: an effective add-on therapy in refractory status epilepticus. Epilepsia. 2015;56(6):e83–9.
201. Webster DL, et al. Status epilepticus: a possible association with human metapneumovirus infection. Pediatrics. 2014;133(3):e747–50.

2 Pathogenesis of Refractory Status Epilepticus

Zhifang Dong and Zhong Chen

Abstract

The most significant characteristic of seizures is self-limitation, which is associated with the postictal refractory period that follows a seizure. The endogenous anticonvulsant mechanism is one of the most important reasons that seizures self-terminate. However, the most significant characteristic of refractory status epilepticus (RSE) is that it is more drug resistant to first-line anti-status epilepticus drugs than are other forms of status epilepticus (SE). In general, RSE represents a severe form of SE. Because it has high mortality and is associated with increased neuronal damage, RSE should be terminated as soon as possible. In this chapter, we discuss a potential mechanism by which SE may transform into RSE, beginning with seizure termination.

2.1 Mechanism of Seizure Termination

2.1.1 The Characteristics of Seizure Self-Limitation

In contrast to the onset of neurological diseases, most seizures are self-limiting. Seizure termination may be caused by activation of the endogenous anticonvulsant system. However, the underlying mechanism for this phenomenon is not completely understood [1, 2]. The mechanism of seizure termination may be more complex than that of the origin or even the seizure itself [1]. The studies of seizure self-limitation are advantageous for seeking new methods to prevent and treat epilepsy. There are three main characteristics of seizure self-limitation: the

Z. Dong
Chongqing Key Laboratory of Translational Medical Research in Cognitive Development and Learning and Memory Disorders, Children's Hospital of Chongqing Medical University, Chongqing 400014, China

Ministry of Education Key Laboratory of Child Development and Disorders, Children's Hospital of Chongqing Medical University, Chongqing 400014, China

Z. Chen (✉)
Department of Neurology and Epilepsy Center, Second Affiliated Hospital, School of Medicine, Zhejiang University, Hangzhou, China
e-mail: chenzhong@zju.edu.cn

X. Wang, S. Li (eds.), *Refractory Status Epilepticus*, DOI 10.1007/978-981-10-5125-8_2

transience of seizures, the postictal refractoriness, and the inhibition after seizures exhibits a synergistic relationship with antiepileptic drugs.

Non-status epilepticus is usually very short in duration. A study of 579 seizures across 159 adults by Jenssen et al. [3] showed that the average duration of simple partial seizures, complex partial seizures, and secondary generalized tonic–clonic seizures were 28 s, 78 s, and 130 s, respectively. In a study of general tonic–clonic seizures, which were first described by Theodore et al. [4], 120 seizures in 47 epileptic patients lasted an average of 62 s. Recently, a large-sample retrospective study showed that the average duration of generalized tonic–clonic seizures was 74.6 s [5]. These results show not only that most seizures are self-limiting in the absence of intervention but also that seizure termination can occur rapidly.

It has long been known that postictal refractoriness following seizures is an important feature of seizure self-limitation. In the treatment of depression, more current stimulation is required after the first electroconvulsive shock (ECS) to trigger the occurrence of the next electric convulsion [6]. This is consistent with a study by Löscher W. and colleagues [7], who found that seizure susceptibility was decreased following a few hours of spontaneous tonic–clonic seizures in an idiopathic generalized epilepsy genetic model. The period of decreased seizure susceptibility is called postictal refractoriness [6, 8]. For a short duration, the threshold for subsequent seizures is increased. Nutt et al. performed ECS daily for 10 days and found that the seizure threshold was increased for 5–60 min after seizures and then returned to normal over a short time [6]. Löscher found that the increased seizure threshold returned to normal within 24 h after seizures [7].

The increase in the threshold for subsequent seizures is called epileptic tolerance, and the effect of antiepileptic drugs will be significantly increased during this time. Using different animal models, Mace et al. compared the curative effects of phenobarbital, phenytoin, and carbamazepine during epileptic tolerance according to different seizure types, and they found that the efficacy of antiepileptic drugs was significantly increased during this period [9]. Löscher et al. found that the efficacy of carbamazepine (15 mg/kg) was significantly increased during epileptic tolerance using four different stimulation methods, which suggested that the inhibition after seizures exhibits a synergistic relationship with antiepileptic drugs [10].

2.1.2 Factors Related to Seizure Self-Limitation

Seizure self-limitation is related to many factors. At present, a tendency exists to consider that age, sex hormones, structure, and gene abnormalities will affect the duration of seizures, and disruption of the equilibrium state will lead to repeated occurrence of epileptogenesis.

A study by Jenssen et al. on adult patients with epilepsy found that the average durations of complex partial seizures and secondary generalized tonic–clonic seizures are 78 s and 130 s, respectively [3]. However, a study by Shinnar et al. on 407 children with epilepsy found that 50% experienced a seizure lasting no less than 5 min, and 29% had a first seizure that lasted no less than 10 min [11]. It is well-established that the seizure termination mechanism is highly correlated with age.

In 1857, a study by Locock et al. of 52 patients with epilepsy suggested that sex hormones might have an effect on seizures. In addition, different hormones had various effects [12]. Estrogen could reduce the seizure threshold, whereas progesterone had an antiepileptic effect. Due to the presence of progesterone and estriol, seizure duration is significantly reduced during pregnancy [12]. Factors affecting epilepsy have been confirmed by patients with menstrual period epilepsy and animal models and were interpreted as evidence of neurotransmitter regulation [13–15]. Kaminski and colleagues [16] found that androgen metabolites can regulate the γ-aminobutyric acid (GABA) receptor and shorten seizure duration.

Investigations of cranial magnetic resonance imaging (MRI) scans of 36 temporal lobe epilepsy patients with cortical atrophy and white matter disruption by Kemmotsu et al. showed that cortical atrophy is closely related to seizure self-limitation, and the severity of white matter integrity damage is closely related to onset age [17]. Meanwhile, these authors found that compared to right temporal lobe epilepsy, left temporal lobe epilepsy produces more severe structural damage. This may be due to the greater susceptibility of the left hemisphere to early damage and seizures [17]. According to a study on children undergoing their first febrile SE episode, the seizure duration is not only influenced by factors including age, temperature, and sex but also temporal lobe structure abnormalities [18].

Single gene interactions can influence the severity and prolong the duration of epilepsy and increase the frequency of seizures. Bergren et al. found that congenic C57BL/6J.Q 54 mice exhibit a decreased incidence of spontaneous seizures, delayed seizure onset, and longer survival than [C57BL/6J × SJL/J]F(1).Q 54 mice [19]. A study of absence seizures using a Gria4 knockout mouse model revealed that the intracisternal A-particle retrotransposon (IAP) of the C3H substrain had a significant effect on the duration and incidence of spike-wave discharges [20].

2.1.3 Potential Mechanism of Seizure Self-Limitation

The ionic environment plays an important role on seizure termination via the accumulation of various factors at an effective concentration over a very short time. Extracellular acidification may contribute to termination of seizure discharges. During the process of seizure discharge, prolonged neuronal activity can lead to an increase in carbon dioxide or anaerobic metabolism, which can cause extracellular or intracellular acidosis [21]. In vitro experiments have illustrated that the hippocampal extracellular can pH reached 6.7 at the termination of seizure-like burst firing. This phenomenon is likely to occur within a few minutes in the case of low pH [22]. In vivo experiments by Caspers et al. also suggest that mechanical ventilation with CO_2 (to ensure acidification) can also terminate seizures [23]. Moreover, our team recently found that extracellular pH-sensitive acid-sensitive ion channels (ASICs) can, through the synaptic mechanisms of interneurons, play an important role in seizure termination in pilocarpine and pentylenetetrazole-induced rat epilepsy models [24]. Velisek et al. found that when the pH was reduced to 7.1, a slight impairment in synaptic transmission and decreased long-term potentiation (LTP) occurred [25]. Inhibition of carbonic anhydrase can also lead to cell acidification and exert an anticonvulsant effect [26].

Intracellular acidification may also contribute to the termination of seizure discharges. Seizures can produce a brain pH ranging from 7.35 to 6.8 by producing lactic acid and utilizing a carbon dioxide retention mechanism, which will terminate seizures [27]. In vitro experiments using hippocampal slices, Xiong et al. found that alkalization can induce seizure discharge [28]. If acidification is increased pharmacologically, the seizure discharge is terminated. Interestingly, this method is also effective in vivo in a febrile convulsion rat model [29]. Ventilation induced by super heating can cause alkalization, seizures, and chronic stress changes. These changes can be terminated by ending mechanical ventilation with CO_2, which will prevent alkali poisoning [29]. However, perfusion with ammonium chloride to prevent intracellular acidification can increase the excitability of neurons, resulting in seizure discharges [29]. In addition, when patients with epilepsy inhaled CO_2 for a few seconds, the brain pH was significantly reduced, resulting in an antiepileptic effect [27]. Recently, some researchers have found that treatment with CO_2 can not only terminate seizures but also prevent long-term damage to the hippocampus during febrile seizures [29]. This rapid and simple method of carbon dioxide inhalation may be an interesting anticonvulsant treatment. Therefore, it is possible to provide an effective method for the prevention and treatment of seizures and SE that is focused on the mechanism related to acidification after seizures [30].

Heinemann et al. found that focal seizure activity results in an approximately 50% decline in extracellular calcium activity [31]. Because synaptic vesicle fusion and neurotransmitter release are dependent on calcium inward current, extracellular Ca^{2+} depletion has an antiepileptic effect. Using functional multi-neuron calcium-imaging technology in animal models, Hongo found that the antiepileptic drug phenytoin can significantly reduce the peak and amount of calcium influx, which plays an important role in the seizure termination [32]. Furosemide can terminate seizure discharges by regulating the chloride ion concentration. Some researchers have suggested that furosemide blocks neuronal action potentials by affecting chloride ions. Lado stated that the reduced level of intracellular chloride ions can increase the GABA function in an activity-dependent manner [2]. Thus, disrupted regulation of intracellular chloride ions may cause antiepileptic drugs that act via GABA, such as phenobarbital, to be ineffective.

Neuromodulators are likely the most interesting part of the seizure termination mechanism. They are substances that are released endogenously and act as nonclassical transmitters or alter synaptic transmission. In contrast to extracellular K+ and pH, they are easily subjected to drug interventions. Among them, adenosine and neuropeptide Y (NPY) have most extensively been addressed [2, 33–35]. Adenosine is thought to be a type of endogenous neural modulator with an anticonvulsive effect, and it is also a type of seizure terminator [33, 34, 36]. Increasing the level of adenosine can prevent seizures, inhibit seizure discharge, and exert a protective effect in neurons, whereas reducing the level of adenosine can increase seizure discharge and neuronal death. If its function is altered, adenosine may promote SE [37]. In a study of epilepsy patients and animal models by Gompel Van et al., the average concentrations of adenosine in the extracellular environment were increased up to 260%, indicating that adenosine plays an important role in seizure termination [36]. During et al. investigated changes in adenosine using microdialysis probes implanted in the hippocampus of patients with intractable complex partial epilepsy and showed that reduced levels of adenosine in hippocampal epileptic foci result in a lower seizure threshold than in the contralateral hippocampus during the interictal period; the level of adenosine was significantly increased in the onset period during seizure activity, and it remained higher than baseline during the postictal refractory period [38]. The level of adenosine is regulated by adenosine receptors and adenosine kinase in vivo. A study using electrical stimulation of a rat model by Young et al. showed that adenosine plays a role in neuroprotection and improves the threshold of epilepsy by activating adenosine receptors [39]. Adenosine kinase is a key enzyme in the regulation of the adenosine level [40]. Boison et al. indicated that increased expression of adenosine kinase (ADK) in the hippocampus is an important reason for decreases in the adenosine level. Adenosine receptor agonists, adenosine transport inhibitors, and adenosine kinase inhibitors play an important role in the process of seizure termination, which may provide a new field for the treatment of epilepsy [40].

NPY is the most abundant peptide in the central nervous system. It is enriched in GABAergic interneurons and can regulate seizure termination and the electrical activity of neurons [2, 35, 41]. A study by Marksteiner et al. in 1989 found that endogenous NPY release was increased during seizures and played a role in seizure termination [42]. The activity of NPY is regulated by five types of NPY receptors. Using animal models of epilepsy, Meurs et al. [35] suggested that the activation of Y2 and/or Y5 receptors, in addition to blocking the Y1 receptor in the central nervous system, can terminate seizures.

Synchronization over the short distance between neurons and interneurons plays an important role in the initiation of seizures and may lead to seizure termination. The core mechanism of seizures is highly synchronized abnormal discharges by tens of thousands of neurons. The premise of highly synchronized abnormal discharges is that the epileptic signal is passed on to other neurons quickly, and, if signaling is interrupted, the seizure is terminated. As a gap junction, the electrical synapse plays an important role in seizure termination. Gap junctions are formed by the connection protein, which exists in different subtypes in inhibitory neurons [43]. The opening and closing of gap junctions is regulated by various forms of proteins. Connexins are separated at an acidic pH, leading to reduced conductance of the gap junction, while a pH level corresponding to alkali poisoning can promote connexin binding to increase gap junction conductance [44]. In vitro experiments illustrate that gap junctions are in a state of decoupling when the paroxysmal discharge is stopped [45]. In vivo experiments based on a 4-aminopyridine cortex injection-induced epilepsy model suggests that gap junction-blocking agents (including nonspecific blockers such as raw stomach ketone, octanol, and the connection protein 36-specific blocker quinine) may inhibit seizure discharge [46]. In vitro experiments by Jahromi verified that gap junction-blocking agents, such as gastric ketone, can terminate seizures in the hippocampal CA1 region [47], suggesting that gap junctions play a role in the maintenance and termination of seizures.

One of the mechanisms that limit synaptic transmission during epileptiform activity is the loss of synaptic vesicles containing the neurotransmitter glutamate. In vitro experiments in a hippocampal slice model of high-K+-induced activity by Staley et al. investigated the correlation of seizure-like burst duration with the subsequent interburst interval length. Based on the results, they hypothesized that the duration of the seizure discharge depends on the new release of glutamate. In the same article, they showed that interburst intervals of 3 s or longer may ensure maximum discharge duration (more than 420 ms). Even when the GABA-A and GABA-B were blocked, this phenomenon still occurred [48]. By replacing Ca^{2+} in the extracellular solution with Sr2+, Jones et al. found that the rate of glutamate release at CA3 axon terminals was reduced, which prolonged bursts in a concentration-dependent manner [49]. Therefore, the supply of releasable glutamate is an important stimulant that maintains the process of epileptiform activity. In the clinical situation, although the interval of bursts (e.g., clonic in tonic–clonic seizures) is regulated by vesicular recovery, the duration of the seizure might not be regulated. Other reports using the same model have also shown that in different regions of the hippocampus, although action potential bursts had a long duration (10–20 min), it was not possible to induce an increase in postsynaptic glutamate transmission [50]. The most likely possibility for this phenomenon is that another antiepileptic mechanism is initiated, which increases of the storage of glutamic acid during the process of epileptiform discharge. Therefore, the role of glutamatergic failure in seizure termination requires further study.

GABAergic inhibition continues during epileptic activity. Epileptic foci produce both recurrent and surround inhibition of neighboring areas, and, in the long term, this activity appears to be unable to effectively limit seizures, either temporally or spatially [51]. It is well established that synaptic inhibition is regulated by the presynaptic neurotransmitter GABA, which acts on postsynaptic neurons via GABA-A and GABA-B receptors. Chen et al. suggested that seizure activity is suppressed by a GABA-B receptor agonist (baclofen), and it is reversed by a GABA-B receptor antagonist in the pentylenetetrazole (PTZ)-kindled epilepsy model [52]. This phenomenon has also been confirmed by in vitro experiments [52]. A report by Zivanovi et al. showed that GABA-B receptor antagonists reduce the after-discharge threshold in an electrical stimulation model, which indicates that GABA-B receptors play an important role in seizure arrest [53]. However, Vergnes et al. found that GABA-B receptor antagonists microinjected in the thalamus can suppress absence seizures, whereas microinjection of antagonists in cortical and limbic structures can promote seizures in a spontaneous nonconvulsive absence seizure model [54]. Therefore, it is difficult to determine the effect of GABA-B receptor activation on seizure arrest due to the mixed findings involving anticonvulsive and proconvulsive activity [52]. GABA-A receptors are closely related to seizure termination. In epilepsy animal models, the electroconvulsive shock threshold is enhanced by microinjection of GABA-A receptor agonists, such as muscimol, into the subthalamic nucleus [55], which is consistent with the results found in a substantia nigra reticular nucleus-kindled model by Iadarola et al. [56]. Chen et al. found that the sensitivity of GABA-A receptors is decreased during SE, resulting in seizure termination [57]. Changes in subunit composition may also lead to decreased GABA-A receptor sensitivity [58]. Chudomel et al. suggested that changes in the maturation of extrasynaptic GABA-A receptors can lead to changes in seizure susceptibility [59]. In vivo experiments by Stell et al. have shown that mutation of the GABA-A receptor delta subunit plays an important role in preventing the occurrence and termination of epileptic seizures by affecting the tonic GABA current [60]. Inhibitory activity is similar to the glutamate release involved in the formation of the discharge rhythm [61] that maintains epileptic activity [62]. The finding that electrical activity begins only when the inhibitory current is not active has been affirmed using a kainic acid-induced epilepsy model [61]. A study of brain tissue in patients with temporal lobe epilepsy found that spontaneous activity was blocked when the GABA-A receptor was dysfunctional [63]. In a mild, single seizure model (such as the kindling model), it was found that the inhibition after a double pulse (i.e., inhibition of 50–500 ms after the second action potential) was increased, indicating that GABA activity is upregulated after epilepsy [64]. Consistent with the in vivo study of Lawrence et al. [65], researchers have also found that endogenous neurosteroids can terminate seizures by strengthening GABA-mediated inhibitory transmission [60].

Some researchers believe that a decreased level of extracellular glucose and hypoxia can terminate seizure activity [66, 67]. A study of Doman et al. found that energy failure caused by lack of glucose or hypoxia can lead to ion pump dysfunction and then seizure termination [67]. In a model using hippocampal slices without magnesium, Kirchner et al. found that the use of artificial cerebrospinal fluid with low glucose can decrease the discharge frequency by 50% and the discharge amplitude by 25% in 24 min. When using solution with normal blood glucose levels, the effects on both the frequency and amplitude were reversed [66]. These findings showed that hypoglycemia has a significant but not immediate effect on seizure discharges. A study by Namba et al. also found that the glucose disposal rate in most brain areas is decreased after seizure kindling in rats, which indicates that energy failure may be related to seizure arrest [68]. However, energy failure caused by hypoxia or hypoglycemia often leads to coma and neuronal necrosis. Therefore, it is possible that energy failure may be more closely related to the onset of the seizure activity than seizure termination [69].

Presynaptic glutamate uptake by astrocytes is the main mechanism for the accumulation of glutamate at the synapse [70]. A study by Tian showed that glial release of glutamate contributes to the maintenance of the paroxysmal depolarizing shift that is the hallmark of "epileptic" neurons [71].

The remote interaction between neurons is closely related to the increased synchronization of the cerebral cortex, and the long-term effects may include changes in the regulation loop of the subcortical nuclei that affect the seizure threshold, duration, severity, and termination of epileptic seizures. Studies of patients with epilepsy suggest that vagal nerve stimulation can activate certain nuclei in the brainstem such as the nucleus of the solitary tract, reduce the frequency of seizures, and promote seizure termination [72]. On July 16, 1997, the Food and Drug Administration (FDA) approved the neurocybernetic prosthesis as refractory adjuvant treatment of refractory partial seizures for adults and children 12 years of age or older. However, the mechanism of seizure reduction is still unclear. Theoretically, the treatment affects vagal nerve stimulation of cortical activity and brainstem nuclei (such as blue spots) that contain catecholamine. Albala et al. [73] found that the depletion of norepinephrine in the forebrain can contribute to seizures, which indicates that the release of norepinephrine can lead to seizures. Blue spot stimulation can spread to the thalamus, amygdala, hippocampus, and cerebral cortex, resulting in termination of seizures [72]. Vagal nerve stimulation increases the levels of catecholamine metabolites and GABA in cerebrospinal fluid [74], which affects the synchronization of the cerebral cortex [75]. An increase in cerebral cortical synchronization can activate sodium- and calcium-activated potassium channels and silence electrical activity in neurons, resulting in termination of seizures [76].

Numerous subcortical anatomical regions mediate anticonvulsant effects, such as the substantia nigra pars reticulata (SNR) and the subthalamic nucleus (STN). Anticonvulsant circuits may limit seizures by reducing the recruitment and spread of seizure activity from the seizure onset zone to "naive" areas of the brain by decreasing excitatory feedback and amplification [2]. The SNR is a key area for GABA-mediated anticonvulsant activity and affects activity in the brain via the brainstem, thalamus, superior colliculus, and pedunculopontine nucleus [56]. In a pentylenetetrazole-induced epilepsy model, Okada et al. found that the SNR could be silenced by microinjection of the GABA antagonist muscimol, which suppressed epileptic seizure occurrence and development; microinjection of the GABA antagonist bicuculline also produced a similar anticonvulsant effect [77]. The regulation of excitation and inhibition by subcortical nuclei appears to vary with sex and developmental age. SNR is an example of a subcortical region that is capable of modulating seizure thresholds. Application of GABA agonists to the substantia nigra can induce anti- or proconvulsant effects that vary by sex and developmental age [78]. Male rats have two regions in the SNR, the anterior and posterior regions, which produce anticonvulsant and proconvulsant effects in seizures, respectively [79]. However, female rats have no equivalent proconvulsant posterior region [2]. A study found that three episodes of SE in the anterior region of the SNR of rats within 6 days of birth indicate an abnormality [79]. During development and maturation, the SNR loses its anticonvulsant effects, which indicates that this area is mainly involved in seizure control. Shinnar et al. suggested that during the development of the brain, the effect of the SNR on seizures can be explained by the reduced ability to increase or decrease seizure susceptibility in early childhood epilepsy. This finding indicates that the SNR not only exerts an anticonvulsive effect but also produces differences in the seizure termination effect between mature and immature brains [11].

Several studies have shown that the STN, which is adjacent to the SNR, is also capable of modulating seizure activity. In an electrical stimulation animal model, Lado found that electrical stimulation of the subthalamic nucleus increases the seizure threshold and has an anticonvulsant effect [80], which is consistent with a study conducted in epileptic patients by Chabardes [81]. A recent small sample study of patients with medial temporal lobe epilepsy showed that coordination of the thalamus and cortex through the regulation of cortical synchronization leads to seizure termination. One of the possibilities is that the subthalamic nucleus receives inhibitory GABA input from spiral efferents [82].

2.1.4 Conclusion

Postictal refractoriness has been widely studied in variety of epilepsy animal models (such as electric/chemical-induced and kindling models). During this period, the threshold of recurrence and the effect of antiepileptic drugs are increased. Age, sex hormones, and structural and genetic abnormalities are closely related to seizure termination. The self-limiting characteristic of seizures indicates that the mechanism of seizure termination is likely to be established in a relatively short time. Endogenous anticonvulsant mechanisms, including the ionic microenvironment, various endogenous neuromodulators, gap junctions, synaptic transmission (including depletion of glutamate and increased inhibition), energy failure, glial buffering of glutamate, and remote interaction of neurons, are likely to be new treatment strategies for seizures. In particular, pH changes, adenosine, and NPY are the most promising pharmacological therapeutic targets. Changes in pH can occur in a short time, while the exogenous pH can affect the endogenous environment. Therefore, although the alteration of pH may have no significant effect on preventing or prolonging postictal refractoriness, it is likely to play a decisive role in the seizure termination. The release of adenosine and NPY occur during seizure activity (NPY can have an effect even after a few months); however, these substances can regulate the excitability of neurons. Therefore, pharmacological intervention based on adenosine and NPY may also reduce the frequency of spontaneous seizures and prolong postictal refractoriness. The next step will focus on the temporal and spatial changes of these mechanisms and the signaling pathways involved in them.

2.2 The Pathogenesis of SE

2.2.1 Changes in the Internal Environment During SE

Over the past 20 years, a number of studies have elucidated a series of changes that are involved in the progression from a single seizure to SE. These changes can be divided into the four stages.

The main manifestations of SE stage 1 (from a few milliseconds to seconds) are abnormal phosphorylation of proteins, the opening and closing of ion channels, and the release of neurotransmitters [57]. Using an SE animal model induced by kainic acid, Yamagata et al. found that during the process of SE, the phosphorylation level of synaptic protein 1 decreased rapidly. After the cessation of SE, the level of phosphorylation returned to normal [83]. Lee et al. also found that the phosphorylation of p65-Ser276 NFκB in the piriform cortex decreased rapidly in a rat SE model [84]. Moreover, Oliveira et al. found that in a pilocarpine-induced acute epilepsy animal model, small-conductance (SK) Ca(2+)-activated K+ channels are dysfunctional [85]. Wu et al. showed that in the acute stage following SE, the acid-sensing ion channels (ASICs) of the piriform cortex cannot be regulated normally in animal models [86]. A study found that the expression of Na (V) 1.2 and Na (V) 1.6 subunits declines continuously for 30 days after SE [87]. Certain evidence has shown that in an animal model of SE induced by pilocarpine, the increased release of GABA and glutamate (120% and 182%, respectively) in the hippocampus were closely related to SE. They also found that transcranial electrical stimulation at low current intensities (<2800 A) will increase the release of GABA and decrease glutamate release in basal cells [88].

The main manifestation of SE stage 2 (from seconds to minutes) is the change in receptor composition, including a reduction of inhibitory GABA-A receptor subunits regulated by endocytosis and an increase in excitatory *N*-methyl-D-aspartic acid (NMDA) and α-amino-3-hydroxy-5-methyl-4-isoxazole-propionic acid (AMPA) receptors. A study found that the aggregation of GABA-A receptors in cells is increased following SE [89], but the expression of GABA-A on the cell surface is reduced [90], which was consistent with immunofluorescence data [91, 92]. An anatomical study conducted by Naylor et al. in an SE model induced by lithium-pilocarpine showed that the amount of GABA-A β2/3 and γ2 receptor subunits was decreased, and the percentage of these subunits inside dentate gyrus granular cells was increased. Additionally, they found that the amplitude of miniature inhibitory postsynaptic currents (mIPSCs) in GABA-A receptors of dentate gyrus granular layer cells was decreased. This is not consistent with the amplitude of mIPSCs at the synapses; the extrasynaptic GABA-A current was increased in SE. The establishment of a mathematical model also showed that the change in mIPSCs reflects the decrease in the postsynaptic functional GABA-A receptors in SE [91]. An in vitro study showed that mIPSCs, which reflect the postsynaptic function of GABA, decreased by 20% during SE. Kapur et al. found that recurrent seizures can lead to sustained inhibition of GABA function [93]. Regulation of GABA-A receptors can lead to the tolerance of benzodiazepines, which makes these receptors very important for the regulation of the SE duration [94, 95].

On the other hand, Naylor et al. found that in an SE model induced by lithium chloride and pilocarpine, the re-localization phenomenon, in which the NMDA receptor subunit NR1 translocates from the inner side of the cell to the cell surface, occurred in dentate gyrus granular cells and CA3 pyramidal cells at 1 h following SE. They also found NMDA miniature excitatory postsynaptic currents (mEPSCs) were increased in hippocampal slices following SE, and during the process of SE, the amount of the functional postsynaptic NMDA receptors increased by 38% per synapse [96].

SE stage 3 (from a few minutes to day) includes the increased expression of excitatory neuropeptides and decreased expression of inhibitory neuropeptides; thus, the hyperexcited state is maintained [97]. Liu et al. found that SE significantly increased substance P and mRNA levels of the substance P precursor (preprotachykinin A) in hippocampal mossy fibers. They also found that in brain slices, substance P accelerated the release of glutamate. An increasing number of researchers believe that increasing the level of substance P may promote hippocampal excitability and maintain SE [97]. On the other hand, inhibitory NPY is present in inhibitory GABAergic interneurons and is a regulator of neuronal excitability. NPY plays an important role in the pathogenesis of SE [98]. O'Loughlin et al. found that the expression of NPY was decreased following SE in animal models [99].

Genetic and epigenetic analyses show that the expression of many genes changes during SE stage 4 (from a few days to weeks) [100, 101], which may lead to epilepsy. Studies of an SE animal model showed that the epigenetic changes occurred in the fourth stage of SE episodes and included whole-genome changes in DNA methylation of hippocampal cells [102]. Reschke et al. found that the regulation of micro RNA plays an important role in epilepsy and neuronal injury-induced by SE [103].

2.2.2 The Pathogenesis of SE

The persistence of seizures is due to an imbalance in neuronal excitability and inhibition or inhibitory mechanism abnormalities [104]. Pharmacological studies of animal models show that SE has two distinct phases: the initial and maintenance periods. The refractory period occurs during the late stage of the maintenance period. During the initial and the early maintenance period, protein phosphorylation, changes in ion channels, neurotransmitter release, and changes in receptor transport provide the foundation for long-term seizures [57]. The pathogenesis of the refractory period will be discussed in detail in the next section of this chapter.

Protein phosphorylation is involved in the pathogenesis SE. Using a pilocarpine-induced SE animal model, Kim et al. found that NF-κB phosphorylation regulates SE-induced astrocyte reactive hyperplasia and neuronal degeneration in the hippocampus [105]. Using the same model, one study found that the enhancement of p65-Ser536 NF-κB phosphorylation in the hippocampus may increase the susceptibility to SE [106].

Moreover, Lerche et al. found that voltage and ligand-gated ion channel dysregulation (deficiency of sodium ion channels in inhibitory neurons and dysfunction of different types of ion channels in the initial part of the axon) led to increased excitability of neurons and plays an important role in SE [107]. In vivo and in vitro data show that silencing K+ channels reduces neuronal excitability and alleviates the development of SE [108]. Kv4.2 is the most important type A potassium channel in the hippocampus and cortex. Much evidence suggests that Kv4.2 is an important regulator of neuronal excitability, and Kv4.2 abnormalities are found in different types of human epilepsy or epileptic animal models. Studies have shown that decreased function of Kv4.2 may be an important mechanism of increases in local neuron loop excitability [109]. Some researchers have established an in vitro spontaneous epileptic brain slice model using 4-AP and magnesium-free artificial cerebrospinal fluid. They found that sodium ion-gated channel changes affect neuronal depolarization and neuronal excitability and may also play an important role in SE [110].

Release of presynaptic neurotransmitters also has an effect on SE. Upreti et al. showed using FM1–43 two-photon imaging, electron microscopy, and other techniques that increased presynaptic transmitter release and increased release area accelerate SE in hippocampal slices [111]. Studies have confirmed that extrasynaptic NMDA receptors rarely open in the physiological state and can abnormally open in pathological states such as SE. Glutamate secreted by astrocytes may lead to synchronous neuronal discharge by activating synaptic NMDA receptors. Activation of extracellular NMDA receptors can mediate excitotoxicity and may result in neuronal death after SE [112]. It has been suggested that extracellular NMDA receptor abnormalities may be involved in the pathogenesis of SE. At present, some researchers have confirmed that dysfunction of the entire GABA transmitter system can lead to abnormal neuronal excitation, which can then progress to SE [113]. Volgushev et al. found that different temperatures have various effects on neurotransmitter release; the release of excitatory neurotransmitters in the presynaptic membrane is reduced at low temperature [114]. Motamedi et al. found that sustained hypothermia can affect the development of SE through the release and transmission of GABA in interneurons, which can explain the current clinical application of mild hypothermia during SE [115].

With respect to receptor transport, some researchers have found that short-term changes in classical receptors can lead to inhibition and imbalances in excitatory neuropeptides after SE [116]. Vadillo et al. proposed that glutamate-mediated excitability is the initiation factor of SE [117]. Using an SE model, Grosshans et al. found that NMDA receptors in the cytoplasm translocated to the surface of the neuronal membrane, which led to SE [118]. In addition, studies have shown that calmodulin kinase II can regulate glutamate and GABA receptor transport [119], and this process is closely related to the neuropathology of SE [120]. The increase in the number of glutamate receptors on the cell surface and the reduction of GABA receptors during SE [121, 122] leads to a decrease in GABAergic activity. Previous studies have shown that the transport of GABA receptors is reduced in both in vivo and in vitro models of SE [119, 123]. Reducing GABA receptor sensitivity and decreasing chloride influx by activating chloride ion channels accelerates SE [123]. Using a self-sustaining SE model, some researchers found that repeated activation of GABA-A receptors in dentate granulosa cells and interneurons leads to GABA-A receptor endocytosis in the synaptic loop of the hippocampus, which plays an important role in SE [116].

SE is the result of highly synchronized neuronal firing. At present, an increasing number of studies have found that maximum synchronization of neurons on a micro- and macroscopic level may result in seizure termination. Thus, failure to achieve sufficiently high synchronization may cause SE or transition from SE to postictal refractoriness [124]. Schindler et al. evaluated synchronous electroencephalograms (EEG) of six patients with SE and found that the pre-SE EEG showed a gradual increase in neuronal synchronous discharges, which was highly consistent with SE [125]. They suggested that the enhancement of neuronal synchronization might be a self-regulating mechanism for the initiation of SE.

2.2.3 Conclusions

Self-limitation is the most significant characteristic of a seizure. However, in contrast to most seizure types, the self-limiting ability of SE disappears. Most researchers speculate that the main causes for seizures to develop into SE include the failure of the endogenous mechanism of seizure termination, the disappearance of postictal refractoriness following seizures, and a mechanism that causes seizures to be sustained in humans. The key factor is the change in neurotransmitters on the membrane, which changes the excitatory and inhibitory process of neurons and causes seizures to be sustained. Additionally, other mechanisms of human SE, such as abnormal protein phosphorylation, abnormal ion channels, and the release of neurotransmitters, are the basis of long-term epilepsy. Understanding of the significance of the SE mechanism lies in the identification of new targets for potential anti-status epilepticus drugs and is conducive to improving SE control.

2.3 The Pathogenesis of RSE

There are two main characteristics of SE: the persistence and the time-dependent drug resistance. Most seizures are self-limiting. However, SE rarely undergoes spontaneous termination before the onset of fatigue and brain damage, which is called self-persistence. One study found that in a SE model induced by electrical stimulation and drug administration, the seizures could be sustained even when predisposing factors are removed, and RSE could occur. Clinical research has shown that seizures lasting for more than 30 min rarely exhibit spontaneous termination [57].

On the other hand, drug resistance during SE development is time-dependent. Pharmacological studies in animal models have suggested that two distinct phases are present in SE, the initial and maintenance phases. In the late maintenance phase, a refractory period may emerge. In the early stages of SE, many drugs that can increase inhibition or reduce excitability may prevent epilepsy from developing [116]. However, once RSE occurs, only a few drugs that inhibit glutamate neurotransmitter can effectively terminate this condition [91]. Studies have found that in the RSE model, the antiepileptic effect of the same dose of benzodiazepines was significantly decreased in the late stage of SE. A study using an animal model showed that when SE lasted for 30 min, the therapeutic effect of the benzodiazepines was 20 times lower. The effect was reduced more slowly for phenytoin [126]. However, NMDA blockers are continuously effective for preventing SE [127]. The critical transformation from SE to RSE occurs at 30–60 min after the beginning of SE, and a delay in treatment of SE is an important risk factor in this transition [128].

2.3.1 Translocation of GABA and Glutamate Receptors

SE is continuous and uninterrupted, which can be explained by receptor transport. During this period, the number of glutamate receptors on the cell surface increases, and the number of GABA receptors decreases [121, 129], which causes the GABAergic activity decrease. Many studies have suggested that the internalization of GABA-A receptors in the hippocampus plays an important role in the transformation from a single seizure to RSE. GABA is the most common inhibitory neurotransmitter, preventing hyperexcitability of neurons by activating GABA-A receptors. Due to GABA inhibition, patients with SE show partial or complete resistance to benzodiazepines [130]. Naylor et al. studied a SE model induced by pilocarpine and found that the number of GABA-A receptors in the synapses of the granule cells located in the dentate gyrus was significantly reduced [91]. Goodkin found the activity-dependent rapid internalization of the β2/β3 subunit of GABA-A receptor occurred in the hippocampal neuron model; therefore, they proposed that the increase in activity-dependence of GABA-A receptor internalization in the synapses during SE causes decreased inhibitory transmission [131]. Prolonged SE can quickly change the function of GABARs in granule cells in the hippocampal dentate gyrus [132]. Studies have found that the decrease in expression of the β2/β3 subunit of GABA-A receptors on the cell surface leads to RSE [90]. To a certain extent, the internalization and reduction of GABA-A receptors in the synaptic cleft can explain the lack of GABA-A inhibition in RSE and the progressive and time-dependent drug resistance of benzodiazepines [126, 132].

Glutamate is the most common excitatory neurotransmitter, and it modulates neuronal excitability through the NMDA receptor. Aggregation of AMPA and NMDA receptors occurs on the synaptic membrane [133], resulting in epilepsy. This will further increase excitability during epileptic seizures. Immunohistochemical data have shown that the NR1 subunit of NMDA receptors is transported from the subsynaptic area to the synaptic surface at 1 h after SE, and physiological data have also shown that the number of functional NMDA receptors in dentate gyrus granule cell synapses increases during this phase.

GABA and glutamate receptor transportation are important for drug effects on SE [90]. First-line antiepileptic drugs such as benzodiazepines interact with GABA-A receptors, and the therapeutic effect decreases when status is prolonged. Drugs that are effective for RSE, such as propofol, interact with another binding site that differs from the site of benzodiazepines and barbiturates [134]. Isoflurane is associated with the suppression of inward flow of ions through postsynaptic GABA-A receptors [135].

2.3.2 Neuronal Injury and Death

The state of SE is continuous and uninterrupted, and the accompanying neuron damage and drug resistance are obvious when SE lasts more than 30 min. Fujikawa DG evaluated the percentage of eosinophils in a pilocarpine-induced animal model and found that if SE lasts for 40 min or longer, mild or more irreversible injury can occur in hippocampal neurons. This view is also consistent with the results of an animal model study by Mazarati [136]. Consistent with the results of a study by Sloviter [137], Meldrum et al. found that epilepsy itself can lead to neuronal death [138], and neuronal necrosis caused by SE is an important factor for recurrent epileptic seizures [139]. In the past century, mild hypothermia has been found to have a protective effect on neurons and has been used for the treatment of brain injury in perinatal infants with hypoxic-ischemic encephalopathy. Subsequent investigations have shown that this protective effect induced by mild hypothermia has an inhibitory effect on early seizures [140].

A wide range of neuronal necrosis caused by RSE occurs in the form of "programmed necrosis" [141]. Apoptosis occurs in the immature brain. One of the major genes that promote apoptosis is Bax, and Bcl-X is a gene that inhibits apoptosis. In RSE, the expression of Bcl-X is decreased, and Bax expression is increased in hippocampal neurons, which induces apoptosis [142]. A study on humans found that the density of hippocampal neurons in the brain of patients who died from RSE was reduced [143]. This study showed that the expression of neuron-specific enolase, a marker of neuronal death, was increased in the serum of patients with SE [144]. In vivo data from Cock et al. showed that neuronal death is closely related to the mitochondrial dysfunction after SE [145]. A study using MRI found that patients have brain edema and chronic brain atrophy after SE [146], and the area where epileptic activity was strongest shows local brain atrophy [147]. This evidence further supports a causal relationship between seizures and neuronal loss. J. Nixon also reported brain atrophy on MRI findings in patients with SE, and the autopsy reports showed that neurons were decreased in the brain [148]. Cendes et al. reported a decrease in neurons in an 84-year-old male with SE induced by domoic acid poisoning [149]. Therefore, drug resistance in RSE can also be explained by the loss of normal physiological function after neuronal injury.

2.3.3 Changes in the Expression of Neuropeptides

RSE is related to brain neuropeptides in the hippocampus; for example, it is closely related to a decrease in the expression levels of galanin [150], dynorphin [151], somatostatin, and NPY [152] and an increase in the expression of substance P, tachykinin, and neurokinin [97]. These changes may play an important role in the maintenance of RSE. One study showed that hippocampal fibers rich in galanin were decreased 3 h after the initiation of RSE [153]. Galanin and its agonist effectively prevent RSE via galanin receptor 1 (GalR1) and galanin receptor 2 (GalR2), and a galanin antagonist accelerates the development of RSE [154]. A study using animal models showed that rats in which galanin was overexpressed do not develop RSE, and galanin knockout mice exhibited increased susceptibility to RSE [155].

NPY is expressed in GABAergic inhibitory interneurons and is a regulator to neuronal excitability [98]. In a transgenic mouse model of RSE induced by kainic acid, the lack of NPY significantly increased the mortality [98] and spontaneous seizures after initiation of RSE [156]. A study on isolated rat hippocampal nerve terminals found that blocking NPY could promote neuronal excitability by the release of glutamate [157].

Injection of substance P in the hippocampus can lead to RSE, and substance P antagonists can block RSE [158]. Glutamate release was exacerbated by substance P in hippocampal slices. An increasing number of researchers have proposed that the increased levels of substance P in refractory status epilepsy may promote excitability of the hippocampus and maintain SE [97].

A previous study also found that preprotachykinin mRNA that encodes substance P is expressed in dentate gyrus granule cells in patients with RSE, while it is almost undetectable in normal subjects [159]. Compared to the receptor transport mentioned previously, these peptide networks change more slowly, but they tend to promote excitability in the balance between excitability and inhibition in the hippocampus: therefore, these peptides may be involved in the occurrence and development of RSE.

2.3.4 Inflammatory Process

Studies have shown that inhibiting the inflammatory process can promote the integrity of the blood brain barrier and reduce the severity of SE [160]. Friedman A. and Dingledine R. found that inflammatory factors, such as IL-1-beta, TNF-alpha, and toll-like receptor 4, were involved in the occurrence of RSE [161]. Juhász et al. reported that in a 56-year-old male patient with new onset RSE, in addition to the seizures being controlled by surgical removal of the epileptic foci, the inflammatory foci, which were not removed, also disappeared [162]. These data illustrate the relationship between the inflammatory process and RSE. However, the role of inflammation in the pathophysiology of refractory epilepsy is still unclear.

2.3.5 Changes in Gene Expression

Studies have confirmed that changes in the expression of genes associated with epileptogenesis play a role in the pathogenesis of RSE. Serial analysis of gene expression (SAGE) showed that 92 genes were differentially expressed in the hippocampus in a SE model. These genes are closely related to ribosomal proteins, protein processing, axon growth, and proliferation of proteins in glial cells [114]. Barnes et al. used in situ hybridization in a kainic acid-induced SE model to examine changes in semaphorin gene expression, which was confined to neurons [163].

2.3.6 Conclusions

Epilepsy induced by RSE is a widespread phenomenon that occurs in different species and at different ages. However, less research has been conducted on humans. A retrospective study showed that 31–43% of patients with SE developed RSE [128]. In a prospective study of RSE, approximately 23% of patients with SE become nonresponsive to first-line and second-line antiepileptic drugs and developed RSE [128]. Therefore, some cases of RSE evolve from SE, while other RSE cases directly evolve from a single seizure, without a transitional period of SE, and may progress to epileptogenesis. Existing studies have found that translocation of GABA and glutamate receptors, neuronal injury and death, changes in the expression of neuropeptides, inflammatory process, and changes in gene expression are related to the development of RSE, which may play an important role in the understanding of the pathogenesis of RSE and in preventing or reversing the development of RSE.

References

1. Dragunow M. Endogenous anticonvulsant substances. Neurosci Biobehav Rev. 1986;10(3):229–44.
2. Lado FA, Moshe SL. How do seizures stop? Epilepsia. 2008;49(10):1651–64.
3. Jenssen S, Gracely EJ, Sperling MR. How long do most seizures last? A systematic comparison of seizures recorded in the epilepsy monitoring unit. Epilepsia. 2006;47(9):1499–503.
4. Theodore WH, et al. The secondarily generalized tonic-clonic seizure: a videotape analysis. Neurology. 1994;44(8):1403–7.
5. Pan S, et al. Factors influencing the duration of generalized tonic-clonic seizure. Seizure. 2016;34:44–7.
6. Nutt DJ, Cowen PJ, Green AR. Studies on the post-ictal rise in seizure threshold. Eur J Pharmacol. 1981;71(2–3):287–95.
7. Loscher W, Frey HH. Postictal refractoriness associated with reduction of glutamic acid decarboxylase in discrete brain regions in epilepsy-prone gerbils. Biochem Pharmacol. 1987;36(16):2695–9.
8. Reisner AD. The electroconvulsive therapy controversy: evidence and ethics. Neuropsychol Rev. 2003;13(4):199–219.
9. Mace JA, Burnham WM. The effect of repeated seizures on anticonvulsant drug response in the kindling model.

Electroencephalogr Clin Neurophysiol. 1987;67(2):171–5.
10. Loscher W, Honack D. The effect of interstimulation interval on the assessment of anticonvulsant drug potency in fully kindled rats. Epilepsy Res. 1990;7(3):182–96.
11. Shinnar S, et al. How long do new-onset seizures in children last? Ann Neurol. 2001;49(5):659–64.
12. Locock C. Discussion of paper by EH Sieveking: analysis of 52 cases of epilepsy observed by the author. Lancet. 1857;1:527.
13. Alam MN, Ahmad A, Al-Abbasi FA. Female ovarian steroids in epilepsy: a cause or remedy. Pharmacol Rep. 2013;65(4):802–12.
14. Harden CL, et al. Seizure frequency is associated with age at menopause in women with epilepsy. Neurology. 2003;61(4):451–5.
15. Harden CL, et al. The effect of menopause and perimenopause on the course of epilepsy. Epilepsia. 1999;40(10):1402–7.
16. Kaminski RM, et al. Anticonvulsant activity of androsterone and etiocholanolone. Epilepsia. 2005;46(6):819–27.
17. Kemmotsu N, et al. MRI analysis in temporal lobe epilepsy: cortical thinning and white matter disruptions are related to side of seizure onset. Epilepsia. 2011;52(12):2257–66.
18. Hesdorffer DC, et al. Risk factors for febrile status epilepticus: a case-control study. J Pediatr. 2013;163(4):1147–51.e1.
19. Bergren SK, et al. Genetic modifiers affecting severity of epilepsy caused by mutation of sodium channel Scn2a. Mamm Genome. 2005;16(9):683–90.
20. Frankel WN, et al. Unraveling genetic modifiers in the gria4 mouse model of absence epilepsy. PLoS Genet. 2014;10(7):e1004454.
21. Chesler M, Kaila K. Modulation of pH by neuronal activity. Trends Neurosci. 1992;15(10):396–402.
22. Velisek L, et al. Lowering of extracellular pH suppresses low-Mg(2+)-induces seizures in combined entorhinal cortex-hippocampal slices. Exp Brain Res. 1994;101(1):44–52.
23. Caspers H, Speckmann EJ. Cerebral pO2, pCO2 and pH: changes during convulsive activity and their significance for spontaneous arrest of seizures. Epilepsia. 1972;13(5):699–725.
24. Cao Q, et al. Elevated expression of acid-sensing ion channel 3 inhibits epilepsy via activation of interneurons. Mol Neurobiol. 2016;53(1):485–98.
25. Velisek L. Extracellular acidosis and high levels of carbon dioxide suppress synaptic transmission and prevent the induction of long-term potentiation in the CA1 region of rat hippocampal slices. Hippocampus. 1998;8(1):24–32.
26. Thiry A, et al. Carbonic anhydrase inhibitors as anticonvulsant agents. Curr Top Med Chem. 2007;7(9):855–64.
27. Tong CK, Chen K, Chesler M. Kinetics of activity-evoked pH transients and extracellular pH buffering in rat hippocampal slices. J Neurophysiol. 2006;95(6):3686–97.
28. Xiong ZQ, Saggau P, Stringer JL. Activity-dependent intracellular acidification correlates with the duration of seizure activity. J Neurosci. 2000;20(4):1290–6.
29. Schuchmann S, et al. Experimental febrile seizures are precipitated by a hyperthermia-induced respiratory alkalosis. Nat Med. 2006;12(7):817–23.
30. Ziemann AE, et al. Seizure termination by acidosis depends on ASIC1a. Nat Neurosci. 2008;11(7):816–22.
31. Heinemann U, Lux HD, Gutnick MJ. Extracellular free calcium and potassium during paroxsmal activity in the cerebral cortex of the cat. Exp Brain Res. 1977;27(3–4):237–43.
32. Hongo Y, et al. Heterogeneous effects of antiepileptic drugs in an in vitro epilepsy model—a functional multineuron calcium imaging study. Eur J Neurosci. 2015;42(2):1818–29.
33. Boison D. Adenosinergic signaling in epilepsy. Neuropharmacology. 2015;104:131–9.
34. Lewin E, Bleck V. Electroshock seizures in mice: effect on brain adenosine and its metabolites. Epilepsia. 1981;22(5):577–81.
35. Meurs A, et al. Clinical potential of neuropeptide Y receptor ligands in the treatment of epilepsy. Curr Top Med Chem. 2007;7(17):1660–74.
36. Van Gompel JJ, et al. Increased cortical extracellular adenosine correlates with seizure termination. Epilepsia. 2014;55(2):233–44.
37. Ault B, Wang CM. Adenosine inhibits epileptiform activity arising in hippocampal area CA3. Br J Pharmacol. 1986;87(4):695–703.
38. During MJ, Spencer DD. Adenosine: a potential mediator of seizure arrest and postictal refractoriness. Ann Neurol. 1992;32(5):618–24.
39. Young D, Dragunow M. Status epilepticus may be caused by loss of adenosine anticonvulsant mechanisms. Neuroscience. 1994;58(2):245–61.
40. Boison D. Adenosine and epilepsy: from therapeutic rationale to new therapeutic strategies. Neuroscientist. 2005;11(1):25–36.
41. Vezzani A, Sperk G. Overexpression of NPY and Y2 receptors in epileptic brain tissue: an endogenous neuroprotective mechanism in temporal lobe epilepsy? Neuropeptides. 2004;38(4):245–52.
42. Marksteiner J, Sperk G, Maas D. Differential increases in brain levels of neuropeptide Y and vasoactive intestinal polypeptide after kainic acid-induced seizures in the rat. Naunyn Schmiedeberg's Arch Pharmacol. 1989;339(1–2):173–7.
43. Hestrin S, Galarreta M. Electrical synapses define networks of neocortical GABAergic neurons. Trends Neurosci. 2005;28(6):304–9.
44. Valiunas V. Biophysical properties of connexin-45 gap junction hemichannels studied in vertebrate cells. J Gen Physiol. 2002;119(2):147–64.
45. De Curtis M, Manfridi A, Biella G. Activity-dependent pH shifts and periodic recurrence of spontaneous interictal spikes in a model of focal epileptogenesis. J Neurosci. 1998;18(18):7543–51.

46. Gajda Z, et al. Quinine, a blocker of neuronal cx36 channels, suppresses seizure activity in rat neocortex in vivo. Epilepsia. 2005;46(10):1581–91.
47. Jahromi SS, et al. Anticonvulsant actions of gap junctional blockers in an in vitro seizure model. J Neurophysiol. 2002;88(4):1893–902.
48. Staley KJ, et al. Presynaptic modulation of CA3 network activity. Nat Neurosci. 1998;1(3):201–9.
49. Jones J, et al. Desynchronization of glutamate release prolongs synchronous CA3 network activity. J Neurophysiol. 2007;97(5):3812–8.
50. Lopantsev V, Both M, Draguhn A. Rapid plasticity at inhibitory and excitatory synapses in the hippocampus induced by ictal epileptiform discharges. Eur J Neurosci. 2009;29(6):1153–64.
51. Dorn T, Witte OW. Refractory periods following interictal spikes in acute experimentally induced epileptic foci. Electroencephalogr Clin Neurophysiol. 1995;94(1):80–5.
52. Chen L, Chan YS, Yung WH. GABA-B receptor activation in the rat globus pallidus potently suppresses pentylenetetrazol-induced tonic seizures. J Biomed Sci. 2004;11(4):457–64.
53. Zivanovic D, et al. Action of GABA-B antagonist on cortical epileptic afterdischarges in rats is similar to that of GABA-A antagonist. Physiol Res. 2003;52(5):651–5.
54. Vergnes M, et al. Opposite effects of GABAB receptor antagonists on absences and convulsive seizures. Eur J Pharmacol. 1997;332(3):245–55.
55. Shehab SA, et al. Experimental manipulations of the subthalamic nucleus fail to suppress tonic seizures in the electroshock model of epilepsy. Exp Brain Res. 2006;173(2):274–81.
56. Iadarola MJ, Gale K. Substantia nigra: site of anticonvulsant activity mediated by gamma-aminobutyric acid. Science. 1982;218(4578):1237–40.
57. Chen JW, Naylor DE, Wasterlain CG. Advances in the pathophysiology of status epilepticus. Acta Neurol Scand Suppl. 2007;186:7–15.
58. Brooks-Kayal AR. Rearranging receptors. Epilepsia. 2005;46(Suppl 7):29–38.
59. Chudomel O, et al. Age- and sex-related characteristics of tonic GABA currents in the rat substantia nigra pars reticulata. Neurochem Res. 2015;40(4): 747–57.
60. Stell BM, et al. Neuroactive steroids reduce neuronal excitability by selectively enhancing tonic inhibition mediated by delta subunit-containing GABAA receptors. Proc Natl Acad Sci U S A. 2003;100(24):14439–44.
61. Khazipov R, Holmes GL. Synchronization of kainate-induced epileptic activity via GABAergic inhibition in the superfused rat hippocampus in vivo. J Neurosci. 2003;23(12):5337–41.
62. Cohen I, et al. On the origin of interictal activity in human temporal lobe epilepsy in vitro. Science. 2002;298(5597):1418–21.
63. Kohling R, et al. Spontaneous sharp waves in human neocortical slices excised from epileptic patients. Brain. 1998;121(Pt 6):1073–87.
64. Tuff LP, Racine RJ, Adamec R. The effects of kindling on GABA-mediated inhibition in the dentate gyrus of the rat. I. Paired pulse depression. Brain Res. 1983;277(1):79–90.
65. Lawrence C, et al. Endogenous neurosteroid synthesis modulates seizure frequency. Ann Neurol. 2010;67(5):689–93.
66. Kirchner A, Veliskova J, Velisek L. Differential effects of low glucose concentrations on seizures and epileptiform activity in vivo and in vitro. Eur J Neurosci. 2006;23(6):1512–22.
67. Doman G, Pelligra R. A unifying concept of seizure onset and termination. Med Hypotheses. 2004;62(5):740–5.
68. Namba H, et al. Local cerebral glucose utilization in the postictal phase of amygdaloid kindled rats. Brain Res. 1989;486(2):221–7.
69. Patrick AW, Campbell IW. Fatal hypoglycaemia in insulin-treated diabetes mellitus: clinical features and neuropathological changes. Diabet Med. 1990;7(4):349–54.
70. Benarroch EE. Neuron-astrocyte interactions: partnership for normal function and disease in the central nervous system. Mayo Clin Proc. 2005;80(10):1326–38.
71. Tian GF, et al. An astrocytic basis of epilepsy. Nat Med. 2005;11(9):973–81.
72. Groves DA, Brown VJ. Vagal nerve stimulation: a review of its applications and potential mechanisms that mediate its clinical effects. Neurosci Biobehav Rev. 2005;29(3):493–500.
73. Albala BJ, et al. Unilateral peri-substantia nigra catecholaminergic lesion and amygdala kindling. Brain Res. 1986;370(2):388–92.
74. Carpenter LL, et al. Effect of vagus nerve stimulation on cerebrospinal fluid monoamine metabolites, norepinephrine, and gamma-aminobutyric acid concentrations in depressed patients. Biol Psychiatry. 2004;56(6):418–26.
75. Marrosu F, et al. Increase in 20-50 Hz (gamma frequencies) power spectrum and synchronization after chronic vagal nerve stimulation. Clin Neurophysiol. 2005;116(9):2026–36.
76. Timofeev I, Grenier F, Steriade M. Contribution of intrinsic neuronal factors in the generation of cortically driven electrographic seizures. J Neurophysiol. 2004;92(2):1133–43.
77. Okada R, Negishi N, Nagaya H. The role of the nigrotegmental GABAergic pathway in the propagation of pentylenetetrazol-induced seizures. Brain Res. 1989;480(1–2):383–7.
78. Veliskova J, et al. The expression of GABA (A) receptor subunits in the substantia nigra is developmentally regulated and region-specific. Ital J Neurol Sci. 1998;19(4):205–10.
79. Veliskova J, Moshe SL. Sexual dimorphism and developmental regulation of substantia nigra function. Ann Neurol. 2001;50(5):596–601.
80. Lado FA, Velisek L, Moshe SL. The effect of electrical stimulation of the subthalamic nucleus on seizures is frequency dependent. Epilepsia. 2003;44(2): 157–64.

81. Chabardes S, et al. Deep brain stimulation in epilepsy with particular reference to the subthalamic nucleus. Epileptic Disord. 2002;4(Suppl 3):S83–93.
82. Evangelista E, et al. Does the thalamo-cortical synchrony play a role in seizure termination? Front Neurol. 2015;6:192.
83. Yamagata Y, Nairn AC. Contrasting features of ERK1/2 activity and synapsin I phosphorylation at the ERK1/2-dependent site in the rat brain in status epilepticus induced by kainic acid in vivo. Brain Res. 2015;1625:314–23.
84. Lee SK, Kim JE, Kim YJ, et al. Hyperforin attenuates microglia activation and inhibits p 65-Ser 276 NFkappaB phosphorylation in the rat piriform cortex following status epilepticus. Neurosci Res. 2014;85:39–50.
85. Oliveira MS, Skinner F, Arshadmansab MF, et al. Altered expression and function of small-conductance (SK) Ca(2+)-activated K+ channels in pilocarpine-treated epileptic rats. Brain Res. 2010;1348:187–99.
86. Wu H, Wang C, Liu B, et al. Altered expression pattern of acid-sensing ion channel isoforms in piriform cortex after seizures. Mol Neurobiol. 2016;53(3):1782–93.
87. Ellerkmann RK, Remy S, Chen J, et al. Molecular and functional changes in voltage-dependent Na(+) channels following pilocarpine-induced status epilepticus in rat dentate granule cells. Neuroscience. 2003;119(2):323–33.
88. Santana-Gomez CE, Alcantara-Gonzalez D, Luna-Munguia H, et al. Transcranial focal electrical stimulation reduces the convulsive expression and amino acid release in the hippocampus during pilocarpine-induced status epilepticus in rats. Epilepsy Behav. 2015;49:33–9.
89. Goodkin HP, Yeh JL, Kapur J. Status epilepticus increases the intracellular accumulation of GABA-A receptors. J Neurosci. 2005;25(23):5511–20.
90. Goodkin HP, Joshi S, Mtchedlishvili Z, et al. Subunit-specific trafficking of GABA (A) receptors during status epilepticus. J Neurosci. 2008;28(10):2527–38.
91. Naylor DE, Liu H, Wasterlain CG. Trafficking of GABA (A) receptors, loss of inhibition, and a mechanism for pharmacoresistance in status epilepticus. J Neurosci. 2005;25(34):7724–33.
92. Naylor DE, Wasterlain CG. GABA synapses and the rapid loss of inhibition to dentate gyrus granule cells after brief perforant-path stimulation. Epilepsia. 2005;46(Suppl 5):142–7.
93. Kapur J, Stringer JL, Lothman EW. Evidence that repetitive seizures in the hippocampus cause a lasting reduction of GABAergic inhibition. J Neurophysiol. 1989;61(2):417–26.
94. Delorenzo RJ, Garnett LK, Towne AR, et al. Comparison of status epilepticus with prolonged seizure episodes lasting from 10 to 29 minutes. Epilepsia. 1999;40(2):164–9.
95. Ure A, Altrup U. Block of spontaneous termination of paroxysmal depolarizations by forskolin (buccal ganglia, Helix pomatia). Neurosci Lett. 2006;392(1–2):10–5.
96. Naylor DE, Liu H, Niquet J, Wasterlain CG. Rapid surface accumulation of NMDA receptors increases glutamatergic excitation during status epilepticus. Neurobiol Dis. 2013;54:225–38.
97. Liu H, Mazarati AM, Katsumori H, et al. Substance P is expressed in hippocampal principal neurons during status epilepticus and plays a critical role in the maintenance of status epilepticus. Proc Natl Acad Sci U S A. 1999;96(9):5286–91.
98. Baraban SC, Hollopeter G, Erickson JC, et al. Knock-out mice reveal a critical antiepileptic role for neuropeptide Y. J Neurosci. 1997;17(23):8927–36.
99. O'Loughlin EK, Pakan JM, Mcdermott KW, et al. Expression of neuropeptide Y1 receptors in the amygdala and hippocampus and anxiety-like behavior associated with Ammon's horn sclerosis following intrahippocampal kainate injection in C57BL/6J mice. Epilepsy Behav. 2014;37:175–83.
100. Elliott RC, Miles MF, Lowenstein DH. Overlapping microarray profiles of dentate gyrus gene expression during development- and epilepsy-associated neurogenesis and axon outgrowth. J Neurosci. 2003;23(6):2218–27.
101. Pulido Fontes L, Quesada Jimenez P, Mendioroz IM. Epigenetics and epilepsy. Neurologia. 2015;30(2):111–8.
102. Miller-Delaney SF, Das S, Sano T, et al. Differential DNA methylation patterns define status epilepticus and epileptic tolerance. J Neurosci. 2012;32(5):1577–88.
103. Reschke CR, Henshall DC. micro RNA and epilepsy. Adv Exp Med Biol. 2015;888:41–70.
104. Fountain NB, Lothman EW. Pathophysiology of status epilepticus. J Clin Neurophysiol. 1995;12(4):326–42.
105. Kim JE, Kim DS, Jin Ryu H, et al. The effect of P2X7 receptor activation on nuclear factor-kappaB phosphorylation induced by status epilepticus in the rat hippocampus. Hippocampus. 2013;23(6):500–14.
106. Ryu HJ, Kim JE, Yeo SI, et al. ReLA/P65-serine 536 nuclear factor-kappa B phosphorylation is related to vulnerability to status epilepticus in the rat hippocampus. Neuroscience. 2011;187:93–102.
107. Lerche H, Shah M, Beck H, et al. Ion channels in genetic and acquired forms of epilepsy. J Physiol. 2013;591(4):753–64.
108. Dey D, Eckle VS, Vitko I, et al. A potassium leak channel silences hyperactive neurons and ameliorates status epilepticus. Epilepsia. 2014;55(2):203–13.
109. Barnwell LF, Lugo JN, Lee WL, et al. Kv4.2 knockout mice demonstrate increased susceptibility to convulsant stimulation. Epilepsia. 2009;50(7):1741–51.
110. Hill MW, Wong M, Amarakone A, et al. Rapid cooling aborts seizure-like activity in rodent hippocampal-entorhinal slices. Epilepsia. 2000;41(10):1241–8.
111. Upreti C, Otero R, Partida C, et al. Altered neurotransmitter release, vesicle recycling and presynaptic structure in the pilocarpine model of temporal lobe epilepsy. Brain. 2012;135(Pt 3):869–85.

112. Szczurowska E, Mareš P. NMDA and AMPA receptors: development and status epilepticus. Physiol Res. 2013;62(Suppl 1):S21–38.
113. Kaminski RM, Fu Z, Venkatesan K, et al. 11-Deoxycortisol impedes GABAergic neurotransmission and induces drug-resistant status epilepticus in mice. Neuropharmacology. 2011;60(7–8):1098–108.
114. Volgushev M, Kudryashov I, Chistiakova M, et al. Probability of transmitter release at neocortical synapses at different temperatures. J Neurophysiol. 2004;92(1):212–20.
115. Motamedi GK, Gonzalez-Sulser A, Dzakpasu R, et al. Cellular mechanisms of desynchronizing effects of hypothermia in an in vitro epilepsy model. Neurotherapeutics. 2012;9(1):199–209.
116. Wasterlain CG, Mazarati AM, Naylor D, et al. Short-term plasticity of hippocampal neuropeptides and neuronal circuitry in experimental status epilepticus. Epilepsia. 2002;43(Suppl 5):20–9.
117. Vadillo FJ, Noya M. Concept, classification and pathophysiology of status epilepticus. Neurologia. 1997;12(Suppl 6):2–9.
118. Grosshans DR, Clayton DA, Coultrap SJ, et al. LTP leads to rapid surface expression of NMDA but not AMPA receptors in adult rat CA1. Nat Neurosci. 2002;5(1):27–33.
119. Kochan LD, Churn SB, Omojokun O, et al. Status epilepticus results in an N-methyl-D-aspartate receptor-dependent inhibition of Ca2+/calmodulin-dependent kinase II activity in the rat. Neuroscience. 2000;95(3):735–43.
120. Gurd JW, Rawof S, Zhen Huo J, et al. Ischemia and status epilepitcus result in enhanced phosphorylation of calcium and calmodulin-stimulated protein kinase II on threonine 253. Brain Res. 2008;1218:158–65.
121. Nair PP, Kalita J, Misra UK. Status epilepticus: why, what, and how. J Postgrad Med. 2011;57(3):242–52.
122. Abend NS, Loddenkemper T. Pediatric status epilepticus management. Curr Opin Pediatr. 2014;26(6):668–74.
123. Kapur J, Coulter DA. Experimental status epilepticus alters gamma-aminobutyric acid type A receptor function in CA1 pyramidal neurons. Ann Neurol. 1995;38(6):893–900.
124. Cash SS. Status epilepticus as a system disturbance: is status epilepticus due to synchronization or desynchronization? Epilepsia. 2013;54(Suppl 6):37–9.
125. Schindler K, Elger CE, Lehnertz K. Increasing synchronization may promote seizure termination: evidence from status epilepticus. Clin Neurophysiol. 2007;118(9):1955–68.
126. Mazarati AM, Baldwin RA, Sankar R, et al. Time-dependent decrease in the effectiveness of antiepileptic drugs during the course of self-sustaining status epilepticus. Brain Res. 1998;814(1–2):179–85.
127. Mazarati AM, Wasterlain CG. N-methyl-D-asparate receptor antagonists abolish the maintenance phase of self-sustaining status epilepticus in rat. Neurosci Lett. 1999;265(3):187–90.
128. Hocker S, Tatum WO, Laroche S, et al. Refractory and super-refractory status epilepticus—an update. Curr Neurol Neurosci Rep. 2014;14(6):452.
129. Abend NS, Bearden D, Helbig I, et al. Status epilepticus and refractory status epilepticus management. Semin Pediatr Neurol. 2014;21(4):263–74.
130. Reddy DS, Kuruba R. Experimental models of status epilepticus and neuronal injury for evaluation of therapeutic interventions. Int J Mol Sci. 2013;14(9):18284–318.
131. Goodkin HP, Sun C, Yeh JL, et al. GABA(A) receptor internalization during seizures. Epilepsia. 2007;48(Suppl 5):109–13.
132. Kapur J, Macdonald RL. Rapid seizure-induced reduction of benzodiazepine and Zn2+ sensitivity of hippocampal dentate granule cell GABA-A receptors. J Neurosci. 1997;17(19):7532–40.
133. Rajasekaran K, Joshi S, Kozhemyakin M, et al. Receptor trafficking hypothesis revisited: plasticity of AMPA receptors during established status epilepticus. Epilepsia. 2013;54(Suppl 6):14–6.
134. Prasad A, Worrall BB, Bertram EH, et al. Propofol and midazolam in the treatment of refractory status epilepticus. Epilepsia. 2001;42(3):380–6.
135. Kofke WA, Young RS, Davis P, et al. Isoflurane for refractory status epilepticus: a clinical series. Anesthesiology. 1989;71(5):653–9.
136. Mazarati AM, Wasterlain CG, Sankar R, et al. Self-sustaining status epilepticus after brief electrical stimulation of the perforant path. Brain Res. 1998;801(1–2):251–3.
137. Sloviter RS. Decreased hippocampal inhibition and a selective loss of interneurons in experimental epilepsy. Science. 1987;235(4784):73–6.
138. Meldrum BS, Horton RW. Physiology of status epilepticus in primates. Arch Neurol. 1973;28(1):1–9.
139. Pitkanen A, Lukasiuk K. Mechanisms of epileptogenesis and potential treatment targets. Lancet Neurol. 2011;10(2):173–86.
140. Brown GC. Nitric oxide and neuronal death. Nitric Oxide. 2010;23(3):153–65.
141. Pollard H, Charriaut-Marlangue C, Cantagrel S, et al. Kainate-induced apoptotic cell death in hippocampal neurons. Neuroscience. 1994;63(1):7–18.
142. Tian R, She Y, Jia Y, et al. Effect of pingxian granules on protein expression of apoptosis regulatory genes in hippocampus of pentylenetetrazol-induced epileptic model rats. China J Chin Mater Med. 2012;37(9):1307–10.
143. Corsellis JA, Bruton CJ. Neuropathology of status epilepticus in humans. Adv Neurol. 1983;34:129–39.
144. Degiorgio CM, Heck CN, Rabinowicz AL, et al. Serum neuron-specific enolase in the major subtypes of status epilepticus. Neurology. 1999;52(4):746–9.
145. Cock HR, Tong X, Hargreaves IP, et al. Mitochondrial dysfunction associated with neuronal death following status epilepticus in rat. Epilepsy Res. 2002;48(3):157–68.
146. Lazeyras F, Blanke O, Zimine I, et al. MRI, (1) H-MRS, and functional MRI during and after

prolonged nonconvulsive seizure activity. Neurology. 2000;55(11):1677–82.
147. Morimoto T, Fukuda M, Suzuki Y, et al. Sequential changes of brain CT and MRI after febrile status epilepticus in a 6-year-old girl. Brain Dev. 2002;24(3):190–3.
148. Nixon J, Bateman D, Moss T. An MRI and neuropathological study of a case of fatal status epilepticus. Seizure. 2001;10(8):588–91.
149. Cendes F, Andermann F, Carpenter S, et al. Temporal lobe epilepsy caused by domoic acid intoxication: evidence for glutamate receptor-mediated excitotoxicity in humans. Ann Neurol. 1995;37(1):123–6.
150. Wasterlain CG. Inhibition of cerebral protein synthesis by epileptic seizures without motor manifestations. Neurology. 1974;24(2):175–80.
151. Mazarati A, Liu H, Wasterlain C. Opioid peptide pharmacology and immunocytochemistry in an animal model of self-sustaining status epilepticus. Neuroscience. 1999;89(1):167–73.
152. Sperk G, Marksteiner J, Gruber B, et al. Functional changes in neuropeptide Y- and somatostatin-containing neurons induced by limbic seizures in the rat. Neuroscience. 1992;50(4):831–46.
153. Mazarati AM, Liu H, Soomets U, et al. Galanin modulation of seizures and seizure modulation of hippocampal galanin in animal models of status epilepticus. J Neurosci. 1998;18(23):10070–7.
154. Mazarati A, Wasterlain CG. Anticonvulsant effects of four neuropeptides in the rat hippocampus during self-sustaining status epilepticus. Neurosci Lett. 2002;331(2):123–7.
155. Mazarati A, Lu X, Shinmei S, et al. Patterns of seizures, hippocampal injury and neurogenesis in three models of status epilepticus in galanin receptor type 1 (GalR1) knockout mice. Neuroscience. 2004;128(2):431–41.
156. Erickson JC, Clegg KE, Palmiter RD. Sensitivity to leptin and susceptibility to seizures of mice lacking neuropeptide Y. Nature. 1996;381(6581):415–21.
157. Silva AP, Lourenco J, Xapelli S, et al. Protein kinase C activity blocks neuropeptide Y-mediated inhibition of glutamate release and contributes to excitability of the hippocampus in status epilepticus. FASEB J. 2007;21(3):671–81.
158. Loscher W. Mechanisms of drug resistance in status epilepticus. Epilepsia. 2007;48(Suppl 8):74–7.
159. Liu H, Sankar R, Shin DH, et al. Patterns of status epilepticus-induced substance P expression during development. Neuroscience. 2000;101(2):297–304.
160. Marchi N, Granata T, Freri E, et al. Efficacy of anti-inflammatory therapy in a model of acute seizures and in a population of pediatric drug resistant epileptics. PLoS One. 2011;6(3):e18200.
161. Friedman A, Dingledine R. Molecular cascades that mediate the influence of inflammation on epilepsy. Epilepsia. 2011;52(Suppl 3):33–9.
162. Juhasz C, Buth A, Chugani DC, et al. Successful surgical treatment of an inflammatory lesion associated with new-onset refractory status epilepticus. Neurosurg Focus. 2013;34(6):E5.
163. Barnes G, Puranam RS, Luo Y, et al. Temporal specific patterns of semaphorin gene expression in rat brain after kainic acid-induced status epilepticus. Hippocampus. 2003;13(1):1–20.

Brain Damage Caused by Status Epilepticus

3

Zhen Hong

Abstract

In this chapter, we describe the results of clinical studies and animal model experiments aimed at exploring brain damage induced by status epilepticus (SE). Evidence from autopsies has indicated that epileptic brains exhibit morphological abnormalities, including neuronal injury, glial activation, disruption of the blood-brain barrier (BBB), mossy fiber sprouting, and vascular injury. Many affected individuals also exhibit behavioral abnormalities. The molecular mechanisms and related signaling pathways that potentially underlie SE-induced brain damage are also discussed. Several hypotheses have been proposed to explain these effects of SE. These include but are not limited to an imbalance between the excitatory and inhibitory transition systems, disturbances in brain metabolism and inflammation, dysfunction of the mTOR pathway, and the regulation of the renin-angiotensin system (RAS). These detailed investigations will accelerate the development of promising strategies to treat SE in the future.

3.1 Introduction

Status epilepticus (SE) becomes a life-threatening neurological emergency if treatment at the neurological unit is delayed. SE usually leads to long-term, significant, complex, and extensive brain damage that includes neuronal death, nerve damage, and other changes in neuronal networks. The severity of damage depends on several factors, including the type, intensity, duration of attack and the age of patient. SE has a sustained onset that alters GABAergic neuron-based inhibitory systems and other neurochemical synaptic transmission. Here, a number of studies aimed at clarifying mechanism underlying these changes and exploring target-specific drugs to improve the prognosis of SE.

Z. Hong
Department of Neurology, Huashan Hospital, Fudan University, 12 Wulumuqi Zhong Road, Shanghai 200040, China
e-mail: hongzhen@medmail.com.cn

X. Wang, S. Li (eds.), *Refractory Status Epilepticus*, DOI 10.1007/978-981-10-5125-8_3

3.2 Clinical Evidence and the Chronology of Brain Damage During and After SE

As early as 1825, Bouchet provided an autopsy report that described 18 epileptic cases in which 8 of the patients exhibited hippocampal injury and 4 experienced cerebellar softening. In 1880, Sommer and Pfleger firstly described the pathological changes observed in the autopsy epileptic brain, especially damage to the hippocampus and limbic system in detail. Their study marked an important milestone in the history of epilepsy, and the results have been broadly confirmed lately. They identified hippocampal sclerosis as the pathological hallmarks of refractory temporal lobe epilepsy (TLE).This type of neuropathological damage includes segmental loss of pyramidal neurons, granule cell dispersion, and gliosis. These changes were thought to result from epileptic seizure which has a significant effect on the mortality and morbidity, and the neuronal loss was attributed to disturbances in local metabolism and circulation caused by seizures [1].

In 1966, Margerison and Corsellis [2] found that in 55 autopsies performed in patients with epilepsy, approximately 70% exhibited hippocampal CA1 neuronal loss and gliosis. It was reported that in patients with SE, there was significant acute neural damage in the CA1 area, thalamus, the corpus callosum, and cerebellar Purkinje cells. They defined two types of hippocampal damage. The first was "classical" Ammon's horn sclerosis, which was described previously, and the second was neuronal loss confined in the hilus of the dentate gyrus, which is termed "end folium sclerosis."

In 1992, DeGiorgio [3] and his colleagues found that typical pyramidal neuronal necrosis and loss were observed in the hippocampal CA1 and CA3 areas in patients who died suddenly from generalized clonic status epilepticus, and these patients exhibited progressive hippocampal atrophy and sclerosis in addition to clear damage in the temporal lobe area on imaging.

In 1997, Meierkord [4] showed that on MRI, patients with SE exhibited a significant increase in T2 signaling that was associated with seizure-induced cytotoxicity and vasogenic edema. This result was subsequently confirmed by Kim [5]. In 8 patients with SE, MRI showed that signal intensity and swelling in the cortical gray matter, subcortical white matter, or hippocampus on periictal T2-weighted and diffusion-weighted images transiently increased.

In 1999, Oe [6] reported that at 10 months after SE, a patient showed gradual hemiplegia and mental retardation. MRI of this patient revealed high signals in T2-weighted images that were indicative of lesions representing atrophy in the cortex, white matter, caudate nucleus, and hippocampus. SPECT imaging showed the presence of reduced blood flow lesions, which may be related with cytotoxic injury and vascular edema caused by SE.

In 2003, Fujikawa [7] demonstrated that 3 post-mortem patients with NCSE who had no history of seizures exhibited cell death in the hippocampus, amygdala, piriform cortex, dorsomedial nucleus, and cerebellum. These neuronal cell deaths were mainly distributed in the glutamate receptor-dense region of the limbic system, suggesting that excitotoxic injury may be involved in brain injury mechanisms caused by SE.

3.3 Animal Experimental Evidence of Brain Damage During and After SE

In addition to autopsies in patients who died from SE, studies of brain damage in SE have principally involved the use of animal experiments which focused on several characteristics of the central nervous system, as described below.

3.3.1 Injury Sites

As early as 1994, J. M. Petras [8] described a mechanism by which SE could induce extensive brain damage in the piriform cortex, striatum, fornix fibers, hypothalamic cortical projection fibers, and spinal cord. These findings were confirmed in MRI studies later. Catherine Roch [9] found that at 2 days after pilocarpine-induced SE, the T2 relaxation time was significantly increased in the ventral and dorsal hippocampus, amygdala, thalamus, entorhinal cortex, and piriform cortex. Moreover, the change in hippocampal volume was consistent with the change in the T2 signal. In the chronic phase following SE, open-field tests confirmed that the T2 relaxation time in the amygdala was closely related with locomotor activity, suggesting that the T2 signal in the amygdala may be an early imaging marker of epileptogenesis. Nevertheless, quantitative MRI analysis revealed that a high T2 signal in the parietal cortex and hypothalamus on day 2 after SE was strongly linked with animal mortality [10, 11]. Interestingly, using a 2.35-T MRI system, Choy [12] found that T2 signal in the parietal cortex increased only during the very early stages of SE, restabilized after 2 days, and exhibited no further changes.

3.3.2 Neuronal Damage

3.3.2.1 Neuronal Loss

In pilocarpine or kainic acid-induced SE, silver staining showed prominent neuronal loss in the amygdala, hippocampal CA1 and CA3 areas, entorhinal cortex, and hypothalamus that was closely associated with the duration of epileptic seizures [13]. At 24 h after SE induced by an intra-hippocampal injection of pilocarpine, Fluoro-Jade staining revealed the neurodegeneration in the hilus and CA3 and CA1 pyramidal cell subfields [14]. In pentylenetetrazole (PTZ)-induced SE, the same reduction in neurons was observed at 24 h after SE and maintained for 10 weeks [15].

3.3.2.2 Influencing Factors

Many factors have been implicated in the neuronal loss in the hippocampus following SE. (1) Latency and methods of injection: In a kainic acid (KA)-induced SE model, latency period was different between animals administered intraperitoneal and tail-vein injections. Intraperitoneal injections provoked long-latency SE and induced the increased expression of caspase-generated markers, whereas tail-vein injections resulted in short-latency SE and predominantly necrotic cell death. To some extent, these data indicated that latency to the onset of SE determined the apoptotic or necrotic mechanisms following SE [16]. (2) Spontaneous recurrent seizures (SRSs): Animals exhibited latency after SE. In addition, SRSs, including secondary generalized tonic-clonic seizures, occurred in most animals [17]. Neuronal loss in the hippocampus was usually involved with the occurrence of SRSs. In the pilocarpine-induced SE model, significant neuronal loss was observed in the dentate gyrus and the CA1 and CA3 regions of the hippocampus. Animals that exhibited a greater degree of cell loss in the CA3 region of the hippocampus had a later onset of chronic epilepsy [18]. (3) Neurogenesis: The role of neurogenesis in SE is complex and controversial. In SE, neurogenesis may be a mechanism that contributes to self-repair after injury. However, the recombination of neural network during the process of self-repair may result in neuronal over-excitation and thereby promote epileptogenesis. The data suggested that SE could induce axon sprouting in the hippocampus, especially in the intramolecular layer which takes part in the generation of SRS. In the pilocarpine and KA-induced SE model, granule cells proliferated with long dendrites, more dendritic spines were observed in the dentate gyrus, a small number of neuronal cell bodies were large, and there was a reduction in the number of newborn neuronal dendritic spines rather than regular neurons. Moreover, approximately 14% of proliferating cells differentiated into inhibitory GABA energy basket cells [19]. These evidences suggested that neurogenesis may play a neuroprotective role in the early stage of SE. Nevertheless, these generated neurons may promote the development of chronic epilepsy after SE.

3.3.3 Glial Cell Injury

SE induces the abnormal activation of glial cells, and activated glial cells play an extensive and complex role following SE. On the one hand, activated astrocytes release a variety of pro-inflammatory cytokines, including IL-1β and TNF-α, which increase neuronal excitability, leading to neuronal loss [20, 21]. On the other hand, glutathione is synthesized mainly by astrocytes. During the early stages of SE, glutathione levels significantly increase and then gradually decrease. However, there is no clear relationship between the synthesis of glutathione in hippocampal astrocytes, neuronal loss, and frequency of SRS in chronic stage during epileptogenesis. To a certain extent, the EPO produced by astrocytes may serve as neuroprotective factors in SE by delaying neuronal cell death [22].

In addition, microglial cells are the prominent mediators for phagocytic cell activities in CNS. Here, activated microglia has been shown to induce inflammatory response, which could play a key role in a variety of encephalopathies. There is a study demonstrated the changes of somatostatin receptor (SSTR) in the hippocampus of pilocarpine-induced SE model. SSTR2B and SSTR4 immunoreactivity were significantly increased in microglial cells after epilepsy, and the expression of SSTR was unregulated evidently in the hippocampal microglial cells. Increased expression levels of SSTR in neurons and glia may due to the enhanced inhibition of the dentate gyrus and the regulation of reactive microgliosis in the hippocampus [23].

However, another study found that the level of PLPP/CIN protein was significantly upregulated in astrocytes and granule cells. High levels of PLPP/CIN protein participate in the regulation of acid detergent fibers (ADFs) and F-actin, leading to excitability and pulse suppression. These results indicate that the loss of astrocytes during SE may partly result from a synergistic effect involving PLPP/CIN-mediated actin kinetics [24].

3.3.4 Blood-Brain Barrier Injury

The main function of the BBB is to maintain the stability of the brain environment, to participate in regulation in cerebral blood flow and material transport, and to protect the brain from inflammatory factors and other macromolecular damage. Disruption of BBB leads to increased excitability in the brain. It is a chronic process that involves in increased interstitial protein concentrations, the activation of astrocytes, and an imbalance in K^+ and Ca^{2+} homeostasis [25]. In the early stage of epileptic seizure, there is substantial albumin extravasation by astrocytes and neurons after SE [26], suggesting that the BBB was impaired during epileptic seizures. This result was confirmed in electrical stimulation-induced SE animal models. During the chronic period after an epileptic seizure, the degree of BBB structural damage was positively correlated with the frequency of SRS. Moreover, artificially opening the BBB during the chronic epileptic phase induced a persistent increase in the number of seizures in a majority of epileptic rats. These findings indicate that BBB leakage occurs during epileptogenesis and the chronic epileptic phase, suggesting that dysfunction of BBB contributes to the progression of epilepsy. After 1–2 days of SE, albumin had begun to exude from the piriform cortex, entorhinal cortex, hippocampus, hypothalamus, striatum, and olfactory bulb, and this change in BBB permeability was sustained for 1 week after the initiation of SE. These data suggest that the structural integrity of BBB plays a crucial role in SE-induced brain injury.

In addition, the destruction of BBB structural integrity in SE leads to changes in the local blood pressure, the formation of oxidative-free radicals, the immune response, and the loss of tight junction proteins.

3.3.5 Mossy Fiber Sprouting (MFS)

MFS is one of the most important morphological features of hippocampal plasticity in temporal lobe epilepsy. It was observed in several SE animal models, including kainic acid model [27], pilocarpine models [28, 29], and the kindling model [24]. Sprouted mossy fibers diffuse longitudinally along the hippocampus, which increases longitudinal linking of their lamellae. There is no clear evidence of the relationship between mossy fibroblast sprouting and the severity of SRS during the chronic phase. But in SRS phase, mossy fibroblast buds exhibit abnormal excitatory associations between granule cells and increased susceptibility to seizure. Studies have shown that the intra-cerebroventricular injection of nerve growth factor (NGF) accelerates the processes underlying the epileptic kindling model, increases mossy fiber sprouting in the molecular layer of the CA3 region, and protects against SE after hippocampal neuronal loss. These data suggest that MFS may be a direct consequence of SE rather than a compensatory response to neuronal death. Data support the notion that seizure-induced MFS can be primarily attributed to the combined effects of neuronal activation and the activation-induced upregulation of growth factors [30]. However, more studies are needed to determine whether MFS is a common cause of SE seizures and neuronal loss [31]. It has been speculated that in granule cells, MFS not only establishes an excitatory loop but also restores excitability in inhibitory interneuron afferents during SE. Moreover, the increased inhibition of granule cells enables the brain to restore itself to the homeostasis after injury [32].

3.3.6 Brain Function and Cognitive Behavioral Injury

In epileptic animal models, SE leads to a short-term decrease in activities which is accompanied by impaired learning and memory. In amygdala-kindled SE animal model, electrical stimulation resulted in impaired spatial cognitive ability (Morris water maze test) in adult epileptic animals. The pilocarpine-induced SE model mimicked the behavioral and cognitive impairments which was directly observed in SE patients [33]. Additionally, in open-field tests, SE rats exhibited a significant increase in excessive activity and decrease in behavioral habituation, suggesting that their spatial exploratory and spatial cognition abilities were impaired [10, 34]. In PTZ-induced SE rats, T-maze and open-field tests showed that the number of fecal boli increased, and one-way escape latency was long after SE, implying the emotional memory, learning, and behaviors were impaired which are related to unconditional fear. However, the abnormalities were not persistent [35].

3.3.7 Vascular Injury

One study about lithium-pilocarpine-induced SE model found that in the hippocampus, certain treatment resulted in a significant reduction in SRS. This effect was mediated by an increase in the transcription of hypoxia stress factor 1α (hypoxia-inducible factor-1α, HIF- 1α) after seizure and the regulation of the expression of erythropoietin and vascular endothelial growth factor (VEGF). They also found that at 7 days after the termination of SE, recombinant human erythropoietin (rhEPO) significantly decreased BBB leakage, neuronal death, and microglial activation in the dentate hilus and in the CA1 and CA3 subfields and inhibited the generation of ectopic granule cells in the hilus [36]. VEGF is the key signal molecule that promotes angiogenesis. It not only changes the permeability of BBB but also increases the infiltration of monocytes into the brain parenchyma. These effects directly or indirectly regulate the excitability and plasticity of neurons. The expression of VEGF rapidly increased during the early stages of SE, and this effect lasted through the chronic stages of epileptogenesis.

In addition, activated TrkB significantly promoted epileptogenesis, and the frequency of SE induced by chemoconvulsant was significantly reduced in TrkB knockout mice. Interestingly, in post-SE model, sustained selective inhibition of TrkB for 2 weeks using a chemical-genetic method significantly reduced both the frequency of SRS and hippocampal neuronal loss during the chronic stages of epileptogenesis and alleviated anxiety in the mice [37]. These data suggested that the BDNF-TrkB signaling pathway is involved in the mechanism underlying SE-induced neuronal injury.

3.3.8 Others

Tau protein, phosphorylated microtubule-associated protein is abundant in neurons, which stabilize microtubules in the CNS. High concentration of total tau and phosphorylated tau in the cerebrospinal fluid is likely to indicate axonal and neuronal damage. Currently, Tau protein is used as a core biomarker for AD diagnosis in clinical trials [38]. An analysis of cerebrospinal fluid in 20 patients with SE showed that in 14 of the patients, levels of tau protein were evidently increased and 6 patients have high levels of CSF phosphorylated-tau protein. Moreover, levels of total-tau protein in the CSF were significantly higher in patients who developed to refractory SE in comparison to patients with drug-controlled seizure. Patients were inclining to develop to chronic epilepsy when the CSF total-tau level is high. These results suggest that CSF total-tau values were positively correlated with the duration of SE, and it may therefore serve as a clinical biomarker for assessing the severity and prognosis of SE [39].

3.4 Brain Damage Mechanisms During and After SE

The pathophysiology of SE remains poorly understood. The pathogenic mechanisms underlying SE-induced brain damage are investigated primarily using animal models, which induced by chemoconvulsion (e.g., pilocarpine with or without lithium or using kainic acid) and electrical stimulation, as well as organotypic slice culture. However, animal models used currently rarely replicate the characteristics of NCSE. It is of importance that numerous molecular and cellular pathways should be paid attention when studying the initiation, maintenance, and development of SE.

Several studies have confirmed that in SE, phosphorylation of protein occurs during "on-off" changes of ion channel, and neurotransmitters are released over a very short period of time and then followed by synaptic receptor trafficking. This process includes an increase in excitatory synaptic receptors and a decrease in inhibitory transmission. During the first week after the onset of SE, a large number of neurons are lost in the hippocampus and other fields of limbic system. The structural destruction of the BBB results in vasogenic edema [40, 41], glial activation, and inflammatory response [42]. It manifested that a series of pathological changes occur during the early stages of SE and promote epileptogenesis.

3.4.1 Metabolic Disturbance

In SE, both energy consumption and glucose utilization are significantly increased, and the oxygen demands of the brain consequently outstrip the supply [43]. Under physiological conditions, the cerebrovascular system is self-regulatory, and cerebral blood flow therefore does not fluctuate with significant changes in blood pressure. During the early stage, SE interrupts this self-regulation. In SE, there is initially a sharp increase in arterial blood pressure. It produces a significant increase in cerebral blood flow, which aimed at bringing more oxygen and glucose to the brain to compensate for its excessive oxygen demand. However, as SE developed, lactic acidosis and a lack of sensitivity in peripheral blood vessels to plasma catecholamine induce continuous decline in blood pressure that ultimately results in ischemia and hypoxia in the brain, leading to damage including neuronal necrosis and glial activation.

3.4.1.1 Mitochondria

Mitochondria are the "power stations" of most cells, and their functions include supplying energy to cells, maintaining calcium homeostasis, generating reactive oxygen species (ROS), and regulating apoptotic cells. In the brain, mitochondria are mainly responsible for supplying ATP and regulating ROS signaling pathways and Ca^{2+} concentration in the synapse. Within a few hours to several days following the onset of SE, mitochondrial dysfunction induces the activation of caspase, which results in programmed cell death (including apoptosis, pyroptosis, and necroptosis), leading directly to brain damage.

In brain slices, SE was induced by perfusing Mg^{2+}-free medium. This caused the supply of NADH to neurons to be inconsistent with cellular electrical activity and the generation of free radicals, resulting in neuronal death in the hippocampus. In vivo, it has been suggested that a large amount of ROS is produced during chronic epileptic seizures and SE, leading to neuronal death [44]. NADPH oxidase is the main ROS component generated during this pathophysiology. AEBSF, an NADPH inhibitor, significantly reduced cell death. Furthermore, ROS produced by NADPH contributes to seizure-induced cell death, which is accompanied by the release of glutamate and the activation of NMDA receptors [45]. NADPH is the main source of superoxide production following NMDA receptor activation [46], but the relationship between ROS production and mitochondria in SE remains unclear. Recently, a number of studies suggested that mitochondrial dysfunction-induced brain injury played an important role in SE and might affect the activation of the excitatory neurotransmitter system, which consequently induced epileptogenesis in the CNS.

3.4.1.2 Endoplasmic Reticulum

The endoplasmic reticulum (ER) is an organelle that is important in protein synthesis and directly contributes to cell survival by correctly folding and classifying proteins. When calcium homeostasis is disturbed, unfolded proteins aggregate, and this can cause the ER to experience stress (characterized by eNOS activation), potentially resulting in its destruction [47]. In SE, ER stress-induced brain injury may be mediated by the PERK-Eif2α-CHOP signal transduction pathway [48]. In a pilocarpine-induced SE model, SE-induced eNOS activation induces BBB disruption through the upregulation of GRP78 expression in piriform cortex [49]. These finding suggested that modulating ER stress may be a potential therapeutic strategy for impaired endothelial cell function resulting from vasogenic edema during SE.

3.4.2 Neurotransmission-Induced Brain Damage During and After SE

3.4.2.1 Reduced GABAergic Neurotransmission During and After SE

GABA is the most important inhibitory transmitter in the CNS. Benzodiazepines are first-line drugs used to control SE, and they mainly affect GABAA receptors (GABAARs), which themselves play central roles in inhibitory neurotransmission in the forebrain [50]. Recently, extensive studies have linked SE to GABA receptors. In the hippocampus, GABAR-mediated inhibition is decreased during SE. The imbalance between excitatory and inhibitory transmission plays an important role in epileptogenesis after SE.

In SE animal models, it has been shown that GABA receptor-mediated neuroprotection effects are significantly attenuated in the hippocampus. In hippocampal slices obtained from animals undergoing prolonged SE, the amplitudes of the mIPSCs in the pyramidal neurons of DGCs and CA1 were significantly lower than controls at 30–60 min after SE [51–53]. The amplitude of mIPSCs decreased prior to the forelimb convulsions in SE animals. Besides, the frequency of mIPSC was similarly reduced, suggesting that GABA receptor-induced currents reacted rapidly upon SE initiation and it may be due to the reduction of cell membrane expression of GABAA receptor subunits. Similar results have also been reported in cultured primary hippocampal neurons. These findings indicated that GABA receptor-mediated synaptic inhibition was reduced during the very early stage of SE.

Although changes were observed in GABA receptor-mediated currents and the magnitude of mIPSCs is known to be closely linked with the number of receptors in the synapse, the mechanism underlying the trafficking of surface receptors during SE should be further clarified. Data from biotinylation assays have implied that in the hippocampus, the distributions of GABA receptor subunits, including the γ2, β2/3, and α1 subunits, are significantly reduced in SE model. Alterations of these subunits may result from regulation of the receptors at the transcription or translation level or the abnormal transport of receptors. The rapid response of GABA receptor subunits indicated that the differential modulation of the surface expression of GABA receptors might play a central role in the brain damage caused by SE.

Culturing primary neurons on glass coverslips with Mg^{2+}-free or high-potassium buffer induces SE-like burst discharges. During this process, the endocytosis of γ2 and β2/3 subunits was significantly increased [54], but there was no change in the δ subunit. These changes may have resulted from the depolarization of neurons, the activation of NMDA receptors, or the ligand binding. Moreover, endocytosis of the GABA receptor reduces the expression of GABA receptors on the cell membrane. Nevertheless, it remains unclear whether the assembly of GABA receptors and their anchorages on the cell membrane are also affected.

In addition, the phosphorylation and dephosphorylation of GABA receptors determines the stability and trafficking of GABA receptors on the cell membrane, which in turn affects the expression of GABA receptors on cells. When the ionotropic NMDA receptor is activated, the resulting influx of Ca^{2+} activates the second messenger protein kinase C (PKC) and calcineurin, which regulates GABA receptor phosphorylation [55, 56]. The expression of PKCα, PKCβ, and PKCγ were significantly reduced, and the phosphorylation of the β3 subunit was greatly downregulated in SE animal model. Zn^{2+} is an allosteric regulatory factor of the GABAA receptor in hippocampal dentate granule cells. In whole-cell patch clamp, GABA receptor currents from hippocampal dentate granule cells were acutely altered in rats undergoing SE.

Additionally, GABA receptor-induced currents were less sensitive to diazepam, and Zn^{2+} retained their sensitivity to GABA and pentobarbital [57]. It concluded that prolonged SE rapidly mediated the plasticity of GABAA receptors in hippocampal dentate granule cell.

3.4.2.2 Excitatory Neurotransmission

Glutamate is the most important excitatory neurotransmitter in the CNS and plays important roles in synaptic plasticity, neurogenesis, and neurodegeneration. There are two classes of glutamate receptors, including ionotropic receptors and metabotropic receptors. The ionotropic receptors form the ion channel pore opens when glutamate binds to its receptor. These receptors are divided into NMDA receptors, KA receptors, and AMPA receptors according to their selective agonist. Metabolic receptors are divided into many types, including mGluR1-8, which primarily couple with G proteins and function via intracellular secondary messenger systems, such as PLC (phosphatase C) and AC (adenylate cyclase).

A large body of evidence confirms that NMDA receptors and AMPA receptors are involved in generating and maintaining SE [58, 59]. The excessive activation of NMDA receptors results in increased neuronal damage and apoptosis during SE and modulates SE-associated epileptogenesis. NMDA receptor antagonists significantly decrease excitotoxicity-induced neuronal damage in CA1 and CA3 areas, as well as the mossy fiber sprouting in KA-induced SE model. In vitro, repeatedly stimulating glutamatergic neuronal transmission pathways leads to cell death and sustained epileptiform activity in SE brain slices.

In organotypic hippocampal slice cultures, SE was associated with an increase in the surface expression of NR1-containing NMDAR, and an increase of NMDA synaptic and extrasynaptic currents indicated functional NMDA receptor accumulation to the cell surface in dentate granule cells. This coincides with the internalization of synaptic GABAA receptors [60]. NMDA receptors were recruited to the postsynaptic membranes of granule cells in the DG and to pyramidal neurons in the CA3 area at 1 h after the induction of pilocarpine-induced SE. An NMDA-mEPSC variance analysis suggested that NMDA receptors in the cell membrane were increased by approximately 38% during SE. In this study, SE-induced neuronal death was found to be dependent on extracellular Ca^{2+} entry that entered primarily through the NMDA receptor channel subtype [61]. Moreover, activated astrocytes mediated the release of glutamate, resulted in the induction of slow inward currents in neurons. These currents are essential for neuronal synchronization and the triggering of action potentials (APs).

GluA2-containing AMPAR is not permeable to Ca^{2+}. Rajasekaran and colleagues showed that in acute isolated hippocampal slices, at 10 and 60 min after SE induction, there was a significant reduction in the GluA2 subunit, and AMPA receptors in CA1 of the hippocampus exhibited inwardly rectifying currents. These effects were also observed in the dentate gyrus region at 10 min, but not 60 min after SE. These finding suggest that AMPA receptor blockade may be a possible anticonvulsant alternative for SE [62].

In addition, these results suggest that glutamatergic neuronal excitability and excitotoxic effects play important roles in initiation and maintenance of SE. It could be proposed that inactivation of the GABAA receptor initiates SE, whereas rapid surface accumulation of NMDA receptors promotes an abnormal increase in excitotoxicity during SE, thereby contributing to chronic epileptic seizure [51, 52, 63].

3.4.3 Inflammation

3.4.3.1 ATP Pathway

In the central and peripheral nervous system, ATP is released in an activity-dependent manner from different cell types and plays different roles as either a neurotransmitter or a neuromodulator in astrocyte-to-neuron communication to propagate astrocytic responses and regulate microglial responses [64]. Under normal physiological conditions, the extracellular concentration of ATP is very low. The over-excitement of neurons acts as a "danger signal," causing concentration of extracellular ATP increased and ATP-gated purinergic receptor (P2) activation in the CNS.

In KA- and pilocarpine-induced SE models, P2X7R receptors were significantly increased at both the transcription and translation level on the hippocampal microglia but not astrocytes and oligodendrocytes [65, 66]. P2X7R receptor activation is an essential step in microglial activation and proliferation. P2X7R may affect neuronal cell death by regulating the release of the pro-inflammatory cytokine interleukin-1beta (IL-1β) [67, 68]. Moreover, the P2X7R inhibitor A-438079 produced an anticonvulsant effect during SE. It not only reduced electrographic and seizure severity during SE but also seizure-induced neuronal death in the neocortex and hippocampus [69]. During ATP signaling, adenosine, a product of the breakdown of ATP, plays an important role in terminating epileptic seizures [70].

3.4.3.2 Interleukin-1β Pathway

The interleukin-1β/Toll-like receptor pathway indirectly regulates NMDA receptors in epileptic seizures. VX-765 is an inhibitor of IL-converting enzyme, which induces a potent anti-inflammatory effect. In kainic acid-induced SE rats, VX-765 inhibited seizure-induced secretion of IL1β from astrocytes in organotypic slices and led to delay of seizure initiation and 50% reduction of seizure duration [71]. These data indicated that interleukin-activated IL1β/Toll-like receptor pathway was closely associated with SE.

Furthermore, the mechanism underlying IL1β participates in SE including activation of neuronal sphingomyelinase and Src kinase which induced by IL1β, as well as the phosphorylation of NR2B and NMDA receptor-induced Ca^{2+} influx.

3.4.3.3 COX2

In both KA- and pilocarpine-induced SE models, COX2 expression was significantly unregulated. COX2 is involved in a variety of neuroinflammatory pathways, including the activation of microglia. The upregulation of COX2 is closely associated with the regulation of apoptosis in excitotoxicity-induced injuries. Cultured microglial treated with EP2 (PGE2) subtype antagonist showed neuroprotective effects. These small molecular compounds could permeate BBB and significantly inhibit the upregulation of COX2 mRNA. In SE animal model, administration of COX2 inhibitor after SE significantly increased the survival rate of hippocampal neurons and reduced the duration of SRS for 28–42 days. It has been showed that COX2-selective inhibitors significantly increase the risk of cardiovascular disease. It proposed that combination of anti-inflammatory factors and COX-2 and IL-1β inhibitors may be an effective strategy to treat SE in the future.

Furthermore, IL-18 was predominantly expressed in the endothelial cells and astrocytes of injured neurovascular units, and IL-18 levels in the piriform cortex, the hippocampus, and the hypothalamus were significantly increased in SE animal models [72]. However, the inflammatory response initiated by epilepsy is strongly influenced by the age of the animal.

3.4.4 The Mammalian Target of Rapamycin (mTOR) Pathway

mTOR, an atypical serine/threonine protein kinase, is a member of the phosphatidylinositol kinase-related kinase (PIKK) protein family. mTOR is evolutionarily conserved and involves in many aspects of cellular proliferation and growth, including gene transcription, protein translation, ribosome synthesis, apoptosis, neurite growth, and synaptic plasticity. Over-activation of the mTOR pathway is involved in the over-excitability of neurons and also plays a critical role in the development, migration, and function of GABAergic neurons. In pilocarpine-induced SE, rapamycin was shown to reduce axon sprouting by increasing the survival of somatostatin-positive interneuron [73]. Moreover, BDNF-mediated stimulation of neurons led to an increase in the levels of mTOR pathway-mediated mRNAs, including LIMK-1, eNOS, Pyk2, Homer2, GluR1, NR1/3, and DLG2 [74].

3.4.5 Others

It has been reported that angiotensin (AT1) receptor subtypes are involved in regulating brain excitability, LTP, and susceptibility to epilepsy. AT1 is an important component of the renin-angiotensin-aldosterone system (RAAS). An independent local brain RAS composed of the necessary functional components (i.e., angiotensinogen, peptidases, angiotensin, and specific receptor proteins) significantly improved a variety of physiological and pharmacological functions including memory, cerebral blood flow and cerebroprotection, stress, depression, alcohol consumption, seizure, Alzheimer's and Parkinson's diseases, and diabetes [75].

In KA-induced SE, the osmotic pumping of angiotensin II significantly shortened the latency and increased the frequency of chronic-stage SRS. However, the roles played by the AT1 and AT2 receptors in activating epileptogenesis require further study [76]. The second messenger Ca^{2+} has been shown to be involved in a variety of signaling pathways, including the activation of G-protein-coupled receptors, which have recently been focused on as a novel target for anticonvulsants. The anticonvulsant drug levetiracetam was shown to regulate intracellular Ca^{2+} influx. What's more, single seizure resulted in continuous increase of T-type calcium channel activity, suggesting that the continuous discharge observed in epileptic seizures could be enhanced and maintained by the activation of calcium channel.

Finally, DNA methylation, microRNA regulation, post-gene transcriptional modifications, A-type K^+ channels, HCN channels, and chloride ion transporters have also been implicated in the mechanisms underlying SE-induced brain damage and epileptogenesis. In conclusion, further studies are necessary to solve this puzzle. Understanding of these pathophysiology will provide new strategies to treat SE.

References

1. Wasterlain CG, Fujikawa DG, Penix L, Sankar R. Pathophysiological mechanisms of brain damage from status epilepticus. Epilepsia. 1993;34(Suppl 1):S37–53.
2. Margerison JH, Corsellis JA. Epilepsy and the temporal lobes. A clinical, electroencephalographic and neuropathological study of the brain in epilepsy, with particular reference to the temporal lobes. Brain. 1966;89:499–530.
3. DeGiorgio CM, Tomiyasu U, Gott PS, Treiman DM. Hippocampal pyramidal cell loss in human status epilepticus. Epilepsia. 1992;33:23–7.
4. Meierkord H, Wieshmann U, Niehaus L, Lehmann R. Structural consequences of status epilepticus demonstrated with serial magnetic resonance imaging. Acta Neurol Scand. 1997;96:127–32.
5. Kim JA, et al. Transient MR signal changes in patients with generalized tonicoclonic seizure or status epilepticus: periictal diffusion-weighted imaging. Am J Neuroradiol. 2001;22:1149–60.
6. Oe H, Yuasa R, Tsuchiyama M, Kitamura K. Neuroimaging findings of hemiconvulsions, hemiplegia, epilepsy (HHE) syndrome. Rinsho Shinkeigaku. 1999;39:485–8.
7. DeGiorgio CM, et al. Serum neuron-specific enolase in human status epilepticus. Neurology. 1995;45:1134–7.
8. Petras JM. Neurology and neuropathology of Soman-induced brain injury: an overview. J Exp Anal Behav. 1994;61:319–29.

9. Roch C, Leroy C, Nehlig A, Namer IJ. Magnetic resonance imaging in the study of the lithium-pilocarpine model of temporal lobe epilepsy in adult rats. Epilepsia. 2002;43:325–35.
10. Suleymanova EM, Gulyaev MV, Abbasova KR. Structural alterations in the rat brain and behavioral impairment after status epilepticus: an MRI study. Neuroscience. 2016;315:79–90.
11. Nairismagi J, et al. Progression of brain damage after status epilepticus and its association with epileptogenesis: a quantitative MRI study in a rat model of temporal lobe epilepsy. Epilepsia. 2004;45:1024–34.
12. Choy M, et al. Quantitative MRI predicts status epilepticus-induced hippocampal injury in the lithium-pilocarpine rat model. Epilepsy Res. 2010;88:221–30.
13. Covolan L, Mello LE. Temporal profile of neuronal injury following pilocarpine or kainic acid-induced status epilepticus. Epilepsy Res. 2000;39:133–52.
14. Furtado MA, Castro OW, Del Vecchio F, de Oliveira JA, Garcia-Cairasco N. Study of spontaneous recurrent seizures and morphological alterations after status epilepticus induced by intrahippocampal injection of pilocarpine. Epilepsy Behav. 2011;20:257–66.
15. Franke H, Kittner H. Morphological alterations of neurons and astrocytes and changes in emotional behavior in pentylenetetrazol-kindled rats. Pharmacol Biochem Behav. 2001;70:291–303.
16. Kondratyev A, Gale K. Latency to onset of status epilepticus determines molecular mechanisms of seizure-induced cell death. Brain Res Mol Brain Res. 2004;121:86–94.
17. Stafstrom CE, Chronopoulos A, Thurber S, Thompson JL, Holmes GL. Age-dependent cognitive and behavioral deficits after kainic acid seizures. Epilepsia. 1993;34:420–32.
18. Mello LE, et al. Circuit mechanisms of seizures in the pilocarpine model of chronic epilepsy: cell loss and mossy fiber sprouting. Epilepsia. 1993;34:985–95.
19. Liu H, et al. Suppression of hippocampal neurogenesis is associated with developmental stage, number of perinatal seizure episodes, and glucocorticosteroid level. Exp Neurol. 2003;184:196–213.
20. Vinet J, et al. Microglia are less pro-inflammatory than myeloid infiltrates in the hippocampus of mice exposed to status epilepticus. Glia. 2016;64:1350–62.
21. Avignone E, Lepleux M, Angibaud J, Nagerl UV. Altered morphological dynamics of activated microglia after induction of status epilepticus. J Neuroinflammation. 2015;12:202.
22. Filibian M, et al. In vivo imaging of glia activation using 1H-magnetic resonance spectroscopy to detect putative biomarkers of tissue epileptogenicity. Epilepsia. 2012;53:1907–16.
23. Kwak SE, et al. The expression of somatostatin receptors in the hippocampus of pilocarpine-induced rat epilepsy model. Neuropeptides. 2008;42:569–83.
24. Kim JE, et al. Pyridoxal-5′-phosphate phosphatase/chronophin induces astroglial apoptosis via actin-depolymerizing factor/cofilin system in the rat brain following status epilepticus. Glia. 2010;58:1937–48.
25. Seiffert E, et al. Lasting blood-brain barrier disruption induces epileptic focus in the rat somatosensory cortex. J Neurosci. 2004;24:7829–36.
26. van Vliet EA, et al. Blood-brain barrier leakage may lead to progression of temporal lobe epilepsy. Brain. 2007;130:521–34.
27. Routbort MJ, Bausch SB, McNamara JO. Seizures, cell death, and mossy fiber sprouting in kainic acid-treated organotypic hippocampal cultures. Neuroscience. 1999;94:755–65.
28. Shibley H, Smith BN. Pilocarpine-induced status epilepticus results in mossy fiber sprouting and spontaneous seizures in C57BL/6 and CD-1 mice. Epilepsy Res. 2002;49:109–20.
29. Watanabe Y, et al. Null mutation of c-fos impairs structural and functional plasticities in the kindling model of epilepsy. J Neurosci. 1996;16:3827–36.
30. Adams B, et al. Nerve growth factor accelerates seizure development, enhances mossy fiber sprouting, and attenuates seizure-induced decreases in neuronal density in the kindling model of epilepsy. J Neurosci. 1997;17:5288–96.
31. Vaidya VA, Siuciak JA, Du F, Duman RS. Hippocampal mossy fiber sprouting induced by chronic electroconvulsive seizures. Neuroscience. 1999;89:157–66.
32. Riban V, et al. Evolution of hippocampal epileptic activity during the development of hippocampal sclerosis in a mouse model of temporal lobe epilepsy. Neuroscience. 2002;112:101–11.
33. Loscher W, Brandt C. Prevention or modification of epileptogenesis after brain insults: experimental approaches and translational research. Pharmacol Rev. 2010;62:668–700.
34. Brandt C, Gastens AM, Sun M, Hausknecht M, Loscher W. Treatment with valproate after status epilepticus: effect on neuronal damage, epileptogenesis, and behavioral alterations in rats. Neuropharmacology. 2006;51:789–804.
35. Erdogan F, Golgeli A, Arman F, Ersoy AO. The effects of pentylenetetrazole-induced status epilepticus on behavior, emotional memory, and learning in rats. Epilepsy Behav. 2004;5:388–93.
36. Chu K, et al. Erythropoietin reduces epileptogenic processes following status epilepticus. Epilepsia. 2008;49:1723–32.
37. Liu G, et al. Transient inhibition of TrkB kinase after status epilepticus prevents development of temporal lobe epilepsy. Neuron. 2013;79:31–8.
38. Frisoni GB, Blennow K. Biomarkers for Alzheimer's: the sequel of an original model. Lancet Neurol. 2013;12:126–8.
39. Monti G, et al. Cerebrospinal fluid tau proteins in status epilepticus. Epilepsy Behav. 2015;49:150–4.
40. Turski L, Ikonomidou C, Turski WA, Bortolotto ZA, Cavalheiro EA. Review: cholinergic mechanisms and epileptogenesis. The seizures induced by pilocarpine: a novel experimental model of intractable epilepsy. Synapse. 1989;3:154–71.
41. Sheen SH, et al. Decrease in dystrophin expression prior to disruption of brain-blood barrier within the

rat piriform cortex following status epilepticus. Brain Res. 2011;1369:173–83.
42. Friedman A, Kaufer D, Heinemann U. Blood-brain barrier breakdown-inducing astrocytic transformation: novel targets for the prevention of epilepsy. Epilepsy Res. 2009;85:142–9.
43. Yamada A, et al. Glucose utilization in the brain during acute seizure is a useful biomarker for the evaluation of anticonvulsants: effect of methyl ethyl ketone in lithium-pilocarpine status epilepticus rats. Nucl Med Biol. 2009;36:949–54.
44. Bruce AJ, Baudry M. Oxygen free radicals in rat limbic structures after kainate-induced seizures. Free Radic Biol Med. 1995;18:993–1002.
45. Williams S, Hamil N, Abramov AY, Walker MC, Kovac S. Status epilepticus results in persistent overproduction of reactive oxygen species, inhibition of which is neuroprotective. Neuroscience. 2015;303:160–5.
46. Brennan AM, et al. NADPH oxidase is the primary source of superoxide induced by NMDA receptor activation. Nat Neurosci. 2009;12:857–63.
47. Verkhratsky A. Physiology and pathophysiology of the calcium store in the endoplasmic reticulum of neurons. Physiol Rev. 2005;85:201–79.
48. Chen J, Zheng G, Guo H, Shi ZN. Role of endoplasmic reticulum stress via the PERK signaling pathway in brain injury from status epilepticus. J Mol Neurosci. 2014;53:677–83.
49. Ko AR, Kim JY, Hyun HW, Kim JE. Endothelial NOS activation induces the blood-brain barrier disruption via ER stress following status epilepticus. Brain Res. 2015;1622:163–73.
50. Lowenstein DH, Alldredge BK. Status epilepticus. N Engl J Med. 1998;338:970–6.
51. Goodkin HP, Joshi S, Mtchedlishvili Z, Brar J, Kapur J. Subunit-specific trafficking of GABA(a) receptors during status epilepticus. J Neurosci. 2008;28:2527–38.
52. Naylor DE, Liu H, Wasterlain CG. Trafficking of GABA(a) receptors, loss of inhibition, and a mechanism for pharmacoresistance in status epilepticus. J Neurosci. 2005;25:7724–33.
53. Terunuma M, et al. Deficits in phosphorylation of GABA(a) receptors by intimately associated protein kinase C activity underlie compromised synaptic inhibition during status epilepticus. J Neurosci. 2008;28:376–84.
54. Goodkin HP, Yeh JL, Kapur J. Status epilepticus increases the intracellular accumulation of GABAA receptors. J Neurosci. 2005;25:5511–20.
55. Fukunaga K, Soderling TR, Miyamoto E. Activation of Ca2+/calmodulin-dependent protein kinase II and protein kinase C by glutamate in cultured rat hippocampal neurons. J Biol Chem. 1992;267:22527–33.
56. Bannai H, et al. Activity-dependent tuning of inhibitory neurotransmission based on GABAAR diffusion dynamics. Neuron. 2009;62:670–82.
57. Kapur J, Macdonald RL. Rapid seizure-induced reduction of benzodiazepine and Zn2+ sensitivity of hippocampal dentate granule cell GABAA receptors. J Neurosci. 1997;17:7532–40.
58. Delgado-Escueta AV, Bajorek JG. Status epilepticus: mechanisms of brain damage and rational management. Epilepsia. 1982;23(Suppl 1):S29–41.
59. Mazarati AM, Wasterlain CG. N-methyl-D-asparate receptor antagonists abolish the maintenance phase of self-sustaining status epilepticus in rat. Neurosci Lett. 1999;265:187–90.
60. Wasterlain CG, Naylor DE, Liu H, Niquet J, Baldwin R. Trafficking of NMDA receptors during status epilepticus: therapeutic implications. Epilepsia. 2013;54(Suppl 6):78–80.
61. Deshpande LS, et al. Time course and mechanism of hippocampal neuronal death in an in vitro model of status epilepticus: role of NMDA receptor activation and NMDA dependent calcium entry. Eur J Pharmacol. 2008;583:73–83.
62. Rajasekaran K, Todorovic M, Kapur J. Calcium-permeable AMPA receptors are expressed in a rodent model of status epilepticus. Ann Neurol. 2012;72:91–102.
63. Naylor DE, Liu H, Niquet J, Wasterlain CG. Rapid surface accumulation of NMDA receptors increases glutamatergic excitation during status epilepticus. Neurobiol Dis. 2013;54:225–38.
64. Rodrigues RJ, Tome AR, Cunha RA. ATP as a multi-target danger signal in the brain. Front Neurosci. 2015;9:148.
65. Avignone E, Ulmann L, Levavasseur F, Rassendren F, Audinat E. Status epilepticus induces a particular microglial activation state characterized by enhanced purinergic signaling. J Neurosci. 2008;28: 9133–44.
66. Dona F, et al. Alteration of purinergic P2X4 and P2X7 receptor expression in rats with temporal-lobe epilepsy induced by pilocarpine. Epilepsy Res. 2009;83:157–67.
67. Monif M, Burnstock G, Williams DA. Microglia: proliferation and activation driven by the P2X7 receptor. Int J Biochem Cell Biol. 2010;42:1753–6.
68. Skaper SD, Debetto P, Giusti P. The P2X7 purinergic receptor: from physiology to neurological disorders. FASEB J. 2010;24:337–45.
69. Jimenez-Pacheco A, et al. Increased neocortical expression of the P2X7 receptor after status epilepticus and anticonvulsant effect of P2X7 receptor antagonist A-438079. Epilepsia. 2013;54:1551–61.
70. Boison D. Adenosinergic signaling in epilepsy. Neuropharmacology. 2016;104:131–9.
71. Ravizza T, et al. Inactivation of caspase-1 in rodent brain: a novel anticonvulsive strategy. Epilepsia. 2006;47:1160–8.
72. Johnson EA, Guignet MA, Dao TL, Hamilton TA, Kan RK. Interleukin-18 expression increases in response to neurovascular damage following soman-induced status epilepticus in rats. J Inflamm (Lond). 2015;12:43.
73. Russo E, Citraro R, Constanti A, De Sarro G. The mTOR signaling pathway in the brain: focus on

epilepsy and epileptogenesis. Mol Neurobiol. 2012;46:662–81.
74. Schratt GM, Nigh EA, Chen WG, Hu L, Greenberg ME. BDNF regulates the translation of a select group of mRNAs by a mammalian target of rapamycin-phosphatidylinositol 3-kinase-dependent pathway during neuronal development. J Neurosci. 2004;24:7366–77.
75. Wright JW, Harding JW. Brain renin-angiotensin—a new look at an old system. Prog Neurobiol. 2011;95:49–67.
76. Ivanova NM, et al. Long-term intracerebroventricular infusion of angiotensin II after kainate-induced status epilepticus: effects on epileptogenesis, brain damage, and diurnal behavioral changes. Epilepsy Behav. 2015;51:1–12.

Clinical Features of Refractory Status Epilepticus in Various Conditions

4

Xuefeng Wang, Yuehua Zhang, and Howan Leung

Abstract

Refractory status epilepticus (RSE) is a group of clinical manifestations that are caused by a variety of pathologies. Some cases of RSEs have no clear underlying cause, and these include some hereditary epilepsy syndromes in which the cause of RSE is unknown or has not yet been identified. Some cases of RSE occur in patients with pre-existing epilepsy, and these may represent epilepsy progression that occurs without disease-modifying interventions. In children, epilepsy syndromes manifest in a diversity of ways, including as RSE. Most cases of RSE involve multiple underlying causes, and most result from acute serious brain injury, such as hypoxic ischemic encephalopathy, autoimmune encephalitis, and infectious encephalitis. RSE is associated with different clinical features under different conditions, and different treatments are therefore required to treat each patient. Additionally, prognoses in RSE are related to its underlying cause.

In this chapter, we describe the manifestations and summarize the clinical features of RSE under a variety of conditions with the aim of improving the prevention and timely diagnosis of RSE.

X. Wang (✉)
Chongqing Key Laboratory of Neurology, Department of Neurology, The First Affiliated Hospital of Chongqing Medical University, 1 YouYi Road, Chongqing 400016, China
e-mail: xfyp@163.com

Y. Zhang
Department of Pediatrics, Peking University First Hospital, No. 1, Xi'anmen Street, Xicheng District, Beijing 100034, China

H. Leung
Division of Neurology, Department of Medicine and Therapeutics, The Chinese University of Hong Kong, Prince of Wales Hospital, Hong Kong Special Administrative Region, Hong Kong, China

4.1 New-Onset Refractory Status Epilepticus (NORSE)

4.1.1 Definition

Refractory status epilepticus is usually developed as a result of acute brain injury [1–3] such as infection, trauma, or stroke [4]. However, RSE also occurs in the population without a history of epilepsy or obvious causes. NORSE is used to describe patients who develop RSE with no prior history of epilepsy or identifiable causative factors. Wilder-Smith et al. [4] described

X. Wang, S. Li (eds.), *Refractory Status Epilepticus*, DOI 10.1007/978-981-10-5125-8_4

patients who develop RSE with no prior history of epilepsy or identifiable causative factors as having NORSE. The term has been used to describe a group of diseases with similar clinical characteristics.

Kortvelyessy et al. [5] further described NORSE and noted that NORSE has often been described as RSE in healthy adult patients (18–53 years), which included more women (20–32 years) than men (4:1). Although patients may have a fever, in some cases, no febrile illness was present prior to the seizures. Electroencephalogram (EEG) shows multifocal seizures, suggesting that the discharge originates from a non-specific location. More researchers have used fever-induced refractory epileptic encephalopathy syndrome (FIRES) to describe a group of diseases with the characteristics described above in school-aged children 2–17 years old. In addition to the difference in the age of onset, the incidence of FIRES in males (57%) was slightly higher than in females. Based on EEG results, epileptic discharges mainly originate from focal seizures in the frontal and temporal lobes.

4.1.2 Historical Evolution

In 1961, Lyon et al. [6] described patients without previous seizures or a family history of epilepsy who had refractory seizures. The authors reviewed 47 cases and described 16 cases of children who experienced acute-onset refractory seizures and consciousness disorder in the absence of obvious causative factors after a febrile illness. As shown in the prospective and epidemiological population-based study by Delorenzo and colleagues [7], 58% of patients with SE had no history of epilepsy, indicating that healthy people can experience SE in the absence of a history of epilepsy. Subsequently, many similar cases have been reported with different names, including de novo cryptogenic refractory multifocal febrile status epilepticus [8], idiopathic catastrophic epileptic encephalopathy [9], severe refractory status epilepticus owing to presumed encephalitis [10], devastating epilepsy in school-aged children (DESC) [11], acute encephalitis with refractory repetitive partial seizures (AERRPS) [12], and FIRES [13].

According to Ismail et al. [14], these reports may be describing the same entity and reflect the same disease phenomenon, despite the differences in terminology. In 2005, Wilder-Smith et al. [4] published a descriptive, semi-prospective review of all cases of NORSE syndrome that were monitored at a tertiary care public hospital in Singapore between 2000 and 2004. Initially, seven patients with NORSE syndrome were identified and were young females in previously good health with a precedent febrile illness (in five) and extraordinarily prolonged intractable SE (average 32 days). A large number of negative investigations and catastrophic outcomes were the characteristic features. Although five patients presented with a fever-like infection before seizure onset, the etiology and immunology tests were negative, and the results of brain autopsies of two cases showed a lack of evidence of an inflammatory infection. Subsequently, many case reports of NORSE have been published. In 2008, Costello et al. [15] explored the cause of the disease in six patients with NORSE and proposed the possibility of noninfectious causes. NORSE is etiologically heterogeneous, with a proportion of cases caused by noninfectious factors. In 2010, Mathieu et al. [16] reported a case of a school-aged child who suffered from severe new-onset SE a few days after a common viral infection, which confirmed that some NORSE cases are associated with serum neuropil autoantibodies. In 2012, Claire and colleagues [17] assessed the results of five patients with NORSE who had used immunotherapy early in the seizure course and confirmed that early immunotherapy is associated with good outcomes in patients with NORSE. In the same year, Judy et al. [18] proposed the early use of plasma exchange (PE) therapy in patients with NORSE of an unknown etiology to prevent the complications of SE and prolonged hospitalization.

4.1.3 Prevalence

Although many studies and cases of NORSE have been reported, the limited diagnostic ability and number of NORSE patients, difficulty in performing prospective studies, uncertain treatment, removal of the patient from intensive care by family members, and cessation of treatment have greatly increased the number of uncertain factors, hindering our understanding of NORSE epidemiology. Therefore, the exact incidence is still unknown. Jayalakshmi et al. [19] performed a retrospective analysis of patients with new-onset SE who were admitted between May 2005 and October 2013. Among the 114 patients with new-onset SE, 52 patients (45%) progressed to RSE. A cryptogenic etiology was the most significant determinant of the progression of new-onset SE to RSE. Gaspard et al. [20] examined 675 patients with RSE between January 1, 2008, and December 31, 2013, in a retrospective study, and 130 cases were identified as NORSE. The incidence was 19.3%.

4.1.4 Potential Etiology and Possible Pathogenesis

The etiology of NORSE is unknown, and a definite etiology has not been defined in a clinical reference for diagnosing the disease. In the study by Vivek et al. [21], no cause was identified for 11 patients who had serious seizures among 67 patients with super RSE. Gaspard et al. [20] conducted a retrospective study. Of the 130 cases, 52% remained cryptogenic. Jayalakshmi et al. [19] studied 52 patients with NORSE. A cryptogenic etiology accounted for 63.5% of the cases. When the cause remains unknown following extensive laboratory tests and imaging analyses, this type of NORSE is designated as cryptogenic RSE; epidemiological surveys have reported that approximately 10% of patients with SE are diagnosed with cryptogenic RSE.

Although the extensive laboratory and imaging examinations performed at the first visit may not clearly define an etiology, NORSE has causes. According to a large series of investigations of patients with NORSE, NORSE is most likely associated with encephalopathy or some infection.

Encephalitis is defined as encephalopathy (depressed or altered level of consciousness lasting for over 24 h, with mental and behavioral abnormalities), and one or more of the following clinical or diagnostic findings, fever, focal neurological findings, seizures, cerebrospinal fluid (CSF) alteration, an EEG abnormality, a neuroimaging alteration, and screening tests, exclude systematic autoimmune disorders, metabolic encephalopathy, and intoxication [22].

According to published reports, autoimmune encephalitis exhibits a substantial association with NORSE [15, 23, 24]. In the analysis of NORSE causes by Gaspard et al. [20], the most commonly identified etiologies were autoimmune (presence of an autoantibody in the absence of a neoplasm) and paraneoplastic (newly diagnosed neoplasm, with or without the presence of an antibody) encephalitis, which accounted for 19 and 18% of patients, respectively. Encephalitis with anti-*N*-methyl-D-aspartic acid receptor (NMDAR) antibodies was the most frequent etiology, of which half of the cases were related to an ovarian teratoma, and anti-voltage-gated potassium channel (VEKC) complex antibodies, of which a third of the cases were paraneoplastic. Other antibodies may also be involved, such as anti-glutamate decarboxylase 65 kDa (GAD65), anti-α-amino-3-hydroxy-5-methyl-4-isoxazole-propionic acid receptor (AMPAR), anti-γ-aminobutyric acid receptor (GABAR), anti-Hu, anti-voltage-gated calcium channel (VGCC), anti-collapsing response mediator protein 5 (CRMP5), anti-Ro, etc. Hainsworth et al. [23] reported a case study of a 23-year-old, previously healthy patient with bilateral temporal lobe epilepsy (TLE) who was ultimately diagnosed with GABA receptor limbic encephalitis; the patient presented super refractory epilepsy SE. Killian Hurley [25] reported a case study of a 64-year-old patient with pulmonary squamous cell carcinoma who exhibited personality changes, cognitive impairment, complex partial seizures, ataxia, and language barriers to movement 2 weeks prior to being admitted to the hospital for generalized tonic-clonic seizures (GTCS) and decreased consciousness. The serum tests did not detect immune antibodies. The disease may be paraneoplastic encephalitis.

Infection-related factors account for 16% of the NORSE causes. Herpes viruses, excluding herpes simplex virus 1, were the most frequent infectious agents (50%). In addition, Epstein-Barr virus (EBV), cytomegalovirus (CMV), varicella-zoster virus (VZV), and West Nile virus (WNV) have been detected. Rajesh et al. [26] described a woman who presented with NORSE. Investigations confirmed the diagnosis of herpes simplex encephalitis, and she exhibited a dramatic response to acyclovir and complete control of her seizures.

The possible mechanisms underlying NORSE are not clear. Costello et al. [15] contend that NORSE is etiologically heterogeneous. To explain the pathogenesis of NORSE, a large number of hypotheses have been proposed, but none have proven to be conclusive. Tests of the CSF from patients with SE detect oligoclonal bands and anti-glutamic acid decarboxylase (GAD) and anti-glutamic acid receptor 3 (GluR-3) antibodies, and anti-GluRε-2 and anti-voltage-gated potassium channel complex antibodies are detected in some patients [12, 27]. NORSE may be associated with immune disorders, similar to acute disseminated encephalomyelitis and Guillain-Barre syndrome. NORSE may result in an abnormal immune response produced by molecular stimulation by a benign infectious disease. The effectiveness of immunotherapy in some patients supports this hypothesis [28–30]. However, these autoimmune antibodies are detected in some patients with epilepsy, which suggests that it is not a unique feature of NORSE. Thus, the presence of autoimmune antibodies does not support the NORSE immune hypothesis.

Nabbout et al. [31] proposed "the acute encephalopathy induced by inflammation" hypothesis that inflammatory factors (such as IL-1, TNF-α, and IL-6) induce the occurrence of NORSE in different stages of brain development. When inflammatory mediators cause patients to enter the proconvulsive state, IL-1β and TNF-α block glutamate reuptake by astrocytes and increase the extracellular glutamate concentrations [32, 33]. Simultaneously, both cytokines affect GABA receptor endocytosis, block the GABA-mediated chloride ion current, and increase the Ca2+ permeability of *N*-methyl-D-aspartic acid (NMDA) and α-amino-3-hydroxy-5-methyl-4-isoxazole-propionic acid (AMPA) receptors to enhance neuronal excitability [12].

On the other hand, seizures lead to the formation of an aseptic inflammatory state, thus promoting repeated epileptic seizures. The rise of the body temperature of the animal can increase seizure susceptibility, and drug intervention or knock of IL-1β expression in young rats decreases epilepsy susceptibility. These support the view of Nabbout et al. [34]. Unfortunately, van Baalen et al. [13] did not report pathological changes in the inflammatory response in autopsy specimens of brain tissue. The inflammatory mechanism that induces NORSE remains to be discussed.

4.1.5 Clinical Features

4.1.5.1 Prodromal Symptoms

In the study by Gaspard et al. [20], 75 of the 125 cases (60%) exhibited prodromal symptoms preceding the onset of NORSE, including fever (34%), confusion (45%), headache (22%), fatigue (26%), symptoms of a gastrointestinal (18%) or upper respiratory (13%) tract infection, and behavioral changes (16%). In addition, some patients may experience the following symptoms: memory complaints, language difficulties, hallucinations, rash, and arthralgia.

4.1.5.2 Seizure Types

Gaspard et al. [20] analyzed 125 patients with NORSE, and 90% had seizures before admission, of which 13 patients (10%) experienced simple partial seizures, 36 (29%) experienced complex partial seizures, and 83 (67%) experienced tonic-clonic seizure. Thirty-five patients (28%) presented SE before admission, 16 (15%) presented complex/simple partial SE, and 19 (13%) presented generalized convulsive SE. According to the reported cases and studies, the patient's seizure type is complicated and changeable during the progression of NORSE. Simple partial seizures can develop into complex partial seizures, and simple or complex partial seizures may be generalized to tonic-clonic seizures (Table 4.1).

Generalized Tonic-Clonic Seizures

Patients can show generalized tonic-clonic seizures (GTCS) in the first episode. Of all types of SE, generalized convulsive status epilepticus

Table 4.1 Clinical characteristics of NORSE

Authors/years	No. of cases	Age (years)	Prodromal symptoms	Seizure type	Duration (days)
Van Lierdo/ 2003 [13]	6	18–30	Febrile illness (6)	Multifocal seizures and refractory partial seizures	6–191
Wilder-Smith/ 2005 [4]	7	20–52	Antecedent febrile illness (5)	Multifocal/GTCS (6) Multifocal/nonconvulsive status epilepticus (NCSE) (1)	7–92
Costello/ 2009 [15]	6	24–36	Mild febrile illness (4), fever, and coryzal (nasal congestion, sore throat, myalgias)	Serial convulsive seizures (4), abrupt onset of nonconvulsive complex partial SE (2)	9–76
Claire/2012 [17]	5	22–34	Headache (3), vomiting (2), myalgia (1), acute confusion (2), and pyrexia (2)	GTCS interspersed with complex partial seizures	Unknown
Judy/2012 [18]	3	39–51	Two patients had a preceding flu-like illness, 1 presented with a febrile illness	GTCS (2), complex partial seizure (1)	Unknown
Khawaja/ 2015 [35]	11	21–90	Fever(3), encephalopathy (7)	GTCS (10) NCSE (1)	12–110

(GCSE) is most urgent and serious type, presenting persistent limb rigidity and clonic or tonic-clonic seizures with dysfunction of consciousness. Judy et al. [18] described two patients who initially presented GTCS. One was a 43-year-old woman with no history and risk factors for epilepsy who experienced an antecedent flu-like illness and initially presented GTCSs. The initial EEG showed background slowing, and the brain magnetic resonance imaging (MRI) was normal. She was discharged with phenytoin treatment and allowed to return home, but was readmitted with increased seizure frequency within 3 days. The initial EEG showed bitemporal independent focal seizures. The other patient was a 39-year-old, previously healthy woman who presented with a flu-like illness 5 days prior to her first GTCS. Wilder-Smith et al. [4] reported six cases among seven patients who presented a generalized seizure-type status, and the EEG showed multifocal seizures. In the study by Khawaja et al. [35], 90% of patients experienced GTCS.

Simple Partial Seizures

This type of seizure is described as a part of the body or side that presents tonic-clonic seizures with clear consciousness. Peter et al. [9] reviewed six children aged 5 months to 6 years who presented with focal seizures that progressed to intractable multifocal seizures with or without secondary generalization within days; the seizures recurred every few minutes and persisted for weeks. Four patients displayed simple partial seizures with twitching/rotation of their arms; the seizure frequency increased within 1–3 days and ultimately resulted in erratic myoclonus and tonic seizures. The patients developed RSE. Van Lierde et al. [8] reported a study of a 30-year-old woman who presented a simple partial seizure, including right facial twitching, left eye deviation, blinking and hypersalivation, and clear consciousness. The EEG showed right temporal lobe seizures.

Complex Partial Seizures

Mathieu et al. [16] reported a study of a 5-year-old patient with NORSE who experienced an upper respiratory tract infection with fever 3 days before the occurrence of the first epileptic seizure. Clinical manifestations were characterized by a disturbance of consciousness and abnormal EEG. Seizures were initially brief (1–2 min), but their frequency gradually increased. The patient was eventually diagnosed with refractory TLE associated with serum neuropil autoantibodies. A 51-year-old Hispanic male presented a suspected complex partial seizure and a preceding febrile illness. However, his CSF findings and routine EEG were normal. He was initially treated with carbamazepine, but 2 weeks later, he stopped the medication on his own. Four months later, he returned with a 5-day history of confusion and lethargy [18]. Costello et al. [15] reported a case study of six patients with NORSE. Two patients showed an abrupt onset of nonconvulsive complex partial SE without generalized convulsive activity. Confused behavior with obtundation and intermittent focal motor seizure activity were the main clinical manifestations.

Secondary GTCS

Many publications have described patients with NORSE who initially present partial seizures, followed by GTCS that are designated as secondary GTCS. Van Lierde et al. [8] examined six young patients and showed that five patients exhibited partial seizures, such as head and eye deviation, facial twitches, aphasia, blinking, and hypersalivation. Later, the patients developed secondary GTCS.

Gianfranco et al. [36] described a 41-year-old man who presented with a parainfectious syndrome characterized by a low-grade fever and vomiting. Within 3 days, the patient experienced increasingly complex partial epileptic seizures that rapidly changed from tonic-clonic seizures to generalized SE.

Absence Seizures

Absence seizures have not been reported in the literature to date.

4.1.5.3 Related Factors

Age

Jayalakshmi et al. [19] analyzed 52 patients with NORSE and the average age was 28.7 + 20.2 years old. Individuals less than 18 years old, adults, and elderly people (greater than or equal to 60 years old) accounted for 28.8%, 57.7%, and 13.5% of the population, respectively. The average age of adult sufferers is 28.3 years [15]. This promoted NORSE mainly appeared in adults.

Gender

Costello et al. [15] summarized the clinical features of cryptogenic new-onset RSE in adults. Among 23 patients, the ratio of males and females was 4:19, suggesting that adult women are more likely to develop NORSE. As shown in the study by Jayalakshmi et al. [19], women accounted for 51.5% of 33 patients with cryptogenic NORSE. However, men accounted for 63.2% of patients with symptomatic NORSE.

Main Concomitant Symptoms

Patients with NORSE not only have various types of seizures but can also present many concomitant symptoms, including affective disorders such as apathy, obtuseness, and anger. In the study by Khawaja et al. [30], one patient had seizures accompanied by an excited state.

4.1.6 Disease Evolution

Figure 4.1.

4.1.7 Auxiliary Examination

4.1.7.1 Laboratory Examination

Metabolic and infectious investigations should be considered for all patients who are suspected of having NORSE.

Routine examinations include blood, urine, electrolyte, and blood biochemical tests. CSF examinations include leukocyte counts and protein levels. Infection-related tests include bacterial and fungal blood cultures and viral polymerase chain reaction to determine the levels of herpes simplex virus (HSV), EBV, VZV, CMV, WNV, and human immunodeficiency virus (HIV). Immune-related tests include measurements of the serum levels of immunoglobulins (EBV, VZV, WNV, HSV, and CMV), autoantibodies (antithyroid peroxidase and antithyroglobulin), and paraneoplastic autoantibodies (anti-NMDA receptor, anti-VGKC complex, anti-Hu, anti-VGCC, and anti-Ro).

Gaspard et al. [20] studied 125 patients with NORSE and 91 presented abnormal CSF, which accounted for 73% of the population. CSF pleocytosis was observed 52%, and the CSF leukocyte counts were 5 mμ/L (1–14 mμ/L) on average. Increased CSF protein levels were observed in

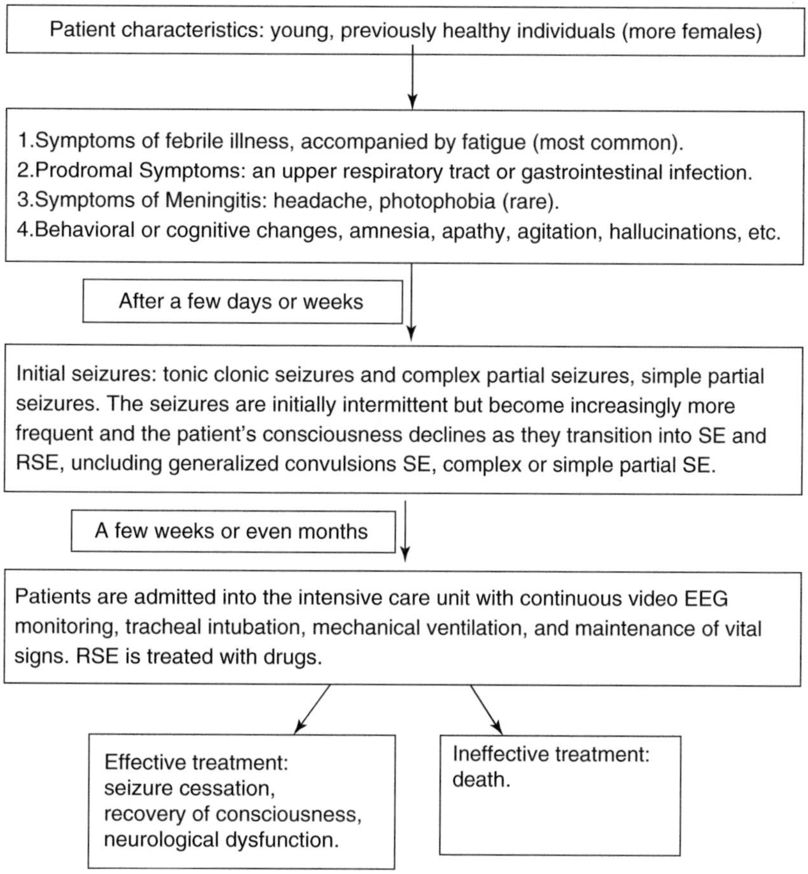

Fig. 4.1 Disease evolution of NORSE

64% of the patients, and the CSF protein levels were 39 mg/dL (26–91 mg/dL).

4.1.7.2 Image Examination

Most of the early magnetic resonance imaging (MRI) are normal, but then brain structural damage appears. In retrospective review by Gaspard et al. [20], 62% of the patients had an abnormal MRI. The statistical analysis identified dominant abnormalities in limbic (19%) and neocortical structures (22%) or both (16%).

4.1.7.3 Electrophysiological Examination

In the retrospective review by Gaspard et al. [20], 88% of patients undergoing continuous EEG monitoring exhibit epileptiform discharges: 46% exhibit unilateral, 24% exhibit bilateral, 15% exhibit complete, and 8% exhibit multifocal discharges. Periodic or epileptiform discharges are observed in 72% of patients. Lateralized discharge (39%) is more common than the bilateral independent (24%), generalized (22%), or multifocal discharge (2%).

4.1.8 Treatments

Due to the complexity of the NORSE condition and unknown mechanism, an effective and specific treatment is not available for patients. Currently, the conventional treatments include seizure control, vital sign support, and treatments for related complications. Candidate antiepileptic drugs (AEDs) for seizure control include pentobarbital, midazolam, propofol, ketamine, and inhalation anesthetics. In addition, considering the causal role of inflammation in NORSE, researchers have attempted to use various methods to regulate the immune system, including intravenous steroids, intravenous immunoglobulin, plasma exchange therapy, and a number of inflammatory cell monoclonal antibodies (such as rituximab). Steroids reduce intracranial pressure, and the use of large doses of steroids may be justified when the patient is unable to determine the cause and rule out an infection. Some cases and clinical trials support the use of immunotherapy. However, treatments that increase the permeability of the blood brain barrier and GABA inhibition of cholesterol may affect the maintenance of seizures.

Judy et al. [18] described three cases of NORSE. All patients received an extensive evaluation, including brain MRI, CSF studies, radiological scans for malignancy, and serological autoimmune and infectious investigations, but no clear causes were identified. The use of various anticonvulsants and general anesthetics for at least 5 days was ineffective. Each patient began to use plasma exchange therapy, and SE ceased on the fourth day. Based on this case series, plasma exchange may be a beneficial treatment for patients with NORSE, even when etiology is unclear and anti-neuronal antibodies or typical paraneoplastic are not detected. Plasma exchange may reduce the serum drug concentrations, and the drug concentrations should be monitored as necessary.

Claire et al. [17] reported the outcomes of patients with NORSE who were treated with immunotherapy early in the course of the disease. Three of the five patients received the immunotherapy, all of whom recovered without significant neuropsychological deficits. Two patients returned to full-time employment, and the other patient experienced a mild decrease in cognitive function. One patient who did not receive immunotherapy died of five intensive care unit (ICU)-related complications after 3 weeks, and the outcome of the other patient was not known. Thus, immunotherapy appears to be associated with good neurological outcomes. Khawaja et al. [30] analyzed the potential effect of immunotherapy on NORSE. Of the 11 patients, eight were treated with IT (immunoglobulins, intravenous steroids, plasmapheresis, or a combination), and four received chemotherapy. Of the eight patients treated with IT, six experienced favorable outcomes (defined as any outcome other than death, a vegetative state, or an inability to care for oneself) compared with zero of the three patients who did not receive immunotherapy. The authors believed that although the efficacy of immunotherapy in randomized controlled trials of patients with NORSE is difficult to verify, early use of immunotherapy in patients with NORSE of an unknown etiology may prevent the incidence and mortality of the associated complications.

4.1.9 Prognosis

Generally, patients with NORSE have poor outcomes. The use of multiple AEDs and general anesthetics may lead to severe cardiac, respiratory, and hemodynamic complications. One large series reported poor outcomes in approximately half of the patients with RSE, including death (35%), severe neurological deficits (13%), and mild neurological deficits (13%); a minor fraction of the patients recovered to baseline levels (35%) [37]. The retrospective review of patients with RSE by Gaspard et al. [20] analyzed the prognosis of 125 patients with NORSE. Seventy-seven of the 125 patients (62%) experienced poor outcomes, and 28 (22%) died. The duration of SE, use of anesthetics, and medical complications are the predictors of poor outcomes. In addition, 63 patients were followed for an average of 9 months; 57% patients exhibited an improved functional status, and 79% had good or fair outcomes at the last follow-up, but 37% developed epilepsy, with most survivors (92%) remaining on antiseizure medications.

4.2 Refractory Status Epilepticus in Pre-Existing Epilepsy

4.2.1 Definition

NORSE is usually associated with an uncertain or cryptogenic etiology [35]. Refractory status epilepticus in patient with pre-existing epilepsy (PERSE) refers to the RSE occurred in patients with pre-existing epilepsy who come into SE that is usually resistant to the initial treatment failure

RSE [3, 38–40]. The occurrence of PERSE is attributed to genetic factors, drug resistance, improper treatments with AEDs, new-onset systemic infection or metabolic disorders, and inappropriate initial treatment regimens [41–44].

4.2.2 Historical Evolution

As early as 1980, Young et al. [45] described five adult patients (19–62 years) with SE. The early use of first-line and/or second-line AEDs (e.g., phenytoin, diazepam, clonazepam, phenobarbital) was ineffective at controlling SE. Two of the patients in this study had a history of epilepsy. One 19-year-old female patient had congenital right hemiparesis and underwent left hemisphere resection. She began to present seizures at the age of two. She experienced repeated generalized seizures for 5 consecutive days, which was proven to be caused by phenytoin poisoning (serum concentration: 50 μg/mL). The seizures rapidly developed into SE, which continued for 3 h before she was admitted to the hospital. After admission, the patient was administered diazepam, phenobarbital, phenytoin, and polyacetaldehyde, but SE was not terminated. Another 62-year-old patient suffered from meningitis 20 years ago and experienced recurrent lateral or generalized seizures in subsequent years. Before admission, he experienced 4 days of continuous seizures. The phenytoin serum concentration was 16.2 μg/mL at admission. Diazepam, phenobarbital, and paraldehyde treatments failed to stop the seizures. The other three patients with no previous history of epilepsy experienced RSE after acute inflammatory brain damage. SE was quickly controlled in five patients with an esthetic barbiturate (pentobarbital or thiopental). Meanwhile, the intravenous barbiturate treatment must be maintained for a few days, otherwise the SE would quickly recur. In 1985, Nouailhat et al. [46] retrospectively analyzed 192 adult patients with SE who were consecutively admitted to two ICUs over 7 years. Fifty (26%) patients had a history of epilepsy. Two-thirds of the 192 patients were admitted to the ICU because the initial treatment with benzodiazepines and/or phenobarbital failed; 52% of the patients required respiratory support, and 36% died. In 1996, Walker et al. [47] studied 26 patients with RSE (15 males and 11 females) who were referred to an ICU and whose seizures continued for more than 30 min. The median age of the patients was 33 (17–73) years old. Before referral, these patients were treated with benzodiazepines or phenytoin and other drugs. All drugs failed to terminate SE. Among the 16 patients who were treated with phenytoin, seven definitively had a deficient loading dose of phenytoin, and four possibly had a deficient loading dose. Eighteen (69.2%) of the 26 patients had a previous history of epilepsy. The etiology of five patients with RSE was an AED dose reduction or withdrawal. Two of the five cases were caused by poor compliance. More studies of PERSE have been published since then, but it was not classified as a special type of RSE and was not researched in depth. Anesthetic drugs are required to control PERSE in a growing number of patients, some of whom even developed super-RSE. The disability rate and mortality were quite high [40, 43].

4.2.3 Prevalence

Patients with pre-existing epilepsy often present with SE, which is often associated with treatment regimen. Although many cases have been published [21, 43, 48, 49], PERSE has not been completely examined, and a specific, unified definition has not been reported. Specific statistical data for PERSE are not available; thus, the exact morbidity is unknown. The overall curative effect of treatments for PERSE is also unclear.

The retrospective cohort study by Pugin et al. [40] included patients with SE from May 1997 to April 2010, who were treated with continuous intravenous pentobarbital infusions. Overall, 116 patients with RSE (61 ± 17 years, 38 males and 78 females) and 31 patients with super-RSE (48 ± 20 years, 14 males and 17 females) who were refractory to the initial treatment (first- and second-line AEDs) were included. Of these patients, 38/116 (33%) with RSE and 8/31 (26%) with super-RSE had a previous history of epilepsy.

The super-RSE group included two patients with Lennox-Gastaut syndrome and one patient with cortical dysplasia. The etiologies of 22 (19%) patients with RSE and five (16%) patients with super-RSE were defined as epilepsy. The authors concluded that 31.3% of patients with RSE and an initial treatment failure were PERSE. The retrospective open cohort study by Jayalakshmi et al. [43] included 177 patients (31.6 ± 19.2 years, 104 males and 73 females) with convulsive SE in a neurology intensive care unit (NICU) from 2005 to 2013. Of these patients, 105 (33.8 ± 19 years) cases were non-RSE, 42 (30.7 ± 14.8 years) cases were RSE, and 30 (24.6 ± 23.6 years) cases were super-RSE. Patients with pre-existing epilepsy accounted for 41% (43/105) of the non-refractory SE group, 35.7% (15/42) of the RSE group, and 16.7% (5/30) of the super-RSE group. In conclusion, the occurrence of PERSE was 11.3% in all patients with convulsive SE. The occurrence of PERSE was 27.8% in all patients with initial treatment failure SE. The international multicenter study by Ferlisi et al. [50] included 413 patients with RSE from 44 different cities, 181 (38%) of whom had pre-existing epilepsy.

4.2.4 Potential Risk Factors

4.2.4.1 AED-Related Factors

AED-related factors include nonadherence, AED withdrawal, below-reference AED serum concentrations, and drug poisoning [43, 44, 51]. In patients with pre-existing epilepsy, AED-related factors are very common precipitating factors of SE [51]. Lie et al. [41] retrospectively analyzed consecutive admissions for 124 patients with SE who had pre-existing epilepsy from January 1999 to August 2012. One inclusion criterion was that the patients should be treated with AEDs. In this study, 52 patients with 64 episodes of SE used an objective evaluation index, therapeutic drug monitoring (TDM), to measure AED nonadherence. The patients were designated as AED nonadherence when concentration/dose (C/D) ratios were <75% compared to the drug fasting control value. AED nonadherence was observed in 24 (38%) SE episodes, of which seven (11%) episodes were definite and 17 (27%) episodes were probable. Among the 24 SE episodes that demonstrated AED nonadherence, 4/24 (16.7%) episodes were RSE and 1/24 (4.2%) was super-RSE.

Jayalakshmi et al. [43] analyzed 177 patients with convulsive SE. Among the 105 patients with non-RSE, 43 (41%) patients had pre-existing epilepsy, and in 16/105 (18.1%) patients, SE was attributed to AED withdrawal. Among the 42 patients with RSE, 15 (35.7%) patients had pre-existing epilepsy, and 3/42 (9.5%) cases of RSE were attributed to AED withdrawal. Among the 30 patients with super-RSE, 5 (16.7%) patients had pre-existing epilepsy, and 2/30 (13.3%) super-RSE cases were attributed to AEDs withdrawal.

Hocker et al. [44] studied 63 episodes of RSE in 54 adult patients (18–93 years old) from January 1999 to August 2011. Thirty-seven (59.7%) patients had history of seizures. Low AED levels or missed doses caused eight (12.7%) RSE episodes. A change in medication caused two (3.2%) RSE episodes. Drug intoxication or withdrawal caused two (3.2%) RSE episodes. Congenital or hereditary factors caused three (4.8%) RSE episodes.

4.2.4.2 Delays in the Initial Treatment of SE

Delays in the initial treatment (including prehospital, diagnosis, and medication delays) of SE resulted in AED-resistant SE, and the delays were associated with a poor prognosis for these patients [52, 53]. Kamppi et al. [53] retrospectively studied 82 adult patients (16–85 years old, 42 males and 40 females) with SE, of whom 51 (62.2%) had previously diagnosed epilepsy. Twenty-nine (35.4%) of 82 patients had symptomatic epilepsy, 14 (17.1%) had idiopathic epilepsy, and eight (9.8%) had cryptogenic or unclassified epilepsy. The median time of the delay in SE treatment before admission was 2 h 4 min. The median time of delay in treatment after a clear diagnosis of SE was made was 2 h 10 min. The median delay between the diagnosis and the first medication was 35 min. The long delay before the initial SE treatment (first- or second-line drugs) resulted in treatment failure in 86.6% (n = 71) of patients with SE that subsequently developed into RSE or super-RSE. The incidence rate of super-RSE was 48.8% ($n = 40$) in this study.

The prospective cohort study by Sanchez et al. [52] included 81 pediatric patients (0.2–19.3 years old, 44 males and 37 females) with refractory convulsive SE in whom the initial treatment (benzodiazepines in 78 patients, levetiracetam in two patients, phenobarbital in one patient) failed. Thirty-eight patients had pre-existing epilepsy, and 14 patients had a previous history of SE. Before admission, 27 patients with pre-existing epilepsy exhibited continuous seizures. Only 12 (44.4%) patients received the first dose of AEDs (benzodiazepines) before arriving at the hospital: the family administered the treatment to 7/12 patients, and the emergency medical services administered the treatment to 5/12 patients. The median time from the start of SE to the first, second, and third doses of AEDs was 28 (6–67) min, 40 (20–85) min, and 59 (30–120) min, respectively. The delay in SE treatment before admission, the time at which the first dosage of AEDs was administered after admission, and the delay time when changing to different AEDs are all reasons for the failure of the initial treatment for RSE.

4.2.4.3 Other Factors

Other factors included systemic infection, metabolic disorders, cerebral vascular disease, and hypoxia. Power et al. [54] retrospectively analyzed the inducement of 20 RSE episodes in 13 patients who had pre-existing epilepsy. Two RSE episodes in two patients were caused by mitochondrial disease, seven episodes in four patients were caused by pneumonia, five episodes in three patients were caused by AED treatment failure, one episode was caused by cerebral hemorrhage, one episode was caused by upper airway infection, one episode was caused by hypoxia/aspiration, and three episodes in three patients were caused by unknown causes. Lie et al. [41] studied 64 SE episodes in 52 patients with a pre-existing epilepsy diagnosis who were treated with AEDs. With the exception of RSE induced by treatment nonadherence in 24 patients, 17% of the SE attacks were induced by other factors, such as alcohol withdrawal, excessive stress, sleep deprivation, and fever.

4.2.5 Clinical Features

4.2.5.1 Onset Age

Patients with PERSE had large range of onset ages. Children, adults, and the elderly can all experience PERSE. Power et al. [54] retrospectively analyzed 13 adult patients with RSE and a history of epilepsy ranging in age from 19.5 to 65 years old. Miyahara et al. [55] retrospectively analyzed nine patients (six males and three females) with progressive myoclonus epilepsy who had previous history of epilepsy, and the age at the onset of RSE ranged from 3 to 28 years. Sanchez et al. [52] studied 81 children with refractory convulsive SE, and the onset age was 0.2–19.3 years old. Of these patients, 38 children had a previous history of epilepsy. Lie et al. [41] studied 64 admissions for SE in 52 patients who were previously diagnosed with epilepsy and treated with AEDs. The study included ten children under the age of 16, five (50%) of whom were included in the AED nonadherence group. Among the 17 elderly patients over 60 years old, 7 (44%) patients were included in the AED nonadherence group. However, of the 37 adult patients between 16 and 59 years old, 12 (32%) were included in the AED nonadherence. Children and elderly patients with SE and pre-existing epilepsy represented the largest proportion of the AED nonadherence group.

4.2.5.2 Seizure Types

Patients with RSE who had a pre-existing epilepsy diagnosis might experience a variety of seizure types. Miyahara et al. [55] retrospectively analyzed nine patients with RSE who were diagnosed with progressive myoclonus epilepsy before and had a pre-existing epilepsy diagnosis. The RSE types included in the study were myoclonic SE ($n = 3$), myoclonic generalized SE ($n = 4$), and generalized SE ($n = 2$). Tassinari et al. [56] studied five patients with Lennox-Gastaut syndrome (8–17 years old, three males and two females) who had pre-existing epilepsy. After intravenous benzodiazepine (diazepam or nitrazepam) treatment, all these patients immediately experienced tonic SE. In these patients, SE was thought to be precipitated by benzodiazepine. The patients were then refractory to a variety of drug therapies, such as the barbiturates, primidone, and ethosuximide. Nobutoki et al. [57] reported seven refractory nonconvulsive SE episodes in five patients who had a history of epilepsy. Two patients were diagnosed with Lennox-Gastaut syndrome. The other three patients were diagnosed with symptomatic generalized epilepsy, continuous spike-waves during slow-wave sleep, and ring chromosome 20 syndromes, respectively.

4.2.6 Treatments

Data describing special treatment options for PERSE are currently lacking. The main treatment is the use of AEDs, anesthetics, and nonconventional treatments to terminate the seizures as soon as possible. The incidence rate of complications in patients with PERSE is higher than that in patients who effectively responded to the initial treatment. Patients with PERSE often require treatment in an ICU or even ventilation. These patients subsequently exhibit arrhythmia, respiratory failure, hypotension, pulmonary infection, and multiple organ dysfunction, significantly affecting the prognosis [54, 58]. The specific treatment scheme is described in Chaps. 6 and 7.

4.2.7 Prognosis-Related Factors

The retrospective cohort study by Pugin et al. [40] analyzed 31 adults with super-RSE (48 ± 20 years old) who were intravenously administered pentobarbital for treatment. Of these patients, eight (26%) had a previous history of epilepsy, and the etiology of super-RSE was epilepsy in five (16%) patients. The analysis of the clinical data did not identify a correlation between the patients' previous history of epilepsy and the outcome upon hospital discharge. Hocker et al. [44] studied 63 RSE episodes in 54 adult patients (18–93 years old, 36 males and 57 females). Thirty-seven (59.7%) patients had a previous history of epilepsy, and 17 (27.9%) patients had previous episodes of SE. Fifty-five (87.30%) RSE episodes were treated with anesthetic drugs. The statistical analysis of the data identified that a previous history of epilepsy, age, a previous history of SE, SE type, and the anesthetic drug treatment had little connection with the patients' prognoses.

An observational retrospective study by Lie et al. [41] analyzed patients with SE who had a pre-existing epilepsy diagnosis and were being treated with AEDs. The study analyzed the AED nonadherence of 52 patients with 64 SE episodes using the TDM index. Among the 24 SE episodes observed in patients with identified AED nonadherence, 4/24 (16.7%) episodes were RSE and 1/24 (4.2%) episode was super-RSE. All patients with AED nonadherence (n = 24) eventually survived, including 21 patients with a complete recovery and three patients with sequelae (including cognitive impairment and malignant epilepsy). Among the patients with SE in the AED adherence group, 4/40 (10%) episodes were RSE and 3/40 (7.5%) were super-RSE. Ultimately, six patients died (nonadherence group, zero; adherence group, six) due to the etiology, such as juvenile neuronal ceroid lipofuscinosis. The prognosis of patients with PERSE was related to the underlying etiology, and AED nonadherence might not affect the patients' prognoses.

Poweret et al. [54] studied 20 RSE episodes in 13 patients with pre-existing epilepsy. Three RSE episodes left the patients with minor sequelae. Two RSE episodes left the patients with severe sequelae. Fourteen RSE episodes left the patients without sequelae and one patient died. Of the five episodes observed in five patients without pre-existing epilepsy, two episodes had severe sequelae, one episode had no sequelae, and one episode had mild sequelae, and one patient died. Compared with patients without pre-existing epilepsy, treatment was easier in patients with pre-existing epilepsy, the required time for the treatment was shorter, and the prognosis was better. Half of the patients' sequelae were related to the basic etiology of RSE [54, 59].

4.3 Refractory Status Epilepticus in Children's Epilepsy Syndrome

Currently, more than 30 kinds of epilepsy syndromes have approved by the International League Against Epilepsy (ILAE), and different syndromes have different ages of onset [60]. The ILAE task force published a report describing the definition and classification of SE in 2015 that listed SE in epileptic syndrome according to age [61]. In this paper, we describe SE course which easily appears in some specific epilepsy syndromes. RSE occurs readily apparent in epilepsy in infancy with migrating focal seizures, Dravet syndrome (DS), epilepsy with myoclonic-atonic seizures, and progressive myoclonus epilepsy. All of the syndromes have their own clinical and EEG characteristics; the types of SE and their relations with the prognoses of these epilepsy syndromes are also different.

4.3.1 Epilepsy in Infancy with Migrating Focal Seizures (EIMFS)

4.3.1.1 Historical Evolution

EIMFS, which was previously called migrating partial seizures in infancy (MPSI), was first proposed by Coppola in 1995 [62]. In this study, 14 babies (both boys and girls) had epileptic seizures that never been reported previously. The average age of the first attack occurred at a mean age of 3 months. The major clinical manifestations were new, persistent, and multifocal seizures and multiple irrelevant wandering epileptic discharges that persisted in an EEG. From 1 to 10 months, seizures occurred frequently, and their clinical/EEG manifestations were variable. A clear etiology cannot be determined, and the overall prognosis was poor. Since then, patients with the same type of seizures have been gradually reported [63–66]. In 2010, the ILAE classified the disease as children's epilepsy syndrome and renamed it as EIMFS [67].

4.3.1.2 Potential Causes

The underlying causes of this syndrome are considered to be caused by genetic factors. Currently, researchers have identified eight pathogenic genes that lead to the disease: KCNT1, SCN1A, SCN2A, SCN8A, PLCB1, SLC25A22, TBC1D24, and SLC12A5 [68–75]. As shown in the 2016 study by Saitsu and colleagues [74], mutations in the SLC12A5 gene damage neuronal KCC2 function and disrupted neuronal Cl^- extrusion to cause EIMFS.

4.3.1.3 Clinical Manifestations

Age of Onset

According to the studies [62], the age of onset was within 6 months after the birth and in newborns at the earliest. The peak age was 3 months. In 2012, Barcia and colleagues [76] examined the EIMFS data from a hospital over nearly a decade and found that the average age of onset was 2 months (2 h–7 months).

Seizure Types

Additional reports of multiple continuous wandering focal seizures have been published [76]. McTague and colleagues [77] conducted a two-year follow-up of 14 children with EIMFS. It is found that most children (64%) exhibited focal motor seizures, 59% exhibited focal seizures affecting alternating sides of body, 17% exhibited secondary generalization, 8% exhibited GTCS, 43% exhibited autonomic features, and 7% exhibited epileptic spasms.

Progression

Coppola [67] summarized the natural course of EIMFS and divided it into approximately three stages. (1) The first stage usually starts within 6 months after birth. Sporadic epileptic seizures can appear at weeks or months after birth, even appeared within 1 day after birth. These patients are mostly characterized by focal motor with secondary generalization seizures and autonomic symptoms, such as apnea, a flushed face, or cyanosis. (2) The second stage has been described as "stormy phase," ranging from 1 month to 1 year of age. The clinical features include various forms of focal seizures that occur in clusters of attacks 5–30 times a day, even a few days in a row; these children may readily develop SE. Clinical manifestations include head and eyes turn to one side, eyelid blinking, one or both sides of the body clonus or tonic-closure seizures, flushing and/or cyanosis of face, chew swallow, and secondary tonic-clonic generalization. (3) In the third stage, the age span is larger, ages 1–5 years and over. At this stage, seizures generally do not occur. Alternatively, patients experience occasional clusters of epileptic seizures or SE caused by spontaneous intercurrent disease.

4.3.1.4 Auxiliary Examination

EEG

As reported in the study by Barcia et al. [76], the EEG showed multiple focal wandering epilepsy discharges on the side of the affected hemisphere or between bilateral hemispheres that involve multiple sites, and the timing and location of the clinical seizures and the EEG epilepsy discharge were closely related. Coppola [67] divided the natural course of EIMFS into approximately three phases. The first phase of the EEG shows a diffuse slowing of the background activity at the interphase of the attack, and the slow waves easily proceed from one brain hemisphere to the other. In the second phase, the ictal and interictal EEG performances always overlap. It can be the wandering focal discharge, but it can also simultaneously show local fixed discharge and new discharge in other areas. The third stage of EEG does not show special features.

Head MRI

The initial head MRI performed at onset is normal, but gradually becomes abnormal and is characterized by gradual cortical and subcortical atrophy. In the study by McTague and colleagues [77], the abnormal MRI findings were found in 8/14 patients, and the scan was normal in 4/8 at first. Seven cases of children (4 months–3.5 years) were characterized by diffuse cerebral atrophy, five cases of myelination delay were characterized by T2 hyperintensity of the deep white matter, and one case was characterized by symmetrical abnormal signals in the bilateral putamen and caudate nuclei.

4.3.1.5 Treatments

AEDs

EIMFS is an intractable epilepsy syndrome. Most children do not respond to many types of AEDs, either single drugs or a combination of old and new AEDs. Thus, the attacks are not easily controlled, particularly in the "flurry stage" [76].

Drug Combination Therapy

Bromide

Clinicians have utilized a combination of AEDs and bromide. The therapeutic dosage is 30–80 mg/kg/d, and the best bromide treatment concentration is 75–125 mg/dL [78]. The side effects mainly include vomiting, drowsiness, and skin rashes, but a reduction in the bromide dosage can eliminate these side effects. Caraballo et al. [78] examined six patients with drug-resistant EIFMS who suffered from daily attacks and were treated with the combination of potassium bromide with AEDs for 0.5–5 years. The seizure frequency was significantly reduced in four children, and two cases were invalids. After an average follow-up of 3.5 years, the seizure frequency did not change in the four children, and good nerve examination results were obtained.

Quinidine

The most common etiology of EIFMS is that a KCNT1 mutation enhances channel activity. The anti-arrhythmic drug of quinidine is partial KCNT1 antagonists; thus, quinidine significantly reduces the seizure frequency and improves mental and motor development. Bearden and colleagues [79] reported one case study of a 3-year-old child with drug-resistant EIFMS who was still suffering from uncontrollable and suffocating attacks after being treated with a variety of AEDS and a ketogenic diet. Without changing the original treatment, the addition of quinidine dosages that gradually increased from 2 to 33 mg/kg/d stopped the attacks after 1 week of maintenance dose treatment. The seizure cessation persisted for 6 months. When seizures recurred, the child was treated with 42 mg/kg/d quinidine for 7 months and was again seizure free and did not experience side effects. As shown in the study by Milligan and colleagues [80], quinidine significantly decreases the increased KCNT1 function, supporting the hypothesis that quinidine effectively inhibits KCNT1 and treats EIFMS.

Ketogenic Diet

In addition, early ketogenic diet therapy may help reduce the seizure frequency and severity in children and control SE, thus avoiding progressive cognitive impairment. Caraballo and colleagues [81] treated three sick children with a ketogenic diet over 7 months. The seizure frequency was reduced obviously, including one child with a seizure reduction of 75–99%, one child with a seizure reduction of <50%, and one child with seizure-free. Their neuropsychological performance also improved significantly.

4.3.1.6 SE in EIMFS

Age of SE Onset

SE is most commonly present in the "stormy phase" from 1 month to 1 year of age in patients with EIMFS. SE also occasionally occurs in other stages. Cilio and colleagues [75] reported a case study of two children with EIMFS whose RSE onset ages were 2 months and 9 months, respectively.

Types of SE

Patients with EIMFS SE experience various types of attacks and often present a variety of overlapping attack types, including generalized tonic-clonic SE, laterality clonic SE, myoclonus SE, partial SE, and mixed seizures SE [75, 82].

Treatment

Children with EIMFS readily develop RSE that failed to respond to traditional AEDs such as clonazepam, phenobarbital, phenytoin, midazolam, and lamotrigine. Cilio and colleagues [75] reported a case study of two children with EIMFS occurred RSE which did not respond to a variety of AEDs, including sedation anesthetic drugs, biotin, and hormones. After an intravenous loading dose of 60 mg/kg levetiracetam for 30 min and a subsequent intravenous administration of 30 mg/kg levetiracetam for 15 min twice a day, the seizure was controlled. The infusions were gradually replaced by an oral levetiracetam treatment and maintained for a long time. Ultimately, the two patients did not present with SE in the follow-up. Shein et al. [82] reported one case in which SCN1A mutations caused EIMFS in children with RSE against midazolam, levetiracetam, barbitone, pyridoxal, and folic acid. Then the child gradually used unconventional treatments. The patient firstly used a low-temperature treatment that maintained the target rectal temperature (target temperature 33.0–34.0 °C) and the seizures terminated after 43 h. However, 10 h after the return to the normal temperature, seizures recurred and have been ineffective to the low-temperature treatment. The following treatment of bumetanide did not show an obvious curative effect. Within 48 h after the initiation of a ketogenic diet, the attacks were controlled. Based on this case report, low-temperature treatments and ketogenic diets are effective treatments for RSE.

4.3.1.7 Prognosis

Generally, the short- and long-term prognosis of children with EIMFS is poor. Children with EIMFS tend to develop SE which the traditional AEDs and narcotic drugs are ineffective. The disease is not easily controlled and ultimately develops into RSE, which has a high mortality rate. Most surviving children have a gradual regression of intelligence and motor development. The psychomotor ability is poor in many children, and they inevitably develop disturbance intelligence [67, 76].

4.3.2 Dravet Syndrome

4.3.2.1 Historical Evolution

Dravet syndrome was previously designated severe myoclonic epilepsy in infancy (SMEI); the disease was first reported in 1978 by the

French doctor Dravet. It is an infantile form of epileptic encephalopathy and a type of refractory epilepsy syndrome [83, 84].

4.3.2.2 Potential Etiology

Mutations in the SCN1A gene cause Dravet syndrome in approximately 70–80% of children [83]. A few, restricted cases were reported in children from a few women with disease-causing mutations in genes encoding the original calcium mucin PCDH19. The other genes as well as the SCN2A, GABRG2, GABRA1, and STXBP2 genes are also discovered in a few patients [85–89].

4.3.2.3 Clinical Features

The onset time is within 1 year after birth and the peak age at 6 months. After childhood, the seizure frequency and severity are significantly reduced. The first attack is often associated with persistent fever or febrile convulsion. Various types of attacks are present, including generalized seizures, laterality clonic seizures, tonic-clonic seizures, myoclonic seizures, atypical absence seizures, and partial seizures [83, 84, 90–92].

4.3.2.4 Progression

Dravet et al. [93] summarize the natural course of Dravet syndrome, which is divided into approximately three stages. (1) The first stage is the "febrile stage" within 1 year old. It usually occurs at 4–8 months in a baby experiencing a fever or a normal baby. Typical attacks are tonic seizures; the duration is usually long for more than 15 min. The attacks can develop into SE. Two weeks to 2 months after the initial attack, other seizures occur and are repeated, even in statuses. (2) The second stage is the "worsening stage." More of these types of seizures occur in 1- to 4-year-olds and present as many types of frequent epileptic seizures and statuses: transient myoclonus seizures, atypical absence seizures, focal seizures, and autonomic nerve symptoms. Then, psychomotor development began to slow, and attention deficits, hyperactivity, and autism can also appear. This stage lasts from 1 to 5 years old approximately. (3) The third stage is the "stabilization stage." It typically occurs in children older than 5 years of age. The convulsive epilepsy frequency reduces and occurs mainly in sleep. Simultaneously, motor development and behavior improve, but the cognitive impairment continues.

4.3.2.5 Auxiliary Examination

An EEG performed before the age of 1 year appears grossly normal; after the age of 1 year, multiple atypical EEG patterns appear. The interictal background activity can be normal or slow. The ictal EEG performances are variable and they depend on the seizure type. The performances include generalized spike-waves, poly-spike-waves, focal waves, and multifocal waves. Photosensitivity is also frequent in patients with Dravet syndrome [84, 90, 93, 94]. Speechio and colleagues [95] studied the EEG performances of 22 children with Dravet syndrome over the first 5 years of diagnosis; the initial EEG background activities were normal in all patients. Twenty-seven percent of the children with Dravet syndrome exhibited a slowing of their EEG background activities after 6 months. The EEG appeared to show epileptic discharge at seizure onset in 27% of the patients. Sixty-four percent exhibited seizure discharges within 5 years of follow-up, 57% of children exhibited multifocal epilepsy discharges during follow-up, 28.5% exhibited focal epilepsy discharges, and 14% exhibited generalized epilepsy discharges.

4.3.2.6 Treatments

Most children do not respond to a variety of single or combinations of AEDs [91, 92, 96].

Drug Treatment

Drug treatment often requires several medicines. Wallace et al. [97] summarized the drugs used to treat Dravet syndrome, and the main first-line drugs are listed below. (1) Valproic acid is typically at an initial dosage of 10–15 mg/kg/day and gradually increased to 30–60 mg/kg/day for maintenance treatment. Liver enzyme levels, routine blood tests, and blood lipid levels should be examined periodically during treatment. Common side effects include hair loss, thrombocytopenia, pancreatitis, and high blood ammonia levels. (2) Clobazam is usually used at an initial dosage of 0.2–0.3 mg/kg/day. Within 2–3 weeks, the dosage is gradually increased to 0.5–1.0 mg/kg/day, with a maximum dosage of 1.5–2.0 mg/kg/day, but the side effects (e.g., sedation, ataxia, increased saliva secretion) also increase as the dosage is increased. When used in conjunction with stiripentol, the clobazam dosage must usually be reduced to 0.20–0.4 mg/kg/day. In addition, second-line drugs include topiramate, stiripentol, levetiracetam, and bromide.

Ketogenic Diet

For GTCS and myoclonic seizures, a ketogenic diet can significantly reduce the frequency of attacks, and children had similar reactions to stiripentol, a ketogenic diet, clobazam, and valproic acid. Dressler and colleagues [98] who retrospectively analyzed 39 children with Dravet syndrome who used a ketogenic diet reported that the 3-month treatment response was 70%, the GTCS and myoclonic seizures occurred in children less frequently, and SE was not observed. The children generally had a good tolerance, with no obvious side effects.

Surgery

Vagus nerve stimulation (VNS) and corpus callosum dissection can effectively reduce the attack frequency in patients with Dravet syndrome, and the sooner operation occurs, the greater benefit to the patients. Dlouhy and colleagues [99] retrospectively investigated patients with Dravet syndrome who underwent VNS or corpus callosum dissection therapy in hospital from 2001 to 2014.VNS reduced the seizure frequency by more than 50% in 4/6 patients, and corpus callosum dissection reduced the frequency of attacks by over 50% in 2/6 patients, indicating that VNS and corpus callosum dissection therapies effectively reduce the frequency of attacks.

4.3.2.7 Prognosis

The overall morbidity and mortality is high. Normal intelligence and motor development are observed during the first year after birth. However, psychomotor development is gradually delayed and regresses, and ataxia and pyramidal tract occur. According to the study of Shmuely et al., the mortality of patients with Dravet syndrome was 80% (142/177). The death occurs at a mean age of 8.7 ± 9.8 years in 142 patients, and 73% death occurs before 10 years. Epilepsy-associated (sudden unexpected death in epilepsy and SE) deaths accounted for 81% of all deaths [84].

4.3.2.8 SE in Patients with Dravet Syndrome

Patients with Dravet syndrome readily develop SE. Most infants and young children with Dravet syndrome experience febrile or nonfebrile SE. In cases with fever, repeated attacks occur and RSE and super-RSE typically develop, which have a high mortality rate [90, 91].

Prevalence

According to the literature, the morbidity of SE in patients with Dravet syndrome is approximately 70–90% [83, 90, 94]. Tanabe and colleagues [90] retrospectively analyzed 109 patients with SMEI (male/female = 51:58), aged 1–37 (10.7 ± 6.53) years in two medical centers, including 99 patients with convulsive status epilepticus (CSE), and reported a morbidity of 90.8%.

Onset Age

The majority of patients developed SE during infancy or early childhood. Ragona et al. studied 26 patients of Dravet syndrome, and 21occured SE. The number of episodes of SE was 0–7 (1.8 ± 1.7) before 18 months. The peak age of onset of SE is 6–18 months [100]. SE was reduced in older children and teenagers [101]. Tanabe and colleagues [90] retrospectively analyzed 99 patients with SMEI. The first onset of CSE was 1–15 years old (4.25 ± 3.79), and repeated episodes were subsequently observed. The vast majority of SE cases were induced by fever and readily developed into RSE, nonfebrile SE was observed rarely.

Seizure Types

Generalized tonic-clonic SE, laterality clonic SE, atypical absence SE, myoclonic SE, and NCSE can all occur, but the first two attack forms are the most common [91]. NCSE was not frequently observed; it is generally not life-threatening, but it does cause obvious brain damage. Once a definitive diagnosis is made, the seizures should be able to be controlled immediately [83].

Auxiliary Examination

In head MRIs, children with Dravet syndrome who repeatedly present with SE may show an involvement of the hippocampus and non-specific brain atrophy [90].

Treatments

In patients with Dravet syndrome, particularly effective, targeted therapies are not currently available for SE and RSE, and the traditional treatments are still being utilized to control seizures, support vital signs, and manage related complications simultaneously. Tanabe and colleagues [90] retrospectively analyzed the SE of 99 patients with an SMEI. The authors believed that once SE occurred, an intravenous antiepileptic medicine should be rapidly administered whether a fever is observed. The most effective drug is barbitone (including phenobarbital, thiopental sodium, and pentobarbital), and its efficiency can reach 75–100%. Benzodiazepines, such as midazolam and diazepam, are the second effective, with efficacies of 68.8 and 54.3%, respectively. Sometimes, various drugs must be combined to treat RSE. Fever-induced SE tends to develop into RSE, the attacks persist for a long time, and treatments such as benzodiazepines do not prevent its occurrence [90]. A variety of AEDs or anesthetics are ineffective. Coma is often observed after seizures are controlled, and this type of SE may cause acute encephalopathy [90, 102, 103].

Prognosis

The overall prognosis of SE in patients with Dravet syndrome is poor, due to the inefficiency of drug control; the frequent development of RSE and super-RSE can be seen. Fever-induced SE is particularly easy to be resistant to treatment. Serious brain damage, mental decline, and even death often occur [90, 104]; however, some patients in recovery stages show different sequelae, like serious disturbances in eye contact and active language and loss of self-care ability. According to a previous study [105], the causes of death in 59 patients with SE were studied. The cause of 21 (36%) children was acute encephalopathy with SE, with the complications of multiple organ failure, DIC, and other severe complications. The duration and frequency of the early onset of SE are extremely important factors that influence the prognosis of children with Dravet syndrome [85, 105].

4.3.3 Genetic Generalized Epilepsy (GGE)

4.3.3.1 Definition

Genetic generalized epilepsy, also known as idiopathic generalized epilepsy (IGE), is a series of epilepsy syndrome that does not present damage to the brain structure or other symptoms and signs of nerve damage; clinical manifestations and EEG changes show the initiation of bilateral seizures. It is considered a genetic disease that often depends on age [106–111]. The ILAE [60, 107] lists the following syndromes that are consistent with the IGE standards:(1) juvenile myoclonic epilepsy (JME), (2) benign myoclonic epilepsy in infancy (BMEI), (3) childhood absence epilepsy (CAE), (4) epilepsy with myoclonic absences (EMA), (5) epilepsy with generalized tonic-clonic seizures (EGTCS) alone, and (6) juvenile absence epilepsy (JAE). Of course, some epilepsy syndromes are consistent with IGE but might not have been recognized by ILAE [112]. Different syndromes exhibit different clinical characteristics (e.g., onset age, type of epilepsy, treatment), EEG, and imaging findings. Each syndrome has strict clinical and EEG diagnostic criteria, but the outbreak types of this syndrome and onset age can overlap; thus, the syndrome may be difficult to distinguish in the early stage as the absence of characteristic manifestations [106, 110, 111].

4.3.3.2 Prevalence

Jallon et al. [113] summarize the IGE epidemiological data and reported an all-estimate incidence of IGE in epilepsy of 15–20%. Asadi-Pooya and colleagues [111] retrospectively analyzed the data of 2190 patients with epilepsy, including 442 diagnosed with IGE, at a school of medicine from September 2008 to May 2011. IGE morbidity was 20.2% in this study.

4.3.3.3 Onset Age

IGE has a wide range of age of onset and includes infants, children, adolescents, and adults. Different IGE syndromes are often age dependent. Asadi-Pooya and colleagues [111] retrospectively analyzed 442 patients with IGE (190 males and 252 females). The onset age ranged from 6 months to 54 years old, and the average age was 12.4 ± 6.9 years.

4.3.3.4 Seizure Types

The seizure types include GTCS, myoclonic seizures, absence seizures, clonic seizures, and myoclonic-astatic seizures [106]. IGE has different attack types in different syndromes, but attack types may also overlap. One large clinical study [111] described a retrospective analysis of 442 patients with IGE of the epileptic seizure type, of which 375 (84.8%) patients experienced GTCS, 250 patients (56.6%) developed myoclonic seizures, 211 (47.7%) patients presented absence seizures, and rare attack types included three myoclonic-astatic seizures and one clonic seizure.

4.3.3.5 SE in Patients with GGE

SE can occur in all seven syndromes of IGE, and different syndromes have different types of attacks, but the type of the SE attack can overlap. Studies examining the SE-induced morbidity of different syndromes of IGE [114] are currently lacking.

Prevalence

The overall SE-induced morbidity of patients with IGE is not clear, but the morbidity of tonic-clonic SE in patients with IGE is significantly lower than in patients with symptomatic epilepsy [114]. In the retrospective study by Asadi-Pooya et al. [111] of 442 patients with IGE from 2008 to 2011, only 16 (3.6%) patients presented with GCSE, and one patient presented with NCSE; thus, the morbidity of SE was lower.

Triggers

Sometimes SE in patients with IGE is induced by external environmental factors, such as inappropriate medication, drug withdrawal, or poisoning; this state is mainly typical absence SE [115]. In the study by Thomas and colleagues [116], SE was caused by the inadequate use of AEDs in 14 patients with IGE (15–46 years old, seven males and seven females). Before referral, all patients had taken carbamazepine for treatment and recently suffered seizure aggravation or emerging seizure type. Seven patients were taking carbamazepine combined with other drugs, including phenytoin, gabapentin, and vigabatrin. The potential induced factors included: increasing the dose of carbamazepine or the doses of carbamazepine together with phenytoin; initiation of carbamazepine, gabapentin, or vigabatrin; or decreasing the dose of phenobarbital. Finally, ten patients presented with absence SE and four with myoclonus SE. After adjusting the therapeutic schedule and drug dosages, SE was completely controlled in all patients. Thus, patients with IGE who use AEDs inappropriately can aggravate their seizures and even present SE.

SE Types and Characteristics

The three types of epilepsy in IGE include myoclonic seizures, GTCS, and absence seizures, which can present as acute SE and require emergent treatment [117].

Typical Absence SE

This seizure type belongs to NCSE, is the most common form of SE in patients with IGE, and often occurs in normally developing children. Different subtypes of IGE have different occurrence rates of typical absence SE. Typical absence SE occurs among JAE and JME in particular. The incidence of absence SE in JME was 1.2–6.7% [118, 119]. Typical absence SE should be distinguished from atypical absence SE and complex partial SE. The three kinds of SE symptoms overlap, but the episodes have different EEG findings, reactions to drugs, and prognoses [114]. (1) The pathogenesis of absence SE is currently unknown, but genetic factors and environmental factors may have roles. Clear evidence supporting the hypothesis that absence SE can lead to brain damage is not available [114], and studies have reported that absence SE was not detected of brain injury in animal models; thus, excessive interventions are not performed [120, 121]. However, clinical researchers postulate that absence SE presents as acute SE requires emergent treatment [117]. (2) Predisposing factors include a strong light stimulus, fatigue, mood changes, reducing the dosage or stopping the use of AEDs, and inappropriate medication (e.g., carbamazepine, sabril, thiamethoxam) [114, 116]. Absence SE can appear after seizures, and GTCS can interrupt or terminate a typical absence SE [114]. (3) The clinical manifestations include confusion, decreased activity, open silence, and disorientation. Patients may experience other concomitant symptoms, such as slight myoclonic seizures, rhythmic eyelid blinking, facial and oral jitter, and attacks. Absence SE lasts more than 30 min and sustains for several hours or even days [114, 115, 117]. (4) The ictal EEG performances are characterized by trains of 3 Hz spike and waves; the interictal background activity can be normal.

Myoclonus SE

This type is rarely observed in patients with IGE [122]; it mostly occurs in patients with JME and always in the waking state and relatively in patients with EMA [122, 123]. Myoclonus SE usually adopts the form of a myoclonic seizure storm, with an aggravated severity and an increased frequency of myoclonus, and finally SE is achieved. The seizures are sustained for a few minutes to several hours, and myoclonus SE is often terminated by a tonic-clonic seizure. The incidence rate of myoclonus SE in patients with IGE is not yet clear, but we assume that it is significantly lower than the incidence rate in Dravet syndrome, Doose syndrome, and progressive myoclonus epilepsy [114].

Tonic-Clonic SE

This type is rarely observed in IGE but is more common in secondary generalized epilepsy. If a sudden drug withdrawal occurs, SE may be induced [114]. The incidence of tonic-clonic SE in patients with IGE in clinical practice has not been reported, and published data are lacking. In a study of 554 patients with tonic-clonic SE, obvious acute cause was not found in 11% of the patients. However, in the 11% cases, most would not now be diagnosed as IGE.

Treatments

Regardless of the SE type, benzodiazepines should be used as first-line treatments and often work [124].

Typical Absence SE Therapy

Bilo et al. [125] reviewed previous studies of patients with a diagnosis of IGE and presented with absence SE. Good curative effects of intravenously administered benzodiazepines were observed in patients with absence SE. The initial treatment was diazepam with a conventional dose of 0.2–0.3 mg/kg, clonazepam 1 mg in adult and 0.25–0.5 mg in children, or lorazepam 0.07 mg/kg in adult and 0.1 mg/kg in children. If needed, the drugs may be repeatedly administered. If the patient becomes an invalid, 20–40 mg/kg valproic acid was intravenously administered. If children experience repeated seizures at home, benzodiazepines should be administered orally or rectally to the terminate attacks. Patients should be seen by a doctor in the hospital when necessary [114, 118, 125].

Therapy for Myoclonus SE

Badhwar et al. [122] reviewed previous studies of patients diagnosed with IGE presented with myoclonic SE and suggested that benzodiazepines, such as clonazepam, should be used as the initial therapy. If SE was not terminated, the efficiency of secondary use of benzodiazepines was not sufficient. Then the authors recommended a high loading dose of intravenous valproic acid to quickly achieve the therapeutic level [126]. Sheth and colleagues [124] reported two cases of female patients with JME (15 and 28 years); myoclonic SE was finally terminated with a slow intravenous injection of 500 mg of valproic acid in 30 min. After this treatment, SE was terminated in both patients within 5 min, and the EEG performance returned to normal.

Therapy for Tonic-Clonic SE

In patients with IGE, the frequency of myoclonic seizures often increases before the onset of tonic-clonic SE. The emergency administration of benzodiazepines will often prevent the development of SE. Tonic-clonic SE is usually easily controlled in patients with IGE compared with patients with other types of epilepsy, and an aesthetic therapy is rarely needed [114].

Prognosis

Although the clinical symptoms of the same type of SE attacks in different types of IGE can be similar, the curative effects on different syndromes are different, and thus the patients' prognoses are different [106, 110, 114]. In general, benzodiazepines effectively prevent SE, with less morbidity of refractory SE.

4.3.4 Panayiotopoulos Syndrome

4.3.4.1 Historical Evolution

PS is an age-related benign focal epilepsy occurring in childhood that primarily manifest as autonomic seizures. Relevant studies of the disease were reported as early as 1989, but the ILAE formally accepted it as a separate electroclinical syndrome in 2001 [127]. The early stage of PS is also known as benign occipital lobe epilepsy in children, but for some children with epilepsy, EEG discharge does not occur in occipital region. Therefore, the ILAE officially changed its name to Panayiotopoulos syndrome in 2010 [60].

4.3.4.2 Clinical Manifestation

Onset Age

The age of onset is generally 1–14 years old, the age of highest morbidity is 4–5 years old, and 76% of children have an age of onset of 3–6 years old [128]. Degerliyurt and colleagues [129] conducted a follow-up study of 38 patients with Panayiotopoulos syndrome and showed that 87% of children had an age of onset before the age of 8, and the average age at first onset was 4.6 years old.

Seizure Types

This type of seizure is associated with autonomic symptoms. As shown in the study by Degerliyurt et al. [129], the most common symptoms included episodic vomiting, eye or head deviation, and altered consciousness. Twenty-six percent of children had rolandic features, 5% had visual symptoms, and 81.5% had sleep-related seizures.

Seizure Characteristics

Seizures mainly occur in sleep, particularly in the early stage of the sleep cycle, and seizures only occur during sleep in two-thirds of patients. Febrile convulsions are relatively typical characteristics of attacks. Patients start with cluster of vomiting, accompanied by changes in the face (e.g., pale, cyanosis, and blush), pupil changes (see scattered mostly), cardiopulmonary and thermoregulatory anomalies (such as difficulty in breathing and changes in the heart rate and rhythm), cough, bowel function changes, incontinence, headache, eye skewed to one side, and side deflection of the head. Children are conscious in the early stage of the attack. With the development of epilepsy, confusion and dullness can occur in children [127–136].

4.3.4.3 Auxiliary Examination

Interictal EEG showed multifocal or wandering discharges, with a significant occipital feature; sleep can induce seizures or seizures may only appear during sleep [127, 128, 136]. However, with increasing age, the discharge is moved forward, and the parietal, frontal, and temporal lobes may be involved [137]. Diffuse discharge may also be the only EEG performance observed throughout the course of the disease or develop into focal discharge gradually. Carabolla and colleagues [138] retrospectively analyzed nine cases with typical clinical manifestations of Panayiotopoulos syndrome and found that the EEG performances of all children during the initial awake period and sleep stage were diffuse spike and slow waves. During sleep, three patients presented focal spikes in the occipital, frontal, and temporo-occipital regions, respectively.

4.3.4.4 Treatments

No widely accepted therapy guidelines exist, and sufficient evidence about the effectiveness of specific AEDs is not available. As Panayiotopoulos syndrome is a benign syndrome, drug therapy should mainly pay attention to avoiding the side effects of drugs. Fewer studies of multidrug treatments have been reported [127, 136]. Carbamazepine and valproic acid therapies are more common in the clinic, but carbamazepine has also been reported to aggravate the patient's condition. Kikumoto and colleagues [139] reported one case study of a 4-year-old boy with Panayiotopoulos syndrome who experienced a newly developed myoclonic seizures and absence seizures after treatment with carbamazepine. His EEG began to deteriorate as well. The absence seizure stopped, and the EEG returned to normal after he stopped the carbamazepine treatment. Levetiracetam is also a potentially effective AED. Garcia et al. [140] reported a study of three patients with Panayiotopoulos syndrome treated with levetiracetam. The three patients had autonomic symptoms for 2–6 years and relapsed quickly after seizures were controlled with valproic acid. However, after the administration of an initial dosage of 1000–2000 mg/d levetiracetam followed by a gradual increase in dosage and a subsequent change to a single-drug treatment of levetiracetam, the children did not experience seizures for 2–3 years, and one patient did not experience seizures when the drug was withdrawn after 2-year treatment of levetiracetam.

4.3.4.5 SE in Panayiotopoulos Syndrome

Definition

In Panayiotopoulos syndrome, SE is called "autonomic status epilepticus" and belongs to NCSE. Experts have recently agreed that autonomic SE is defined as a seizure lasting for more than 30 min characterized by a change in any form of autonomic function in the early stage or a change in autonomic function that did not exist in the onset of the attack, but priority is given to autonomic function changes during the attack [133].

Duration

The outbreak of Panayiotopoulos syndrome usually lasts for 5–15 min; on average, 44% of the seizures last for 30 min to several hours (mean, 2 h) and up to 12 h. Therefore, nearly half of all attacks conform to autonomic SE [127, 128, 132, 135, 136]. Lada and colleagues [132] retrospectively analyzed 43 patients with Panayiotopoulos syndrome; the epileptic seizure lasted for more than 30 min in 46.5% of patients who were diagnosed with autonomic SE. The same children may exhibit brief attacks and can present longstanding seizures; the autonomic symptoms may or may not be obvious. However, even when experiencing the most severe and longest attack, children will fully recover to normal after a few hours of sleep [133].

Seizure Types

Most of these seizures exhibit autonomic symptoms. Studies have proposed that CSE is a manifestation of Panayiotopoulos syndrome. CSE mainly occurs at the beginning of Panayiotopoulos syndrome and is a rare type. Verrotti and colleagues [141] compared patients without CSE with patients with CSE and found that patients with Panayiotopoulos syndrome exhibited an average age of CSE onset of 6.5 years and that generalized tonic seizures were the most common type. One-third of the patients with CSE were admitted to the ICU, but the overall prognosis of patients is good, and the children's epilepsy was ultimately terminated at the last follow-up.

Treatments

Panayiotopoulos syndrome in which autonomic SE occurs should be treated [128, 134, 136] and terminated as early as possible. According to Lada and colleagues [132], intravenous, rectal, or oral benzodiazepines (such as diazepam, etc.) are an acceptable therapeutic method to stop attacks. Family therapy early after onset might be more effective than emergency room treatment. Therefore, parents should place children in a side-lying position, maintain airway patency, and administer benzodiazepines via the oral or rectal route. The efficacy of anti-nausea drugs for recurrent vomiting is not clear. Dehydration due to repeated vomiting should be corrected [136].

Prognosis

Although automatic SE of Panayiotopoulos syndrome has a high morbidity, Panayiotopoulos syndrome still is a benign form of epilepsy, and the general prognosis is good [127, 136]. However, a few patients still exhibit neuropsychological damage, and thus SE should be terminated as soon as possible to obtain a better prognosis. Kanemura and colleagues [142] prospectively studied six patients with Panayiotopoulos syndrome and found that after SE the children's frontal lobe and prefrontal lobes grew more slowly, the ratio of the prefrontal/frontal lobe volumes stagnated for some time, and performance on neuropsychological tests was reduced in the SE group, suggesting that in some patients with Panayiotopoulos syndrome, SE is related to a developmental delay of the prefrontal lobe and causes neuropsychological problems.

4.3.5 Epilepsy with Myoclonic-Atonic Seizures (EMAS)

4.3.5.1 Historical Evolution

EMAS was first reported by the German doctor Hermann Doose in 1970; thus, EMAS is also known as Doose syndrome. It was formerly designated as myoclonic-astatic epilepsy or myoclonic-atonic epilepsy (MAE), and ILAE renamed the disease EMAS in 2010 [143].

4.3.5.2 Potential Etiology

The etiology is related to heredity mainly, and the pathogenic genes include SCN1A, SCN2A, SCN1B, GABRG2, SLC2A1, CHD2, and SLC6A1 [144–148].

4.3.5.3 Clinical Manifestations

Onset Age

This disease primarily occurs in children between 7 months and 6 years old, generally between 3 and 4 years. The incidence is significantly higher in boys than in girls. In this disease, children always exhibit normal development before disease onset, without organic nervous system diseases [143, 149]. Kilaru et al. [150] conducted a follow-up study of 23 children with EMAS (19 males), with an average follow-up time of 38 months. Thirty-nine percent of the children had a history of febrile convulsions and a family history of epilepsy. The average onset age of seizures was 36 (2–86) months.

Seizure Types

The types of seizures include GTCS, myoclonic seizures, atonic seizures, myoclonic-atonic seizures, atypical absence seizures, tonic seizures, and clonic seizures. Most children initially present with GTCS at the onset, followed by other types of seizures. In the first few months, seizures are very frequent and primarily occur in the daytime [143, 149].

Progression

Febrile seizures can occur a few months before nonfebrile seizures. The seizure frequency gradually increases within an average time of 3 months, and then a variety of types of seizures occur. Children may have ataxia, but show no abnormalities in a neurological examination. Myoclonic-atonic seizures and mild clonic seizures primarily occur over the next few months. One-third of children still experienced a large number of myoclonic seizures and GTCS during puberty. Although these children exhibit good cognitive function, dyspraxia with poor manual dexterity still occurs [151].

4.3.5.4 Auxiliary Examination

The EEG is normal (or a θ rhythm is observed in the background) in the early stage, and then 2–3 Hz spike-waves and poly-spike-waves are observed at every lead, but focal discharges are not observed [143, 149]. Oguni et al. [149] conducted a case study of 30 patients with MAE who were divided into clonus and atonic groups. The ictal EEG showed generalized spike-waves and poly-spike-waves in all patients. In the atonic group, the morphological characteristics of the spike-waves are positive-negative-deep-positive waves and later with large negative slow waves, but no significant difference in EEG characteristics was observed between the two groups.

4.3.5.5 Treatments

EMAS is difficult to treat. Thus, clinicians strive for early detection and early treatment.

AEDs

In single-drug treatments, valproic acid is the first-line drug. If valproic acid is invalid, other drugs could replace it according to the seizure types. The combination drug therapies of valproic acid combined with lamotrigine or valproic acid combined with ethosuximide are effective [144]. Lamotrigine should be avoided when myoclonic seizures are the main type of seizures because it may exacerbate the condition. In addition, the concentration of lamotrigine should be increased slowly to avoid rash, and patients should be observed for at least 6 weeks [152]. Levetiracetam and zonisamide are also potentially effective drugs but have not been tested in experiments [151]. Levetiracetam has not been extensively studied as a treatment for EMAS. In the study by Kilaru et al. [150], only one patient treated with levetiracetam was seizure-free for less than 6 months. When using AEDs, clinicians should pay attention to carbamazepine, phenytoin, oxcarbazepine, and aminocaproic acid, because these drugs may exacerbate the seizures [152].

Ketogenic Diet

The most effective treatment is thought to be the ketogenic diet, followed by ACTH and ethosuximide. Oguni et al. [153] conducted a retrospective investigation of 81 patients with EMAS, and when a ketogenic diet was used to treat EMAS in 26 patients, 58% ($n = 15$) of the patients were seizure-free, 35% ($n = 9$) of the patients experienced at least 50% relief, and the remaining patients ($n = 2$) experienced slight relief. The early implementation of the ketogenic diet can exert greater benefits on EMAS. However, it is still very effective as a final step.

Hormone Therapy

Glucocorticoids, particularly ACTH and dexamethasone, were the first reported treatment. Doose et al. [154] first proposed that 1 mg/kg dexamethasone or 80 IU of ACTH could be used to control seizures. Oguni et al. [153] conducted a retrospective investigation of 81 patients with EMAS, and when ACTH was used to treat EMAS in 22 patients, eight patients were seizure-free, five patients experienced at least 50% relief, and the remaining patients ($n = 8$) experienced slight relief. The main limitations of hormone therapy are recurrence after withdrawal and side effects after long-term use.

4.3.5.6 SE in EMAS

Types of SE

Atypical Absence SE

Atypical absence SE is the most common type and manifests prolonged chaotic consciousness, indifferent expression, reduced movements lasting for hours to days or even weeks, or recurrence within 1–2 years [143].

Mixed SE

When a typical SE occurs, myoclonus or frequent atonic seizures may occur simultaneously [143]. Deng et al. [155] summarized the clinical features of 48 children with EMAS, seven (14.6%) of whom had a history of SE, and six patients had mixed atypical absence and myoclonic SE that manifested as prolonged chaotic consciousness, indifferent expression, reduced movements, and multifocal, nonrhythmic facial or limb muscle twitching, such as blinking, arched eyebrow, or sudden jitter of limbs.

NCSE

Caraballo et al. [156] reported a case study of 69 children with EMAS, 20 (29%) of whom had NCSE characterized by trance and indifferent expression that was accompanied by facial and limb myoclonus lasting for 2 h to several days. Trivisano et al. [157] reported a case study of 18 children with this disease, and three (16.7%) had NCSE.

Others

Grande-Martin et al. [158] reported a case in which valproic acid induced tonic SE in one child with this disease. Deng et al. [155] summarized the clinical features of 48 children with EMAS, and one child had atonic SE, which was manifested as frequent falls and an inability to maintain the standing posture.

Treatments

The most effective treatment for persistent myoclonus is the ketogenic diet, followed by glucocorticoid therapy. Benzodiazepines are effective, particularly in an acute administration, but the drug should be slowly withdrawn to prevent relapse [151]. Based on the study by Oguni et al. [159], the most effective treatment for EMAS was the ketogenic diet, followed by ACTH and ethosuximide. This study also supports the hypothesis proposed by Doose that ethosuximide is the most favorable AED for EMAS, and ethosuximide combined with valproic acid can better control EASM.

Prognosis

The course of EMAS is difficult to predict, and its prognosis thus changes substantially. Cognition may be normal, but serious mental impairments may also occur. In general, 30–50% of patients have a good prognosis [157]. The frequent occurrence of SE is one of the important factors affecting the prognosis of EMAS [152]. In the study by Oguni et al. [153], 18% (15/81) of children with incomplete control exhibited a cognitive impairment. Half of the patients with a poor prognosis had recurrent NCSE with nocturnal tonic seizures. A family history of epilepsy and NCSE were risk factors for a poor prognosis.

4.3.6 Progressive Myoclonic Epilepsy (PME)

4.3.6.1 Definition

PME is a group of rare neurodegenerative diseases characterized by myoclonus, epilepsy, and progressive neurological deterioration. The etiology is a group of progressive neurological diseases [55, 160]. The disease first appeared in a case report by Lafora G. R. and Glueck B. published in 1911, the patient experienced disease onset as an adolescent, and development before onset was normal. After the onset, a progressive development of myoclonus and cognitive decline occurred, and this patient was ultimately confirmed to have autosomal recessive inherited progressive myoclonic epilepsy [161].

4.3.6.2 Common Etiology

Neuronal ceroid lipofuscinoses (NCLs), myoclonic epilepsy with ragged red fibers (MERRFs), Niemann-Pick disease type C (chronic neurological type), Gaucher disease type III (neuropathy type), sialic acid deposition disease (cherry erythema myoclonic syndrome), dento-rubro-pallido-luysian atrophy (DRPLA), Lafora disease, Unverricht-Lundborg disease (ULD), and the action myoclonus-renal failure (AMRF) syndrome are common forms of this disease. In these diseases, epilepsy is currently thought to be due to the accumulation of abnormal metabolites in cortical neurons [160, 162, 163].

4.3.6.3 Clinical Manifestations

Onset Age

This disease occurs from childhood to adolescence, and the age of onset of PME due to different causes may differ. For example, ULD begins at an age of 6–16 years, and AMRF syndrome begins at an age of 15–25 years [160, 162].

Seizure Types

These seizures are mainly generalized or partial myoclonic seizures that are manifested as irregular, non-synchronous, asymmetric seizures. Other types may include atonic seizures, GTCS, and absence seizures [160].

Common Clinical Manifestations

The majority of patients are healthy people with normal intelligence before disease onset. Neurological deterioration occurs during the course of the disease, including progressive cognitive decline, ataxia, neuropathy, and muscle lesions [160, 162].

4.3.6.4 Treatment and Progress

In the early stage of the disease, AEDs, such as valproic acid, clonazepam, and zonisamide, are effective at treating seizures. However, as the disease progresses, drug efficacy decreases, resistance to AEDs occurs, and this disease can develop into refractory epilepsy [55, 160–162, 164, 165].

4.3.6.5 Prognosis

Of the types of epilepsy, PME has a high morbidity and mortality. The prognosis depends on the specific disease, such as Lafora disease, NCL, and Gaucher disease type III. In the courses of these diseases, patient mortality is high and the prognosis is poor. In ULD, which progresses slowly, appropriate treatment can allow many patients to achieve a normal life [160].

4.3.6.6 SE in PME

Based on some cases and series of reports [55, 161, 162], the initial onset of SE in patients with PME usually occurs when patients gradually achieve drug resistance. At this time, SE readily recurs and drug-resistant SE is commonly observed.

Age of Onset

PME is a group of rare genetic diseases. Currently, a small number of reports of SE in patients with PME have been published; therefore, the statistical data for the age of onset are not available. In these patients, SE appears more frequently after the first epileptic seizure and tends to occur in patients with drug-resistant epilepsy. Miyahara et al. [55] retrospectively analyzed nine patients with PME (six males and three females) with RSE. All patients with PME were treated with AEDs in the early stage, and a good effect was achieved. Subsequently, PME was progressed to drug-resistant epilepsy and recurrent SE; continually RSE developed. The age of RSE onset in these nine patients was 3–28 years, all within 2–21 years after the onset of the initial seizure in patients with PME.

Seizure Types

Myoclonic SE is the main type, but NCSE, generalized CSE, myoclonic-generalized SE, etc. can also occur [55, 164–166]. Miyahara et al. [55] retrospectively analyzed nine patients with PME and RSE. The etiology was two NCL, one MELAS, one Gaucher disease type III, two DRPLA, and three with unknown etiology. The SE types included three cases of myoclonic SE, four cases of myoclonic-generalized status epilepticus (MGSE), and two cases of generalized SE. Lopez-Meza et al. [166] reported two patients with PME caused by Lafora disease, all of which manifested as NCSE. Before admission to the hospital, these two female patients experienced repeated myoclonic seizures, complex partial seizures, generalized seizures, and a continuous deterioration neuropsychological function lasting for 2 and 8 years, respectively. After admission, EEG showed signs of NCSE. In one patient, SE was controlled by a single-drug treatment and neuropsychological function recovered. The other patient gradually progressed from NCSE to generalized CSE during hospitalization and became resistance to anticonvulsant drugs; this patient required long-term treatment in the ICU.

Treatment

Because of the multiple etiologies and complexity of PME [160], only a few reported case studies of SE in patients with PME are available [55, 161, 165, 166]. Currently, a specific, effective treatment for PME is not available. Clinically, the treatment includes AEDs to control SE, life support, and prevention and treatment of complications.

Miyahara et al. [55] retrospectively analyzed nine patients with PME and RSE (11–34 years, six males and three females), all of whom were in the progressive phase of PME, indicating a decrease in the efficacy of AEDs and the emergence of drug-resistant epilepsy. In these patients, persistent myoclonic and/or generalized seizures lasted for more than 30 min. All patients were administered an intravenous bolus or continuous intravenous infusion of benzodiazepines or barbiturates, but seizures were not terminated and developed into RSE. After the failure of the BDZ and barbiturate treatment, nine patients were administered a slow intravenous injection of 10–15 mg/kg phenytoin. For patients who were orally administered phenytoin, the intravenous injection dose should be 100–250 mg (<3 mg/kg). Phenytoin was effective in seven patients, and the other two patients continued using midazolam or barbiturate before SE terminated (one patient required assisted ventilation). All patients with SE were orally administered phenytoin (5–14 mg/kg/d) after the termination of SE to prevent recurrence. In the follow-up, SE did not recur in three patients, and SE was not observed in two patients within 4 years. The seizure frequency was significantly reduced in two patients, and phenytoin was effective in six patients. Significant side effects were not observed. Based on this clinical study, phenytoin may be used to treat patients with PME who do not respond to adequate doses of benzodiazepines or barbiturates, and phenytoin is effective at alleviating SE in patients in the progressive stage of PME. Phenytoin may also be used as a prophylactic treatment for SE in patients with PME. Patients who do not respond to phenytoin require additional AEDs and anesthetic drugs that are commonly used to treat RSE, such as levetiracetam, valproic acid, and midazolam, and may be administered other nontraditional treatments such as a ketogenic diet and hypothermia therapy [164, 165, 167].

Prognosis

In PME, patients may present a progressive aggravation of myoclonus, recurrent epilepsy, early dementia, and even death. SE and RSE are the main causes of death in these patients. PME is caused by many factors, but few cases and studies of SE in patients with PME are available. Thus, the overall prognosis of patients with PME cannot be assessed [55, 160].

4.3.7 Electrical Status Epilepticus in Sleep (ESES)

4.3.7.1 Definition

ESES is a special EEG phenomenon that refers to almost sustained spike-waves discharges evoked by sleep that occurs in the interictal period rather than ictal period [168]. The ILAE definition does not clearly determine the number of spike-wave discharges released in the EEG that are defined as ESES. Therefore, the criteria used in different studies are different. The first reported study utilized the spike and waves duration in the total non-rapid eye movement (NREM), that is, a "spike-wave index" (SWI) of 85–100% as the criterion for the definition of ESES. However, in subsequent reports, an SWI greater than 50% was the diagnostic criterion for ESES [169, 170].

4.3.7.2 Historical Evolution

Electrical SE during sleep is a special EEG phenomenon associated with epileptic seizures, language disorders, cognitive impairment, and other clinical manifestations. This progressive cognitive and language disorder with persistent bioelectrical epilepsy was first described in pediatric patients by Kennedy and Hill in 1942 [171]. In 1971, Patry and Tassinari [169] studied six children with sleep-induced electrical SE. For the first time, epileptic seizures, ESES, and disorders of cognition and speech were linked. These authors defined ESES as diffuse, sustained 1–3 Hz outbreak activity at the beginning of sleep that continued throughout the slow-wave period of sleep, which accounted for at least 85% of the activity in continuously monitored EEG. Since then, reports and studies of children with this disease have emerged. Clinicians have gradually begun to understand and focus on the relationship between ESES and epilepsy syndrome in children [170, 172, 173].

4.3.7.3 Major Types of ESES-Related Epilepsy Syndromes

The major types of ESES include: Landau-Kleffner syndrome, benign childhood epilepsy with centrotemporal spike (BECTS) variants, and syndrome of continuous spikes and waves during slow-wave sleep (CSWS) [170].

4.3.7.4 Common Features of ESES-Related Epilepsy Syndromes

Onset Age

These syndromes begin in preschool to school-aged children [170]. Su et al. [174] analyzed the efficacy of the levetiracetam + clonazepam treatment in 15 patients (nine males and six females) with BECTS variants. The age of the first epileptic seizure in these children ranged from 2.6 to 11.8 (6.7 ± 2.6) years, and the age of ESES onset was 4.5–13.5 (8.0 ± 2.5) years. Chen et al. [168] retrospectively analyzed 82 patients (39 males and 43 females) with ESES, including 49 patients with BECT variants, 27 patients with CSWS, and 6 patients with Landau-Kleffner syndrome (LKS). The first epileptic seizure in these patients occurred from 1.4 to 11 years, and the age of ESES onset was 2–10.8 years old.

Seizure Types

Partial motive seizures can occur during sleep, and generalized seizures, such as atypical absence, atonic seizure, and GTCS, can occur during the lucid period [170]. Chen et al. [168] retrospectively analyzed 82 patients (39 males and 43 females) with ESES. Patients with BECT variants ($n = 49$) exhibited an early manifestation of partial seizures, mainly during sleep. In the course of BECT variants, 33 patients gradually developed epileptic negative myoclonus, and 19 patients developed atypical absence seizures. All patients with CSWS ($n = 27$) experienced partial seizures, mainly during sleep. Five patients had GTCS during the lucid period, accompanied by atypical absence or myoclonic seizures. Four patients experienced atonic seizures. Patients with LKS ($n = 6$) experienced nocturnal dominant partial seizures, and two experienced atypical absence and myoclonic seizures.

EEG Features

The EEG is characterized by spike-waves mainly in the rolandic area or frontal area. The EEG is significantly increased and diffused in sleep and exhibits an almost sustained release during NREM [170].

4.3.7.5 Features of Different Subtypes

Benign Childhood Epilepsy with Centrotemporal Spike Variants

Benign childhood epilepsy with centrotemporal spike variants, also known as atypical benign partial epilepsy of childhood, received its name due to the early course of this disease and because it conforms to the clinical characteristics of BECT. In the course of the disease, new types of seizures that differ from BECTS seizure types can occur (i.e., epileptic negative myoclonus and atypical absence), and oropharyngeal dyskinesia can occur. Mild cognitive impairment can occur after the disease [172, 173, 175, 176].

According to the clinical manifestations, BECTS variants are divided into two subtypes: type I and type II. These two types have different clinical characteristics with some level of overlap.

Type I

The clinical manifestations are often unstable motion, trembling of hands, dropping objects being held, coarse tremor, and other symptoms that belong to the manifestation of epileptic negative myoclonus. Clinically, epileptic negative myoclonus can involve one or both limbs, resulting in a short-term loss of muscle tone and interference with the coordination of movement, causing movement instability. When an upper limb is involved, the manifestation is trembling of hands and dropping objects being held. When the trunk is involved, the manifestation is nod and the tilt of body. When a lower limb is involved, the manifestation is standing or walking instability and falling [172, 175, 177–179].

Type II

The clinical features of type II BECTS variants are speech disorders and oropharyngeal apraxia manifested as dysarthria, aphasia, frequent salivation, inflexible tongue movement, and a loss of mixing function when eating. The tongue cannot be stretched out of the mouth in severe conditions, and the patient may exhibit dysphagia and choking when drinking or other manifestations of operculum syndrome. However, these children have a normal level of intelligence and a normal understanding of language. In severe cases leading to aphasia, the patients can answer questions or express their wishes by gesturing. Symptoms may fluctuate and last for several weeks to several months. The persistence of a large number of epileptiform discharges can damage the low rolandic area and the mouth and facial representation areas around the lateral fissure, causing operculum dysfunction leading to oropharyngeal apraxia. Some researchers have described the phenomenon as acquired epileptic opercular syndrome [173, 180].

Mixed Type

Type I and Type II symptoms can occur in the same child, which is known as the mixed type, suggesting that the range of epileptic functional impairments is more extensive and more serious. Clinically, the mixed type is more common [176, 181].

EEG

The EEG shows a significant increase in the number of local discharges in the rolandic area in both conscious and sleep periods, and the discharge in sleep meets the diagnostic criteria for ESES.

Type I EEG manifestations: Children have frequent spike-waves released in the lucid period, and discharge significantly increases during sleep, which often reaches to 50–80% or more of NREM. Clinically, type I is often accompanied by varying degrees of slow language expression, a lack of smooth expression, etc. [172, 175, 177–179].

Type II EEG manifestations: Frequent spike-waves are released in the rolandic area during the lucid period that is often accompanied by ESES phenomena during sleep [173].

Epilepsy with Continuous Spike and Wave During Slow-Wave Sleep (CSWS)

CSWS is an age-dependent childhood epilepsy syndrome, and the children usually have neuropsychological injury and/or motor regression [170].

Onset Age

The age of onset ranges from 2 to 12 years of age, and the peak age is 4–5 years. ESES often appears 1–2 years after the first epileptic seizures. The age of onset of ESES is 3–14 years old, and the peak age is 8 years [182]. Herguner et al. [183] studied ten patients with CSWS for whom the age of onset was 1.5–4 years and the mean age of onset was 2.25 ± 1.27 years.

Seizure Types

CSWS is mainly manifested as partial motive seizures during sleep and generalized seizures in the lucid period [183, 184]. Nineteen to forty percent of patients may have partial SE. Absence seizures are the most common type of generalized seizures, and a drop attack accounts for 44.5% of seizures in the lucid period [183, 185].

Clinical Features

(1) Level of mental and motor development before disease onset: Two-thirds of children exhibit normal mental and motor development before disease onset, and one-thirds of the children were diagnosed with mental retardation, and the most obvious delay occurred in language development [183, 184]. (2) After disease onset, patients exhibit cognitive and motor dysfunction [183, 184]. Most of the children exhibited progressive neuropsychological damage during ESES that was observed on the EEG. The main manifestations were comprehensive cognitive regression and motor regression, which were common and manifested as ataxia, poor fine motor control, spastic quadriplegia, hemiplegia, hypotonia, and other abnormal nervous system signs in half of the children [185]. (3) Language disorders were mainly manifested as language expression disorders, which are different from typical acoustic agnosia of children with LKS. The manifestations and degree of neuropsychological injury in children with CSWS are related to the severity, site of involvement, and duration of ESES [182, 183].

EEG

Focal paroxysmal spike and slow waves are observed in frontal areas, rolandic areas, frontotemporal areas, and centrotemporal areas during the lucid stage [184]. Extensive and continuous 1.5–4.0 Hz spike-waves are released during sleep, and a small number of focal abnormalities are occasionally observed in the frontal or frontotemporal area [186]. ESES occurs during sleep, and ESES is strongly associated with neuropsychological impairments [183, 187]. Cognitive and motor regression occurs after ESES [184]. The ESES phenomenon observed on EEG is required to diagnose CSWS.

Landau-Kleffner Syndrome (LKS)

LKS, which is also known as acquired epileptic aphasia, is one of the common causes of acquired speech disorders in children [170, 188].

Pathogenesis

Currently, certain causal relations between EEG abnormalities and aphasia have been postulated, namely, a prolonged continuous discharge involving the speech center or the combined cortex can damage or disrupt processes of creation and modify brain circuitry during development, producing a "functional excision" of the cortical language function area that leads to language dysfunction [170, 189].

Main Features

Language ability is normal before disease onset. Patients start to acquire aphasia at the age of 2–7 years, accompanied by behavioral changes manifested as hyperactivity, irritability, aggression, and autism [170, 172, 188]. Tsuru et al. [190] reported a case study of a patient with LKS who began to have generalized seizures at the age of 3 years 10 months, and speech gradually began to deteriorate. Subsequently, spoken language deteriorated and the right hand was clumsy at the age of 4 years 4 months. This patient lost the ability to understand language at the age of 6 years 5 months and became extremely active, completely aphasic, and unresponsive to language commands.

EEG

Background activities are normal or exhibit mild, non-specific abnormalities. The release of 1.5–2.5 Hz paroxysmal spike-waves from the temporal area is the main observation during the lucid period, which can spread to the parieto-occipital area and to the frontal area. In the NREM sleep period, generalized or focal frequent spike and slow waves may occur, which are often persistent and defined as ESES. The spike-waves index varies greatly in different individuals and in each night of same individual's sleep. Epileptiform discharges on EEGs are required to diagnose LKS [182, 188, 190].

4.3.7.6 Treatments

In children with ESES, cognitive impairment resulting from persistent discharges is a more serious problem than the epileptic seizures, and the primary goal of treatment is to improve the EEG discharges and eliminate ESES as soon as possible. The treatment options for this particular group of children are controversial, and the current treatment options are described below [189].

AEDs

AEDs, such as benzodiazepines, levetiracetam, and valproic acid, are the first choice treatments for ESES-related epilepsy syndrome. Su et al. [174] analyzed 15 children (nine males, six females) with BECTS variants. These children were treated with levetiracetam in the early stage, but the EEG did not show an improvement or the seizures persisted. Then, these children were treated with oral levetiracetam (20–40 mg/kg/d) combined with 2 months of short-term oral clonazepam before bed (once a day for the first month, 0.02–0.03 mg/kg; once every other day in the second month, 0.02–0.03 mg/kg). Of the 15 patients, only one had recurring ESES and seizures. The remaining patients had no clinical seizures, and the sleep EEG suggested normal range or only a small amount of low-amplitude discharges in the centrotemporal area. Thus, levetiracetam combined with short-term clonazepam was more effective in controlling the patients' clinical seizures and reducing epileptiform discharges during sleep compared with clonazepam or levetiracetam monotherapy; moreover, the combination produced fewer adverse events [189].

Steroid Hormones

A combination of corticosteroids and ACTH could be considered as a treatment for patients with poorly controlled seizures or who show an improvement in the persistent discharge on the EEG. Corticosteroids and ACTH have been reported to effectively control seizures, eliminate electrical SE, and improve neuropsychological damage. However, the long-term use of steroid hormones can produce serious side effects [188, 190–192].

Sinclair et al. [191] studied ten patients with CSWS or LKS (2–11 years, seven males and three females), eight of whom had seizures, and the EEG showed ESES. Prednisone was continuously administered at a dosage of 1 mg/kg/

day for 6 months. The follow-up periods were 6 months, followed by continuous annual visits for 1–10 years. With the exception of one patient, the other patients exhibited significant improvements in language, cognition, and motor function. The patients' EEGs were all completely normal within 3–6 months after treatment, but clinical recurrence still existed. Transient drug side effects were observed in four children, including two patients with weight gain, one patient with behavioral changes, and one patient with hypertension. Based on this study, steroid hormones are safe and effective in patients with CSWS and LKS syndrome, with few and reversible side effects. Chen et al. [168] retrospectively analyzed 82 patients (39 males and 43 females) with ESES phenomena. All patients were treated with methylprednisolone at a dosage of 15–20 mg/kg/d, and each course is 3 days followed by a 4-day interval. During the interval, oral prednisone was administered at a dosage of 1–2 mg/kg/d. Three continuous courses were administered. Continuous prednisone therapy was administered after discharge, and 2 weeks later, the prednisone dosage was gradually reduced. The total course was 6 months. The authors defined a reduction of the SWI on EEG from 85% to less than 50% as having a significant effect and a decrease (>20%) but still > 50% was effective. The total rate of significantly effective and effective SWI was 83% (62/82) within 1 month after treatment with methylprednisolone, and the seizure frequency was significantly reduced in all patients within 1 month.

Immunoglobulin

Arts et al. [189] studied the efficacy of intravenous administration of high-dose immunoglobulin at treating LKS (n = 3) and CSWS syndrome (n = 3) in children, including six children with ESES (4–9 years old, 2 females). Intravenous immunoglobulin (IVIG) of 400 mg/kg/day for the first 5 days, followed by one dose of 400 mg/kg every 3 weeks, i.e., 4, 7, 10 weeks, etc. until week 25, was used as the administration method. During the IVIG treatment and 12-month follow-up period, none of these children experienced epileptic seizures, but no significant improvement was observed in the EEG. Neuropsychological function was improved in one patient with CSWS syndrome. Three patients without an improvement in neuropsychological function were subsequently treated with steroid therapy, which was very effective in one patient. According to previous studies, IVIG is occasionally effective in patients with ESES, but the onset time and efficacy cannot be assessed due to individual differences [189]. Thus, high-dose IVIG may be administered to patients who exhibit an ineffective response to corticosteroid treatments.

4.3.7.7 Prognosis

Although epileptic seizures and EEG discharges in children with ESES often disappear after puberty, these patients are often left with permanent neuropsychological dysfunction. The cognitive deficits are comprehensive or selective. Thus, early recognition and termination of ESES is the most important prognostic factors [170]. Overall, the disability rate of children with ESES is extremely high.

4.3.8 Lennox-Gastaut Syndrome (LGS)

4.3.8.1 Definition

LGS is a common age-related epileptic encephalopathy in clinical, the onset time usually occurs in childhood, and the syndrome gradually worsens until adulthood. Resistance to AEDs occurs and patients often exhibit cognitive deficits and behavioral changes. The etiology is complex and diverse, including cryptogenic and symptomatic etiologies. The symptomatic etiologies include prenatal and intrapartum infection and hereditary diseases such as tuberous sclerosis [193, 194]. The attack pattern of LGS onset is similar to Dravet syndrome and Doose syndrome; thus, these diseases may have overlapping features in the early stage. Some LGS cases may have evolved from infantile spasms and West syndrome. Some LGS cases may also evolve into West syndrome. Therefore, early differential diagnosis is relatively difficult [193–196].

4.3.8.2 Historical Evolution

The formation and development of a definition and classification for LGS have been the work of many authors over many years. In 1935, Gibbs et al. [197] reported the clinical presentation of the patients who were described by Lennox and Davis, and these patients presented with cognitive impairment and multiple types of seizures, accompanied by specific spike and slow wave patterns on the EEG. Then, Gastraut et al. [198] described 100 cases of this type of patient in 1966 and their common characteristics were spike and slow wave release on EEG, cognitive impairment, and multiple types of seizures, including myoclonus seizures and atypical absence seizures. This type of disease was officially named Lennox-Gastaut syndrome at a European conference in 1968 [194, 199].

4.3.8.3 Clinical Manifestations

Onset Age

The age of onset is in the first 10 years of life and the peak age is 3–5 years. Male are more common [194, 199]. Kumar et al. [200] studied 31 patients with LGS who had an onset age of 8.757 ± 2.05 (1–11) years.

Seizure Types

LGS manifests as various types of seizures [193, 201], including tonic seizures, atypical absence seizures, atonic seizures, and myoclonic and focal seizures. Tonic seizure is the most typical type of LGS seizure, and tonic seizures are the reference for diagnosing the disease. In the study by Kumar et al. [200], the most common seizure type in 31 patients with LGS was myoclonic seizures, which was observed in 25 patients (80.6%), followed by atonic seizures (64.5%). GTCS were observed in 16 patients (51.6%), atypical absence seizures in 10 patients (32.3%), and complex partial seizures in 11 patients (35.5%). Chevrie et al. [201] studied 80 patients with LGS and found that 75% of these patients have two or more types of seizure.

4.3.8.4 EEG

In the interictal period, the 1.5–2.5 Hz spike and slow waves are observed, which last for a few seconds to a few minutes. This seizure pattern often shows a maximum voltage in the frontal regions [198]. However, this EEG manifestation is not the absolute standard for an LGS diagnosis. The EEG performance in the ictal period is related to the seizure type; for example, the manifestation of tonic seizures, which are commonly observed in LGS, may initially be present as a low-amplitude, fast frequency (10–13 Hz) discharge that subsequently develops into a full outbreak of slow wave or slow sharp wave patterns, followed by a continuous attenuation of discharges on EEG lasting for 1–3 s [202].

4.3.8.5 SE in LGS

Prevalence

The incidence of SE in patients with LGS is extremely high, and some studies have reported that 50–75% of children with LGS have a history of NCSE, whereas tonic SE is rare [56, 193, 195, 203]. Hoffmann-Riem et al. [195] studied 101 patients with LGS (5–34 years, 57 males and 44 females). The authors regarded the repeated or persistent nonconvulsive epilepsy and persistent bilateral spike-waves on the EEG that lasted for more than 6 h as NCSE. Eighty-two (85%) patients experienced NCSE in the course of disease, and 64 patients (67%) experienced CSE.

Seizure Types and Manifestations

The seizure types include NCSE, tonic SE, and CSE, of which the most common type is NCSE [193, 195, 203]. NCSE often alternates with tonic seizures, is manifested as behavioral disorders, and is accompanied by abnormal myoclonus of the face and upper limbs. Sometimes the NCSE lasts for several hours to several weeks, and this type is often refractory SE. Hoffmann-Riem et al. [195] retrospectively analyzed 101 patients with LGS and showed that 82 patients (85%) had NCSE and 64 patients (67%) had CSE. The age at first onset of NCSE was 1–12 (4.3 ± 2.0) years old, and NCSE occurred in 60% of children less than 5 years old.

In the study by Tassinari et al. [56], five patients with LGS had refractory tonic SE. In the initial stage, the patients with tonic SE had no loss of consciousness and were able to speak and eat. Subsequently, the level of consciousness gradually decreased into a confused state, and the patients experienced difficulties in swallowing and respiration. Then, a series of tonic seizures occurred. However, life-threatening autonomic dysfunctions (e.g., respiratory failure, high fever, tachycardia) are not common [56, 204].

Treatments

Markand et al. [196] postulated that intravenous injections of benzodiazepines are still the most effective treatment for children with SE. However, Tassinari et al. [56] reported that five children with LGS developed refractory tonic SE after an intravenous administration of benzodiazepines (diazepam or nitrazepam) and had a poor response to many drugs (e.g., barbiturates, primidone, ethosuximide). These five children exhibited a confused state with repeated tonic seizures or sustained discharge on EEG before the administration of benzodiazepines. Based on this study, if children with LGS in this state are administered benzodiazepines, the tonic seizures may worsen or tonic SE may even be induced.

Hoffmann-Riem et al. [195] found that NCSE is difficult to treat and is often refractory. The authors included 101 patients with LGS in their study, 62 of whom had clear etiologies. Eighty-two patients had NCSE in the course of the disease. Even if children with NCSE received the comprehensive standard treatment in a timely manner, the therapeutic effect was still poor, particularly for children with a clear etiology, and the underlying diseases should be treated first. Nobutoki et al. [57] reported seven episodes of refractory NCSE in five patients, two of whom were diagnosed with LGS and had three episodes of NCSE. All patients were treated with midazolam after they did not respond to the initial benzodiazepine treatment. Midazolam was administered intravenously at a loading dose of 0.15–0.3 mg/kg, followed by a continuous infusion of 0.1–0.2 mg/kg/h. The infusion rate was increased by 0.1 mg/kg/h every 0.5–1 h until the NCSE was controlled. The maximum dose of midazolam was 0.4 mg/kg/h. Eventually, five episodes of NCSE were terminated completely within a few hours after the administration of midazolam, without significant side effects.

Prognosis

According to Hoffmann-Riem et al. [195], the prognosis and the development and severity of mental retardation in children with LGS are related to the etiology. Patients who experienced their first epileptic seizures prior to the age of 3 years developed West syndrome, CSE or NCSE occured, and experienced continuous tonic seizures would have a poor prognosis. The occurrence of NCSE, particularly in the early stage, was highly associated with severe mental retardation in later stages ($p < 0.001$, OR = 25), whereas CSE exhibited a lower association with the severity of mental retardation. Therefore, the early termination of NCSE significantly improves patients' prognosis [193, 196, 205].

4.4 Refractory Status Epilepticus in Hypoxic Ischemic Encephalopathy

Hypoxic ischemic encephalopathy (HIE) is caused by various factors that lead to a partial or total reduction cerebral blood flow or a pause in cerebral blood flow, which subsequently induces cerebral ischemia and hypoxia-induced neurological damage. According to the age of onset, HIE is divided into neonatal HIE and adult HIE. Neonatal HIE is a common neurological disease caused by perinatal asphyxia, a term that is used to describe brain damage in newborns caused by partial or complete hypoxia or a reduction in or suspension of cerebral blood flow. Neonatal hypoxic brain damage is caused by many factors, such as perinatal asphyxia, recurrent apnea, severe respiratory disease, and right to left shunt congenital heart disease. One to eight in 1000 newborns will have HIE [206]. Adult HIE is divided into two subgroups. One group is caused by cardiac arrest, and HIE occurs after successful cardiopulmonary resuscitation (CPR). Cardiac arrest has different causes in these patients, such as heart disease, anesthesia, drug poisoning, shock, surgical accidents, shock, and hypokalemia. The brain is extremely sensitive and exhibits poor tolerance to ischemia and hypoxia even after the spontaneous recovery of CPR. Therefore, the majority of patients develop brain injury, which can easily develop a persistent vegetative state. Another subgroup is ischemic hypoxia caused by other factors, such as asphyxia, CO poisoning, pulmonary failure, acute severe asthma, and foreign bodies in the trachea, but not cardiac arrest [206].

4.4.1 Historical Evolution

The RSE in HIE was firstly described in 1987 by Simpson et al. [207] who reported a case study of a young male who died from an RSE due to an HIE caused by hanging suicide. In 1990, Jumao et al. [208] reviewed 23 cases of myoclonic SE in patients and found that HIE was the cause in 15 patients. In 2008, Sirsi et al. [209] reported a study of a neonate who developed RSE due to HIE, which was not sensitive to first-line AEDs. The administration of midazolam ultimately controlled the symptoms. In 2013, Sutter et al. [210] summarized the medical histories of all patients with RSE in an ICU at a health center from 2005 to 2011 and determined that RSE caused by ischemic anoxic encephalopathy was an independent cause of death.

4.4.2 Prevalence

Based on a literature review, Rittenberg et al. [211] analyzed 80 patients who experienced cardiac arrest outside the hospital and found that the incidence of RSE was 12–19%. Legriel et al. [212] studied 89 patients with ischemic encephalopathy and found that the incidence of RSE was 22%. Krumholz et al. [213] summarized the data for 114 patients with HIE who had an RSE incidence of 32%. In summary, 12–32% of HIE patients can manifest as RSE. In addition, Sutter et al. [210] studied 260 patients with SE and found that HIE was the cause in 23% of patients. Buttram et al. [214] studied 59 patients with RSE, and 22% of patients were diagnosed with HIE. In summary, the proportion of patients with an etiology of HIE is 22–23% [210, 214, 215].

4.4.3 Potential Mechanisms

4.4.3.1 Cell Energy Metabolism

Critical cerebral ischemia results in reduced delivery of energy substrates (i.e., oxygen and glucose) to the brain. Anaerobic metabolism during HIE rapidly depletes the stores of glucose and high-energy phosphates (ATP and phosphocreatine) in the neonatal brain, resulting in the accumulation of lactate and inorganic phosphate [216–218]. Patients with HIE experience a delayed or "secondary" energy failure that occurs 1–2 days later, and the energy failure eventually leads to neuronal apoptosis or death [219]. Neuronal apoptosis is considered to underlie the pathological changes and may be a potential pathogenic mechanism of epilepsy and RSE.

4.4.3.2 Eurotoxicity of Excitatory Amino Acids (EAA)

EAA receptor hyperactivation is strongly implicated in the pathogenesis of perinatal HIE injury. Glutamate is not degraded, but instead is removed from the synaptic cleft by energy-dependent neuronal and glial uptake transporters [220]. EAA receptors are widely expressed throughout the neonatal gray matter, which are divided into NMDA and AMPA receptors. In patients with HIE, energy depletion affects glutamate uptake, leading to extracellular glutamate accumulation, which can cause SE and even RSE [221]. As shown in the 1996 study by Cataltepe et al. [222], elevated glutamate levels are detected in the CSF after HIE. In the 2015 study by Zanelli et al. [223], depolarized neurons in CA1 region were hypoxic, the action potential (AP) threshold decreased, the AP amplitude increased, and Na^+ channels were confirmed to be involved in the process.

4.4.3.3 Intracellular Calcium Accumulation and Oxygen Free Radicals

As a consequence of cerebral HIE, multiple mechanisms contribute to the increased intracellular calcium levels by releasing the sequestered stores from the endoplasmic reticulum and mitochondria and by inducing calcium influx. Sustained depolarization and platelet-activating factor receptor hyperactivation lead to an influx of extracellular calcium. Failure of oxidative phosphorylation induces the release of intracellular calcium stores from the mitochondria and ER. Deleterious consequences of increased intracellular calcium levels include the activation of phospholipases, endonucleases, proteases, and nitric oxide synthase [224]. Activated phospholipase A2 generates arachidonic acid, and activated phospholipase C produces inositol-1,4,5-triphosphate, both of which trigger calcium release from the ER. Proteases and endonucleases damage cytoskeletal proteins and DNA, respectively [225].

Increased production of reactive oxygen species contributes to the pathogenesis of neonatal HIE-induced brain injury. Under normal conditions, low concentrations of superoxide anion and hydrogen peroxide are produced as a by-product of mitochondrial electron transport [226]. These radicals are scavenged enzymatically by superoxide dismutase (SOD), catalase, and glutathione peroxidase and nonenzymatically by reaction with antioxidant molecules, such as alpha-tocopherol and ascorbic acid. Oxygen free radicals directly damage DNA, proteins, and membrane lipids and initiate apoptosis [227]. Based on accumulating evidence, the newborn brain is vulnerable to oxygen free radical-induced damage. Two recent clinical studies suggested beneficial effects of allopurinol therapy. In a preliminary study of asphyxiated human infants, allopurinol treatment improved cerebral hemodynamics and electrical activity. Calcium influx led to the formation of a large number of free radicals, triggering cascade biochemical reactions that may lead to SE [227].

4.4.3.4 Inflammation

Cytokines generally include interleukins (ILs), interferons (IFs), tumor necrosis factor (TNF), chemokines, and growth factors. According to relevant clinical data, immune mediators play important roles in the pathogenesis of HIE [228]. IL-1β promotes the occurrence and development of HIE in neonatal and adult brain injury. Ischemia and hypoxia can promote the expression of the IL-1β gene and its biological activity [229]. TNFα is also a cytokine that plays a key role in HIE. Under hypoxic conditions, the expression of the TNF gene rapidly increases. IL-1β and TNFα inhibitors have been applied in the clinic to treat connective tissue disease, but these inhibitors are ineffective treatments for encephalopathy [230]. Based on recent studies of refractory epilepsy, the levels of IL-1β and TNFα and other proinflammatory factors are obviously increased, suggesting that the inflammatory pathway may promote the occurrence and development of SE [231].

4.4.4 Clinical Features

4.4.4.1 Onset Time

The duration of RSE (myoclonic seizures) after CPR in adults may be within 24 h (acute phase) or a few days to several weeks (chronic phase). In 1980, Snyder et al. [232] studied 63 adult survivors of cardiac arrest after resuscitation. Eight patients experienced myoclonic seizures within 12 h, and four patients developed seizures after 3 days. Thus, we suggest that partial seizures often begin within 12 h. Rittenberger et al. [211] also believe that NCSE always occurs within 12 h after cardiac arrest. In 1990, Jumao et al. [208] proposed that myoclonic SE caused by hypoxic encephalopathy often occurs within 14 h. In 1988, Morris et al. [233] reported three cases with RSE caused by HIE, two cases occurred within 24 h after HIE, and the other occurred within 30 h after CPR. According to the 1995 study by Arnoldus et al. [234], RSE occurred within 4 h after CPR; other scholars also believe that the acute onset should occur within 4 h. In 2005, Hui et al. [235] reported a case study of 18 patients with myoclonic SE due to HIE, which occurred within 1–38 h after CPR; similar cases were reported by McGinn et al. [236] in 2016. In summary, RSE most likely occurs within 4–24 h after CPR but can also occur after 3 days.

4.4.4.2 Seizure Types

NCSE

Sutter et al. [210] reported that the most common type of RSE occurring after HIE is NCSE (65%); simple partial seizures, complex partial seizures, and absence seizure account for 29.26% of NCSE.

CSE

In 1987, Simpson et al. [206] reported a case study of patients who were unconscious due to hanging and the symptoms manifested as tonic-clonic RSE; an intravenous injection of pentobarbital was used to control the seizures. The head CT scan showed only mild cortical edema, but 2 days later, the head CT scan showed diffuse cortical edema with bilateral basal ganglia infarcts. During the hospital stay, the EEG still showed epileptic discharge. Five months later, the patients died of pneumonia, and the autopsy showed severe brain softening lesions and multiple infarcts.

4.4.4.3 Complications

Most patients with SE or RSE after HIE also exhibit heart, lung, and multiple organ failure, hypoxemia, acidosis, and other complications [237]. In the 2013 study by Sutter et al. [210], most patients with RSE after HIE were in a coma (76%). In addition, seizures and other neurological symptoms may also occur, such as cognitive dysfunction and muscle weakness.

4.4.5 Auxiliary Examinations

4.4.5.1 Examination of HIE

Routine blood tests, urinalysis, electrolyte levels, blood gas analysis, liver and kidney function tests, and autoimmune antibody levels are also helpful in diagnosing HIE. An arterial blood gas analysis shows different degrees of acidosis. Neuron-specific enolase (NSE) may be helpful in diagnosing the disease. Thomke et al. [238] examined neuron enolase levels in 50 patients and detected high levels of NSE expression in 27 patients.

Neuroimaging is important for HIE diagnosis. CT scans of patients in whom the myoclonic state emerged after CPR reveal cerebral edema, ischemic cortical lesions, cerebral hemorrhage, cerebral infarction, or subarachnoid hemorrhage. Early CT scans suggest mild cerebral edema; 3–5 days later, CT scans display diffuse cortical swelling and highly intense signals for the bilateral basal ganglia. At the 1 month CT examination, diffuse cerebral infarction and compensatory hydrocephalus are observed [239]. MRI imaging of HIE-induced brain injury is divided into different types, including the cerebral edema type, cerebral hemorrhage type, secondary cerebral hemorrhage type, and cerebral white matter damage type. (1) Brain edema type: (1) Localized cerebral edema with basal ganglia injury is displayed as a low lamellar T1 signal and high T2 signal in lesions in the temporal cortex, parietal cortex, or single lobular white matter. High T2 signals are observed for lesions in the basal ganglia. (2) Extensive cerebral edema with basal ganglia injury: The MRI shows unclear gray matter and white matter boundaries in the occipital lobe, temporal lobe, and frontal lobes in the T1- and T2-weighted images. The signal for the T1-weighted image of the gray matter increases, whereas the signal for the T2-weighted image of the white matter decreases. The frontal lobes and periventricular white matter displays lamellar T1 hypointensity and T2 hyperintense lesions, and the basal ganglia display abnormal T2 hypointensity. (3) Simple brain edema: (1) The MRI shows lamellar T1 hypointense and T2 hyperintense lesions in the white matter of the bilateral, occipital, or parietal lobes. (2) Cerebral hemorrhage type: Spot or sheet bleeding is observed, and the MRI shows T1 hypointensity or slight hypointensity and T2 hypointensity in the brain parenchyma. (3) Secondary cerebral hemorrhage type: The MRI shows a nonuniform signal for the white matter adjacent to the ventricles, including a high T1 signal and low T2 signal, as well as a low T2 signal and high T2 signal in the lesions. (4) Cerebral white matter damage type: The MRI shows low T1 signals in the lesions and high T2 signals in the lesions in the lateral ventricle anteroposterior angle and semioval white matter. According to some studies of children with HIE, the early and late MRIs revealed that focal white matter abnormalities in children tend to return to normal, but extensive white matter abnormalities in children tend to lead to permanent brain damage accompanied by basal ganglia atrophy, cystic degeneration, and other serious sequelae. In the 2013 study by Akman et al. [239], patients with RSE caused by HIE showed high fluid-attenuated inversion recovery (FLAIR) signals in white matter, gray matter, and deep nuclei and high T2 signals in the hippocampus and parahippocampal gyrus, and the pia mater signal increased.

4.4.5.2 Examination of SE

Long-term digital video EEG is widely used in the ICU to monitor the status of epilepsy, recurrent seizures, encephalopathy, and other diseases. In 2004, Pandian et al. [240] reviewed the long-term digital video EEG data for 612 patients and suggested a relationship between the EEG data and the clinical prognosis. A digital EEG is more likely to detect epileptic seizures than an EEG, and digital video EEG can maintain a high capture rate of abnormal waveforms, burst suppression, spike slow waves, and three-phase waves. In 2005, Thomke et al. [238] described the EEG features of 50 patients with myoclonic SE after CPR. Most of these patients showed EEG suppression, and 12 had 10–55 s epileptiform discharges in their EEGs. As shown in the study in 2013 by Akman et al. [239], patients with HIE often have generalized periodic epileptiform discharges (GPEDs), which are both an EEG manifestation of severe encephalopathy and an indicator of RSE after HIE [241]. In 2003, Bensalem et al. [242] reported a case study of a patient with RSE caused by ischemic hypoxic encephalopathy, and the EEG showed explosive suppression with a comprehensive rhythm of epilepsy-like sharp wave discharge. In 2005, Hui et al. [235] reported a study of 18 patients with HIE who experienced myoclonic SE; the EEGs of ten patients showed comprehensive paroxysmal spikes, cluster spikes, or diffuse low voltage. The RSE after HIE sometimes presents a rare three-phase wave, typical spike-and-wave activity (TSWA), suggesting that benzodiazepine-type AEDs are not effective [243].

Amplitude integrated electroencephalogram (aEEG) is a simple operation with less interference from the external environment that is easy to interpret and can be implemented for long-term, continuous bedside monitoring; aEEG also displays other characteristics that not only reflect changes in the background activity on the EEG but also reflect the epileptic activity. aEEG has great value in monitoring brain function [235, 236].

In patients with HIE, cortical somatosensory evoked potentials show a bilateral disappearance of cortical response N20 and the presence of a P14 reaction, indicating a very poor prognosis [244].

CSF examination can be abnormal. The CSF glutamate levels are increased in patients with HIE, and the ratio of the glutamate and GABA levels in the CSF is significantly decreased over a long time. In SE, we can exclude HIE-induced brain damage if the CSF glutamate levels and glutamate/GABA ratio did not change.

4.4.6 Treatments

4.4.6.1 Treatment for HIE

Any cause of HIE results in a poor prognosis, but early treatment is better than late treatment. In the 2016 study by Youn et al. [206], early treatment of children with HIE (within 1 h) significantly reduced the mortality and morbidity.

Symptomatic Supportive Treatment

Conventional treatment is mainly utilized to increase cerebral blood flow, control and eliminate brain edema, and restore the function of living neurons that survive in the hypoxic ischemic area. The goal of early treatment is to maintain good ventilation, PaO_2 > 60–80 mmHg, and $PaCO_2$ and pH in the normal ranges, which are key measures of the ability of the treatment to maintain good cerebral and systemic blood perfusion. Clinicians should avoid treatments that induce a cerebral perfusion pressure that is too low or too high. An appropriate blood glucose level should be maintained to provide the energy required for nerve cell metabolism. Early treatment also aims to control seizures and treat brain edema. Posttreatment measures mainly include rehabilitation and training; the earlier the physical rehabilitation training is implemented, the more conducive it is to the recovery of brain function and to reducing sequelae.

Mild Hypothermia Treatment

Mild hypothermia therapy may be considered the most useful treatment, particularly in adults with severe HIE [245]. Polderman and Herold [246] believe that the hypothermia treatment, which reduces the core body temperature to 32–35 °C, may be the standard treatment for HIE.

The effectiveness of mild hypothermia therapy has been confirmed in preclinical animal experiments. In the study by Atkins et al. [247], a 33–36 °C mild hypothermia treatment was confirmed to significantly reduce traumatic brain injury-induced seizures in animals compared with the control group. D'Ambrosi et al. [248] also confirmed this result. As shown in the study by Schmitt et al. [249], a mild hypothermia treatment also improved the pathological changes related to epileptiform discharges in epileptic seizures and SE in animal models of SE, including neuronal necrosis and apoptosis as well as brain edema [250, 251].

Hyperbaric Oxygen Therapy

In the late 1960s, some researchers began to rescue patients with HIE using hyperbaric oxygen. Hyperbaric oxygen therapy increases the partial oxygen pressure in the alveoli, elevates the oxygen content, and improves aerobic metabolism to combat HIE caused by partial or complete hypoxia [252]. In addition, hyperbaric oxygen increases the number of microvascular openings to maintain appropriate tissue metabolism and nutrient level. Furthermore, hyperbaric oxygen reduces HIE-induced brain injury by inhibiting the expression of inflammatory factors, inhibiting neuronal apoptosis, and promoting the expression of brain-derived neurotrophic factor (BDNF) in response to reperfusion after ischemia [253].

4.4.6.2 Treatment for RSE

AEDs

SE is still the primary cause of death and should be terminated as soon as possible. The most commonly used AEDs include midazolam, pentobarbital, metamine, propofol, and valproic acid (seeing Chap. 6).

In 2012, Mader et al. [243] reported a case with NCSE after CPR. The EEG showed typical spike-and-wave activity (TSWA). The patient was administered 10 mg of lorazepam, but the seizures were not sensitive to phenytoin, levetiracetam, and other drugs; ultimately midazolam was administered. First, the patient received an intravenous infusion of 0.2 mg/kg, and then the intravenous infusion was maintained at 0.05 mg/kg/h. The clinical symptoms disappeared, but the EEG still showed TSWA. The clinical symptoms and EEG discharges disappeared when the intravenous infusion was maintained at 20 μg/kg/min. Pentobarbital can control the seizures in most patients with RSE caused by HIE. Young et al. [254] do not recommend the use of pentobarbital to treat patients with bilateral facial muscle syncope spasm, bilateral pupil disappearance, or disappearance of the vestibular reflex accompanied by burst suppression in EEG.

Non-pharmacological Treatments for RSE

For controlling RSE, non-pharmacological treatments can be used, e.g., VNS, deep brain stimulation (DBS), etc. VNS was reported to treat RSE in HIE. VNS was approved by the US FDA in 1997 for the non-pharmacological treatment of refractory epilepsy in children aged 12 years or older and adults, with the aim of reducing seizures in patients with drug-resistant epilepsy. In 2008, Zamponi et al. [255] reported a case with RSE caused by HIE. The child received a single cervical incision implanted VNS at 26 months of age. Three days later, the stimulus started at 0.25 mA and gradually increased from 0.25 mA to 1.5–20.25 mA at a stimulation frequency of 30 C/s; the vagus nerve was stimulated for 30 s and then stopped for 5 min. The child's symptoms improved significantly.

4.4.7 Prognosis

The American Academy of Neurology suggested that myoclonus after a cardiac arrest tends to lead to a poor prognosis [256]. In 1994, Wijdicks et al. [257] reported a study of 107 patients who were in a coma after CPR; 37% of these patients developed myoclonic SE, all of whom died. In 2005, Hui et al. [235] reported a case study of 18 patients with refractory clonic SE after hypoxia. The myoclonic SE duration was 30 min–31 days (average 14 h). Of these patients, 16 died, one was in a vegetative state, and one experienced severe disability. In 2005, Thomke et al. [238] reported a poor prognosis for patients with generalized myoclonus after CPR, as 15 patients died within 24 h, nine patients died 4 days after CPR, 21 patients died within the next 5–12 days, and the remaining patients were in a vegetative state. In 2013, Akman et al. [239] reported a study of 21 patients with GPDs; five patients died, only seven patients had a better prognosis, and the rest of the children presented with moderate to severe neurological sequelae. According to the relevant literature, the mortality of RSE was 16–39%, and children with HIE which was the cause have a poor prognosis.

In 1994, Towne et al. [258] proposed that HIE is an independent risk factor for death in patients with SE. In 2007, Rossetti et al. [259] also proposed that SE after hypoxia is an independent risk factor for death. Generally, patients with HIE-induced RSE have irreversible brain damage, and disability and mortality is extremely high. The majority of surviving patients are in a persistent vegetative state. When HIE is the cause of secondary SE or RSE, clinicians should take measures to improve the patients' survival rates.

4.5 Refractory Status Epilepticus in Autoimmune Encephalitis

Generally, autoimmune encephalitis (AE) includes paraneoplastic encephalitis (such as anti-Hu antibody-mediated encephalitis, anti-Ma2/Ta antibody-mediated encephalitis, and anti-CV2/CRMP5 antibody-mediated encephalitis), anti-cell surface antigen antibody-mediated encephalitis or anti-synaptic antibody-mediated encephalitis (a narrower definition of AE), and encephalitis associated with other systemic autoimmune diseases (such as systemic lupus erythematosus (SLE)-associated encephalopathy and Hashimoto's encephalitis) [260]. Based on the lesion involved, AE is usually divided into limbic encephalitis and diffuse encephalitis, with or without a potential tumor. According to recent clinical studies, a large proportion of patients with AE may have epilepsy and SE [261–263]. Generalized seizures or SE may be the initial symptom of the disease, often requiring urgent medical intervention, such as deep sedation or even drug-induced coma. These treatments for epilepsy or SE may mask other symptoms of AE, such as movement disorders or mental disorders, leading to delayed identification and diagnosis of the disease [261].

4.5.1 Prevalence

With the progress of science and technology over the last decades, more and more newly valuable anti-intracellular antigen antibodies and anti-cell surface antigen antibodies have been identified. AE has become an increasingly studied disease in neurological clinical research, and data for cases of clinically diagnosed with AE have gradually accumulated, but clinicians still have a limited ability to identify the AE. Most clinical publications are case reports or series of case reports of a small number of patients, which increases the uncertainty of the morbidity of RSE in AE; therefore, statistical data on the incidence of RSE in AE are not available [264]. Gaspard et al. [20] retrospectively analyzed 130 adult patients (18–81 years, 83 females, 47 males) with RSE of an unknown etiology within 48 h of admission from 13 academic medical centers from 2008 to 2013, and 67 (52%) cases remained unexplained at the end of the study. The most common identified etiologies are non-paraneoplastic autoimmune (19%, $n = 25$) and paraneoplastic (18%, $n = 23$) etiologies. AE (non-paraneoplastic or paraneoplastic) is the most common cause of new-onset RSE. Baysal-Kirac et al. [265, 266] retrospectively analyzed the clinical manifestations and laboratory features of seven patients diagnosed with AE (22–76 years, four females, three males) whose autoantibodies included anti-Hu ($n = 1$), anti-GAD ($n = 2$), anti-NMDA receptor ($n = 3$), and anti-amphiphysin antibodies ($n = 1$). Four patients (57%) manifested RSE during the course of disease. Among these patients, two patients developed NCSE that could not be controlled by AEDs. After immunotherapy (methylprednisolone and IVIg), the EEG discharges and clinical manifestations improved significantly. In addition, one patient manifested as NCSE and one manifested as focal motor SE died eventually.

Cyril et al. [267] reported a study of 39 patients (14 males, 25 females) who were clinically diagnosed with AE from December 2009 to June 2013 at a NICU in a tertiary care center in southern India, whose ages ranged from 2 to 55 years (mean age of 15.95 years). SE occurred in 23 patients (60.5%), including 14/23 (35.9%) patients who were positive for anti-NMDA receptor antibodies but negative for other autoimmune antibodies.

4.5.2 Clinical Features

4.5.2.1 Time to RSE Onset

Most patients with AE display a subacute onset, whereas a small number manifests an acute or chronic onset; however, SE can occur at any stage of the disease [267, 268]. The retrospective multicenter study by Holzer et al. [268] analyzed 13 patients with immune-mediated RSE whose ages ranged from 17 to 69 years old (average age of 32.5 years). The proportion of female patients was as high as 92% (12/13). Eight of 13 patients had anti-NMDA receptor antibody-mediated encephalitis. In seven patients, SE was insensitive to multiple AEDs and anesthetics, and in the other six patients, SE was controlled by multiple combinations of AEDs. The authors prescribed immunotherapy to 11 patients, but not to two patients who were refractory to AEDs and anesthetics. The duration of AE was 10 days to 12 years (mean time of 2 months). The latency from the initial symptom to SE ranged from 0 to 11 months. In seven (53%) patients, SE occurred within 1 week, and in the other six (47%) patients, the elapsed time from the manifestation of the initial symptoms to the onset of SE varied between 1 week and 11 months (average time of 3.3 months, median time 1 month). The course of SE ranged from 2 h to 12 years; three cases lasted for less than 1 month (2 h, 10 days, and 18 days, respectively), one case lasted for as long as 12 years, and most of the cases (nine cases) lasted for 1–4 months. In an observational study, Petit-Pedrol et al. [261] examined six patients (three children and three adults) with anti-GABA receptor antibody-mediated encephalitis (five males, one female) whose ages ranged from 3 to 63 years old (mean age of 22 years). Five patients (four males, one female) developed SE that ultimately progressed into RSE during the course of the disease. The elapsed time from the manifestation of the initial symptoms to SE varied from several days to several months (24 h, 48 h, 5 days, 2 months, and a few months, respectively).

4.5.2.2 Types of RSE

Holzer et al. [268] distributed 12 questionnaires to 12 experienced European neurological medical institutions and obtained data for 13 adult patients who were diagnosed with antibody-mediated status epilepticus from seven neurological centers. In seven patients, SE was insensitive to multiple AEDs and anesthetics, and SE was only controlled by the administration of multiple combinations of AEDs to the other six patients. Seven patients presented complex partial seizures, five presented generalized seizures, and only one presented simple partial seizures. Sarria-Estrada et al. [269] retrospectively analyzed five patients with paraneoplastic AE (49–77 years, four males, one female). All of these patients exhibited RSE: four cases presented NCSE, two cases presented simple partial SE, and one case presented generalized tonic-clonic SE (two cases experienced two episodes of SE). Baysal-Kirac et al. [265] reported a study of seven adult patients with AE: one patient was positive for anti-Hu antibodies and one was positive for anti-amphiphysin antibodies, two were positive for anti-GAD antibodies, and three were positive for anti-NMDA receptor antibodies. Four patients progressed to RSE: the two anti-GAD antibody-positive patients presented NCSE, and two anti-NMDA receptor antibody-positive patients presented NCSE and focal motor SE.

4.5.3 SE in Different Types of AE

4.5.3.1 Paraneoplastic Autoimmune Encephalitis

Based on recent clinical reports [269–273], the main type of RSE observed in patients with paraneoplastic autoimmune encephalitis is partial

SE. Jacobs et al. [274] reported a study of one 53-year-old female patient with anti-Hu-limbic encephalitis who was also diagnosed with a poorly differentiated mediastinal tumor. The patient manifested refractory complex partial SE during the course of disease, which was ineffectively treated by the initial lorazepam, carbamazepine, and topiramate therapy, and high doses of phenytoin, phenobarbital, and propofol were still unable to terminate the seizures. Moreover, the seizures were not sensitive to immunotherapy or tumor resection. Sarria-Estrada et al. [269] reported a case study of five patients with SE caused by paraneoplastic encephalitis; the average age of onset was 60 years, male to female ratio was 4:1. Two patients presented with simple partial SE, two patients manifested complex partial SE, and one patient presented with GTCS. The duration of SE ranged from 24 h to 8 weeks. One patient was diagnosed with anti-Hu antibody-mediated encephalitis and small cell lung cancer. The first episode of SE was simple partial seizures. The seizures were controlled by intravenous immunoglobulin and chemotherapy. However, 4 months later, SE recurred as the tumor size increased and was manifested as complex partial or secondary GTCS. The patient died 6 months later of complex partial SE. Therefore, the authors postulated that the occurrence and recurrence of SE in patients with paraneoplastic autoimmune encephalitis are related to the persistent release of paraneoplastic antibodies by the tumor itself, and the prognosis of SE in paraneoplastic encephalitis depends on the prognosis of the tumor. The recurrence of SE indicates progression of the malignant tumor [269, 274, 275].

4.5.3.2 Anti-Cell Surface Antigen Antibody-Associated Encephalitis

Encephalitis Associated with Anti-VGKC Antibodies

The voltage-gated potassium channel is a transmembrane protein composed of three proteins: contactin-associated protein-like 2 (CASPR2), leucine-rich glioma inactivated factor-1 (LGI1), and contactin-2 complex. VGKC modulates membrane excitability by regulating the resting potential and repolarization of the cell membrane [276, 277]. VGKC antibody-associated encephalitis is a common form of AE. In two large epilepsy center cohort studies, VGKC antibodies were detected in 5% of patients [278]. Suleiman et al. [279] retrospectively studied ten children with encephalitis who showed SE and refractory epilepsy between 2003 and 2009 in a department of Pediatrics, and they examined a variety of autoimmune antibodies using serological testing. The patient's serum was negative for the anti-LGI-1, anti- CASPR2, anti-NMDAR, anti-GAD, and anti-GlyR antibodies. Four patients (40%) were positive for VGKC-Ab (1–14 years, one male, three females). All patients were healthy before disease onset, but experienced CSE over the course of the disease. The duration of SE was 30–60 min (n = 1), 60 min to 24 h (n = 1), and more than 24 h (n = 2). The four patients suffered from clusters of refractory seizures (15 episodes per day) persisting for 5–20 days, and all of the patients were transferred to ICU (2–18 days). In the acute phase, the patients were not treated with immunotherapy, but ultimately, only one patient fully recovered, one patient exhibited a cognitive impairment, and the remaining two patients exhibited left TLE, neuropsychological changes, and cognitive impairments. Kotsenas et al. [280] summarized the seizures in 42 patients with VGKC-limbic encephalitis. Eight patients (19%) presented with GTCS, and only one (2.38%) 46-year-old female who was an alcoholic progressed to SE. Ramanathan et al. [281] reported a case study of a 35-year-old female patient with CASPR2 antibody-mediated AE who had a family history of autoimmune disease. As the disease progressed, the patient gradually developed myoclonic SE. The EEG showed diffuse periodic discharges and a rhythmic 2 Hz spike-wave. The serum CASPR2 autoantibody levels were 909 pmol/L (normal range 0–100 pmol/L), the LGI-1 antibody was negative, and the GAD antibody levels were also increased (148 U/mL, the normal range of 0–5 U/mL). The CSF analysis suggested lymphocytosis and intrathecal oligoclonal band synthesis. The patient achieved burst suppression in EEG by being sedated with thiopental, and continuous sedation with propofol and midazolam ultimately controlled SE. While concurrent with the discontinuation of propofol and midazolam, the authors administered a combination of a variety of AEDs, including valproic acid, phenytoin, levetiracetam, ethosuximide, lacosamide, topiramate, and clomipramine, which failed to control the seizures. After immunotherapy, the seizures were alleviated. Based on previous studies, myoclonic SE suggests a poor prognosis [37, 281], but in this case, immunotherapy effectively controlled refractory myoclonic SE.

Anti-NMDA Antibody-Associated Autoimmune Encephalitis

Anti-NMDA receptor-mediated encephalitis is one of the most common types of AE observed in women, children, and adolescents [282, 283]. Dalmau et al. [282] studied the clinical manifestation and features of 100 patients with anti-NMDA receptor-mediated encephalitis (5-76 years, average age of 23 years) and found that 76% of the patients with NMDA receptor-mediated encephalitis had epileptic seizures and only 6% had SE in the acute phase. Florance NR et al. [283] studied 81 patients (69 females, 12 males) with anti-NMDA receptor-mediated encephalitis, including 32 (40%) children (23 months–18 years, 26 females, four males), and only two cases developed SE. Holzer et al. [268] studied 13 patients with antibody-mediated RSE (17–69 years, 12 females, one male) that exhibited the highest detection rate of NMDA-Ab. The sera from eight patients (17–58 years, seven females, one male) were positive for the NMDA-Ab, and this antibody was also detected in the CSF from seven of these patients. Multiple AEDs, including phenytoin, valproate, midazolam, topiramate, phenobarbital, propofol, and other drugs, were ineffective at treating RSE in the four patients with anti-NMDAR antibody-mediated encephalitis; in the other four patients with anti-NMDAR antibody-mediated encephalitis, RSE was eventually controlled by a combination of a variety of AEDs and immunotherapy, rather than more than two kinds of drugs. Johnson et al. [284] reported a case study of a 35-year-old female who primarily suffered from persistent NCSE but was previously physically healthy. She was admitted to hospital after experiencing progressive headache with short-term memory loss and irritability for 3 weeks. After 1 week, the patient lost consciousness, the EEG showed NCSE, and the NCSE was resistant to phenytoin, levetiracetam, and valproate and couldn't be completely controlled by benzodiazepine drugs as well. Subsequently, propofol terminated the periodic NCSE discharges on the EEG, which was followed by a sequential pentobarbital treatment to maintain the burst suppression of the EEG, but each attempt to minimize the depth of pentobarbital anesthesia led to the recurrence of SE. Anti-NMDA receptor antibodies against NR1 and NR2B were detected in CSF, and an ultrasound showed a hemorrhagic ovarian cyst. The authors successively prescribed immunoglobulin, rituximab, cyclophosphamide, and other immunosuppressive agents, but no improvement was noted. After using phenobarbital to control the seizures for 5 months, the patient underwent ovariectomy, and a postoperative biopsy confirmed teratoma. Five weeks after the operation, the EEG showed a faster background rhythm, the epilepsy-like waveform gradually disappeared, and the normal sleep-wake cycle appeared. Seven weeks after the operation, the patient recovered, and her neurophysiological function recovered gradually. The patient continued to experience a slightly depressed mood, hallucinations and anomic difficulty, and memory loss; however, recurrence did not occur in the follow-up. The refractory NCSE in this patient was eventually controlled by effectively treating the primary disease.

Anti-GAD Antibody-Mediated Autoimmune Encephalitis

This kind of AE is as common as anti-LGI1-mediated AE, but the onset age is younger [285, 286]. Glutamic acid decarboxylase (GAD) is the rate-limiting enzyme that catalyzes the decarboxylation of glutamic acid to generate the inhibitory transmitter GABA. According to Vianello et al. [287], anti-GAD antibodies can reduce GABA synthesis and/or interfere with extracellular GABA secretion, which affects GABAergic synaptic transmission, thereby increasing cellular excitability and reducing the seizure threshold. Kanter IC et al. [288] reported a case study of a 21-year-old male patient who was diagnosed with anti-GAD antibody-mediated AE. He was admitted to hospital for a sudden emergence of complex partial SE that progressed into RSE in December 2005, and complex partial seizures and generalized seizures alternated. Neither a combination of a variety of high-dose AEDs (propofol, lorazepam, topiramate, phenytoin, valproate, and lamotrigine) nor GABA drugs achieved the desired effect of seizure-free. The first-line immunomodulatory treatments (glucocorticoid, immunoglobulins, plasma exchange) exhibited no or only short-term effects. In June 2006, the patient was prescribed the experimental treatment cyclophosphamide that subsequently achieved a significant effect; the patient's condition gradually improved, and long-term seizure control was achieved. The development of repeated episodes of refractory epilepsy may be associated with intrathecal GAD synthesis, and cyclophosphamide is an alternative treatment regimen for these patients. Gogi Kumar et al. [289] reported a case study of a 30-year-old female patient whose initial symptom was headache that developed into general tonic-clonic seizures within several days. The seizures were not controlled by a variety of oral and intravenous first- or second-line AEDs, and the patient eventually developed into drug-RSE. The types of SE were complex partial seizures and generalized seizures. Phenytoin, phenobarbital, levetiracetam, lacosamide, and continuous infusions of propofol and other treatments could not terminate the seizures, and immune regulators (glucocorticoids and immunoglobulin) were also ineffective. After palliative resection of the epileptic foci, plasma exchange, and the administration of second-line immunotherapy (cyclophosphamide), the plasma antibody titer began to decrease, and SE was eventually controlled. However, during follow-up, the patient still experienced repeated seizures, including NCSE. Thus, AE is an underlying cause of RSE. The prognosis of patients with anti-GAD-AE is poor, and AEDs and immune regulation cannot achieve the ideal effect of eliminating the seizures. After an intravenous injection of methylprednisolone, the GAD antibody titers remained high, and the seizure frequency was not reduced [286, 290]. Only plasma exchange or cyclophosphamide treatments decreased the antibody titers and seizure frequency and improved the clinical symptoms, but the efficacy was not maintained [288, 291–294]. Therefore, long-term immunosuppressive therapy may be required in these patients.

Anti-GABA Receptor Encephalitis

Boronat et al. [295] reported a case study of 70 patients with autoimmune-mediated limbic encephalitis. Ten patients (14.3%) were positive for an anti-GABA-B receptor antibody, the male to female ratio was 9:1, and the average age was 60 years. The incidence of epilepsy was 80%. GABA receptors inhibit synaptic transmission in the central nervous system (CNS). Anti-GABAR antibodies do not reduce the number of synaptic GABARs, but alter their synaptic function, which leads to seizures [261, 295–298]. Petit-Pedrol et al. [261] studied six patients with GABAB-mediated encephalitis (3–63 years, five males, one female) and showed that abnormally high T2 or FLAIR signals were observed in images of extensive cortical and subcortical regions. Over the course of the disease, all six patients progressed to drug-RSE or partial SE. The elapsed time from the manifestation of the initial symptoms to SE ranged from 24 h to several months. In one patient, SE was terminated by levetiracetam, ultimately resulting in recovery. The other five patients were treated with three or more AEDs (four patients required barbiturate anesthetics for a drug-induced coma) and immunotherapy. Three of five patients achieved SE termination and partial or complete recovery, and two of five patients died of sepsis during the RSE attack, which occurred within 48 h of the onset of disease and persisted until death. The duration of SE was 4 weeks and 8 weeks, respectively. Guan et al. [298] reported a study of 18 ethnic Han patients with GABAB-limbic encephalitis in China. Seventeen patients (94.4%) had new-onset seizures, and 16 patients (88.9%) presented seizures as the initial symptoms. In all patients, the initial AEDs could not control epilepsy, and four patients (22.2%) developed RSE that were resistant to multiple AEDs. The authors hypothesized that high titers of anti-GABAR antibodies in the serum and CSF are associated with seizure severity or RSE in patients with this type of encephalitis. Hinsworth et al. [23] also reported a study of a previously healthy 23-year-old patient with GABA (B)-mediated limbic encephalitis who exhibited refractory bilateral TLE; the seizure was ineffectively controlled by a variety of AEDs and anesthetics and subsequently developed into new-onset super-RSE. SE was not controlled by multiple AEDs (levetiracetam, phenytoin, sodium valproate, topiramate, and lacosamide) and anesthetics (midazolam, propofol, and pentobarbital). Multiple types of immunotherapy (methylprednisolone, intravenous immunoglobulin, plasma exchange, and rituximab) were administered as the principle treatment for AE, and SE was gradually controlled. Six weeks after the onset of the disease, the patient was finally diagnosed with GABA (B)-associated limbic encephalitis by testing the autoantibody levels.

4.5.3.3 Other Systemic Autoimmune Diseases Associated with Encephalitis

Steroid-Responsive Encephalopathy Associated with Autoimmune Thyroiditis

Steroid-responsive encephalopathy associated with autoimmune thyroiditis (SREAT) refers to Hashimoto's encephalopathy (HE). HE is defined as a recurring or progressive encephalopathy associated with Hashimoto's thyroiditis and is characterized by positivity for thyroid autoantibodies in serum and/or CSF and a good response to glucocorticoids. The clinical manifestations are not specific, and a variety of symptoms involving the CNS may be present. The most common features are epileptic seizures and cognitive changes [299]. The incidence of epilepsy in these diseases is as high as 66%, but fewer clinical reports of SE in HE have been published [299, 300]. Seizures in HE perform as progressive myoclonic epilepsy or new-onset SE in childhood. Monti et al. [301] reported a study of two patients with NCSE as the initial manifestation of HE: one patient was a 51-year-old female with Hashimoto's thyroiditis who was admitted for a persistent eye gaze and fluctuating unconsciousness, and the other was a male patient who presented with recurrent absence seizures and sustained eye movement. EEGs for both patients showed long-term bilateral frontal spike slow wave and multi-spike slow wave, which were consistent with the diagnosis of NCSE. Early clinical manifestations of HE vary and lack specificity; the occurrence of the disease is not associated with thyroid function, as normal thyroid function, hyperthyroidism, or hypothyroidism have been observed [302]. Therefore, the misdiagnosis and misdiagnosis rates may be high in patients with SE whose basic etiology is HE.

Systemic Lupus Erythematosus Caused by Encephalopathy

In connective tissue disease, 25–27% of patients with SLE suffer CNS injuries, the incidence of epilepsy in SLE is as high as 7–40%, and epilepsy and SE usually occurs during the disease course [303–305]. Appenzeller et al. [306] followed 159 patients with SLE for 4–7.8 years and found that seizures are relatively common, but SE is rare in these patients with SLE. Sixty patients (11.6%) suffered from seizures, but only two patients (1.26%) developed SE and eventually died due to SE. Park et al. [304] reported a case study of a 17-year-old woman with a first episode of SE whose laboratory tests showed anemia and was positive for lupus anticoagulant. The other laboratory tests, including antinuclear, anti-ds-DNA, and anticardiolipin antibodies, CSF, and blood biochemical examinations, did not show any significant findings and did not find any evidences of viral, bacterial, or fungal infection. The EEG revealed general spike slow waves or multiple spike-waves. A variety of traditional AEDs did not control the SE, and RSE was only terminated by a sulfur infusion. The delayed diagnosis and treatment of this patient was due to the initial negative outcome of the antinuclear antibody test and the initial presentation of symptoms of SE. Although SE rarely appears in patients with SLE, particularly as the initial symptom, the clinicians should still pay attention to its identification, and multiple repeated laboratory tests can improve the detection rate of the disease.

Neuropsychiatric SLE occurred in the significant activity of SLE. According to several publications, patients with SLE developed CSE over the course of the disease, which is common in SLE, whereas complex partial SE is rare and is frequently misdiagnosed or undiagnosed [307–309]. Fernandez-Torre et al. [305] reported a case study of a 23-year-old woman with a 6-year history of SLE who was treated with glucocorticoids. Seizures occurred during the course of the disease and were controlled by AEDs, and the EEG gradually normalized. After several months of gradual discontinuation of the drugs, the patient gradually developed abnormal behaviors and became unconscious. The EEG indicated focal epileptic discharges in the right parietal area and temporo-occipital region that rapidly spread to contralateral side many times; each epileptic discharge lasted for 2–3 min. The clinical manifestations were a rigid left turn of head and fine myoclonus of the left leg, which could not be recalled by the patient. Thus, a diagnosis of complex partial SE was considered. After the administration of the lamotrigine, the seizures did not recur, and positive signs were not observed in the neurological examination. In the 2-year follow-up, the patient achieved seizure-free status. The authors postulate that complex partial SE may be the reasons why patients with SLE present with a sudden, acute coma and changes in the conscious state. Therefore, clinicians should pay special attention to the early EEG.

4.5.4 Diagnosis of RSE in AE

4.5.4.1 Diagnosis of AE

AE typically lacks specific biomarkers and symptoms, making a clinical diagnosis difficult. For patients with the clinical manifestations of acute or subacute onset of new-onset seizures or SE accompanied by significant mental and behavioral abnormalities, such as short-term memory impairment, clinicians must consider that SE may be caused by AE and must perform the video EEG, cerebral MRI, and blood and CSF-related autoimmune antibody tests to confirm the diagnosis. MRI can show specific abnormalities in the unilateral or bilateral limbic system signals, such as a hypointense signal on T1 W1 images and hyperintense signals on T2WI and FLAIR images. Enhanced scans often did not enhance the abnormalities. In the acute phase, the volumes of the amygdala and/or hippocampus increase in most patients and return to normal or decrease further during the recovery period [310]. Structures in addition to the limbic system may be involved in some patients, and the MRI may also be normal in some patients, particularly in the early stages of the disease [279, 311, 312]. CSF analyses show typical inflammatory changes, normal or slightly elevated cerebral pressure, and slightly increased or normal cell numbers and protein levels, and the corresponding antibodies may also be detected. Oligoclonal bands or intrathecal IgG synthesis may also be detected [282, 313]. The CSF protein levels increase in patients with HE, but the white blood cell count is normal, showing a protein-cell separation phenomenon. In approximately 100% of HE patients, the serum TPO-Ab (thyroid peroxidase antibody) or TG-Ab (thyroglobulin antibody) levels increase. However, the titers are not significantly correlated to thyroid function or the clinical manifestations, and glucocorticoids cannot reduce the antibody titer. The sera from patients with SLE-induced encephalopathy may be positive for antinuclear antibodies, anti-dsDNA antibodies, and anti-SM antibodies.

If the patients have been diagnosed with AE, a thorough inspection is required to determine whether a tumor is present.

4.5.4.2 Diagnosis of RSE

SE is defined as a seizure duration that exceeds the duration of the majority of episodes of the same type of seizure, with no sign of cessation or recurrent episodes, during which the state of consciousness does not return to baseline [61]. Currently, an accepted definition for RSE generally refers to the failure of adequate first-line and second-line AED therapies [314]. Patients with AE require long-term video EEG monitoring for a precise diagnosis of SE and to determine the presence of nonconvulsive SE.

4.5.5 Treatments for RSE in AE

RSE is one of the common and urgent symptoms of AE in neurology departments and is a potentially fatal disease with extremely high mortality and disability. It is different from the other neurological emergencies, such as cerebrovascular diseases. The treatment of SE is more similar to the treatments for cardiac arrest or shock. For the treatment of SE, treatments of the initial symptoms usually precede the etiological treatment [315]. Clinicians should administer basic life support with first-line AEDs to terminate the episodes of SE and then treat the etiology. Certain specific etiologies and long-term seizures are significant risk factors for increased mortality in patients with SE [316]. Therefore, a timely diagnosis and treatment of the potential causes of SE have the same critical clinical benefit as the early termination of seizures. Thus, the treatment of RSE caused by AE is divided into two phases: termination of seizures and the treatment of the primary disease and prevention of complications.

4.5.5.1 Termination of SE

Shorvon et al. [317] proposed the concept of phased treatment for RSE (details are provided in Chaps. 6, 7, and 8). Anesthetics are still the preferred treatment for this disease. Before applying anesthetics, good mechanical ventilation and the establishment of rapid intravenous infusion channels to cope with adverse reactions of anesthetics, such as changes in breathing and circulation, are needed. Anesthetics should be maintained until the EEG shows burst suppression; the time of withdrawal of anesthetics is suggested to occur after the patient is seizure-free for at least 24–48 h. If the patient is still in a vegetative state, a variety of comprehensive treatment methods should be used, such as physical therapy (hypothermia and electroconvulsive therapy), the ketogenic diet, and surgery. Currently, a randomized or controlled study of RSE treatments has not been published; thus, the recommended treatment is based on studies of small samples and case reports.

As reported in the study by Holzer et al. [268] of the curative effects of treatments for antibody-mediated SE on 13 patients, an "optimum first-line AED" does not exist, and the combination of different types of AEDs does not show an advantage in controlling epilepsy. Specifically, the use of sodium valproate, phenytoin, and levetiracetam alone or in combination failed to control AE-mediated SE, although the doses and blood concentrations of the drugs reached the recommended therapeutic dose. As shown in a previous report, no AEDs were effective in seven patients (54%), and lorazepam and prednisone were effective in one patient. Furthermore, the symptoms of three patients improved after receiving a combination of four types of AEDs, and one patient's symptoms improved after the administration of a combination of five types of AEDs. Kirkpatrick et al. [318] reported a case study of a patient with NMDA-LE and NCSE who was in a coma. RSE was not controlled by a variety of AEDs and immunotherapy. However, after the addition of felbamate, the rhythmic delta activity wave in the EEG stopped and the patient awoke from coma. Felbamate is an antagonist of the NR2B subunit of the NMDA receptor [319, 320], but its mechanism as a specific treatment for SE in NMDA-LE requires further study. In addition, in patients with SLE, phenytoin should be avoided to control seizures for phenytoin can cause drug-induced lupus [321].

4.5.5.2 Etiological Treatment

Etiological treatment is essential to control SE and RSE in patients with AE. Different treatment methods should be chosen based on the primary disease. First, a thorough inspection of the tumor should be performed to determine whether the patient has paraneoplastic encephalitis. If a tumor is present, tumor resection is necessary because it is the most effective treatment for AE caused by paraneoplastic autoantibodies [322]. Additionally, clinicians must determine the existence of other systemic autoimmune diseases, such as Hashimoto's thyroiditis and SLE, while actively treating the primary disease [301, 304].

When prescribing immunotherapy, such as pulsed methylprednisolone therapy, plasma exchange, or immunosuppressive agents, the side effects need to be assessed during treatment; in particular, patients treated with drugs with a risk of inducing seizures should be carefully monitored [323]. Immunotherapy can be administered according to the protocol described by Ramanathan et al. [324]: intravenous injection of methylprednisolone for 3–5 days (30 mg/kg/day up to 1 g/day), followed by high-dose oral prednisolone (1–2 mg/kg/day). Additionally, clinicians should monitor the occurrence of glucocorticoid-induced epilepsy and SE. In some cases, 2–5 intravenous injections of 2 g/kg immunoglobulin are also needed. If the symptoms do not improve within 1–2 weeks, 3–5 sessions of plasma exchanges should be considered, or patients should start second-line treatments, such as immunosuppressive agents (cyclophosphamide and rituximab) [325]. Researchers have not clearly determined whether rituximab or cyclophosphamide is more effective [326]. Second-line immunotherapy is usually effective when first-line immunotherapy fails [288, 289, 327].

4.5.5.3 Surgical Treatment

When second-line immunotherapy fails, surgery is often considered, such as unilateral temporal lobe resection or selective resection of the amygdala and/or hippocampus. Weimer et al. [328] reported a case study of a 45-year-old female patient with limbic encephalitis and RSE who presented with abnormal T2 and FLAIR signals in images of the right temporal lobe, bilateral frontal lobe, and pons. Continuous EEG monitoring showed continuous epileptic discharges in the right temporal lobe. RSE was effectively controlled after temporal lobe resection. Although abnormal T2 and FLAIR signals have been observed in images of the temporal lobe from patients with limbic encephalitis, some authors postulate that these signals may not be related to seizure frequency. Although few reports have described the improvements of SE following resection of non-epileptic lesions [329–332], more researches are needed to confirm these findings.

4.6 Refractory Status Epilepticus in Central Nervous System Infections

According to the results of one epidemiological survey, most types of RSE are symptomatic SE, and CNS infections are one of the most common causes of RSE [333]. CNS infections are also a common cause of death in patients with RSE, the same as malignant intracranial tumors and large-area stroke [3, 334]. Increasing our understanding of the principles that govern the occurrence and development of RSE will allow clinicians to be better at diagnosing and treating this type of SE.

4.6.1 RSE in Bacterial Meningitis

Bacterial meningitis is a serious type of CNS disease that is caused by a bacterial infection. Common pathogens implicated in these events include *Streptococcus pneumoniae* and *Neisseria meningitidis*. Severe bacterial meningitis is often associated with high mortality and morbidity in patients who develop RSE, and the treatment options available to and prognoses in these patients are poor.

4.6.1.1 Prevalence

Bacterial meningitis and SE are commonly observed in the same patients in the clinic. The bulk of case studies have reported that the incidence of SE is 4.1–53% in patients with bacterial meningitis, a rate that is significantly higher than the incidence of SE in the general population. In a case study of a 3-month-old infant with pneumococcal meningitis and potential congenital immune deficiency, the authors reported that SE continued to occur after the patient was treated with standard antibiotic and anticonvulsive therapy, and the patient subsequently developed RSE [335]. Another case study described 220 patients aged 1 month to 12 years old who had bacterial meningitis. Of these patients, 34 developed RSE [336]. In another study, 31 cases (26.5%) of epileptic seizures and ten cases (32.2%) of SE were observed in a population of 117 adult patients with bacterial meningitis [337]. Finally, in one study of 696 adult patients with meningitis, 121 patients developed epileptic seizures, and 4.1% (5/121) developed SE [338]. Hence, SE has been reported to occur in 4.1–32.2% of patients with bacterial meningitis, and some of these patients will develop RSE.

4.6.1.2 Factors Related to Epilepsy or SE

In patients with bacterial meningitis, SE is associated with the age of the child and the duration of the seizures [339]. Seizures are associated with pathogenic infections in patients with bacterial meningitis, but no prospective studies have explored this issue. As shown in one study of pathogenic infections, partial and partial secondary generalized epilepsy were most common in patients who were infected with *Escherichia coli* or salmonella [340]. An evaluation of 750 patients with seizures that resulted from bacterial meningitis [341] showed that the most commonly implicated pathogens were *Mycoplasma pneumoniae* (84% of positive CSF isolates) and *Neisseria meningitidis* (4%).

4.6.1.3 Clinical Manifestations

Seizure Types

The seizures reported in the literature are primarily partial seizures, partial secondary generalized seizures, and generalized seizures. In one case study, 34 patients with bacterial meningitis presented with seizures in the acute phase [342], and ten of these patients developed SE. Most of the observed seizures were secondary tonic-clonic seizures. In a separate study performed in Spain that included 38 patients [343], eight of the patients had generalized seizures, 23 had partial seizures, and two had partial secondary generalized seizures. Finally, one study of 107 patients with both bacterial meningitis and seizures revealed that 20% had partial seizures, 21% had partial secondary generalized seizures, and 59% had generalized seizures [338].

Time of Epilepsy or SE Onset

Seizures can occur during both the acute phase and the recovery phase in bacterial meningitis. The former is called acute symptomatic epilepsy, and the latter is called delayed epilepsy. Children with bacterial meningitis primarily develop seizures within 48 h of admission [344]. In one study performed in the Netherlands, seizures occurred within 48 h of admission in approximately 75% of 696 patients with bacterial meningitis. Patients with bacterial meningitis who developed seizures in the acute phase experienced severe seizures that readily progressed to SE, and statistical analyses have shown that there is a significant association between delayed epilepsy and epileptic seizures during the acute phase. In a study that included 218 children with SE [345], the initial seizure was SE in 71% of the episodes and was associated with an acute etiology (28% of these patients had bacterial meningitis). A study of 116 patients with bacterial meningitis [340] and seizures, including 17 with SE, showed that the seizures occurred during the acute phase of infection. Sixty-one of the patients did not develop seizures during the acute phase, and these patients did not develop delayed epilepsy. Fifty-five of the patients developed seizures during the acute phase, and 11 of these patients developed delayed epilepsy. Fourteen of the 34 patients who developed seizures in the acute phase and were followed for an additional 18 months also developed delayed RSE [342]. Therefore, SE that occurs during the acute phase is a risk factor for delayed RSE.

4.6.1.4 Auxiliary Examination

CSF

CSF tests are helpful for identifying causal pathogens and provide an important reference for clinical diagnosis and treatment. CSF examinations are the most basic auxiliary examinations in suspected cases of bacterial meningitis. In children with a severe bacterial infection, SE may be associated with abnormal glucose levels and high serum aspartate transaminase or C-reactive protein levels [339].

EEG

When bacterial meningitis occurs with SE, patients often present with an abnormal EEG.

Persistent EEG abnormalities suggest cerebral complications or brain damage. Although EEGs are not specific for bacterial meningitis, they are helpful for diagnosing patients with SE and can help clinicians to monitor a patient's condition and guide decisions regarding therapy. In one study, EEGs were performed on patients with bacterial meningitis [338], and 37 episodes (31%) were recorded, including five SE and six epileptic discharges. Ten of the patients (27%) had mild background abnormalities, 24 (65%) had moderate or severe abnormalities, and 14 (38%) had focal or multifocal abnormalities. In another study, 36 children with pneumococcal meningitis underwent an EEG examination to determine the prognostic value of an initial EEG recording in SE [346], and the results showed that six of the children had a normal or lower than normal initial EEG, and five of these children achieved good progress. Thus, EEGs may have clinical value for determining a prognosis in patients with pneumococcal meningitis.

Neuroimaging

Patients with bacterial meningitis and SE often have abnormal neuroimaging findings on presentation. Performing neuroimaging at an early stage assists with diagnosis and treatment and reduces mortality and morbidity. A prospective study of brain CT scan results in 48 children with purulent meningitis [347] found that 56% (27/48) of the patients presented abnormalities and that hydrocephalus and subdural effusion were the most commonly observed CT abnormalities. Moreover, the incidence of neurological sequelae (e.g., epilepsy or SE) in children with bacterial meningitis was associated with abnormalities on head CT imaging. Children with SE and abnormal neurological examination findings are more likely to have an abnormal MRI.

4.6.1.5 Treatment

The principal treatment for patients with bacterial meningitis and SE is antiepileptic treatment, which should be based on the effective anti-infective therapy (seeing Chaps. 6 and 7).

4.6.1.6 Prognosis

Bacterial meningitis with RSE is commonly observed in a clinical setting, and affected patients are often in serious condition. Limited treatment options are available for these patients, who have a poor prognosis. For example, one study reported an infant with bacterial meningitis and SE who died 1 month after discharge [339]. In another study [336], 88 patients were admitted to ICU and had an average duration of hospitalization of 6.9 days. Thirty-four of these patients (53%) had RSE, and 31 of those cases occurred within 48 h after admission. Four patients who were treated with diazepam for more than 4 days died after 2 weeks of hospitalization, and the mortality rate was significantly higher in patients who had combinations of symptoms that included intracranial hypertension, shock, and respiratory failure. Of the ten patients with SE who were followed, nine of the survivors developed RSE [342]. Although the specific number of children with bacterial meningitis is unknown, in-hospital mortality and long-term morbidity are higher in patients with RSE [348]. Therefore, an early diagnosis and early treatment are essential to reduce mortality and morbidity in RSE in patients with bacterial meningitis.

4.6.2 RSE in Tuberculous Meningitis

Tuberculous meningitis (TBM) is a type of meningitis that is caused by infection with *Mycobacterium tuberculosis* and a common cause of chronic meningitis. TBM is often associated with SE and has a significant impact on a patient's prognosis.

4.6.2.1 Historical Evolution

One case study published in 1953 described a patient with TBM and TLE, and another case study described some treatment of epilepsy [349, 350]. Another study published in 1958 used electricity and clinical radiology techniques to evaluate the changes in epilepsy that were caused by TBM [351]. In a clinical study published in 1989 [352], the authors described 39 cases of nervous system tuberculosis that occurred in Riyadh,

Saudi Arabia. Eleven of the patients (28%) had TBM, and some of these patients had late-stage CSE and a poor prognosis. Patients with TBM are at risk of developing SE as a complication and of then progressing to RSE. In a 2002 study, a continuous infusion of midazolam was used to treat refractory generalized CSE in a patient with TBM. This drug regimen became the precedent for treating patients with TBM and RSE [353]. RSE is a life-threatening disease with a high rate of morbidity and mortality. In 2015, acute nerve injury (such as that observed in TBM and encephalitis) was shown to be a common risk factor for RSE in children [354].

4.6.2.2 Prevalence

In TBM, complications with SE are more common. One report described 76 cases of partial SE [355] in which two cases were caused by TBM. In another study, 20 cases of partial SE were analyzed [356], including four patients with TBM. A separate study examined 147 patients with CNS infections in South Korea [342], including 63 patients with TBM, and found that 6.8% (10/147) of the patients developed SE. Few studies in the literature have evaluated patients with RSE and TBM. The prognosis of patients with TBM who develop SE is good, and only a small number of these patients develop RSE. According to the results of one study, patients who presented with both TBM and SE and were not successfully treated subsequently developed RSE [357].

4.6.2.3 Factors Related to Epilepsy or SE

In patients with SE and TBM, the main symptoms are hydrocephalus, cerebral infarction, tuberculoma, and hyponatremia, and hydrocephalus is the most commonly observed complication. Most complications occur during the middle and late phases of the disease course. Hydrocephalus is more commonly observed in patients who are in the late phase of the disease, with an incidence rate as high as 65% [358]. Severe hyponatremia (<120 mmol/L) can cause patients to enter a deep coma and experience convulsions. If not treated in a timely manner, hyponatremia will aggravate a patient's condition, and electrolyte levels should therefore be promptly checked. In one study of 136 children under 12 years old who were diagnosed with TBM [359], the investigation found that neurological complications (e.g., epilepsy or SE) were attributed to cerebral edema (57%), inappropriate antidiuretic hormone secretion syndrome (35%), hydrocephalus (32%), tuberculosis (27%), abnormal electrical focus (25%), and cerebral infarction (13%). In another case study of 20 patients with TBM in the United States [360], six patients (30%) had seizures, and ten had hyponatremia. Six of the patients experienced repeatedly aggravated seizures during the late phase that potentially resulted from SE. Disturbances in consciousness are a risk factor that may be associated with the development of SE in patients with acute-phase TBM [361].

4.6.2.4 Types of SE

The main clinical manifestations in patients with TBM and SE are partial movement SE and systemic SE. In a case study of 76 patients with partial SE [355], the seizure sites included the upper and lower limbs (41 patients), head and facial muscles (12 patients), simple upper limbs (20 patients), and simple lower limbs (three patients). Forty-eight of the patients (63%) were conscious, and 28 exhibited varying degrees of disturbance of consciousness. Thirty-six of the patients were diagnosed with TBM, including ten patients with SE. The main seizure type was secondary tonic-clonic seizures [342].

4.6.2.5 Auxiliary Examination

CSF

In these patients, most CSF test results are abnormal, and CSF protein levels are generally higher, while glucose levels are lower. Tests of the cells in the CSF have revealed that there are (100–1000) × 10^6 cells/L and that samples consist mainly of lymphocytes. In a study of 61 adult patients [362], 16.3% (10/61) of the subjects experienced seizures, the number of cells, especially lymphocytes, in the CSF was increased, and 77% of the subjects exhibited increased protein levels and increased serum/CSF glucose levels. Acid-fast staining is used to detect pathogens in the CSF, and the presence of *Mycobacterium tuberculosis* in the CSF is the gold standard for diagnosing TBM.

EEG

EEG tracings are important for diagnosing TBM complicated with SE. Abnormalities in EEG background activity may reflect the severity of TBM lesions. Spike-waves, spikes, and slow wave release are important for obtaining a differential diagnosis of TBM complicated with SE. EEG abnormalities may reflect the site of inflammation. When an infection is located in the base of the skull, EEG results may be normal or may show only non-specific abnormalities. Lesions involving only one hemisphere are expressed as moderate to severe diffuse slow waves. Intermittent spikes, spikes, and one-sided periodic epileptiform discharges have been observed in patients with TBM complicated with partial SE [240]. Continuously monitoring EEG results in patients during and after hospitalization may help with documenting disease progression and determining prognoses and outcomes. One study examined EEG findings in patients with TBM [363] and found that although the EEG recordings did not show complete diffuse slowing (a common pattern in TBM), they did show continuous rhythmic sharp wave activity, which has been associated with SE.

Neuroimaging

In patients with TBM complicated by SE, brain CT and MRI will show hydrocephalus, cerebral infarction, basement membrane thickening, edema, and tuberculoma. In 76 patients with TBM and partial SE [355], the main CT finding was brain edema. In a case study of 31 patients with TBM [364], ten patients showed deterioration after treatment and progressed to SE. A review of head CT findings revealed new and (or) progressive signs of hydrocephalus, cerebral infarction, seepage, and tuberculoma. Because multiple factors are involved in generating SE, neuroimaging abnormalities are not yet viewed as an independent risk factor for SE.

4.6.2.6 Treatment

Some of these patients will develop RSE and require long-term antiepileptic treatment (seeing Chaps. 6 and 7). Midazolam has been shown to be effective in 71–97% of patients with RSE. A case study of one patient with TBM and refractory generalized CSE showed that there was a marked reduction in generalized tonic-clonic SE activity after an intravenous infusion of 3 μg/(kg·min) midazolam was administered for 12 h, and this effect began within 45 min. SE was completely controlled after 13 h and left the patient with some neurological sequelae [353]. In the critical state, levetiracetam has been shown to have good efficacy in patients with RSE. In one study of 23 patients with RSE (39% of RSE), injecting levetiracetam via nasogastric tube was effective in 43% of the patients, and SE or RSE was eased within 72 h after the treatment was begun [365]. Patients with TBM with SE have been observed to develop RSE. Hence, in addition to AED treatment, the critical etiology must also be treated [355].

4.6.2.7 Prognosis

In patients with TBM and RSE, the prognosis is poor. According to some studies, gender, latency, and the age of seizure onset are independent prognostic factors in these patients. In a study of 65 patients with TBM [366], 21 of the patients (32.3%) had seizures. The patients were followed for 1 year. The condition in those with SE was severe, and these patients tended to develop delayed epilepsy. In a case study of 63 patients with TBM in South Korea, 23% of the patients presented with seizures in the acute phase, including ten patients who developed SE. After an 18-month follow-up period, the authors determined that experiencing SE during the acute phase is a risk factor for delayed RSE [342]. These data suggested that damage to the brain parenchyma that was caused by a CNS infection is a main cause of SE. Actively controlling long-term, frequent seizures, such as SE, can reduce the incidence of RSE in patients and is therefore the basic strategy for preventing disease progression and improving the prognosis in affected patients.

4.6.3 Other Causes of RSE in Patients with a CNS Infection

4.6.3.1 Parasitic Infection

Parasitic infections of the CNS are associated with a high incidence of mortality in addition to neurological sequelae. Epidemiological evidence indicates that there is a significant correlation between parasitic infections and SE. The high incidence of epilepsy in Africa has been associated with a correspondingly high incidence of parasitic infections of the CNS [367]. In a prospective study of 65 patients with cerebral malaria [368], EEG recordings were performed at 12-h intervals, and continuous recordings were performed using CFAM. Sixty-two percent of the patients experienced seizures after admission, and nearly half had SE.

Common causes of epilepsy or SE in patients with parasitic infections include cerebral cysticercosis and malaria. Falciparum malaria is the most common cause of SE [369], especially in the context of acute symptomatic seizures in children. One patient was described as exhibiting a variety of seizures, including frequent GTCS, partial motor seizures, and complex partial seizures, as a result of a parasitic infection. Because there is a lack of long-term follow-up studies describing SE patients with parasitic infections, it is not clear whether these patients are likely to develop RSE after the first seizure. However, in a study of 65 patients with cerebral malaria [368], eight patients who had neurological sequelae had a poor prognosis, and two patients developed partial SE during the clinical course of the infection. Seven children died in this study, including two patients (29%) who developed SE during the clinical course of the disease. Patients with parasitic infections that were complicated with SE exhibit an exacerbated disease, suggesting that death may be associated with the progression of RSE in patients who exhibit exacerbation.

In SE patients with a parasitic infection, the diagnosis is often based on patient history, epidemiology, and etiology in combination with neurological symptoms and CSF, CT, and other tests. In a study of the EEG findings in 278 patients with a parasitic infection and convulsive SE, 152 (55%) of the patients showed EEG abnormalities, and the performance was similar between children and adults [370].

Patients are usually treated with antiepileptic drugs in the clinic. In a double-blind, placebo-controlled, randomized study of 340 children with cerebral malaria, a single dose of phenobarbital (18 mg/kg) markedly reduced the incidence of SE (from 14 to 5%) [371]. Fosphenytoin has also been suggested as an effective drug because it is administered intramuscularly and has a respiratory depression effect than phenobarbital. However, SE caused by falciparum malaria appears to be resistant to diazepam, likely because of a reduction in the binding capacity of GABA receptors [372]. Deworming, corticosteroid therapy, or both can reduce the risk of seizures in patients with neurocysticercosis, leading to a reduction in the incidence of SE [373]. However, the long-term effects of anti-helminth treatment remain to be further explored. Ultimately, the best way to control parasitic infections of the CNS is to prevent and eliminate the transmission of the parasite. A study of the risk factors for convulsive SE showed that this condition could be prevented in patients with a parasitic infection [370], and effectively preventing and managing an infection reduces the burden of SE in patients, thereby preventing the further deterioration of their condition and reducing the probability of progression to RSE. However, further studies are required to determine whether community interventions aimed at controlling and eliminating parasites will ultimately slow the progression of seizures and reduce the incidence of SE [374].

4.6.3.2 Brain Abscess

A brain abscess refers to suppurative encephalitis, encephalitis, and brain abscess capsule formation, which are caused by purulent bacterial infections. Brain abscesses often cause epilepsy, delirium, paralysis, sensory disturbances, and other symptoms. Seizures may develop when the abscess is located in the dominant hemisphere.

Patients with a brain abscess who develop SE will experience exacerbation and are at increased risk of death. A 22-year study that followed 205 patients with a brain abscess reported that 48 of the patients had seizures during an 18-month follow-up period. The overall mortality rate in the patients was as high as 23% (11/48), possibly because of the presence of SE [375]. Epilepsy is a serious neurological complication of a brain abscess, and it can readily progress to SE, thus exacerbating the patient's condition. Hence, it is necessary to obtain a better understanding of the risk factors in patients with a brain abscess and SE so that we can predict outcomes and guide treatment. In a study of 108 patients with brain abscesses that had an average follow-up of 11 years, the total incidence of epilepsy was 34% [376]. The investigators compared two groups of patients who presented with and without epilepsy after brain abscess therapy, and the difference in morbidity between these groups was used as a parameter to identify potential risk factors for SE. According to this study, a patient's gender and age and local changes and the size of the abscess may be risk factors for SE.

An early diagnosis and an early treatment regimen contribute to the recovery of and prognosis in patients with a brain abscess and SE. CT is highly sensitive (95–99%) to brain abscesses and therefore useful for diagnosing patients with a brain abscess and SE. One report examined 50 children with SE from August 2001 to July 2002. Thirty-four (68%) of the children had brain abnormalities on CT scans, and four of these patients had a brain abscess [377]. A patient's prognosis is mainly determined by the level of consciousness. Actively using antibiotics to control the infection and puncturing the abscess are effective treatments in these patients, and the early use of AEDs can prevent neurological sequelae. One patient with an intracranial infection (possibly a brain abscess) reportedly exhibited a long left seizure after admission, and SE was controlled in this patient using phenytoin and phenobarbital [378]. In another study, a 78-year-old patient was initially diagnosed with SE secondary to a brain abscess [379]. After he underwent surgery and received antiepileptic drugs, antibiotics, and steroids, the brain abscess subsided. In a separate case study [380], a 54-year-old man with a chronic brucellar abscess who had RSE before surgery presented complex partial seizures. His neuroimaging findings revealed extensive lesions in the right temporal lobe. The patient was treated with standard antimicrobial therapy after combination therapy. The patient had a good prognosis at a 1-year follow-up. Because SE can develop after a few years or even decades after a patient has recovered from a brain abscess, such patients may still progress to RSE. Affected patients with SE are in a critical condition and have a high mortality rate, and long-term monitoring is therefore recommended in these patients.

4.7 Refractory Status Epilepticus in Cerebrovascular Disease

Cerebrovascular disease is a common cause of seizures. SE is one of the most serious complications of cerebrovascular disease [381]. SE may be the first sign of stroke, and patients who experience a stroke with SE have a worse prognosis and higher mortality than patients who experience a stroke without SE. Moreover, RSE can lead to a very poor prognosis. Increasing our understanding of RSE in patients with cerebrovascular disease is therefore particularly important [382, 383].

4.7.1 Historical Evolution

As shown in a study by Lowenstein et al. [384] that was published in the 1990s, cerebrovascular disease is associated with a first episode of RSE. Sung et al. [385] subsequently found that cerebrovascular disease was the primary cause of RSE in patients older than 60 years old. Ulvi et al. [353] showed that midazolam effectively controlled RSE secondary to cerebrovascular disease and that its curative effect was superior to that of traditional anesthesia drugs, such as pentobarbital. An increasing number of studies have since explored other methods in addition to anesthetics that can control RSE. Lacosamide has been shown to exert a significant controlling effect, without significant adverse reactions, on RSE in patients with stroke [386–389].

Moreover, some researchers have begun to pay close attention to electric convulsion therapy and the ketogenic diet as treatments for RSE in patients with cerebrovascular diseases [390–393], and these additions have substantially enriched the field.

4.7.2 Classification

In patients with cerebrovascular disease, RSE is divided into NORSE and RSE in pre-existing epilepsy (PERSE).

4.7.2.1 NORSE

NORSE refers to instances in which the disease occurs in a patient with cerebrovascular disease but no history of epilepsy after cerebrovascular disease. Yoshimura et al. [394] studied RSE in patients with cerebrovascular diseases and found that 60% of RSE cases were NORSE.

4.7.2.2 PERSE

Some cerebrovascular diseases coexist with epilepsy. If this pre-existing epilepsy is not effectively treated, the patients may develop RSE. In one study, 38.1% of RSE cases that involved patients with cerebrovascular diseases belonged in this class of patients [394]. Epilepsy caused by cerebrovascular disease was an independent predictor of RSE in patients older than 70 years old [395]. Sudden withdrawal is an important cause of RSE in patients with SE, and delayed treatment is an important factor that contributes to the development of RSE in patients with SE. Pre-hospital emergency treatment can prevent this process.

4.7.3 Epidemiological Investigations

4.7.3.1 Prevalence

Cerebrovascular disease is present in 8–12.8% of all cases of RSE [49, 210]. Of patients with SE occurs and stroke, 44% progress to RSE [2]. Ozdemir et al. [383] investigated 19 patients with stroke and SE and found that five (29.4%) developed RSE. A follow-up survey of 16 in-hospital patients with stroke combined with SE showed that two (12%) of these patients developed RSE. Kalita et al. [396] treated 15 patients who experienced SE after stroke. These treatments were ineffective in seven patients (46%), who subsequently progressed to RSE. The existing data show that 12–46% of SE cases that are caused by cerebrovascular disease will progress to RSE.

4.7.3.2 Mortality Rate

According to one survey, the mortality rate in patients with stroke combined with RSE is 16–23% [397]. Goodwin et al. [389] studied patients who experienced RSE after cerebrovascular disease in an ICU and found that the mortality rate in these patients was 25%. The results of these studies indicate that the mortality rate of RSE after a cerebrovascular disease is clearly correlated with the age at onset, as follows: the greater the age, the more likely the patient is to develop RSE and the higher the mortality rate [48]. In addition, convulsive RSE, which requires mechanical ventilation, has a long duration of SE and coma, both of which increase mortality in these patients [210].

4.7.4 Relative Factors

The condition in patients with cerebrovascular disease complicated by RSE is influenced by many factors. The main influencing factors include the patient's age and physical state, the type of cerebrovascular disease, and the irregular use of AEDs [398].

4.7.4.1 Age

The combination of cerebrovascular disease and RSE most frequently appears in older individuals, especially patients with stroke who are older than 60 years old [399]. This finding may be associated with the age-dependent pathological cerebrovascular changes that cause temporal lobe dysfunction, consequently promoting the development of RSE in older patients [399, 400]. In a study that used the modified Rankin scale to investigate neural functional recovery in patients with stroke, patients who experienced a worse recovery were more likely to develop RSE [401]. Furthermore, Koubeissi et al. [402] determined that age is an independent factor of mortality in patients who develop RSE after stroke.

4.7.4.2 The Type and Location of Cerebrovascular Disease

When a stroke involves a large brain area, a patient is more likely to develop RSE. Patients who experience strokes in the left hemisphere are more likely to be complicated with RSE than patients who experience strokes in the right hemisphere, especially when the stroke involves the left temporal lobe [383]. Central nervous system vasculitis can also lead to the occurrence of RSE. In a survey that tracked 149 patients with pre-existing vasculitis, 10% of patients developed secondary seizures, and a few patients with these seizures developed RSE and had a high mortality rate [306, 403]. According to another study with a small sample size, cerebral hemorrhage, intraventricular hemorrhage, subarachnoid hemorrhage, and subdural hemorrhage can each lead to secondary RSE, usually without prominent motor symptoms [389]. Jeon et al. [404] used head MRI to investigate two patients with RSE and observed brain micro bleeding. The authors hypothesized that the extent of brain micro bleeding may be associated with the occurrence of RSE.

4.7.4.3 Others

When patients with stroke were in poor physical condition, RSE was more likely to develop. Ozdemir et al. [383] investigated 151 patients with stroke and found that of the 19 (12%) patients who were complicated with epilepsy, neurological functional recovery scores of 4–5 were observed in six (4%) patients, five (3%) of the patients suffered from RSE, and two (1%) of the patients died. Moreover, in patients with stroke, the longer the duration of SE, the more likely the patient is to develop RSE [396]. In patients with stroke and RSE, mortality was significantly higher in those who were in a coma (46%) than in those who were not (35%) [403].

4.7.5 Clinical Features

4.7.5.1 Seizure Types

Patients with pre-existing epilepsy and stroke in whom the initial treatment for SE failed may develop RSE. The clinical features in these patients are similar to those in NORSE [405].

RSE Without Prominent Motor Symptoms

Liberalesso et al. [395] performed continuous EEG monitoring and studied the clinical characteristics of 15 male patients with RSE. Fourteen of these cases (93.3%) presented with complex partial SE, and 6.7% presented with myoclonic SE. In the patients with a cerebral hemisphere hemorrhage, RSE usually occurred without permanent motor symptoms while the patient was in a coma state, and only continuous epileptiform discharges were observed during EEG monitoring [406]. Kang et al. [407] used long-term EEG video monitoring to observe 24 patients with disturbances of consciousness that were caused by stroke. Eight of these patients were diagnosed with RSE without prominent motor symptoms, and a disturbance of consciousness was the main presentation. Kennel et al. [408] reported a case study of a patient with sudden partial side limb weakness, a sensory disturbance, and an inability to speak clearly at 3 months after stroke. Head MRI and EEG examinations were performed, and the patient was diagnosed with RSE without prominent motor symptoms in a cerebrovascular disease.

RSE with Prominent Motor Symptoms

General convulsive SE and generalized seizures secondary to complex partial SE are classified as SE with prominent motor symptoms in the new classification for SE published by the ILAE. In a survey by Ozdemir et al. [383], 83% of patients with stroke and general convulsive SE developed general convulsive RSE and had a poor prognosis and a mortality rate of 40%. In a study by Sutter et al. [210], mortality was three times higher in patients with stroke and comprehensive convulsion RSE with prominent motor symptoms than in similar patients without prominent motor symptoms. Lai et al. [49] studied ten patients with RSE with prominent motor symptoms secondary to stroke and found that 52% of these patients exhibited drug resistance and died.

4.7.5.2 Duration

According to a study published by Lai et al. [49], the average duration of RSE after stroke is 7 days. Koubeissi et al. [386] reported a case study of two patients with cerebral hemisphere hemorrhaging and RSE in whom nonconvulsive SE was the main presentation. The duration of SE in these patients was between 30 and 50 h when drugs were administered in a timely manner. A study by Synowiec et al. [409] showed that the average duration of RSE is 101 h, which is longer than the duration reported by Drislane et al. [410]. More patients with a history of epilepsy were included in the latter study, and the duration of RSE in patients who did not respond to the initial treatment was shorter than the duration in patients with NORSE. Lai et al. [49] studied 78 patients with RSE. In all, 12.8% of these cases were caused by stroke, and the average duration of controlled RSE after treatment was 17 days. Based on data from these previous studies, the duration of RSE in patients with cerebrovascular disease is at least 30 h.

4.7.5.3 Onset Time

The onset of SE can occur during the acute period of a cerebrovascular disease. In the acute stage, SE may be used as an onset marker for cerebrovascular disease. It can also appear within a few hours to several days after the development of cerebrovascular disease [411]. In a study reported by Ozdemir et al. [383], 84% of SE episodes appeared within 48 h after stroke. According to a study by Tasker et al. [412], most such attacks are concentrated within the 3–5 days after stroke. SE also occurs during the chronic period of cerebrovascular disease. Long-term repeated epilepsy secondary to cerebrovascular diseases can develop into SE in response to a variety of factors, including irregular treatment with AEDs, and can evolve into RSE. In a study by Sutter et al. [387] that evaluated 111 patients with RSE, 10% of the patients belonged to this class. Lai et al. [49] studied ten patients who developed RSE after stroke and found that 14.1% of the patients who experienced epilepsy after stroke subsequently developed RSE.

4.7.6 Diagnosis

First, a clinician should ensure that a cerebrovascular disease is present. RSE with and without prominent motor symptoms have both been detected in patients with cerebrovascular disease, and the type without prominent motor symptoms is more common, especially in older patients with stroke [393]. RSE can appear during the acute phase of cerebrovascular disease or after repeated episodes of cardiovascular disease-induced epilepsy.

Notably, in stroke patients, it is easier to obtain a diagnosis of RSE with prominent motor symptoms. RSE without prominent motor symptoms is superposed with the symptoms of stroke, making its diagnosis difficult. Limb movement, sensory abnormalities, and abnormal behaviors, such as mental disorder, confusion, and illusions, are likely to be clinically symptomatic of cerebrovascular disease but may also be symptoms of RSE without prominent motor symptoms. Because they lack specificity, these diseases are difficult to distinguish. Currently, it is essential to use continuous EEG monitoring and MRI examinations to ensure that neurological symptoms are caused by SE.

4.7.7 Treatments

Emergency treatment should initially be aimed at maintaining an unobstructed airway. Then, it is important to monitor oxygen partial pressure, establish a venous channel, monitor blood pressure and electrocardiogram results, determine blood glucose levels, and analyze complete blood counts and electrolyte levels. Anesthetics are a generally accepted treatment for RSE in patients with stroke. Anesthetic drugs have been shown to control 90% of episodes in patients with SE. If a patient is resistant to midazolam, other treatments, such as the second-line anesthetic drugs pentobarbital and propofol, should be considered [412]. Additional details are provided in this book.

Recent studies have shown that lacosamide, a new type of AED, may be effective in patients with RSE who are resistant to traditional AEDs and routine anesthetic drugs. Lacosamide is not affected by the type of SE and also does not cause any adverse effects, such as cardiac toxicity, blood pressure fluctuations, and skin rashes [413–415]. Hofler et al. [388] studied 31 patients with RSE and found that nine of the cases were caused by cerebrovascular disease, and 86% of these patients with RSE were effectively controlled by treatment with lacosamide. Koubeissi et al. [386] reported treating a patient who had RSE caused by cerebral hemorrhage. He was treated with an intravenous drip infusion of 100 mg of lacosamide followed by 100 mg twice daily of maintenance treatment, resulting in well-controlled RSE. The other patient was treated with an intravenous drip infusion of 100 mg of lacosamide followed by 200 mg twice per day on the second day, resulting in the effective control of RSE. Legros et al. [414] performed a prospective, randomized controlled study to explore the effect of using lacosamide as an add-on drug in 25 patients from 2010–2012. A dose of either 200 or 400 mg effectively controlled 17 cases (68%), and a distinct effect was also observed in a dose of 400 mg of lacosamide over 15 min (infusion rate of 26.66 mg/min), and the maintenance dose was 200 mg every 12 h (given orally).

In addition to medication, ten children with RSE that was resistant to drugs underwent lesion excision via accurate positioning in a study by Alexopoulos et al. [416]. All of the children experience a good recovery during postoperative follow-up, and RSE was completely controlled in seven of the patients (70%) and significantly improved in three (30%). In another study, patients with RSE caused by CNS vasculitis underwent right TLE lesion resection in the EEG orientation, and a good prognosis was achieved by administering continuous postoperative treatment with immunosuppressant in combination with AEDs [417]. Finally, large doses of hormones and the plasma displacement method have been reported to successfully control RSE [418].

Although there are currently no unified guidance standards for diagnosing and treating RSE, combinations including AEDs, anesthetic drugs, a ketogenic diet, and surgical treatments are the most commonly used treatment options [391, 392, 419, 420].

4.7.8 Prognosis

A retrospective study of 78 patients with RSE showed that 80% of the patients had a poor prognosis, and most died of serious complications [49]. The use of anesthetic drugs increased the chance of infection by 43%, and this effect may have been associated with intubation and disturbances of consciousness [54]. Rossetti et al. [421] performed a follow-up study in 225 hospital patients with SE and found that a patient's prognosis was associated with the patients' age and etiology and the severity of SE and its complications. A multiple factor correlation analysis showed that patients who used vasopressin to lower their blood pressure and presented with secondary complications had a poor prognosis [49]. A retrospective study of 63 patients with RSE showed that more severe arrhythmia and pneumonia and poorer prognoses were observed in patients with longer durations of drug-induced comas [44]. Hence, a variety of methods for treating RSE should be used to change its duration and to reduce brain injury caused by seizures and adverse reactions caused by coma. Cerebrovascular disease should be positively treated because when combined with treatment for RSE, it will not only help control the SE but may also play a key role in determining the prognosis in these patients [422, 423].

4.8 Refractory Status Epilepticus in Infectious Encephalitis

Encephalitis is defined as neurological dysfunction caused by inflammation of the brain parenchyma [424]. In the broad definition, encephalitis includes infectious encephalitis caused by a direct infection of the brain parenchyma, post-infectious inflammatory reactions, such as acute disseminated encephalomyelitis, and autoimmune inflammatory reactions, such as anti-NMDA receptor encephalitis [425]. According to the 2012 criteria of the International Encephalitis Consortium, a diagnosis of encephalitis should include an altered mental status (defined as a decreased or altered level of consciousness, lethargy, or personality change) lasting ≥24 h with no other cause identified and at least two of the following manifestations: (1) documented fever (a temperature higher than 38 °C) within 72 h before or after symptoms appear, (2) generalized or partial seizures that are not fully attributable to a pre-existing seizure disorder, (3) new onset of focal neurological findings, (4) CSF pleocytosis (CSF WBC count ≥5/mm^3), (5) a neuroimaging abnormality in the brain parenchyma suggestive of encephalitis that is either a new onset from previous studies or appears to have an acute onset, and (6) an EEG abnormality consistent with encephalitis that is not attributable to another causes [425]. Thus, seizure is a common clinical sign of encephalitis. According to a case study of 36 patients with RSE by Holtkamp et al. [2], eight cases (22.2%) were caused by encephalitis, indicating that encephalitis is the most common cause of RSE. Since autoimmune encephalitis (AE) has been discussed in another section, we only discuss infectious encephalitis caused by a direct infection of the brain parenchyma in the present chapter.

4.8.1 Historical Evolution

Encephalitis was first introduced by Janz et al. [426] in 1963 as a cause of SE. In 1970, Resnick [427] reported that patients with encephalitis may have severe SE. Encephalitis was found to be a major cause of SE in a 1979 study of 67 cases of SE in children less than 15 years old by Hayakawa et al. [428]. In 1991, Uldry et al. [429] first reported the characteristics of fatal SE caused by HIV encephalitis and attracted researchers' attention. Since then, encephalitis has been recognized as a major cause of SE.

4.8.2 Prevelance

In a study by Vooturi et al. [430], CNS infections were more frequently observed in patients with refractory convulsive RSE than in patients with NORSE. In a study performed in a teaching hospital in India [431], the incidence of SE in patients with CNS infections was 39.8% (37/93). The most frequent causes of the infections were encephalitis (20 patients), including four with Japanese encephalitis, three with herpes simplex encephalitis, one with cerebral malaria, and 12 with non-specific encephalitis; 20% of these patients had RSE. According to a study of 191 patients with encephalitis by Kalita et al. [432], 36 patients had SE, including 11 with RSE (5.8%). In a study of 290 patients with encephalitis by Sonneville et al. [433], 58 (20%) patients developed early-onset SE, including 14 (4.8%) cases of RSE. Coma, non-neurological organ failure(s), and cortical involvement in neuroimaging examinations were independent risk factors for SE in patients with acute encephalitis. In the California Encephalitis Project [434], which was the largest study of encephalitis and included 1151 cases of encephalitis, 502 (44%) patients presented SE, including 43 (4%) patients who developed RSE. Compared to the patients with NORSE or without SE, the patients with RSE were younger, more likely to have a fever (93%) and a prodromal respiratory (57%) or gastrointestinal disorder (64%) and less likely to have CSF pleocytosis (47%) or abnormal neuroimaging (16%). A younger age, prodromal gastrointestinal symptoms, fever, normal CSF WBC, and an initially normal neuroimaging scan were independent risk factors for the development of RSE.

4.8.3 Etiology

Almost all types of infectious encephalitis can cause SE or RSE. Pathogens of encephalitis reported to be associated with RSE include herpes simplex virus, human metapneumovirus, WNV, EBV, *Mycoplasma pneumoniae*, and *Bartonella*. Among the 43 patients with RSE in the California Encephalitis Project, seven patients were diagnosed with viral encephalitis (three confirmed enteroviruses, two probable rotavirus, two probable EBV, one possible HHV6, and one possible adenovirus), and five patients were diagnosed with possible *Mycoplasma pneumoniae* encephalitis [434]. In a retrospective study of 130 cases of NORSE by Gaspard et al. [20], ten cases were caused by infections, among which herpes virus (excluding herpes simplex virus 1) was the most frequent infectious agent (50%). Other causes included cytomegalovirus, EBV, and WNV.

4.8.4 Clinical Features

4.8.4.1 Seizure Types

RSE may present as different seizure types in patients with encephalitis, such as partial seizures or generalized seizures.

Generalized or Primary Partial and Secondary Generalized Seizures

In the study by Lin et al. [435], among the 46 patients with SE caused by encephalitis, 16 (34.8%) patients presented generalized seizures, and 19 (41.3%) patients presented primary partial seizure and secondary generalized seizure.

Partial Seizures

In a case series of *Mycoplasma pneumoniae* encephalitis, all nine patients presented SE, and three of these patients presented complex partial seizures [436]. In a case report by Vehapoglu et al. [437], a patient who was eventually diagnosed with human metapneumovirus (hMPV) encephalitis presented with a coma, paroxysmal right arm twitching, and both eyes turning right, and the EEG showed sharp wave in the right frontal lobe, suggesting a partial seizure. In another case report by Greco et al. [438], a patient who was eventually diagnosed with EBV encephalitis presented a complex partial motor seizure involving the left leg and arm lasting for less than 5 min, followed by a confused state lasting for 3 h, with a generalized high-amplitude slow activity accompanied by unilateral or bilateral spikes and spike slow waves complexes appearing singly or in groups on the EEG.

NCSE

In patients with infectious encephalitis, SE may not only be CSE but also NCSE. In a case report by Bick et al. [439], a patient who presented super-RSE was eventually diagnosed with herpes simplex encephalitis. Initially, the patient presented GTCS and then, after treatment with multiple anti-SE agents, developed NCSE with rhythmic activity in the right central frontal region that occasionally spread to the contralateral frontal region. In a case study of 30 patients with SE caused by encephalitis by Kalita et al. [432], 26 patients presented with GCSE, and four patients presented with NCSE. In another retrospective study of 58 patients with SE caused by encephalitis by Sonneville et al. [433], 46 patients presented with GCSE, whereas another 12 patients presented with NCSE. Because encephalitis is a major cause of NCSE [440, 441], continuous EEG monitoring is required for patients with encephalitis who experience a disturbance of consciousness.

4.8.4.2 Onset Time and Duration

In patients with encephalitis, the onset of SE usually occurs early in the course of the illness, and the duration of the illness is usually protracted. In a retrospective case study of 43 patients with encephalitis who presented with RSE, the median time from the initial symptoms to the onset of SE was 4 days (range 0–41), the median length of the hospital stay for these patients was 47 days (range 9–222), and the median duration of the anesthesia-induced coma was 15 days (range 2–76) [434]. In another retrospective case study of 20 children with encephalitis who presented with RSE by Lin et al., the time from seizure onset to complete clinical seizure control or the appearance of a burst suppression pattern on the EEG was ranged from 1 to 20 days [435].

4.8.5 Auxiliary Examinations

4.8.5.1 EEG

In a retrospective case study of 43 patients with RSE caused by encephalitis, the abnormalities in the EEG included generalized spike discharges, generalized spike and sharp wave activity, multifocal sharp activity, independent bi-hemispheric spike discharges, repetitive sharp waves, focal spike or sharp wave discharges, continuous spike and spike wave activity, right or left temporal spike and sharp activity prior to generalized spread of activity, and rhythmic 2–4 Hz spike wave discharges [434]. However, more multifocal or generalized epileptiform discharges were observed in the patients with RSE than in patients with NORSE in another retrospective study comparing the EEG data from 20 patients with RSE versus 26 patients with NORSE. In the NORSE group, the initial EEG was negative in four patients (15.4%), focal/diffuse cortical dysfunction was observed in nine patients (34.6%), focal epileptiform discharges were observed in eight patients (30.8%), and multifocal epileptiform discharges were observed in five patients (19.2%). In the RSE group, the initial EEG revealed focal epileptiform discharges in one patient (5%), multifocal epileptiform discharges in 14 patients (70%), and generalized epileptiform discharges in five patients (25%) [435].

4.8.5.2 Other Auxiliary Examinations

The initial neuroimaging examinations may be normal in many patients with encephalitis who present with RSE. In a retrospective case study of 43 patients with RSE caused by encephalitis [434], the initial cerebral MRI or CT was normal in 84% of patients, but the subsequent examination showed a focal or multifocal abnormality in the temporal lobe and other cortical, subcortical gray matter or cerebella regions or a hyperintense T2 signal in the mesial temporal region, consistent with herpes encephalitis. In another study of 29 patients with encephalitis-associated SE who accepted the MRI examination [432], 20 patients exhibited abnormalities on the MRI. All four patients with herpes simplex encephalitis showed abnormalities in the temporal lobe. Among the nine patients with Japanese encephalitis, eight patients showed an involvement of the thalamus, the basal ganglion was involved in three patients, the brain stem was involved in five patients, and the cortex was involved in seven patients. Among the 15 patients diagnosed with non-specific encephalitis, the thalamus was involved in three patients, the basal ganglion was involved in one patient, and the cortex was involved in four patients.

In a study of RSE in patients with suspected encephalitis by Glaser et al. [434], three patients received brain biopsies, and another three patients received autopsies. Biopsies from two patients showed mild astrogliosis with no inflammatory cell infiltration and no histopathology suggestive of a neuronal viral infection. The biopsy from the third patient showed microglial nodules and marked lymphocyte infiltration in both the cortex and leptomeninges, suggesting meningoencephalitis. No inclusions indicative of a viral infection were noted and no pathogen was identified. The autopsies of the brains from three other patients showed anoxic-ischemic damage with cerebral edema and neuronal necrosis, but no parenchymal infiltration or other features indicative of encephalitis. Among these patients, one patient had a meningeal lymphocyte infiltration consistent with lymphocytic meningitis.

4.8.6 Treatments

The treatment for SE in patients with infectious encephalitis is similar to the treatment for common SE, but the prognosis is associated with the etiology. Verma et al. [26] reported a case study of a patient with new-onset RSE caused by simplex herpes encephalitis who continued to have electrical SE after treatments with midazoline and propofol. The seizures were eventually controlled after treatment with acyclovir, and the patient had a good prognosis.

Anterior temporal lobectomy (ATL) is an established and effective treatment for patients with medically refractory TLE. In some patients with encephalitis of unknown etiologies and RSE with a clear unilateral origin, ALT should also be considered to assist in the diagnosis, control the seizures, and reduce the mass effect. Bick et al. [439] reported a case study of a 60-year-old man with encephalitis who presented with RSE and displayed a focus of hypoattenuation in the cerebral CT and a hyperintense T2 signal in the right anterior/mesial temporal lobe with associated edema and mass effect. The patient continued to have NCSE after an empirical treatment with the anti-infectious agents including vancomycin, ceftriaxone, ampicillin, and acyclovir and the antiseizure treatments including lorazepam, levetiracetam, propofol, phenobarbital, and phenytoin. His SE was ultimately controlled by ATL and eventually received a good prognosis.

4.8.7 Prognosis

In most patients, RSE is independently associated with a poor prognosis for encephalitis. In a study of encephalitis in 6- to 51-month-old children [435], four of the 26 patients with NORSE died, 16 developed epilepsy and/or a neurological disability, and six returned to baseline. Among the 20 patients with RSE, six died, 13 developed epilepsy and/or a neurological disability, and none returned to baseline. Moreover, the duration from seizure onset to complete clinical seizure control or the appearance of the BS pattern on the EEG was associated with the prognosis. Patients with a duration of less than 3 days showed less cognitive delay at follow-up, and patients with a duration of less than 5 days were less likely to have seizures [435]. In the California Encephalitis Project, 82% of the 43 patients with RSE caused by encephalitis died within 2 years, and the survivors had a severe cognitive or motor disability [434]. Although mortality may be related to an unknown etiology, the mortality within the 90 days after onset was significantly higher in the RSE group than in NORSE group, and the multivariate analysis showed that RSE was a dependent risk factor for patients with encephalitis [433].

The prognosis of RSE in patients with *Mycoplasma pneumoniae* encephalitis is very poor because *Mycoplasma pneumoniae* encephalitis itself is a severe disease with an incidence and mortality that is up to seven times higher than encephalitis caused by other pathogens [442]. In a case series of nine patients with *Mycoplasma pneumoniae* encephalitis, all patients presented with SE. At the end of the study period, none of the patients had returned to baseline, two died (one had RSE), two were in a persistent vegetative state (both had RSE), three had a severe disability (two of them had RSE), and two had a moderate disability (one had RSE) [436].

4.8.8 SE or RSE in Different Types of Encephalitis

4.8.8.1 SE/RSE in Herpes Simplex Encephalitis

Herpes simplex encephalitis (HSE) is the most common type of virus encephalitis. According to different reports, the incidence of seizures in patients with HSE ranges from 75 to 89% [443, 444], including SE or even RSE. The onset of SE not only occurs in the initial stage as new-onset RSE [26] but also occurs after the viral infection as post-infectious autoimmune encephalitis [445] (please see the chapter on RSE in patients with autoimmune encephalitis). Patients with HSE can present with GCSE [26], but more frequently present with NCSE [446, 447]. Since HSE usually affects the limbic system, including the anterior/median temporal lobe, orbital frontal lobe, and insular lobe, the EEGs of patients with HSE are significantly more likely to exhibit periodic discharges and focal slowing in the frontotemporal and occipital regions compared with the EEGs of patients with encephalitis of other etiologies [448, 449]. The neuroimaging data from most patients are abnormal, and the classic presentations on the MRI show asymmetric hyperintense T2 signals in the mesiotemporal and orbitofrontal lobes and the insular cortex, which are corresponding to edema of these regions [450]. Most patients with HSE respond to acyclovir [450] and have a good prognosis after treatment with antiepileptic and antiviral agents [26]. However, malignant RSE has also been observed. Bick et al. [439] had reported a case study of a 60-year-old male patient who developed SRSE caused by HSVE. He continued to have NCSE after empirical treatments with antibacterial and antiviral agents and a three-level anti-SE treatment. His seizures were eventually controlled by ATL.

4.8.8.2 SE/RSE in Japanese Encephalitis

Japanese encephalitis is a common type of encephalitis in Southeast Asia. According to previous reports, the incidence of seizures in patients with Japanese encephalitis was 46–54% [444, 451], which was only second to HSE [444], whereas the occurrence of SE was not common. Patients with Japanese encephalitis predominantly present primary focal seizures with secondary generalization. In a study by Misra et al. [451], 30 of 65 patients with Japanese encephalitis experienced a seizure within a week, including 17 GTCSs and 13 partial motor seizures with secondary generalization. Eleven patients had a single seizure, eight had two seizures, 11 had multiple seizures, and only two patients developed SE, both of whom presented partial motor seizures with secondary generalization and not RSE. However, in a study by Kalita et al., nine of the 30 patients with SE caused by encephalitis were diagnosed with Japanese encephalitis [432]. The interictal EEG more likely showed focal slowing and was less likely to exhibit epileptiform discharges. In a study of 65 patients with Japanese encephalitis by Misra et al. [451], the interictal EEG of the patients with seizures revealed theta to delta slow waves in all patients, but epileptiform discharges were only observed in four patients. The prognosis of the patients with Japanese encephalitis who had seizures was poorer than that of patients without seizures. In a study by Misra et al. [451], three of the 23 patients with Japanese encephalitis and seizures exhibited a complete recovery, eight exhibited a partial recovery, nine exhibited a poor recovery, and three died. Among the 34 patients without seizures, 17 patients exhibited a complete recovery, five exhibited a partial recovery, seven exhibited a poor recovery, and five died. In the study of Kalita et al. [432], four of the nine patients with Japanese encephalitis and seizures died.

4.8.8.3 SE/RSE in Human Metapneumovirus Encephalitis

Since its initial discovery in 2001 [452], human metapneumovirus (hMPV) has been established as a common pathogen of respiratory tract infections with a global distribution. Although most hMPV infections are mild to moderate, several case reports of severe infections, such as encephalitis, have been published. Most patients with hMPV encephalitis had seizures. In the California Encephalitis Project, the nasopharyngeal swabs from five patients were positive, and three of these patients presented seizures [453]. Among the 13 patients included in published case reports, ten patients presented seizures, including three cases of SE [437, 453–459]. HMPV encephalitis often occurs in children and is usually accompanied by severe lung infections. The seizure type may be generalized seizures [455] or partial seizure [437]. The interictal EEG may be normal or exhibit focal sharp waves, and the neuroimaging examinations are usually normal [437, 455]. Most patients with hMPV encephalitis have a good prognosis after treatment with appropriate anti-infectious and antiseizure agents [437, 456]. Webster et al. [455] had reported a case study of two patients with hMPV encephalitis who presented SE accompanied by respiratory failure. Between these patients, one was a previously healthy 15-month-old female who became abnormally excited during the night and then presented uncontrolled full body twitching and eye deviation to the right after 2 days of nausea. After treatment with rectal diazepam followed by intravenous lorazepam, fosphenytoin, and finally phenobarbital, her clinical seizure was eventually controlled 35 min after onset. Another 18-month-old female toddler with a history of one simple febrile seizure presented GTCS after several hours of decreased oral intake and fever. After treatment with midazolam, lorazepam, and fosphenytoin, the patient's SE was eventually controlled 45 min after onset. Both patients had lung infections and gradually developed respiratory failure, but both had a good prognosis after receiving the antiviral and antibacterial treatments. Vehapoglu et al. [437] reported a case study of a 4-month-old male infant who developed hMPV encephalitis and suddenly displayed twitching of the right extremity and eye deviations to the right after 3 days of mild rhinorrhea, cough, and fever. He was somnolent soon after the seizures occurred, with a right frontal sharp wave discharge in the EEG and a normal cerebral

MRI. His seizure was not controlled by AEDs, including levetiracetam, phenytoin, phenobarbital, and midazolam and anti-infectious drugs, including ceftriaxone and acyclovir. Finally, the seizure was gradually controlled by a thiopental sodium infusion, and the infant eventually had a good prognosis.

4.8.8.4 SE/RSE in WNV Encephalitis

WNV is a mosquito-borne subgroup of arboviruses that was, in 1937, first isolated from the blood of a febrile woman in the West Nile province of Uganda in 1937, and WNV began to play a more prominent role in clinical practice since its first outbreak in the US in 1999. According to different reports, the incidence of seizure in patients with WNV encephalitis is approximately 0–9% [460–462]. WNV encephalitis usually symmetrically affects the brain stem and midbrain. The most common type of SE is NCSE; the most frequent abnormality in the EEG is symmetric generalized slowing with a frontal predominance and occasionally with a bilateral or asymmetric temporal predominance. The cerebral MRI often exhibits bilateral symmetrical T2 hypertension in the brain stem and midbrain [463]. Most patients with WNV encephalitis have a good prognosis, with the exception of several severe cases, which have a poor prognosis. Older patients and/or patients in a profound coma tend to have a poor prognosis. During the epidemic of WNV encephalitis in the southeast district of Tunis in 1997, 25 of the 30 patients recovered completely, one had a persistent headache and asthenia, one had persistent arm tremor, and three substantially older (mean age 62 ± 2 vs. 53.3 ± 23.3 years, $p < 0.05$) who were in a profound coma died [464]. However, reports about the relationship between seizures and the prognosis of WNV encephalitis are not available. Bagic et al. [465] reported a case study of a patient with WNV encephalitis who presented RSE. The patient initially experienced chills and fever and gradually experienced asymmetric leg weakness, double vision, and dysphagia and soon had a disturbance of consciousness. On the fourteenth day after onset, the patient began to exhibit "fast eye movements with eyelid flickering." The cerebral MRI exhibited symmetrical abnormalities in the bilateral hippocampus, substantia nigra, central pontine, and dentate nucleus in the cerebellum. The EEG displayed moderate diffuse slowing with a poly-spike wave discharge. After treatment with lorazepam, fosphenytoin, phenobarbital, propofol, valproic acid, and carbamazepine, the electrical SE was eventually controlled. Unfortunately, the patient ultimately died.

4.8.8.5 SE/RSE in Patients with Human Parvovirus B19 Encephalitis

As a pathogen of erythema infectiosum, human parvovirus B19 (hPVB19) usually causes a benign and self-limited disease. However, in immunodeficient subjects or children, it can also cause a severe disease. According to the study by Barah et al. [466], hPVB19 caused 4.3% of cases of undetermined meningoencephalitis during its epidemic outbreak between 1997 and 1998. The incidence of seizure in patients with hPVB19 encephalitis is very low. In a study by Barah et al. [466], only two of the 12 patients with hPVB19 encephalitis presented seizures. According to published reports [466–469], the SE types observed in patients with hPVB19 encephalitis include GTCS, partial seizure, or partial seizure with subsequent generalization. SE may be convulsive SE or NCSE, with diffuse slowing or a focal slow wave with epileptiform discharges. The cerebral MRI usually does not show abnormalities. The pathogenesis is usually considered related to autoimmune inflammatory reactions, and the patient usually has a good prognosis after receiving immunoregulatory, antiviral, and antiepileptic treatments. Erol et al. [469] reported a case study of a 10-year-old girl who was eventually diagnosed with hPVB19 and presented RSE. The patient displayed confusion and GTCS at onset, with diffuse slowing and epileptiform discharges in the left hemisphere in the EEG and a normal cerebral CT/MRI. Her electrical SE persisted after treatment with valproic acid, midazolam, and pentobarbital and was eventually controlled with high-dose corticosteroids. In another case report by Skaff et al. [468], a previously healthy 27-year-old woman initially displayed an erythematous, maculopapular rash over her cheeks, frontal headache with intermittent, low-grade fevers, myalgias, anorexia, and lethargy and developed psychiatric symptoms, including depression, hallucinations, and confusion 5 days after onset. She began to have seizure activity with facial twitching and eye blinking and progressed to CSE, with diffuse slowing on the EEG and no significant abnormalities in the cerebral MRI. She continued to have NCSE after treatment with phenytoin and phenobarbital. A right frontal lobe biopsy was performed 6 weeks after the onset of her illness and showed minimal, chronic, leptomeningeal inflammations and mild, superficial, cortical gliosis. Since the serologic evaluation for HPVB19 on day 53 was positive for both IgM and IgG, she was diagnosed with HPVB19 encephalitis. After multiple treatments, including acyclovir, carbamazepine, lorazepam, topiramate, phenobarbital, VNS, and rehabilitation, she eventually exhibited a near complete recovery. Palermo et al. [467] also reported a case study of a previously healthy 18-year-old male patient who initially presented with headache, fever, sleepiness, and irritability 7 days after an erythematous rash involving all four limbs occurred. Five days later, the patient developed GTCS preceded by auditory sensations, version of the head to the right, and hyperextension of the right arm. The EEG exhibited diffuse and persistent slow delta activity with subcontinuous recruiting sharp theta activity that was prevalent over the right frontotemporal region, whereas the cerebral CT and MRI were normal. After receiving levetiracetam, phenobarbital, and clonazepam treatments, he continued to present eyelid flickering and GTCS. Since the serological tests for the PVB19 DNA, IgG, and IgM were all positive, the patient was diagnosed with HPVB19 encephalitis, and all symptoms, with the exception of ictal epilepsy, recovered after receiving immunoglobulin treatments.

4.8.8.6 SE/RSE in EBV Encephalitis

The Epstein-Barr virus (EBV) is a lymphocyte virus belonging to *Herpesviridae* and is the pathogen responsible for infectious mononucleosis and is closely related to the occurrence of nasopharyngeal carcinoma and childhood lymphoma. It can also lead to acute, severe diseases, such as myocarditis and complications of the CNS, including meningitis, encephalitis, and neuritis. In a study by Mazur-Melewska et al. [470], ten of the 194 patients with EBV infections had infections in the CNS, and five of these patients developed seizures, including four cases of GTCSs and one case of partial seizures. EBV encephalitis often affects the unilateral or bilateral basal ganglion or thalamus [470–472], but it may also affect the temporal and occipital lobes [438] or the brain stem, midbrain, and corpus callosum [473]. The presentations in the EEG include diffuse or focal slow waves, fast beta activity with high-amplitude sharp waves, low-voltage activity with spike-wave discharges, high-amplitude slow waves with unilateral or bilateral spikes, and spike slow waves complexes appearing singly or in a group [438, 470]. The cerebral MRI may show T2 hyperintense in the unilateral or bilateral basal ganglion and thalamus or tempo-occipital region [470–472]. Most patients have a good prognosis after receiving antiviral and antiepileptic treatments; however, a few have a persistent neurological dysfunction [438, 470–473]. Greco et al. [438] reported a case study of a 4-year-old girl who initially presented with NCSE that began with 3 days of fever and sore throat. After 1 month, the patient had a complex motor partial seizure involving the arms and left leg that lasted for less than 5 min and a subsequent acute confused state that lasted for 3 h. The EEG showed a generalized high-amplitude slow wave activity with unilateral or bilateral spikes and spike slow waves complexes that appeared singly or in a group. The cerebral MRI showed subcortical T2 hypertension in the right occipital lobe. Since the patient's serum was positive for IgM and IgG antibodies and the EBV DNA was detected in the CSF using a nested PCR, she was diagnosed with EBV encephalitis and eventually recovered after treatment with acyclovir and other agents. Nishie et al. [474] reported a case study of a 37-year-old female patient with RSE that was thought to be caused by EBV. She initially presented with fever and headache followed by RSE 10 days later, with a diffuse slow-wave outbreak and bilateral paroxysmal diffuse sharp wave on the EEG. She was treated with anesthetic agents for as long as 2 months but ultimately had a good prognosis. Delgado et al. [473] reported a case study of a 55-year-old female patient with EBV encephalitis who had undergone renal transplantation and had been treated with immunosuppressive therapy for more than 7 years. She initially complained of dizziness and influenza-like symptoms and then experienced visual hallucinations, a disturbance of consciousness, and continuous motor partial seizures in the left limbs. The MRI showed T2 hyperintense in the medulla, fornix, midbrain, left thalamus, and around the corpus callosum. Since the serological test for the EBV DNA was negative, the patient was diagnosed with EBV encephalitis and had a good prognosis after treatment with ganciclovir.

4.8.8.7 SE/RSE in Patients with *Mycoplasma pneumoniae* Encephalitis

Mycoplasma pneumoniae (*M. pneumoniae*) is also a common pathogen that causes encephalitis, particularly in children. Among 43 patients with suspected encephalitis who presented with RSE in California Encephalitis Project, five were diagnosed with probable *M. pneumoniae* encephalitis [434]. In a retrospective study by Lin et al. [436], SE was present in all nine cases of *M. pneumoniae* encephalitis occurring in children between 2002 and 2008 (100%), and the most frequent initial seizure type was partial seizure with subsequent generalization (4/9, 44%), followed by complex partial seizures (3/9, 33%) and GTCSs (2/9, 22%). Six patients developed RSE, including four patients with partial seizures and subsequent generalization, one patient with complex partial seizures, and one patient with GTCS. The presentations in the EEG included focal epileptiform discharges in two patients, multifocal epileptiform discharges in three patients, diffuse epileptiform discharges in two patients, and cortical dysfunction in two patients. Cerebral MRI was performed on seven patients, and the abnormalities included atrophy in three patients, T2 hyperintense in the bilateral hippocampus in two patients, acute disseminated encephalitis in one patient, and increased leptomeningeal enhancement at the 6th day from onset in one patient. The overall prognosis was poor. Two patients died (one had RSE), two patients were in a persistent vegetative state (both had RSE), three patients experienced persistent, severe neurological dysfunction (two had RSE), and two patients experienced a mild to moderate neurological dysfunction (one had RSE).

4.8.8.8 SE/RSE in Patients with *Bartonella* Encephalitis

A type of gram-negative bacilli, *Bartonella henselae*, is the etiological agent of cat-scratch disease. It can also infect the CNS and cause neurological symptoms including seizure, encephalopathy, neuroretinitis, and vasculitis. According to published reports [475–478], the incidence of seizure in *Bartonella* encephalitis is approximately 50–79%. It may occur within 6 weeks and may present as GCSE or NCSE, partial seizures, or generalized seizures. The EEG abnormalities include focal slow waves, sharp waves, or spike-waves. The cerebral MRI may exhibit T2 and DWI hypertension in the bilateral pulvinar or tempo-occipital region. If *Bartonella* encephalitis is diagnosed early and effectively treated with antibiotics, such as erythromycin and rifampicin, and antiepileptic agents, most patients have a good prognosis. Singhal et al. [477] reported a case study of two patients with *Bartonella* encephalitis. The first was a 27-year-old female patient with convulsive RSE whose cerebral MRI exhibited T2 and DWI hypertension in the bilateral pulvinar region. The patient had recently received scratches from her pet cat, and her serum and CSF were both positive for anti-*Bartonella* IgG. Thus, she was diagnosed with *Bartonella* encephalitis and gradually recovered after treatment with intravenous erythromycin followed by intravenous trimethoprim. The other case was a 66-year-old female patient who initially presented with sudden right arm clumsiness and developed right arm and facial twitching that gradually progressed to RSE. The cerebral MRI showed T2 and DWI hypertension in the left frontal lobe and parieto-occipital cortices. Based on a cat-scratch history and positive serological anti-*Bartonella* IgG test, she was diagnosed with *Bartonella* encephalitis and was treated with ofloxacin for 2 weeks, followed by minocycline for 3 weeks, multiple antiepileptic agents, corticoids, electrical shock, and eventually underwent surgical resection of the lesions with subpial transections in the left pre- and postcentral gyri. Upon discharge to rehabilitation at 4.5 months, she had recurrent partial and generalized seizures and neurological disabilities, including profound aphasia and right-hand dystonia. Laswell et al. [478] reported a case study of a 28-year-old female patient who presented with new-onset RSE and had a history of recent exposure to a new cat and a positive serological test for *Bartonella*. Thus, the patient was diagnosed with *Bartonella* encephalitis. She continued to experience NCSE after treatment with benzodiazepines, fosphenytoin, propofol, and levetiracetam and eventually recovered after receiving a combination of doxycycline, rifampicin, and high-dose corticosteroids.

4.9 Epilepsy and Refractory Status Epilepticus in Other Diseases

4.9.1 Epilepsy and RSE in Brain Tumors

4.9.1.1 Epilepsy in Brain Tumors

Both primary and secondary brain tumors can cause seizures. Hildbrand et al. [479] showed that in 158 patients with cerebral tumors, 86% of the patients experienced a seizure shortly after receiving a diagnosis of brain tumor, while the remaining patients experienced a seizure during treatment for the tumor. Michelucci et al. [480] showed that in 100 patients with brain tumors complicated with epilepsy, approximately 70% of the patients with brain tumors presented with a seizure before the other symptoms, whereas 12–18% patients with brain tumors had SE. The onset of seizures in patients with brain tumors may be associated with the following two factors: (1) a focal increase in excitatory transmission caused by changes in the local tumor environment that leads to the onset of seizures or (2) seizures may occur because of tumor lesions, such as a high-grade glioma, that grow rapidly and cause severe damage to the local tissue [481, 482].

Prevalence

Epilepsy is associated with cerebral tumors in approximately 4–13% of patients [483]. Benign tumors are more likely to lead to chronic epilepsy that persists for more than 2 years [484]. As shown in a study by Lynam et al. [485], approximately 30% of patients with primary brain tumors present seizures as the main clinical manifestation, and 20% of patients with metastatic tumors present seizures. The incidence of seizures in patients with cerebral tumors is influenced by age, tumor type, tumor location, and other factors. (1) Age: The incidence of seizure is different between adult and pediatric patients with brain tumors. Ullrich et al. [486] conducted a study in 298 pediatric patients with brain tumors. Seizure was a main symptom in 24% of these pediatric patients, and approximately 14% of the patients presented SE, whereas, in a study performed by Lynam et al. [485], 30% of adult patients presented seizures. (2) Tumor type: Among patients with different types of tumors, those with gliomas had the highest incidence of seizure. Gliomas include dysembryoplastic neuroepithelial tumors (DNETs) and gangliogliomas, among others. The remaining tumor types that tend to lead to seizure include metastatic tumors and meningiomas [487]. (3) Tumor location: The location of a tumor is one of the most important factors that affect the incidence of seizure. Patients with tumors in the parietal, frontal, and temporal lobes may have a higher incidence of seizure, and patients with occipital lobe tumors are the least likely to develop seizures [485].

Seizure Types

Partial seizure is the most common seizure type and includes simple partial seizures and CPS [488]. Chang et al. [489] conducted a study in 332 patients with low-grade gliomas and found that approximately 80% of the patients had seizures. The most common type was partial seizure, which was followed by generalized seizure. The type of epileptic seizure was different between children and adults. In a study of adult and pediatric patients with brain tumors that was performed by Wojcik-Draczkowska et al. [490], secondary generalized seizure was the most frequent seizure type in pediatric patients, whereas simple partial seizure or CPS were the most common types in adult patients.

Diagnosis

In patients with brain tumors, seizure is one of the most common clinical symptoms and can occur before or after a brain tumor diagnosis. Gottschalk et al. [491] reported a case study of an old woman with a 60-year history of epilepsy with an unknown cause. Eventually, a cerebral tumor was determined to be the cause of her epilepsy. A complete medical history, a physical examination, a neurological physical examination, an EEG, laboratory examinations, and imaging examinations are required to determine whether the epilepsy is secondary to brain tumor. MRI is essential for obtaining a diagnosis in cerebral tumors because it helps to classify and identify the tumor, both of which can guide subsequent treatment [492].

Treatments

Antiepileptic Treatment

Antiepileptic treatment can be applied in patients who do not conform to surgical indications or whose symptoms must be controlled before surgery to obtain the benefit of the operation. Seizures caused by cerebral tumors are difficult to control. Statistical data show that approximately 24% of patients with brain tumors who present with comorbid epilepsy require more than three types of AEDs [493]. Because few relevant experiments have been published, researchers have not yet determined which drug is the most effective. When choosing a drug, clinicians should consider its tolerance and effectiveness in addition to drug interactions. AEDs, such as valproic acid, lamotrigine, and levetiracetam, are recommended [494]. During chemotherapy, AEDs that can induce the expression of hepatic cytochrome P450 enzyme should be avoided [482]. Accumulating evidence indicates that AEDs may have direct antitumor effects [495]. However, older AEDs, such as phenobarbital and phenytoin, have been shown to promote tumor growth in animal models. These two drugs should therefore be avoided [496]. The American Academy of Neurology has suggested that the prophylactic use of AEDs in patients with brain tumors is not useful [497], and a meta-analysis of a randomized experiment performed in 2015 found that the prophylactic use of AEDs in patients with brain tumors merely decreased the incidence of seizures [498].

Surgery

In general, surgical resection will largely reduce the frequency and severity of seizures [486, 499]. The surgical resection of low-grade gliomas should be conducted as soon as possible because patients with this type of tumor have a good prognosis after surgery [500]. The condition of most patients will clearly improve after surgery, but some patients will continue to experience seizures [501].

Radiotherapy and Chemotherapy

Radiotherapy and chemotherapy are used to prevent the recurrence of a tumor after surgery, and these treatments have recently been suggested for controlling seizures. In a study of patients with low-grade and high-grade gliomas published by Ruda et al. [503], epilepsy was well controlled in patients who received radiotherapy, and after 12 months of radiotherapy, half of the patients had less frequent seizures, and approximately 30% of the patients were seizure-free. In a study of patients with low-grade gliomas published by Sherman et al. [502], temozolomide significantly reduced the frequency of seizures, and 13–55% of the patients were seizure-free. However, chemotherapy may induce epilepsy, and patients should therefore be closely monitored during chemotherapy.

4.9.1.2 RSE in Patients with Brain Tumors

Inducing Factors

(1) The incidence of SE caused by brain tumors varies according to the location of the tumor. Patients with frontal lobe tumors are the most

likely to develop SE, and these patients tend to develop RSE [504]. (2) Improper treatment is one of the common causes of SE or RSE. In a study published by Tiamkao et al. [505], half of the patients with SE had a history of improper therapies. (3) Hormonal abnormalities can also induce SE or RSE. Aladdin et al. [506] reported a case study of a pregnant woman with cavernous angioma who had no history of epilepsy. However, during pregnancy, the patient presented with RSE. Treatment included general anesthesia and appropriate tumor therapy, but these were not effective. After terminating the pregnancy, the patient's seizures eventually stopped. Similarly, Kasai et al. [507] also reported a case study of a pregnant patient with a brain tumor who had secondary SE. The patient's epileptic symptoms gradually disappeared after cesarean section.

Clinical Manifestations

SE or RSE is common among patients with brain tumors. (1) Incidence: Based on previously reported data from patients with brain tumors, the incidence of SE is approximately 15–22% [508, 510]. The location of the tumor affects the incidence of SE, and the incidence is higher in patients with frontal lobe tumors [508]. (2) Time of onset: SE is more likely to occur during the late course of the disease in patients with brain tumors and reflects tumor growth [509]. Moots et al. [510] conducted a study of ten patients with brain tumors to determine when they developed SE. Two patients presented SE when the tumor was diagnosed, four patients presented SE during the period of tumor progression, and only one patient presented SE during radiotherapy. (3) Type: In these patients, the type of SE is similar to seizure caused by brain tumors, but the duration is longer.

Treatments

In patients with brain tumors, diazepam may be the first choice to treat SE. According to Chen et al. [512], general anesthesia can be used to treat patients with RSE, and tumor resection may be conducted after the seizure is controlled. In addition, Swisher et al. [511] proposed that phenytoin, levetiracetam, and pregabalin are useful and safe in patients with cerebral tumors complicated by RSE. Multiple subpial transections and other surgeries may be alternative treatments. In a study by Ng et al. [513], a 48-year-old patient with a brain tumor presented with RSE and then successfully underwent multiple subpial transections under the guidance of subdural grid electrodes. Long-term AED therapy is required in patients with brain tumors who present SE even after the seizures are terminated.

Prognosis

According to Hocker et al. [44], 75% of patients with RSE have a poor prognosis. This is particularly true in patients who are in a drug-induced coma or with severe electroencephalographic suppression. Early diagnosis and good control predict a better prognosis.

4.9.2 Epilepsy and RSE in Diabetes Mellitus

Diabetes mellitus is metabolic disease that influences all systems of the body. Seizures frequently appear in patients with diabetes. In recent years, epilepsy has been considered one of the important neurological complications of diabetes.

4.9.2.1 Epilepsy in Diabetes Mellitus

Pathogenesis

There is no unified conclusion regarding the pathogenesis of epilepsy in patients with diabetes. Several possible etiologies are discussed below.

Immune Abnormity

Glutamic acid decarboxylase antibodies (GAD-Abs) are detected in 60–70% of patients with diabetes who present seizures [514] and are particularly common in patients with type 1 diabetes mellitus (T1DM). As shown in a study by Moloney et al. [515], GAD-Ab levels are higher in patients with T1DM and epilepsy than in patients with T1DM alone, especially in patients who present with epilepsy as the first symptom of T1DM. Glutamic acid decarboxylase (GAD) is expressed in neurons that secrete gamma aminobutyric acid (GABA) and pancreatic beta cells [516], and antibodies against this enzyme can cause seizures [517]. This effect potentially explains the relationship between GAD-Ab and diabetes-associated epilepsy.

Brain Microvascular Lesions

Patients with diabetes, particularly older patients, tend to develop systemic microvascular lesions, and this type of brain lesion can cause a variety of neurological complications. Kashihara et al. [518] reported a case study of a patient with non-insulin-dependent diabetes who presented with seizures. Single photon emission computed tomography images showed a diffuse decrease in cerebral blood flow, and high T2 signals were observed in bilateral hippocampal on the MRI examination, suggesting that seizure may be associated with microvascular lesions in patients with DM.

Gene Mutations

According to recent surveys, gene mutations may be an underlying cause of some syndromes that present as both epilepsy and DM. In a study by Yew et al. [519], two siblings who were diagnosed with young-onset diabetes mellitus exhibited microcephaly, intellectual disability, and epilepsy. This syndrome is caused by a mutation in the TRMT10A gene. In addition, mutations in the ABCC8 and KCNJ11 genes have been shown to be major contributors to developmental delay, epilepsy, and neonatal diabetes syndrome (DEND), which is characterized by diabetes, severe developmental retardation, and epilepsy [520]. Mutations in other genes, such as the ALMS1 splice mutation [521] and IER3IP1 mutations [522], have been observed in other syndromes.

Metabolic Factors

Huang et al. [523] conducted a retrospective study and found that the high blood glucose levels that are observed in patients with diabetes may be associated with seizure. Additionally, low blood glucose levels may increase the risk of seizure in patients with diabetes [524]. In a study by Burns et al. [525], seizures were the most common clinical manifestations in newborns with severe hypoglycemia. When the metabolic disorders mentioned above are corrected, seizures gradually stop.

Others

Based on available evidence, diabetic epilepsy may be associated with focal brain damage [527] and abnormalities in neurotransmitters [528].

Clinical Manifestations

According to statistical data, approximately 25% of patients with diabetes will at some time present seizures [526]. Partial seizure, particularly partial motor seizure, is the most common type of seizure in patients with diabetes [529]. The most common types of epilepsy in pediatric patients with T1DM are non-idiopathic TLE and IGE [530]. Seizure may occur during any stage of diabetes. Seizure may present as the only clinical symptom or after the onset of other diabetic symptoms (such as polydipsia and polyuria). During insulin treatment, epilepsy can also be induced by hypoglycemia [531]. Diabetic seizures have a longer duration and can last approximately 15–30 min [532].

Diagnosis

Currently, there are no unified criteria for diagnosing epilepsy associated with diabetes [514]. First, clinicians must clearly determine whether a patient has experienced a seizure. The clinician must then determine whether the patient has diabetes. Next, the relationship between the seizure and diabetes must be determined using characteristics including incidence, onset time, seizure type, and treatment effect (additional details are presented in Chap. 2).

When a newborn has refractory epilepsy, severe developmental retardation, hypotonia, and DM, DEND syndrome should be considered as potential underlying causes [520]. When a patient with diabetes presents epilepsy, dysaudia, recurrent headache, stroke-like episodes, dementia, hypotension, lactic acidosis, and short stature, clinicians should consider the possibility of MELAS syndrome [533].

Treatments

Controlling Blood Glucose Levels

The goal of treatment should be focused on controlling blood glucose levels and correcting the metabolic disorder. Hypoglycemic drugs may terminate the seizure. If blood glucose levels are ineffectively controlled, epilepsy will recur. However, epilepsy will no longer occur when blood glucose levels return to normal, even if the patient stops using AEDs [514]. Moreover, a low carbohydrate diet may reduce the frequency of seizures by controlling blood glucose levels [514, 534]. In a study by Kim et al. [534], a low glycemic index diet was an effective and tolerable treatment in patients with generalized epilepsy. In addition, an increasing number of clinicians are using the ketogenic diet to treat diabetes-associated epilepsy. Aylward et al. [535] reported a case study of pediatric patients with T1DM who presented with myoclonic astatic epilepsy. After 2 months on a ketogenic diet, seizure frequency was reduced in these patients, indicating that the ketogenic diet has an effect on diabetic epilepsy.

Antiepileptic Treatment

AEDs not only control seizures but also regulate blood glucose levels. A unified perspective of antiepileptic treatments is not currently available. However, drugs such as phenytoin should be avoided because they inhibit insulin secretion, elevate blood glucose levels, and increase the risk of seizure. According to the results of some studies, carbamazepine may be an effective treatment for diabetic epilepsy. Roze et al. [536] reported a case study of diabetic patients who presented SE in whom seizures were terminated following the administration of carbamazepine. Similarly, Batista et al. [537] also reported a case study in which carbamazepine effectively treated patients with diabetes and CPS. Topiramate may be a good alternative because it treats both epilepsy and diabetes [538].

4.9.2.2 RSE in Diabetes Mellitus

Clinical Characteristics

Diabetic seizures are long-lasting and difficult to control. Additionally, they tend to progress to RSE.

Relationship with GAD-Ab Levels

Cikrikcili et al. [266] reported a case study of a 63-year-old patient with Type 2 diabetes mellitus who presented with NCSE and increasing serum GAD-Ab levels. Treatment with methylprednisolone and intravenous immunoglobulin improved the patient's condition and ultimately decreased the patient's GAD-Ab levels. As shown in a study by Kanter et al. [288], GAD-Ab levels are associated with RSE. Baglietto et al. [539] reported a case study of patients with T1DM who presented with epilepsia partialis continua (EPC) and increasing levels of GAD-Ab in the CSF at onset. The epilepsy then became refractory, and during slow sleep periods EEG recordings showed that the patients exhibited continuous spike-waves. Thus, GAD-Ab may participate in the pathogenesis underlying diabetic RSE.

Relationship with Hyperglycemia

Paiboonpol et al. [540] reported a case study of 22 patients with hyperglycemia who presented partial SE. The average duration was 9 days, and the seizures stopped when the patients' blood glucose levels were controlled. Further studies have shown that most of these patients had metabolic disorders, such as high blood glucose levels, low serum sodium levels, and high osmotic pressure.

Types of SE

Schomer et al. [527] noted that focal SE and EPC are the specific manifestation of patients with non-ketonic diabetes. Paiboonpol et al. [540] reported a study of 22 patients with diabetes who presented EPC as the initial symptom. Mukherjee et al. [541] reported a case study of a pediatric patient with T1DM who also showed EPC.

Treatment

Researchers have not yet achieved consensus regarding the optimal treatment for DM-associated RSE. Generally, the treatment should be determined by the symptoms. Phenytoin and phenobarbital should be avoided because they influence insulin secretion. Symptoms should be treated using fluid infusions and strategies that correct electrolyte disturbances and hyperglycemia. When necessary, mannitol should be used to prevent cerebral edema. The treatments used to terminate the seizure are described in Chaps. 6, 7, and 8.

4.9.3 Epilepsy and RSE in Systemic Lupus Erythematosus

Systemic lupus erythematosus (SLE) is a common autoimmune disease that is characterized by multisystem damage caused by autoantibodies and immune complexes. When the CNS is involved, the disease is called neuropsychiatric systemic lupus erythematosus (NPSLE), and its clinical manifestations include epilepsy, cognitive dysfunction, and insanity.

4.9.3.1 Epilepsy in SLE

SLE is common in females. Thus, SLE should be considered when a female presents seizures with an unknown cause.

Prevalence

Tsai et al. [544] conducted a cohort study and found that patients with SLE, especially young patients, are more prone to develop epilepsy, and neurological complications and mental illness increase the risk of epilepsy. The incidence of seizure varies among previous reports. Mikdashi et al. [542] reported an incidence of approximately 14%. However, Ramsey-Goldman [543] conducted a cohort study of 1295 patients with SLE and found that approximately 6% of these patients developed seizures after an SLE diagnosis.

Clinical Manifestations

Seizure Types

SLE can cause a variety of seizure types, including GTCS and partial seizures. Of these, GTCS are the most common [545]. In a study by Mikdashi et al. [542], 28 of 195 patients with SLE presented seizures. According to the international standard for classifying epileptic seizures, three-fourths of patients present generalized seizures, and the remainder present partial seizures. González-Duarte et al. [547] conducted a large-sample cohort study and found that two-thirds of 75 patients with SLE and epilepsy presented tonic-clonic seizures during follow-up.

Onset Time and Disease Course

Seizures can occur at any time in patients with SLE but most frequently occur in its early stage. In a study by González-Duarte et al. [547], approximately half of the patients developed seizures in the early stage of SLE.

In some patients, epilepsy is the only clinical manifestation in the early stage of SLE, and SLE is therefore diagnosed a few years after the appearance of epilepsy [306, 548]. In this situation, epilepsy caused by SLE tends to be misdiagnosed as primary epilepsy.

Patients with SLE who present seizures as the first symptom should be distinguished from patients with SLE induced by AEDs. Degirmencioglu et al. [549] reported a case study of a pregnant woman who was using lamotrigine to treat her epilepsy. In the 36th gestational week, SLE appeared. The symptoms disappeared after the patient stopped using the drugs, and the patient was therefore diagnosed with drug-induced SLE.

Reversible Posterior Encephalopathy and Neonatal Lupus Erythematosus

Reversible posterior encephalopathy (RPE) may be caused by SLE and characterized by headache, vomiting, mental disorders, seizures, and other neurological symptoms. Leroux et al. [550] reported a case study of four patients with RPE caused by SLE. Their MRI results showed edema in the posterior part of the brain. MRI also showed hemorrhagic complications in one patient. Neonatal lupus erythematosus is a rare autoimmune disease characterized by focal seizures, skin lupus, anemia, and thrombocytopenia [551].

Auxiliary Examinations

EEG

Patients with SLE who present seizures usually have obvious abnormalities on an EEG that may be characterized by focal slowing or sharp or spike-waves [552].

Neuroimaging

Imaging is an important auxiliary examination that is used to diagnosis epilepsy caused by SLE. In a study by Ainiala et al. [553], MRI was performed in patients with SLE and epilepsy, and it always showed cortical atrophy and T1- and T2-weighted abnormalities. In a study of 133 patients with NPSLE and epilepsy published by Jeong et al. [554], MRI mainly showed gray matter hyperintensities, suggesting that gray matter hyperintensity on MRI may help to diagnose this disease.

Laboratory Examinations

In patients with SLE and epilepsy, antiphospholipid antibodies (including aCL, LA, and anti-β2GPI) are the most important antibodies. Hawro et al. [555] found that anti-β2GPI is more valuable than aCL and LA antibodies for diagnosing seizures caused by SLE.

Treatments

Treatment for SLE

Studies have demonstrated that treatments for SLE can effectively alleviate epilepsy. Once SLE is diagnosed, an appropriate treatment should be applied. Treatment may include hormones and immunosuppressants. Glucocorticoids or a combination of glucocorticoids and immunomodulators are usually used to treat patients with both SLE and epilepsy [556]. When the disease is acutely exacerbated, a patient should receive large doses of oral or intravenous glucocorticoids [557]. According to one recent study conducted by Barile-Fabris et al. [556], long-term treatment with a combination of cyclophosphamide and methylprednisolone is superior to intravenous methylprednisolone alone in treating refractory epilepsy caused by SLE.

Treatment for Seizures

Most patients with SLE do not require AEDs at the first seizure episode [306], but the long-term use of AEDs should be considered in patients with recurrent seizures [558]. AEDs are selected according to the type of seizure. However, drugs such as lamotrigine [559] and carbamazepine [560] should be avoided because they can cause drug-induced SLE. Antimalarial drugs have been suggested to prevent the recurrence of seizures [561].

4.9.3.2 RSE in SLE

RSE is not common in patients with SLE, but it should receive special attention because it is an urgent and severe condition.

Pathogenesis

In patients with SLE, SE or RSE may be associated with many factors, including cerebrovascular lesions caused by SLE, other neuropsychiatric symptoms, increased disease activity, and positive reactivity to anticardiolipin antibodies [305, 544, 562].

Clinical Manifestations

SE that occurs secondary to SLE can present as multiple types of seizures. The most frequently reported type is CPS. Tsuji et al. [308] reported a case study of a female patient with SLE who initially presented consciousness disorders and in whom the results of CT and MRI indicated brain atrophy. Then, her consciousness got back to normal, and carbamazepine had been given to her because of the abnormality in EEG. Later, she had abnormal consciousness and activity again. This time, her EEG showed continuous diffuse slow waves. The patient was therefore diagnosed with complex partial SE. With the exception of CPS, other seizure types are relatively rare. Nasri et al. [546] reported a case study of a pediatric patient with secondary SLE who presented SE twice over the course of the disease. The first episode involved generalized hypotonic seizures and tonic seizures, while the second episode involved generalized seizure that was secondary to myoclonic seizure.

Diagnosis

When diagnosing SE or RSE induced by SLE, a clinician should determine first whether the patient has experienced a seizure and then whether the cause of epilepsy is SLE. When a diagnosis is difficult, EEG monitoring may provide some useful information.

When patients present abnormal behaviors, clinicians should determine clearly whether the abnormal behavior is a neuropsychiatric symptom of SLE or caused by complex partial SE. Fernandez-Torre et al. [305] reported a case study of a female patient with SLE who had visual hallucination and was eventually diagnosed with complex partial SE using an EEG examination. When diagnosing such a patient, a clinician should always consider the possibility of NCSE because this disorder lacks specific clinical manifestations and can be easily misdiagnosed.

Park et al. [304] reported a case study of a 17-year-old female patient with SLE who presented RSE as the initial symptom. The laboratory examinations performed at admission did not show significant abnormalities, whereas an MRI showed an enhancement of the leptomeninges. During follow-up in the outpatient department, an antinuclear antibody test was positive, and an SLE diagnosis was therefore clear. Similarly, Polychronopoulos et al. [563] reported a rare case study of a patient with SLE combined with refractory epilepsy. This patient showed a typical aura and frequent CPS. Upon admission, the diagnosis was refractory temporal lobe medial epilepsy, but a laboratory examination did not show obvious abnormalities, and no other symptoms of SLE were observed. Therefore, the diagnosis of SLE was delayed. Based on the results of these studies, a diagnosis of SLE should be considered even if laboratory examinations performed at admission showed no significant abnormalities and refractory epilepsy is the only clinical symptom. The appropriate examinations should be repeated to document changes.

Treatments

SLE is an autoimmune disease. Thus, hormone therapy is a suitable and effective treatment option. As shown in a study by Gieron et al. [564], methylprednisolone controlled symptoms and caused the lesions observed on MRI in a patient with SLE and SE to disappear. The principles of treating SE or RSE in patients with SLE are described below. (1) The use of effective AEDs and the timely control of SE are conducive to obtaining a better prognosis. (2) The underlying disease that caused the epilepsy should be positively treated. (3) The treatment should maintain the stability of the patient's internal environment, use strategies including symptomatic treatment and the timely control of complications, and prevent cerebral hernia. (4) Treatments should ensure airway patency and the oxygen supply, and a tracheal intubation or tracheotomy should be conducted, if necessary. If the patient still experiences difficulty breathing, a ventilator can be used. (5) After the seizures have been terminated, appropriate drugs are needed to maintain treatment, and the patient should be monitored carefully throughout this process (additional details are provided in Chaps. 6, 7, and 8).

4.9.4 Epilepsy and RSE in Hepatic Encephalopathy

Hepatic encephalopathy is a syndrome that is based on metabolic disorders caused by hepatic failure or a portosystemic shunt. Hepatic encephalopathy is characterized by personality disorder, dystrophy, asterixis, an altered state of consciousness, coma, and death [565]. Seizure is not common in patients with hepatic encephalopathy, but it does predict a poor prognosis.

4.9.4.1 Epilepsy in Hepatic Encephalopathy

Pathogenesis

Abnormal Neurotransmission

Ardizzone et al. [566] observed that patients with hepatic encephalopathy presented neurological complications, such as seizure, mental disorder, and focal movement disorders. These complications were primarily related to abnormal neurotransmission caused by a toxic substance, such as manganese and ammonium.

Metabolic Disorder

Tanaka et al. [567] found that in patients with hepatic encephalopathy, seizures were associated with hyperammonemia, phenols, short chain fatty acids, and false neurotransmitters. High blood ammonia levels are a risk factor for seizures. As shown in a study by Kumar et al. [568], patients with hyperammonemia (≥122 μmol/L for 3 consecutive days) are more likely to develop seizures.

Others

In patients with acute hepatic failure, seizures may be induced by cerebral edema and hernia [569]. In patients who have undergone a liver transplant, seizures are mainly caused by immunosuppressors and some other drugs [570].

Incidence

The incidence of seizures is approximately 2–33% in patients with hepatic encephalopathy [565]. Ghosh et al. [571] conducted a study involving 65 children who underwent liver transplantation and found that seizures were the most common neurological complication.

Seizure Types

GTCS is the most prevalent type in patients with hepatic encephalopathy. Thabah et al. [572] reported a case study of a patient with Still disease who manifested GTCS and in whom laboratory examinations indicated hepatic dysfunction. The patient was therefore diagnosed with hepatic encephalopathy. Derle et al. [570] conducted a study of patients who received a liver transplant and found that GTCS was the most common seizure type.

Diagnosis

A clear medical history, imaging, electroencephalogram, and laboratory examinations are required to diagnose epilepsy caused by hepatic encephalopathy. In addition, seizure activity may lead to hypoxic brain injury and exacerbate brain edema. Therefore, subclinical seizures should be distinguished when patients with hepatic encephalopathy present an altered state of consciousness [573].

Treatments

The guiding principles of treatment should involve the following: treat the primary disease, correct the inducing factors, complete imaging examinations, choose safe drugs, and perform dynamic electroencephalogram monitoring. It is not necessary to treat a single isolated seizure. Ferro et al. [573] recommend levetiracetam as a first-line drug. However, sedative drugs should be avoided [574]. Additionally, in patients with advanced liver cirrhosis, AEDs that are cleared by the hepatic metabolism, such as carbamazepine or phenytoin, should not be used [575]. Although phenytoin is recommended as a treatment for suspected seizures in patients with acute hepatic failure, Bhatia et al. [576] found that the prophylactic use of phenytoin did not prevent seizures in these patients. Moreover, lactulose may also be an alternative because it can reduce blood ammonia levels and terminate seizures [577].

Moreover, attention should be paid to the management of seizures in patients with hepatic encephalopathy, which is caused by a special etiology. For example, in patients with hepatolenticular degeneration, epilepsy is mainly caused by a vitB6 deficiency that results from penicillamine therapy, which can be controlled by vitB6 or other chelators of copper cations [574].

4.9.4.2 RSE in Hepatic Encephalopathy

SE and RSE are common in patients with hepatic encephalopathy. Eleftheriadis et al. [577] reported a case study of a 54-year-old female patient with liver cirrhosis who had a history of hepatitis B, hepatic encephalopathy, ascites, and spontaneous peritonitis. Upon admission, examination revealed clearly increased blood ammonia levels, and an electroencephalogram showed diffuse sharp waves. According to the patient's medical history and the results of auxiliary examinations, hepatic encephalopathy and SE were considered the diagnosis. AEDs such as clonazepam were ineffective, and the patient was diagnosed with RSE. After the patient was treated with lactulose, SE was controlled, and the patient's blood ammonia levels and electroencephalogram returned to normal. Jo et al. [578] reported a case study of a 52-year-old male patient with liver cirrhosis. He was sent to the emergency room as a result of a change in consciousness but had no history of hepatic encephalopathy, epilepsy, or other diseases. Based on the results of physical and laboratory examinations, the patient was diagnosed with hepatic encephalopathy. The corresponding treatment was administered to the patient, but no obvious improvement in consciousness was observed. Later, MRI and EEG showed that the patient also had NCSE. After the patient was treated with levetiracetam, the seizures were controlled and the EEG returned to normal. Thus, changes in blood ammonia levels and EEG results may be characteristic clinical manifestations that can help diagnose RSE in patients with hepatic encephalopathy.

4.9.5 Epilepsy and RSE in Other Encephalopathy

4.9.5.1 Uremic Encephalopathy

In patients with uremic encephalopathy, seizure may have some relationship with dialysis [579], uremic toxins, and disturbances in the internal environment [580]. RSE is rarely observed in patients with uremic encephalopathy, and its common cause is food poisoning, which may be associated with the neurotoxicity of food. Cassinotto et al. [581] reviewed the literature regarding star fruit intoxication and found that some patients with uremia present RSE after star fruit intoxication. Soliman et al. [582] reported a case study of two patients with chronic renal failure who were poisoned after they ate corrupted salted mullet and showed local twitch and myoclonus. The seizures were not controlled by phenytoin, phenobarbital, and valproic acid. Thus, the patients were diagnosed with RSE. The seizures of one patient were controlled by propofol, but the prognosis of the other patient was poor, and that patient eventually died. Thus, patients with chronic renal failure should avoid eating food that can induce seizures.

4.9.5.2 Carbon Monoxide Poisoning Encephalopathy

Seizure is common in patients with carbon monoxide poisoning. It can be the first symptom or even the only symptom in patients with carbon monoxide poisoning. Some such cases are therefore misdiagnosed [583]. However, RSE is rarely observed in patients with carbon monoxide poisoning. Abdulaziz et al. [584] reported a case study of a 25-year-old patient with carbon monoxide poisoning who presented SE. Benzodiazepines and phenytoin were ineffective. SE was controlled after the administration of thiopentone and the application of positive pressure oxygen therapy. The patient then gradually recovered. In patients with carbon monoxide poisoning, RSE may be associated with extensive cerebral anoxia. Therefore, treatments that protect the brain are crucial, and hyperbaric oxygen therapy is recommended if the patient's medical condition allows it [584].

4.9.5.3 Pulmonary Encephalopathy

Pulmonary encephalopathy can also induce seizures. This may be related to brain anoxia-ischemia [585], respiratory alkalosis [586], and other conditions. We were unable to identify a typical case study involving RSE in patients with pulmonary encephalopathy. However, case studies of patients with myoclonic SE have been published. Zhang et al. [587] reported a case study of a patient who underwent cholecystectomy and presented cardiopulmonary arrest. After cardiopulmonary resuscitation, the patient presented myoclonus, and midazolam only temporarily controlled the symptoms. The patient's condition improved after a continuous intravenous infusion of phenobarbital and valproic acid, which was administered for 4 weeks. The seizures recurred upon withdrawal of the phenobarbital treatment and then stopped after the phenobarbital was readministered.

References

1. Brophy GM, Bell R, Claassen J, Alldredge B, Bleck TP, Glauser T, Laroche SM, Riviello JJ Jr, Shutter L, Sperling MR, et al. Guidelines for the evaluation and management of status epilepticus. Neurocrit Care. 2012;17(1):3–23.
2. Holtkamp M, Othman J, Buchheim K, Meierkord H. Predictors and prognosis of refractory status epilepticus treated in a neurological intensive care unit. J Neurol Neurosurg Psychiatry. 2005;76(4):534–9.
3. Novy J, Logroscino G, Rossetti AO. Refractory status epilepticus: a prospective observational study. Epilepsia. 2010;51(2):251–6.
4. Wilder-Smith EP, Lim EC, Teoh HL, Sharma VK, Tan JJ, Chan BP, Ong BK. The NORSE (new-onset refractory status epilepticus) syndrome: defining a disease entity. Ann Acad Med Singap. 2005;34(7):417–20.
5. Kortvelyessy P, Lerche H, Weber Y. FIRES and NORSE are distinct entities. Epilepsia. 2012;53(7):1276.

6. Lyon G, Dodge PR, Adams RD. The acute encephalopathies of obscure origin in infants and children. Brain J Neurol. 1961;84:680–708.
7. DeLorenzo RJ, Hauser WA, Towne AR, Boggs JG, Pellock JM, Penberthy L, Garnett L, Fortner CA, Ko D. A prospective, population-based epidemiologic study of status epilepticus in Richmond, Virginia. Neurology. 1996;46(4):1029–35.
8. Van Lierde I, Van Paesschen W, Dupont P, Maes A, Sciot R. De novo cryptogenic refractory multifocal febrile status epilepticus in the young adult: a review of six cases. Acta Neurol Belg. 2003;103(2):88–94.
9. Baxter P, Clarke A, Cross H, Harding B, Hicks E, Livingston J, Surtees R. Idiopathic catastrophic epileptic encephalopathy presenting with acute onset intractable status. Seizure. 2003;12(6):379–87.
10. Kramer U, Shorer Z, Ben-Zeev B, Lerman-Sagie T, Goldberg-Stern H, Lahat E. Severe refractory status epilepticus owing to presumed encephalitis. J Child Neurol. 2005;20(3):184–7.
11. Neuwirth M, Paraicz E, Liptai Z. Devastating epileptic encephalopathy-pseudoencephalitis: the new type of catastrophe epilepsy in our department. Ideggyogyaszati Szemle. 2008;61(11–12):391–6.
12. Sakuma H, Awaya Y, Shiomi M, Yamanouchi H, Takahashi Y, Saito Y, Sugai K, Sasaki M. Acute encephalitis with refractory, repetitive partial seizures (AERRPS): a peculiar form of childhood encephalitis. Acta Neurol Scand. 2010;121(4):251–6.
13. van Baalen A, Hausler M, Boor R, Rohr A, Sperner J, Kurlemann G, Panzer A, Stephani U, Kluger G. Febrile infection-related epilepsy syndrome (FIRES): a nonencephalitic encephalopathy in childhood. Epilepsia. 2010;51(7):1323–8.
14. Ismail FY, Kossoff EH. AERRPS, DESC, NORSE, FIRES: multi-labeling or distinct epileptic entities? Epilepsia. 2011;52(11):e185–9.
15. Costello DJ, Kilbride RD, Cole AJ. Cryptogenic new onset refractory status epilepticus (NORSE) in adults-infectious or not? J Neurol Sci. 2009;277(1–2):26–31.
16. Milh M, Villeneuve N, Chapon F, Gavaret M, Girard N, Mancini J, Chabrol B, Boucraut J. New onset refractory convulsive status epilepticus associated with serum neuropil auto-antibodies in a school aged child. Brain Dev. 2011;33(8):687–91.
17. Gall CR, Jumma O, Mohanraj R. Five cases of new onset refractory status epilepticus (NORSE) syndrome: outcomes with early immunotherapy. Seizure. 2013;22(3):217–20.
18. Li J, Saldivar C, Maganti RK. Plasma exchange in cryptogenic new onset refractory status epilepticus. Seizure. 2013;22(1):70–3.
19. Jayalakshmi S, Vooturi S, Sahu S, Yada PK, Mohandas S. Causes and outcomes of new onset status epilepticus and predictors of refractoriness to therapy. J Clin Neurosci. 2016;26:89–94.
20. Gaspard N, Foreman BP, Alvarez V, Cabrera Kang C, Probasco JC, Jongeling AC, Meyers E, Espinera A, Haas KF, Schmitt SE, et al. New-onset refractory status epilepticus: etiology, clinical features, and outcome. Neurology. 2015;85(18):1604–13.
21. Sabharwal V, Ramsay E, Martinez R, Shumate R, Khan F, Dave H, Iwuchukwu I, McGrade H. Propofol-ketamine combination therapy for effective control of super-refractory status epilepticus. Epilepsy Behav. 2015;52(PT A):264–6.
22. Glaser CA, Gilliam S, Schnurr D, Forghani B, Honarmand S, Khetsuriani N, Fischer M, Cossen CK, Anderson LJ. In search of encephalitis etiologies: diagnostic challenges in the California encephalitis project, 1998-2000. Clin Infect Dis. 2003;36(6):731–42.
23. Hainsworth JB, Shishido A, Theeler BJ, Carroll CG, Fasano RE. Treatment responsive GABA(B)-receptor limbic encephalitis presenting as new-onset super-refractory status epilepticus (NORSE) in a deployed U.S. soldier. Epileptic Disord. 2014;16(4):486–93.
24. Bleck TP. Less common etiologies of status epilepticus. Epilepsy Curr. 2010;10(2):31–3.
25. Hurley K, Herron M, McDermott S, Farrell T, O'Riordan D. Squamous cell lung carcinoma presenting with refractory status epilepticus: a case report of paraneoplastic limbic encephalitis. Respir Care. 2015;60(8):e144–7.
26. Verma R, Raut TP, Giri P, Praharaj HN. New onset refractory status epilepticus (NORSE) as the heralding manifestation of herpes simplex encephalitis. BMJ Case Rep. 2013;2013
27. Illingworth MA, Hanrahan D, Anderson CE, O'Kane K, Anderson J, Casey M, de Sousa C, Cross JH, Wright S, Dale RC, et al. Elevated VGKC-complex antibodies in a boy with fever-induced refractory epileptic encephalopathy in school-age children (FIRES). Dev Med Child Neurol. 2011;53(11):1053–7.
28. Jenssen S, Gracely EJ, Sperling MR. How long do most seizures last? A systematic comparison of seizures recorded in the epilepsy monitoring unit. Epilepsia. 2006;47(9):1499–503.
29. DeLorenzo RJ, Garnett LK, Towne AR, Waterhouse EJ, Boggs JG, Morton L, Choudhry MA, Barnes T, Ko D. Comparison of status epilepticus with prolonged seizure episodes lasting from 10 to 29 minutes. Epilepsia. 1999;40(2):164–9.
30. Mazarati AM, Wasterlain CG, Sankar R, Shin D. Self-sustaining status epilepticus after brief electrical stimulation of the perforant path. Brain Res. 1998;801(1–2):251–3.
31. Nabbout R, Vezzani A, Dulac O, Chiron C. Acute encephalopathy with inflammation-mediated status epilepticus. Lancet Neurol. 2011;10(1):99–108.
32. Hu S, Sheng WS, Ehrlich LC, Peterson PK, Chao CC. Cytokine effects on glutamate uptake by human astrocytes. Neuroimmunomodulation. 2000;7(3):153–9.
33. Casamenti F, Prosperi C, Scali C, Giovannelli L, Colivicchi MA, Faussone-Pellegrini MS, Pepeu G. Interleukin-1beta activates forebrain glial cells and increases nitric oxide production and

cortical glutamate and GABA release in vivo: implications for Alzheimer's disease. Neuroscience. 1999;91(3):831–42.
34. Heida JG, Pittman QJ. Causal links between brain cytokines and experimental febrile convulsions in the rat. Epilepsia. 2005;46(12):1906–13.
35. Khawaja AM, DeWolfe JL, Miller DW, Szaflarski JP. New-onset refractory status epilepticus (NORSE)—the potential role for immunotherapy. Epilepsy Behav. 2015;47:17–23.
36. Puoti G, Elefante A, Saracino D, Capasso A, Cotrufo R, Anello CB. New-onset refractory status epilepticus mimicking herpes virus encephalitis. Case Rep Neurol. 2013;5(3):162–7.
37. Ferlisi M, Shorvon S. The outcome of therapies in refractory and super-refractory convulsive status epilepticus and recommendations for therapy. Brain. 2012;135(Pt 8):2314–28.
38. Halawa EF, Draz I, Ahmed D, Shaheen HA. Predictors of outcome of convulsive status epilepticus among an Egyptian Pediatric tertiary hospital. J Child Neurol. 2015;30(13):1736–42.
39. Zeiler FA, Matuszczak M, Teitelbaum J, Kazina CJ, Gillman LM. Plasmapheresis for refractory status epilepticus, part I: a scoping systematic review of the adult literature. Seizure. 2016;43:14–22.
40. Pugin D, Foreman B, De Marchis GM, Fernandez A, Schmidt JM, Czeisler BM, Mayer SA, Agarwal S, Lesch C, Lantigua H, et al. Is pentobarbital safe and efficacious in the treatment of super-refractory status epilepticus: a cohort study. Crit Care. 2014;18(3):R103.
41. Lie IA, Hoggen I, Samsonsen C, Brodtkorb E. Treatment non-adherence as a trigger for status epilepticus: an observational, retrospective study based on therapeutic drug monitoring. Epilepsy Res. 2015;113:28–33.
42. Li Y, Tian L, Zeng T, Chen J, Chen L, Zhou D. Clinical features and outcome of super-refractory status epilepticus: a retrospective analysis in West China. Seizure. 2014;23(9):722–7.
43. Jayalakshmi S, Ruikar D, Vooturi S, Alladi S, Sahu S, Kaul S, Mohandas S. Determinants and predictors of outcome in super refractory status epilepticus—a developing country perspective. Epilepsy Res. 2014;108(9):1609–17.
44. Hocker SE, Britton JW, Mandrekar JN, Wijdicks EF, Rabinstein AA. Predictors of outcome in refractory status epilepticus. JAMA Neurol. 2013;70(1):72–7.
45. Young GB, Blume WT, Bolton CF, Warren KG. Anesthetic barbiturates in refractory status epilepticus. Can J Neurol Sci. 1980;7(4):291–2.
46. Nouailhat F, Levy-Alcover MA, Goulon M. Treatment of status epilepticus in the adult. Retrospective analysis of 192 cases treated in intensive care units. Rev Electroencephalogr Neurophysiol Clin. 1985;14(4):287–92.
47. Walker MC, Howard RS, Smith SJ, Miller DH, Shorvon SD, Hirsch NP. Diagnosis and treatment of status epilepticus on a neurological intensive care unit. QJM. 1996;89(12):913–20.
48. Neligan A, Shorvon SD. Frequency and prognosis of convulsive status epilepticus of different causes: a systematic review. Arch Neurol. 2010;67(8):931–40.
49. Lai A, Outin HD, Jabot J, Megarbane B, Gaudry S, Coudroy R, Louis G, Schneider F, Barbarot N, Roch A, et al. Functional outcome of prolonged refractory status epilepticus. Crit Care. 2015;19:199.
50. Ferlisi M, Hocker S, Grade M, Trinka E, Shorvon S. International steering committee of the StEp A: preliminary results of the global audit of treatment of refractory status epilepticus. Epilepsy Behav. 2015;49:318–24.
51. Alvarez V, Westover MB, Drislane FW, Dworetzky BA, Curley D, Lee JW, Rossetti AO. Evaluation of a clinical tool for early etiology identification in status epilepticus. Epilepsia. 2014;55(12):2059–68.
52. Sanchez Fernandez I, Abend NS, Agadi S, An S, Arya R, Brenton JN, Carpenter JL, Chapman KE, Gaillard WD, Glauser TA, et al. Time from convulsive status epilepticus onset to anticonvulsant administration in children. Neurology. 2015;84(23):2304–11.
53. Kamppi L, Mustonen H, Soinila S. Analysis of the delay components in the treatment of status epilepticus. Neurocrit Care. 2013;19(1):10–8.
54. Power KN, Flaatten H, Gilhus NE, Engelsen BA. Propofol treatment in adult refractory status epilepticus. Mortality risk and outcome. Epilepsy Res. 2011;94(1–2):53–60.
55. Miyahara A, Saito Y, Sugai K, Nakagawa E, Sakuma H, Komaki H, Sasaki M. Reassessment of phenytoin for treatment of late stage progressive myoclonus epilepsy complicated with status epilepticus. Epilepsy Res. 2009;84(2–3):201–9.
56. Tassinari CA, Dravet C, Roger J, Cano JP, Gastaut H. Tonic status epilepticus precipitated by intravenous benzodiazepine in five patients with Lennox-Gastaut syndrome. Epilepsia. 1972;13(3):421–35.
57. Nobutoki T, Sugai K, Fukumizu M, Hanaoka S, Sasaki M. Continuous midazolam infusion for refractory nonconvulsive status epilepticus in children. No To Hattatsu. 2005;37(5):369–73.
58. Jayalakshmi S, Vooturi S, Chepuru R, Sahu S, Surath M. Aetiology and outcome of generalized convulsive status epilepticus in elderly. Seizure. 2015;29:104–8.
59. Kravljanac R, Djuric M, Jankovic B, Pekmezovic T. Etiology, clinical course and response to the treatment of status epilepticus in children: a 16-year single-center experience based on 602 episodes of status epilepticus. Eur J Paediatr Neurol. 2015;19(5):584–90.
60. Berg AT, Berkovic SF, Brodie MJ, Buchhalter J, Cross JH, van Emde BW, Engel J, French J, Glauser TA, Mathern GW, et al. Revised terminology and concepts for organization of seizures and epilepsies: report of the ILAE commission on classification and terminology, 2005-2009. Epilepsia. 2010;51(4):676–85.
61. Trinka E, Cock H, Hesdorffer D, Rossetti AO, Scheffer IE, Shinnar S, Shorvon S, Lowenstein DH.

A definition and classification of status epilepticus—report of the ILAE task force on classification of status epilepticus. Epilepsia. 2015;56(10):1515–23.
62. Coppola G, Plouin P, Chiron C, Robain O, Dulac O. Migrating partial seizures in infancy: a malignant disorder with developmental arrest. Epilepsia. 1995;36(10):1017–24.
63. Gerard F, Kaminska A, Plouin P, Echenne B, Dulac O. Focal seizures versus focal epilepsy in infancy: a challenging distinction. Epileptic Disord. 1999;1(2):135–9.
64. Okuda K, Yasuhara A, Kamei A, Araki A, Kitamura N, Kobayashi Y. Successful control with bromide of two patients with malignant migrating partial seizures in infancy. Brain Dev. 2000;22(1):56–9.
65. Gross-Tsur V, Ben-Zeev B, Shalev RS. Malignant migrating partial seizures in infancy. Pediatr Neurol. 2004;31(4):287–90.
66. Hmaimess G, Kadhim H, Nassogne MC, Bonnier C, van Rijckevorsel K. Levetiracetam in a neonate with malignant migrating partial seizures. Pediatr Neurol. 2006;34(1):55–9.
67. Coppola G. Malignant migrating partial seizures in infancy: an epilepsy syndrome of unknown etiology. Epilepsia. 2009;50(Suppl 5):49–51.
68. Carranza Rojo D, Hamiwka L, McMahon JM, Dibbens LM, Arsov T, Suls A, Stodberg T, Kelley K, Wirrell E, Appleton B, et al. De novo SCN1A mutations in migrating partial seizures of infancy. Neurology. 2011;77(4):380–3.
69. Dhamija R, Wirrell E, Falcao G, Kirmani S, Wong-Kisiel LC. Novel de novo SCN2A mutation in a child with migrating focal seizures of infancy. Pediatr Neurol. 2013;49(6):486–8.
70. Ohba C, Kato M, Takahashi S, Lerman-Sagie T, Lev D, Terashima H, Kubota M, Kawawaki H, Matsufuji M, Kojima Y, et al. Early onset epileptic encephalopathy caused by de novo SCN8A mutations. Epilepsia. 2014;55(7):994–1000.
71. Poduri A, Chopra SS, Neilan EG, Elhosary PC, Kurian MA, Meyer E, Barry BJ, Khwaja OS, Salih MA, Stodberg T, et al. Homozygous PLCB1 deletion associated with malignant migrating partial seizures in infancy. Epilepsia. 2012;53(8):e146–50.
72. Poduri A, Heinzen EL, Chitsazzadeh V, Lasorsa FM, Elhosary PC, LaCoursiere CM, Martin E, Yuskaitis CJ, Hill RS, Atabay KD, et al. SLC25A22 is a novel gene for migrating partial seizures in infancy. Ann Neurol. 2013;74(6):873–82.
73. Milh M, Falace A, Villeneuve N, Vanni N, Cacciagli P, Assereto S, Nabbout R, Benfenati F, Zara F, Chabrol B, et al. Novel compound heterozygous mutations in TBC1D24 cause familial malignant migrating partial seizures of infancy. Hum Mutat. 2013;34(6):869–72.
74. Saitsu H, Watanabe M, Akita T, Ohba C, Sugai K, Ong WP, Shiraishi H, Yuasa S, Matsumoto H, Beng KT, et al. Impaired neuronal KCC2 function by biallelic SLC12A5 mutations in migrating focal seizures and severe developmental delay. Sci Rep. 2016;6:30072.
75. Cilio MR, Bianchi R, Balestri M, Onofri A, Giovannini S, Di Capua M, Vigevano F. Intravenous levetiracetam terminates refractory status epilepticus in two patients with migrating partial seizures in infancy. Epilepsy Res. 2009;86(1):66–71.
76. Barcia G, Fleming MR, Deligniere A, Gazula VR, Brown MR, Langouet M, Chen H, Kronengold J, Abhyankar A, Cilio R, et al. De novo gain-of-function KCNT1 channel mutations cause malignant migrating partial seizures of infancy. Nat Genet. 2012;44(11):1255–9.
77. McTague A, Appleton R, Avula S, Cross JH, King MD, Jacques TS, Bhate S, Cronin A, Curran A, Desurkar A, et al. Migrating partial seizures of infancy: expansion of the electroclinical, radiological and pathological disease spectrum. Brain. 2013;136(Pt 5): 1578–91.
78. Caraballo R, Pasteris MC, Fortini PS, Portuondo E. Epilepsy of infancy with migrating focal seizures: six patients treated with bromide. Seizure. 2014;23(10):899–902.
79. Bearden D, Strong A, Ehnot J, DiGiovine M, Dlugos D, Goldberg EM. Targeted treatment of migrating partial seizures of infancy with quinidine. Ann Neurol. 2014;76(3):457–61.
80. Milligan CJ, Li M, Gazina EV, Heron SE, Nair U, Trager C, Reid CA, Venkat A, Younkin DP, Dlugos DJ, et al. KCNT1 gain of function in 2 epilepsy phenotypes is reversed by quinidine. Ann Neurol. 2014;75(4):581–90.
81. Caraballo R, Noli D, Cachia P. Epilepsy of infancy with migrating focal seizures: three patients treated with the ketogenic diet. Epileptic Disord. 2015;17(2):194–7.
82. Shein SL, Reynolds TQ, Gedela S, Kochanek PM, Bell MJ. Therapeutic hypothermia for refractory status epilepticus in a child with malignant migrating partial seizures of infancy and SCN1A mutation: a case report. Ther Hypothermia Temp Manag. 2012;2(3):144–9.
83. Connolly MB. Dravet syndrome: diagnosis and long-term course. Can J Neurol Sci. 2016;43(Suppl 3):S3–8.
84. Shmuely S, Sisodiya SM, Gunning WB, Sander JW, Thijs RD. Mortality in Dravet syndrome: a review. Epilepsy Behav. 2016;64(Pt A):69–74.
85. Marini C, Scheffer IE, Nabbout R, Suls A, De Jonghe P, Zara F, Guerrini R. The genetics of Dravet syndrome. Epilepsia. 2011;52(Suppl 2):24–9.
86. Depienne C, Bouteiller D, Keren B, Cheuret E, Poirier K, Trouillard O, Benyahia B, Quelin C, Carpentier W, Julia S, et al. Sporadic infantile epileptic encephalopathy caused by mutations in PCDH19 resembles Dravet syndrome but mainly affects females. PLoS Genet. 2009;5(2):e1000381.
87. Shi X, Yasumoto S, Nakagawa E, Fukasawa T, Uchiya S, Hirose S. Missense mutation of the sodium channel gene SCN2A causes Dravet syndrome. Brain Dev. 2009;31(10):758–62.

88. Ishii A, Kanaumi T, Sohda M, Misumi Y, Zhang B, Kakinuma N, Haga Y, Watanabe K, Takeda S, Okada M, et al. Association of nonsense mutation in GABRG2 with abnormal trafficking of GABAA receptors in severe epilepsy. Epilepsy Res. 2014;108(3):420–32.
89. Carvill GL, Weckhuysen S, McMahon JM, Hartmann C, Moller RS, Hjalgrim H, Cook J, Geraghty E, O'Roak BJ, Petrou S, et al. GABRA1 and STXBP1: novel genetic causes of Dravet syndrome. Neurology. 2014;82(14):1245–53.
90. Tanabe T, Awaya Y, Matsuishi T, Iyoda K, Nagai T, Kurihara M, Yamamoto K, Minagawa K, Maekawa K. Management of and prophylaxis against status epilepticus in children with severe myoclonic epilepsy in infancy (SMEI; Dravet syndrome)—a nationwide questionnaire survey in Japan. Brain Dev. 2008;30(10):629–35.
91. Berio A, Piazzi A. Activity of drugs and components of natural origin in the severe myoclonic epilepsy of infancy (Dravet syndrome). Cent Nerv Syst Agents Med Chem. 2015;15(2):95–8.
92. Devinsky O, Marsh E, Friedman D, Thiele E, Laux L, Sullivan J, Miller I, Flamini R, Wilfong A, Filloux F, et al. Cannabidiol in patients with treatment-resistant epilepsy: an open-label interventional trial. Lancet Neurol. 2016;15(3):270–8.
93. Dravet C, Oguni H. Dravet syndrome (severe myoclonic epilepsy in infancy). Handb Clin Neurol. 2013;111:627–33.
94. Shi XY, Tomonoh Y, Wang WZ, Ishii A, Higurashi N, Kurahashi H, Kaneko S, Hirose S. Efficacy of antiepileptic drugs for the treatment of Dravet syndrome with different genotypes. Brain Dev. 2016;38(1): 40–6.
95. Specchio N, Balestri M, Trivisano M, Japaridze N, Striano P, Carotenuto A, Cappelletti S, Specchio LM, Fusco L, Vigevano F. Electroencephalographic features in dravet syndrome: five-year follow-up study in 22 patients. J Child Neurol. 2012;27(4):439–44.
96. Dravet C, Bureau M, Oguni H, Fukuyama Y, Cokar O. Severe myoclonic epilepsy in infancy: Dravet syndrome. Adv Neurol. 2005;95:71–102.
97. Wallace A, Wirrell E, Kenney-Jung DL. Pharmacotherapy for Dravet syndrome. Paediatr Drugs. 2016;18(3):197–208.
98. Dressler A, Trimmel-Schwahofer P, Reithofer E, Muhlebner A, Groppel G, Reiter-Fink E, Benninger F, Grassl R, Feucht M. Efficacy and tolerability of the ketogenic diet in Dravet syndrome—comparison with various standard antiepileptic drug regimen. Epilepsy Res. 2015;109:81–9.
99. Dlouhy BJ, Miller B, Jeong A, Bertrand ME, Limbrick DD Jr, Smyth MD. Palliative epilepsy surgery in Dravet syndrome-case series and review of the literature. Child's Nerv Syst. 2016;32(9):1703–8.
100. Ragona F, Granata T, Dalla Bernardina B, Offredi F, Darra F, Battaglia D, Morbi M, Brazzo D, Cappelletti S, Chieffo D, et al. Cognitive development in Dravet syndrome: a retrospective, multicenter study of 26 patients. Epilepsia. 2011;52(2):386–92.
101. Rilstone JJ, Coelho FM, Minassian BA, Andrade DM. Dravet syndrome: seizure control and gait in adults with different SCN1A mutations. Epilepsia. 2012;53(8):1421–8.
102. Verbeek NE, Wassenaar M, van Campen JS, Sonsma A, Gunning B, Knoers N, Lindhout D, Jansen FE, Leijten F, Brilstra EH, et al. Seizure precipitants in Dravet syndrome: what events and activities are specifically provocative compared with other epilepsies? Epilepsy Behav. 2015;47:39–44.
103. Okumura A, Uematsu M, Imataka G, Tanaka M, Okanishi T, Kubota T, Sudo A, Tohyama J, Tsuji M, Ohmori I, et al. Acute encephalopathy in children with Dravet syndrome. Epilepsia. 2012;53(1): 79–86.
104. Brunklaus A, Ellis R, Reavey E, Forbes GH, Zuberi SM. Prognostic, clinical and demographic features in SCN1A mutation-positive Dravet syndrome. Brain. 2012;135(Pt 8):2329–36.
105. Sakauchi M, Oguni H, Kato I, Osawa M, Hirose S, Kaneko S, Takahashi Y, Takayama R, Fujiwara T. Mortality in Dravet syndrome: search for risk factors in Japanese patients. Epilepsia. 2011;52(Suppl 2):50–4.
106. Gallentine WB, Mikati MA. Genetic generalized epilepsies. J Clin Neurophysiol. 2012;29(5):408–19.
107. Commission on Classification and Terminology of the International League Against Epilepsy. Proposal for revised classification of epilepsies and epileptic syndromes. Epilepsia. 1989;30(4):389–99.
108. Blume WT, Luders HO, Mizrahi E, Tassinari C, van Emde BW, Engel J Jr. Glossary of descriptive terminology for ictal semiology: report of the ILAE task force on classification and terminology. Epilepsia. 2001;42(9):1212–8.
109. Engel J Jr. A proposed diagnostic scheme for people with epileptic seizures and with epilepsy: report of the ILAE task force on classification and terminology. Epilepsia. 2001;42(6):796–803.
110. Nordli DR Jr. Idiopathic generalized epilepsies recognized by the international League against epilepsy. Epilepsia. 2005;46(Suppl 9):48–56.
111. Asadi-Pooya AA, Emami M, Sperling MR. A clinical study of syndromes of idiopathic (genetic) generalized epilepsy. J Neurol Sci. 2013;324(1–2):113–7.
112. Panayiotopoulos CP. The new ILAE report on terminology and concepts for the organization of epilepsies: critical review and contribution. Epilepsia. 2012;53(3):399–404.
113. Jallon P, Latour P. Epidemiology of idiopathic generalized epilepsies. Epilepsia. 2005;46(Suppl 9):10–4.
114. Shorvon S, Walker M. Status epilepticus in idiopathic generalized epilepsy. Epilepsia. 2005;46(Suppl 9):73–9.
115. Genton P, Ferlazzo E, Thomas P. Absence status epilepsy: delineation of a distinct idiopathic generalized epilepsy syndrome. Epilepsia. 2008;49(4):642–9.

116. Thomas P, Valton L, Genton P. Absence and myoclonic status epilepticus precipitated by antiepileptic drugs in idiopathic generalized epilepsy. Brain. 2006;129(Pt 5):1281–92.
117. Wheless JW. Acute management of seizures in the syndromes of idiopathic generalized epilepsies. Epilepsia. 2003;44(Suppl 2):22–6.
118. Agathonikou A, Panayiotopoulos CP, Giannakodimos S, Koutroumanidis M. Typical absence status in adults: diagnostic and syndromic considerations. Epilepsia. 1998;39(12):1265–76.
119. Dziewas R, Kellinghaus C, Ludemann P. Nonconvulsion status epilepticus in patients with juvenile myoclonic epilepsy: types and frequencies. Seizure. 2002;11(5):335–9.
120. Shirasaka Y. Lack of neuronal damage in atypical absence status epilepticus. Epilepsia. 2002;43(12):1498–501.
121. Wong M, Wozniak DF, Yamada KA. An animal model of generalized nonconvulsive status epilepticus: immediate characteristics and long-term effects. Exp Neurol. 2003;183(1):87–99.
122. Badhwar A, Siren A, Andermann E, Andermann F. Myoclonic status epilepticus: video presentation. Mov Disord. 2002;17(2):409–11.
123. Panayiotopoulos CP, Obeid T, Tahan AR. Juvenile myoclonic epilepsy: a 5-year prospective study. Epilepsia. 1994;35(2):285–96.
124. Sheth RD, Gidal BE. Intravenous valproic acid for myoclonic status epilepticus. Neurology. 2000;54(5):1201.
125. Bilo L, Pappata S, De Simone R, Meo R. The syndrome of absence status epilepsy: review of the literature. Epilepsy Res Treat. 2014;2014:624309.
126. Venkataraman V, Wheless JW. Safety of rapid intravenous infusion of valproate loading doses in epilepsy patients. Epilepsy Res. 1999;35(2):147–53.
127. Zaki SA, Verma DK, Tayde P. Panayiotopoulos syndrome in a child masquerading as septic shock. Indian J Crit Care Med. 2016;20(6):361–3.
128. Panayiotopoulos CP, Michael M, Sanders S, Valeta T, Koutroumanidis M. Benign childhood focal epilepsies: assessment of established and newly recognized syndromes. Brain. 2008;131(Pt 9):2264–86.
129. Degerliyurt A, Teber S, Bektas O, Senkon G. Panayiotopoulos syndrome: a case series from Turkey. Epilepsy Behav. 2014;36:24–32.
130. Oguni H, Hayashi K, Imai K, Hirano Y, Mutoh A, Osawa M. Study on the early-onset variant of benign childhood epilepsy with occipital paroxysms otherwise described as early-onset benign occipital seizure susceptibility syndrome. Epilepsia. 1999;40(7):1020–30.
131. Kivity S, Ephraim T, Weitz R, Tamir A. Childhood epilepsy with occipital paroxysms: clinical variants in 134 patients. Epilepsia. 2000;41(12):1522–33.
132. Lada C, Skiadas K, Theodorou V, Loli N, Covanis A. A study of 43 patients with panayiotopoulos syndrome, a common and benign childhood seizure susceptibility. Epilepsia. 2003;44(1):81–8.
133. Ohtsu M, Oguni H, Hayashi K, Funatsuka M, Imai K, Osawa M. EEG in children with early-onset benign occipital seizure susceptibility syndrome: Panayiotopoulos syndrome. Epilepsia. 2003;44(3):435–42.
134. Ferrie CD, Caraballo R, Covanis A, Demirbilek V, Dervent A, Fejerman N, Fusco L, Grunewald RA, Kanazawa O, Koutroumanidis M, et al. Autonomic status epilepticus in Panayiotopoulos syndrome and other childhood and adult epilepsies: a consensus view. Epilepsia. 2007;48(6):1165–72.
135. Panayiotopoulos CP. Autonomic seizures and autonomic status epilepticus peculiar to childhood: diagnosis and management. Epilepsy Behav. 2004;5(3):286–95.
136. Ferrie C, Caraballo R, Covanis A, Demirbilek V, Dervent A, Kivity S, Koutroumanidis M, Martinovic Z, Oguni H, Verrotti A, et al. Panayiotopoulos syndrome: a consensus view. Dev Med Child Neurol. 2006;48(3):236–40.
137. Chahine LM, Mikati MA. Benign pediatric localization-related epilepsies. Part I. Syndromes in infancy. Epileptic Disord. 2006;8(3):169–83.
138. Caraballo RH, Pasteris MC, Portuondo E, Fortini PS. Panayiotopoulos syndrome and diffuse paroxysms as the first EEG manifestation at clinical onset: a study of nine patients. Epileptic Disord. 2015;17(2):143–9.
139. Kikumoto K, Yoshinaga H, Oka M, Ito M, Endoh F, Akiyama T, Ohtsuka Y. EEG and seizure exacerbation induced by carbamazepine in Panayiotopoulos syndrome. Epileptic Disord. 2006;8(1):53–6.
140. Garcia C, Rubio G. Efficacy and safety of levetiracetam in the treatment of Panayiotopoulos syndrome. Epilepsy Res. 2009;85(2–3):318–20.
141. Verrotti A, Sebastiani M, Giordano L, Striano P, Belcastro V, Franzoni E, Parisi P, Pruna D, Spalice A, Vignoli A, et al. Panayiotopoulos syndrome with convulsive status epilepticus at the onset: a long-term study. Seizure. 2014;23(9):728–31.
142. Kanemura H, Sano F, Ohyama T, Aoyagi K, Sugita K, Aihara M. Sequential prefrontal lobe volume changes and cognitive dysfunctions in children with Panayiotopoulos syndrome presenting with status epilepticus. Epilepsy Res. 2015;112: 122–9.
143. Neubauer BA, Hahn A, Doose H, Tuxhorn I. Myoclonic-astatic epilepsy of early childhood--definition, course, nosography, and genetics. Adv Neurol. 2005;95:147–55.
144. Scheffer IE, Wallace R, Mulley JC, Berkovic SF. Clinical and molecular genetics of myoclonic-astatic epilepsy and severe myoclonic epilepsy in infancy (Dravet syndrome). Brain Dev. 2001;23(7):732–5.
145. Wallace RH, Scheffer IE, Parasivam G, Barnett S, Wallace GB, Sutherland GR, Berkovic SF, Mulley JC. Generalized epilepsy with febrile seizures plus: mutation of the sodium channel subunit SCN1B. Neurology. 2002;58(9):1426–9.

146. Mullen SA, Marini C, Suls A, Mei D, Della Giustina E, Buti D, Arsov T, Damiano J, Lawrence K, De Jonghe P, et al. Glucose transporter 1 deficiency as a treatable cause of myoclonic astatic epilepsy. Arch Neurol. 2011;68(9):1152–5.
147. Carvill GL, Heavin SB, Yendle SC, McMahon JM, O'Roak BJ, Cook J, Khan A, Dorschner MO, Weaver M, Calvert S, et al. Targeted resequencing in epileptic encephalopathies identifies de novo mutations in CHD2 and SYNGAP1. Nat Genet. 2013;45(7):825–30.
148. Carvill GL, McMahon JM, Schneider A, Zemel M, Myers CT, Saykally J, Nguyen J, Robbiano A, Zara F, Specchio N, et al. Mutations in the GABA transporter SLC6A1 cause epilepsy with myoclonic-atonic seizures. Am J Hum Genet. 2015;96(5):808–15.
149. Oguni H, Fukuyama Y, Tanaka T, Hayashi K, Funatsuka M, Sakauchi M, Shirakawa S, Osawa M. Myoclonic-astatic epilepsy of early childhood—clinical and EEG analysis of myoclonic-astatic seizures, and discussions on the nosology of the syndrome. Brain Dev. 2001;23(7):757–64.
150. Kilaru S, Bergqvist AG. Current treatment of myoclonic astatic epilepsy: clinical experience at the Children's Hospital of Philadelphia. Epilepsia. 2007;48(9):1703–7.
151. Kaminska A, Oguni H. Lennox-Gastaut syndrome and epilepsy with myoclonic-astatic seizures. Handb Clin Neurol. 2013;111:641–52.
152. Kelley SA, Kossoff EH. Doose syndrome (myoclonic-astatic epilepsy): 40 years of progress. Dev Med Child Neurol. 2010;52(11):988–93.
153. Oguni H, Tanaka T, Hayashi K, Funatsuka M, Sakauchi M, Shirakawa S, Osawa M. Treatment and long-term prognosis of myoclonic-astatic epilepsy of early childhood. Neuropediatrics. 2002;33(3):122–32.
154. Doose H, Gerken H, Leonhardt R, Volzke E, Volz C. Centrencephalic myoclonic-astatic petit mal. Clinical and genetic investigation. Neuropadiatrie. 1970;2(1):59–78.
155. Deng J, Zhang YH, Liu XY, Yang ZX, Xiong H, Wang S, Bao XH, Jiang YW, Qin J, Lin Q, et al. Electroclinical features of myoclonic-atonic epilepsy. Zhonghua er ke za zhi. 2011;49(8): 577–82.
156. Caraballo RH, Chamorro N, Darra F, Fortini S, Arroyo H. Epilepsy with myoclonic atonic seizures: an electroclinical study of 69 patients. Pediatr Neurol. 2013;48(5):355–62.
157. Trivisano M, Specchio N, Cappelletti S, Di Ciommo V, Claps D, Specchio LM, Vigevano F, Fusco L. Myoclonic astatic epilepsy: an age-dependent epileptic syndrome with favorable seizure outcome but variable cognitive evolution. Epilepsy Res. 2011;97(1–2):133–41.
158. Grande-Martin A, Pardal-Fernandez JM, Carrascosa-Romero MC, De Cabo C. Tonic seizure status epilepticus triggered by valproate in a child with Doose syndrome. Neuropediatrics. 2016;47(3):187–9.
159. Oguni H, Hayashi K, Imai K, Funatsuka M, Sakauchi M, Shirakawa S, Osawa M. Idiopathic myoclonic-astatic epilepsy of early childhood—nosology based on electrophysiologic and long-term follow-up study of patients. Adv Neurol. 2005;95: 157–74.
160. Kalviainen R. Progressive myoclonus epilepsies. Semin Neurol. 2015;35(3):293–9.
161. Striano P, Zara F, Turnbull J, Girard JM, Ackerley CA, Cervasio M, De Rosa G, Del Basso-De Caro ML, Striano S, Minassian BA. Typical progression of myoclonic epilepsy of the Lafora type: a case report. Nat Clin Pract Neurol. 2008;4(2):106–11.
162. Frei KP, Schiffmann R. Myoclonus in Gaucher disease. Adv Neurol. 2002;89:41–8.
163. Hayashi M, Kumada S, Shioda K, Fukatsu R. Neuropathological analysis of the brainstem and cerebral cortex lesions on epileptogenesis in hereditary dentatorubral-pallidoluysian atrophy. Brain Dev. 2007;29(8):473–81.
164. Oguz Akarsu E, Tekturk P, Yapici Z, Tepgec F, Uyguner ZO, Baykan B. Eyelid myoclonic status epilepticus: a rare phenotype in spinal muscular atrophy with progressive myoclonic epilepsy associated with ASAH1 gene mutation. Seizure. 2016;42:49–51.
165. Hashmi M, Saleem F, Mustafa MS, Sheerani M, Ehtesham Z, Siddiqui K. Role of levetiracetam in refractory seizures due to a rare progressive myoclonic epilepsy: Lafora body disease. BMJ Case Rep. 2010;2010
166. Lopez-Meza EG, Cerda-Tellez F, Alanis-Guevara IM, Fernandez Gonzalez-Aragon MC, Ruano-Calderon LA. Non-convulsive epileptic status associated with Lafora disease: two case reports. Rev Neurol. 2003;37(10):945–7.
167. Caraballo RH, Valenzuela GR, Armeno M, Fortini S, Mestre G, Cresta A. The ketogenic diet in two paediatric patients with refractory myoclonic status epilepticus. Epileptic Disord. 2015;17(4):491–5.
168. Chen J, Yang Z, Liu X, Ji T, Fu N, Wu Y, et al. [Efficacy of methylprednisolone therapy for electrical status epilepticus during sleep in children]. Zhonghua Er Ke Za Zhi. 2014;52(9):678–82. [Article in Chinese].
169. Patry G, Lyagoubi S, Tassinari CA. Subclinical "electrical status epilepticus" induced by sleep in children. A clinical and electroencephalographic study of six cases. Arch Neurol. 1971;24(3):242–52.
170. Galanopoulou AS, Bojko A, Lado F, Moshe SL. The spectrum of neuropsychiatric abnormalities associated with electrical status epilepticus in sleep. Brain Dev. 2000;22(5):279–95.
171. Doose H, Baier WK. Benign partial epilepsy and related conditions: multifactorial pathogenesis with hereditary impairment of brain maturation. Eur J Pediatr. 1989;149(3):152–8.
172. Aicardi J, Chevrie JJ. Atypical benign partial epilepsy of childhood. Dev Med Child Neurol. 1982;24(3):281–92.

173. Kramer U. Atypical presentations of benign childhood epilepsy with centrotemporal spikes: a review. J Child Neurol. 2008;23(7):785–90.
174. Su TF, Xu SQ, Chen L. Efficacy of levetiracetam combined with short-term clonazepam in treatment of electrical status epilepticus during sleep in children with benign childhood epilepsy with centrotemporal spikes. Zhongguo dang dai er ke za zhi. 2014;16(8):829–33.
175. Doose H, Hahn A, Neubauer BA, Pistohl J, Stephani U. Atypical "benign" partial epilepsy of childhood or pseudo-lennox syndrome. Part II: family study. Neuropediatrics. 2001;32(1):9–13.
176. Cerminara C, Montanaro ML, Curatolo P, Seri S. Lamotrigine-induced seizure aggravation and negative myoclonus in idiopathic rolandic epilepsy. Neurology. 2004;63(2):373–5.
177. Gelisse P, Crespel A, Genton P, Baldy-Moulinier M. Dramatic effect of levetiracetam on epileptic negative myoclonus. Acta Neurol Scand. 2003;107(4):302–3.
178. Capovilla G, Beccaria F, Veggiotti P, Rubboli G, Meletti S, Tassinari CA. Ethosuximide is effective in the treatment of epileptic negative myoclonus in childhood partial epilepsy. J Child Neurol. 1999;14(6):395–400.
179. Parmeggiani L, Seri S, Bonanni P, Guerrini R. Electrophysiological characterization of spontaneous and carbamazepine-induced epileptic negative myoclonus in benign childhood epilepsy with centro-temporal spikes. Clin Neurophysiol. 2004;115(1):50–8.
180. Kramer U, Ben-Zeev B, Harel S, Kivity S. Transient oromotor deficits in children with benign childhood epilepsy with central temporal spikes. Epilepsia. 2001;42(5):616–20.
181. Hamano S, Mochizuki M, Morikawa T. Phenobarbital-induced atypical absence seizure in benign childhood epilepsy with centrotemporal spikes. Seizure. 2002;11(3):201–4.
182. Tassinari CA, Rubboli G, Volpi L, Meletti S, d'Orsi G, Franca M, Sabetta AR, Riguzzi P, Gardella E, Zaniboni A, et al. Encephalopathy with electrical status epilepticus during slow sleep or ESES syndrome including the acquired aphasia. Clin Neurophysiol. 2000;111(Suppl 2):S94–s102.
183. Herguner MO, Incecik F, Altunbasak S, Kiris N. Clinical characteristics of 10 patients with continuous spikes and waves during slow sleep syndrome. Pediatr Neurol. 2008;38(6):411–4.
184. Buzatu M, Bulteau C, Altuzarra C, Dulac O, Van Bogaert P. Corticosteroids as treatment of epileptic syndromes with continuous spike-waves during slow-wave sleep. Epilepsia. 2009;50(Suppl 7):68–72.
185. Praline J, Hommet C, Barthez MA, Brault F, Perrier D, Passage GD, Lucas B, Bonnard J, Billard C, Toffol BD, et al. Outcome at adulthood of the continuous spike-waves during slow sleep and Landau-Kleffner syndromes. Epilepsia. 2003;44(11):1434–40.
186. Scheltens-de Boer M. Guidelines for EEG in encephalopathy related to ESES/CSWS in children. Epilepsia. 2009;50(Suppl 7):13–7.
187. Seri S, Thai JN, Brazzo D, Pisani F, Cerquiglini A. Neurophysiology of CSWS-associated cognitive dysfunction. Epilepsia. 2009;50(Suppl 7): 33–6.
188. Downes M, Greenaway R, Clark M, Helen Cross J, Jolleff N, Harkness W, Kaliakatsos M, Boyd S, White S, Neville BG. Outcome following multiple subpial transection in Landau-Kleffner syndrome and related regression. Epilepsia. 2015;56(11):1760–6.
189. Arts WF, Aarsen FK, Scheltens-de Boer M, Catsman-Berrevoets CE. Landau-Kleffner syndrome and CSWS syndrome: treatment with intravenous immunoglobulins. Epilepsia. 2009;50(Suppl 7):55–8.
190. Tsuru T, Mori M, Mizuguchi M, Momoi MY. Effects of high-dose intravenous corticosteroid therapy in Landau-Kleffner syndrome. Pediatr Neurol. 2000;22(2):145–7.
191. Sinclair DB, Snyder TJ. Corticosteroids for the treatment of Landau-kleffner syndrome and continuous spike-wave discharge during sleep. Pediatr Neurol. 2005;32(5):300–6.
192. Okuyaz C, Aydin K, Gucuyener K, Serdaroglu A. Treatment of electrical status epilepticus during slow-wave sleep with high-dose corticosteroid. Pediatr Neurol. 2005;32(1):64–7.
193. Arzimanoglou A, French J, Blume WT, Cross JH, Ernst JP, Feucht M, Genton P, Guerrini R, Kluger G, Pellock JM, et al. Lennox-Gastaut syndrome: a consensus approach on diagnosis, assessment, management, and trial methodology. Lancet Neurol. 2009;8(1):82–93.
194. Al-Banji MH, Zahr DK, Jan MM. Lennox-Gastaut syndrome. Management update. Neurosciences. 2015;20(3):207–12.
195. Hoffmann-Riem M, Diener W, Benninger C, Rating D, Unnebrink K, Stephani U, Ernst HP, Korinthenberg R. Nonconvulsive status epilepticus—a possible cause of mental retardation in patients with Lennox-Gastaut syndrome. Neuropediatrics. 2000;31(4):169–74.
196. Markand ON. Lennox-Gastaut syndrome (childhood epileptic encephalopathy). J Clin Neurophysiol. 2003;20(6):426–41.
197. Gibbs FA, Davis H, Lennox WG. The electroencephalogram in epilepsy and in conditions of impaired consciousness. Arch Neural Psychiatry.1935;34:1133–48.
198. Gastraut H, Roger J, Soulayrol R, Tassinari CA, Regis H, Dravet C, Bernard R, Pinsard N, Saint-Jean M. Childhood epileptic encephalopathy with diffuse slow spike-waves (otherwise known as "petit mal variant") or Lennox syndrome. Epilepsia. 1966;7(2):139–79.
199. Gastaut H. The Lennox-Gastaut syndrome: comments on the syndrome's terminology and nosological position amongst the secondary generalized

epilepsies of childhood. Electroencephalogr Clin Neurophysiol Suppl. 1982;35:71–84.
200. Kumar A, Paliwal VK, Agarwal V, Neyaz Z, Lal H, Goel G. Relationship of Lennox-Gastaut syndrome with perinatal event: a cross-sectional study. J Pediatr Neurosci. 2015;10(2):98–102.
201. Chevrie JJ, Aicardi J. Childhood epileptic encephalopathy with slow spike-wave. A statistical study of 80 cases. Epilepsia. 1972;13(2):259–71.
202. Crumrine PK. Management of seizures in Lennox-Gastaut syndrome. Paediatr Drugs. 2011;13(2):107–18.
203. Crumrine PK. Lennox-Gastaut syndrome. J Child Neurol. 2002;17(Suppl 1):S70–5.
204. Bittencourt PR, Richens A. Anticonvulsant-induced status epilepticus in Lennox-Gastaut syndrome. Epilepsia. 1981;22(1):129–34.
205. Markand ON. Slow spike-wave activity in EEG and associated clinical features: often called 'Lennox' or "Lennox-Gastaut" syndrome. Neurology. 1977;27(8):746–57.
206. Youn YA, Kim JH, Yum SK, Moon CJ, Lee IG, Sung IK. The hospital outcomes compared between the early and late hypothermia-treated groups in neonates. J Matern Fetal Neonatal Med. 2016;29(14):2288–92.
207. Simpson RK Jr, Goodman JC, Rouah E, Caraway N, Baskin DS. Late neuropathological consequences of strangulation. Resuscitation. 1987;15(3):171–85.
208. Jumao-as A, Brenner RP. Myoclonic status epilepticus: a clinical and electroencephalographic study. Neurology. 1990;40(8):1199–202.
209. Sirsi D, Nangia S, LaMothe J, Kosofsky BE, Solomon GE. Successful management of refractory neonatal seizures with midazolam. J Child Neurol. 2008;23(6):706–9.
210. Sutter R, Marsch S, Fuhr P, Ruegg S. Mortality and recovery from refractory status epilepticus in the intensive care unit: a 7-year observational study. Epilepsia. 2013;54(3):502–11.
211. Rittenberger JC, Popescu A, Brenner RP, Guyette FX, Callaway CW. Frequency and timing of nonconvulsive status epilepticus in comatose post-cardiac arrest subjects treated with hypothermia. Neurocrit Care. 2012;16(1):114–22.
212. Legriel S, Hilly-Ginoux J, Resche-Rigon M, Merceron S, Pinoteau J, Henry-Lagarrigue M, Bruneel F, Nguyen A, Guezennec P, Troche G, et al. Prognostic value of electrographic postanoxic status epilepticus in comatose cardiac-arrest survivors in the therapeutic hypothermia era. Resuscitation. 2013;84(3):343–50.
213. Krumholz A, Stern BJ, Weiss HD. Outcome from coma after cardiopulmonary resuscitation: relation to seizures and myoclonus. Neurology. 1988;38(3):401–5.
214. Buttram SD, Au AK, Koch J, Lidsky K, McBain K, O'Brien N, Zielinski BA, Bell MJ. Feasibility study evaluating therapeutic hypothermia for refractory status epilepticus in children. Ther Hypothermia Temp Manag. 2015;5(4):198–202.
215. Logroscino G, Hesdorffer DC, Cascino G, Annegers JF, Hauser WA. Short-term mortality after a first episode of status epilepticus. Epilepsia. 1997;38(12):1344–9.
216. Laptook AR, Corbett RJ, Nguyen HT, Peterson J, Nunnally RL. Alterations in cerebral blood flow and phosphorylated metabolites in piglets during and after partial ischemia. Pediatr Res. 1988;23(2):206–11.
217. Vannucci RC, Yager JY, Vannucci SJ. Cerebral glucose and energy utilization during the evolution of hypoxic-ischemic brain damage in the immature rat. J Cereb Blood Flow Metab. 1994;14(2):279–88.
218. Younkin DP, Wagerle LC, Chance B, Maria J, Delivoria-Papadopoulos M. 31P--NMR studies of cerebral metabolic changes during graded hypoxia in newborn lambs. J Appl Physiol. 1987;62(4):1569–74.
219. Hope PL, Costello AM, Cady EB, Delpy DT, Tofts PS, Chu A, Hamilton PA, Reynolds EO, Wilkie DR. Cerebral energy metabolism studied with phosphorus NMR spectroscopy in normal and birth-asphyxiated infants. Lancet. 1984;2(8399):366–70.
220. Johnston MV. Excitotoxicity in neonatal hypoxia. Ment Retard Dev Disabil Res Rev. 2001;7(4):229–34.
221. Follett PL, Rosenberg PA, Volpe JJ, Jensen FE. NBQX attenuates excitotoxic injury in developing white matter. J Neurosci. 2000;20(24):9235–41.
222. Cataltepe O, Towfighi J, Vannucci RC. Cerebrospinal fluid concentrations of glutamate and GABA during perinatal cerebral hypoxia-ischemia and seizures. Brain Res. 1996;709(2):326–30.
223. Zanelli SA, Rajasekaran K, Grosenbaugh DK, Kapur J. Increased excitability and excitatory synaptic transmission during in vitro ischemia in the neonatal mouse hippocampus. Neuroscience. 2015;310:279–89.
224. Kristian T, Siesjo BK. Calcium in ischemic cell death. Stroke. 1998;29(3):705–18.
225. Vannucci RC, Brucklacher RM, Vannucci SJ. Intracellular calcium accumulation during the evolution of hypoxic-ischemic brain damage in the immature rat. Brain Res Dev Brain Res. 2001;126(1):117–20.
226. Chan PH. Reactive oxygen radicals in signaling and damage in the ischemic brain. J Cereb Blood Flow Metab. 2001;21(1):2–14.
227. Fullerton HJ, Ditelberg JS, Chen SF, Sarco DP, Chan PH, Epstein CJ, Ferriero DM. Copper/zinc superoxide dismutase transgenic brain accumulates hydrogen peroxide after perinatal hypoxia ischemia. Ann Neurol. 1998;44(3):357–64.
228. Nelson KB, Willoughby RE. Infection, inflammation and the risk of cerebral palsy. Curr Opin Neurol. 2000;13(2):133–9.
229. Yoon BH, Jun JK, Romero R, Park KH, Gomez R, Choi JH, Kim IO. Amniotic fluid inflammatory

cytokines (interleukin-6, interleukin-1beta, and tumor necrosis factor-alpha), neonatal brain white matter lesions, and cerebral palsy. Am J Obstet Gynecol. 1997;177(1):19–26.
230. Eklind S, Mallard C, Leverin AL, Gilland E, Blomgren K, Mattsby-Baltzer I, Hagberg H. Bacterial endotoxin sensitizes the immature brain to hypoxic—ischaemic injury. Eur J Neurosci. 2001;13(6):1101–6.
231. Xu ZH, Wang Y, Tao AF, Yu J, Wang XY, Zu YY, Zhang SH, Chen Z. Interleukin-1 receptor is a target for adjunctive control of diazepam-refractory status epilepticus in mice. Neuroscience. 2016;328:22–9.
232. Snyder BD, Hauser WA, Loewenson RB, Leppik IE, Ramirez-Lassepas M, Gumnit RJ. Neurologic prognosis after cardiopulmonary arrest: III. Seizure activity. Neurology. 1980;30(12):1292–7.
233. Morris HR, Howard RS, Brown P. Early myoclonic status and outcome after cardiorespiratory arrest. J Neurol Neurosurg Psychiatry. 1998;64(2):267–8.
234. Arnoldus EP, Lammers GJ. Postanoxic coma: good recovery despite myoclonus status. Ann Neurol. 1995;38(4):697–8.
235. Hui AC, Cheng C, Lam A, Mok V, Joynt GM. Prognosis following postanoxic myoclonus status epilepticus. Eur Neurol. 2005;54(1):10–3.
236. McGinn KA, Bishop L, Sarwal A. Use of ketamine in barbiturate coma for status epilepticus. Clin Neuropharmacol. 2016;39(1):62–5.
237. Anderson CA, Arciniegas DB. Cognitive sequelae of hypoxic-ischemic brain injury: a review. NeuroRehabilitation. 2010;26(1):47–63.
238. Thomke F, Marx JJ, Sauer O, Hundsberger T, Hagele S, Wiechelt J, Weilemann SL. Observations on comatose survivors of cardiopulmonary resuscitation with generalized myoclonus. BMC Neurol. 2005;5:14.
239. Akman CI, Abou Khaled KJ, Segal E, Micic V, Riviello JJ. Generalized periodic epileptiform discharges in critically ill children: clinical features, and outcome. Epilepsy Res. 2013;106(3):378–85.
240. Pandian JD, Cascino GD, So EL, Manno E, Fulgham JR. Digital video-electroencephalographic monitoring in the neurological-neurosurgical intensive care unit: clinical features and outcome. Arch Neurol. 2004;61(7):1090–4.
241. Drislane FW, Lopez MR, Blum AS, Schomer DL. Detection and treatment of refractory status epilepticus in the intensive care unit. J Clin Neurophysiol. 2008;25(4):181–6.
242. Bensalem MK, Fakhoury TA. Topiramate and status epilepticus: report of three cases. Epilepsy Behav. 2003;4(6):757–60.
243. Mader EC Jr, Villemarette-Pittman NR, Kashirny SV, Santana-Gould L, Olejniczak PW. Typical spike-and-wave activity in hypoxic-ischemic brain injury and its implications for classifying nonconvulsive status epilepticus. Clin Med Insights Case Rep. 2012;5:99–106.
244. Suppiej A, Cappellari A, Cogo PE. Prognostic role of somatosensory and auditory evoked potentials in paediatric hypoxic-ischemic encephalopathy managed with hypothermia: an illustrative case. Clin Neurophysiol. 2009;39(2):101–5.
245. Lemiale V, Huet O, Vigue B, Mathonnet A, Spaulding C, Mira JP, Carli P, Duranteau J, Cariou A. Changes in cerebral blood flow and oxygen extraction during post-resuscitation syndrome. Resuscitation. 2008;76(1):17–24.
246. Polderman KH, Herold I. Therapeutic hypothermia and controlled normothermia in the intensive care unit: practical considerations, side effects, and cooling methods. Crit Care Med. 2009;37(3):1101–20.
247. Atkins CM, Truettner JS, Lotocki G, Sanchez-Molano J, Kang Y, Alonso OF, Sick TJ, Dietrich WD, Bramlett HM. Post-traumatic seizure susceptibility is attenuated by hypothermia therapy. Eur J Neurosci. 2010;32(11):1912–20.
248. D'Ambrosio R, Eastman CL, Darvas F, Fender JS, Verley DR, Farin FM, Wilkerson HW, Temkin NR, Miller JW, Ojemann J, et al. Mild passive focal cooling prevents epileptic seizures after head injury in rats. Ann Neurol. 2013;73(2):199–209.
249. Schmitt FC, Buchheim K, Meierkord H, Holtkamp M. Anticonvulsant properties of hypothermia in experimental status epilepticus. Neurobiol Dis. 2006;23(3):689–96.
250. Yu L, Zhou Y, Chen W, Wang Y. Mild hypothermia pretreatment protects against pilocarpine-induced status epilepticus and neuronalapoptosis in immature rats. Neuropathology. 2011;31(2):144–51.
251. Wang Y, Liu PP, Li LY, Zhang HM, Li T. Hypothermia reduces brain edema, spontaneous recurrent seizure attack, and learning memory deficits in the kainic acid treated rats. CNS Neurosci Ther. 2011;17(5):271–80.
252. Zhu M, Lu M, Li QJ, Zhang Z, Wu ZZ, Li J, Qian L, Xu Y, Wang ZY. Hyperbaric oxygen suppresses hypoxic-ischemic brain damage in newborn rats. J Child Neurol. 2015;30(1):75–82.
253. Yang L, Hei MY, Dai JJ, Hu N, Xiang XY. Effect of hyperbaric oxygenation on mitochondrial function of neuronal cells in the cortex of neonatal rats after hypoxic-ischemic brain damage. Braz J Med Biol Res. 2016;49(5):e5187.
254. Young GB, Gilbert JJ, Zochodne DW. The significance of myoclonic status epilepticus in postanoxic coma. Neurology. 1990;40(12):1843–8.
255. Zamponi N, Rychlicki F, Corpaci L, Cesaroni E, Trignani R. Vagus nerve stimulation (VNS) is effective in treating catastrophic 1 epilepsy in very young children. Neurosurg Rev. 2008;31(3):291–7.
256. Seder DB, Sunde K, Rubertsson S, Mooney M, Stammet P, Riker RR, Kern KB, Unger B, Cronberg T, Dziodzio J, et al. Neurologic outcomes and postresuscitation care of patients with myoclonus following cardiac arrest. Crit Care Med. 2015;43(5):965–72.

257. Wijdicks EF, Young GB. Myoclonus status in comatose patients after cardiac arrest. Lancet. 1994;343(8913):1642–3.
258. Towne AR, Pellock JM, Ko D, DeLorenzo RJ. Determinants of mortality in status epilepticus. Epilepsia. 1994;35(1):27–34.
259. Rossetti AO, Logroscino G, Liaudet L, Ruffieux C, Ribordy V, Schaller MD, Despland PA, Oddo M. Status epilepticus: an independent outcome predictor after cerebral anoxia. Neurology. 2007;69(3):255–60.
260. Yuasa T, Fujita K. Limbic encephalitis—history, symptoms, and the latest classification. Brain Nerve. 2010;62(8):817–26.
261. Petit-Pedrol M, Armangue T, Peng X, et al. Encephalitis with refractory seizures, status epilepticus, and antibodies to the GABA a receptor: a case series, characterisation of the antigen, and analysis of the effects of antibodies. Lancet Neurol. 2014;13(3):276–86.
262. Gagnon MM, Savard M, Mourabit AK. Refractory status epilepticus and autoimmune encephalitis with GABAAR and GAD65 antibodies: a case report. Seizure. 2016;37:25–7.
263. Dalmau J. Status epilepticus due to paraneoplastic and nonparaneoplastic encephalitides. Epilepsia. 2009;50(Suppl 12):58–60.
264. Morbelli S, Arbizu J, Booij J, Chen MK, Chetelat G, Cross DJ, et al. The need of standardization and of large clinical studies in an emerging indication of [18F]FDG PET: the autoimmune encephalitis. Eur J Nucl Med Mol Imaging. 2016.
265. Baysal-Kirac L, Tuzun E, Altindag E, Ekizoglu E, Kinay D, Bilgic B, et al. Are there any specific EEG findings in autoimmune epilepsies? Clin EEG Neurosci. 2016;47(3):224–34.
266. Cikrikcili U, Ulusoy C, Turan S, Yildiz S, Bilgic B, Hanagasi H, et al. Non-convulsive status epilepticus associated with glutamic acid decarboxylase antibody. Clin EEG Neurosci. 2013;44(3):232–6.
267. Cyril AC, Nair SS, Mathai A, Kannoth S, Thomas SV. Autoimmune encephalitis: clinical diagnosis versus antibody confirmation. Ann Indian Acad Neurol. 2015;18(4):408–11.
268. Holzer FJ, Rossetti AO, Heritier-Barras AC, et al. Antibody-mediated status epilepticus: a retrospective multicenter survey. Eur Neurol. 2012;68(5):310–7.
269. Sarria-Estrada S, Toledo M, Lorenzo-Bosquet C, et al. Neuroimaging in status epilepticus secondary to paraneoplastic autoimmune encephalitis. Clin Radiol. 2014;69(8):795–803.
270. Rudzinski LA, Pittock SJ, McKeon A, et al. Extratemporal EEG and MRI findings in ANNA-1 (anti-Hu) encephalitis. Epilepsy Res. 2011;95(3):255–62.
271. Demaerel P, Van Dessel W, Van Paesschen W, et al. Autoimmune-mediated encephalitis. Neuroradiology. 2011;53(11):837–51.
272. Bellaïche Shavit Y, Graus F, Probst A, et al. Epilepsia partialis continua: a new manifestation of anti-Hu–associated paraneoplastic encephalomyelitis. Ann Neurol. 1999;45(2):255–8.
273. Drislane FW. Nonconvulsive status epilepticus in patients with cancer. Clin Neurol Neurosurg. 1994;96(4):314–8.
274. Jacobs DA, Fung KM, Cook NM, et al. Complex partial status epilepticus associated with anti-Hu paraneoplastic syndrome. J Neurol Sci. 2003;213(1):77–82.
275. Gultekin SH, Rosenfeld MR, Voltz R, et al. Paraneoplastic limbic encephalitis: neurological symptoms, immunological findings and tumour association in 50 patients. Brain. 2000;123(7): 1481–94.
276. Irani SR, Alexander S, Waters P, et al. Antibodies to Kv1 potassium channel-complex proteins leucine-rich, glioma inactivated 1 protein and contactin-associated protein-2 in limbic encephalitis, Morvan's syndrome and acquired neuromyotonia. Brain. 2010;133(9):2734–48.
277. Buckley C, Oger J, Clover L, et al. Potassium channel antibodies in two patients with reversible limbic encephalitis. Ann Neurol. 2001;50(1):73–8.
278. Brenner T, Sills GJ, Hart Y, et al. Prevalence of neurologic autoantibodies in cohorts of patients with new and established epilepsy. Epilepsia. 2013;54(6):1028–35.
279. Suleiman J, Brenner T, Gill D, Brilot F, Antony J, Vincent A, et al. VGKC antibodies in pediatric encephalitis presenting with status epilepticus. Neurology. 2011;76(14):1252–5.
280. Kotsenas AL, Watson RE, Pittock SJ, et al. MRI findings in autoimmune voltage-gated potassium channel complex encephalitis with seizures: one potential etiology for mesial temporal sclerosis. Am J Neuroradiol. 2014;35(1):84–9.
281. Ramanathan S, Wong CH, Rahman Z, et al. Myoclonic status epilepticus as a presentation of caspr2 antibody-associated autoimmune encephalitis. Epileptic Disord. 2014;16(4): 477–81.
282. Dalmau J, Gleichman AJ, Hughes EG, et al. Anti-NMDA-receptor encephalitis: case series and analysis of the effects of antibodies. Lancet Neurol. 2008;7(12):1091–8.
283. Florance NR, Davis RL, Lam C, et al. Anti-N-methyl-D-aspartate receptor (NMDAR) encephalitis in children and adolescents. Ann Neurol. 2009;66:11–8.
284. Johnson N, Henry C, Fessler AJ, et al. Anti-NMDA receptor encephalitis causing prolonged nonconvulsive status epilepticus. Neurology. 2010;75(16):1480–2.
285. Frisch C, Malter MP, Elger CE, et al. Neuropsychological course of voltage-gated potassium channel and glutamic acid decarboxylase antibody related limbic encephalitis. Eur J Neurol. 2013;20(9):1297–304.
286. Malter MP, Helmstaedter C, Urbach H, et al. Antibodies to glutamic acid decarboxylase

define a form of limbic encephalitis. Ann Neurol. 2010;67(4):470–8.
287. Vianello M, Tavolato B, Giometto B. Glutamic acid decarboxylase autoantibodies and neurological disorders. Neurol Sci. 2002;23(4):145–51.
288. Kanter IC, Huttner HB, Staykov D, et al. Cyclophosphamide for anti-GAD antibody-positive refractory status epilepticus. Epilepsia. 2008;49(5): 914–20.
289. Kumar G, Mittal S, Moudgil SS, et al. Histopathological evidence that hippocampal atrophy following status epilepticus is a result of neuronal necrosis. J Neurol Sci. 2013;334(1):186–91.
290. Wong SH, Saunders MD, Larner AJ, et al. An effective immunotherapy regimen for VGKC antibody-positive limbic encephalitis. J Neurol Neurosurg Psychiatry. 2010;81(10):1167–9.
291. Finelli PF. Autoimmune limbic encephalitis with GAD antibodies. Neurohospitalist. 2011;1(4):178–81.
292. Mazzi G, De Roia D, Cruciatti B, et al. Plasma exchange for anti GAD associated non paraneoplastic limbic encephalitis. Transfus Apher Sci. 2008;39(3):229–33.
293. Kobayakawa Y, Tateishi T, Kawamura N, et al. A case of immune-mediated encephalopathy showing refractory epilepsy and extensive brain MRI lesions associated with anti-glutamic acid decarboxylase antibody. Clin Neurol. 2010;50(2):92–7.
294. Korff CM, Parvex P, Cimasoni L, et al. Encephalitis associated with glutamic acid decarboxylase autoantibodies in a child: a treatable condition? Arch Neurol. 2011;68(8):1065–8.
295. Boronat A, Sabater L, Saiz A, et al. GABAB receptor antibodies in limbic encephalitis and anti-GAD-associated neurologic disorders. Neurology. 2011;76(9):795–800.
296. Schuler V, Lüscher C, Blanchet C, et al. Epilepsy, hyperalgesia, impaired memory, and loss of pre-and postsynaptic GABA B responses in mice lacking GABA B (1). Neuron. 2001;31(1):47–58.
297. Lancaster E, Lai M, Hughes E, et al. Autoantibodies to the GABA (B) receptor associate with limbic encephalitis and seizures, and alter GABA (B) receptor function [C]. Neurology. 2010; 74(9):A402.
298. Guan HZ, Ren HT, Yang XZ, et al. Limbic encephalitis associated with anti-γ-aminobutyric acid B receptor antibodies: a case series from China. Chin Med J. 2015;128(22):3023.
299. Chong JY, Rowland LP, Utiger RD. HE: syndrome or myth? Arch Neurol. 2003;60(2):164–71.
300. Castillo P, Woodruff B, Caselli R, et al. Steroid-responsive encephalopathy associated with autoimmune thyroiditis. Arch Neurol. 2006;63(2): 197–202.
301. Monti G, Pugnaghi M, Ariatti A, et al. Nonconvulsive status epilepticus of frontal origin as the first manifestation of Hashimoto's encephalopathy. Epileptic Disord. 2011;13(3):253–8.
302. Jellinek EH, Ball K. Hashimoto's disease and encephalopathy. Lancet. 1966;288(7462):512–4.
303. Devinsky O, Schein A, Najjar S. Epilepsy associated with systemic autoimmune disorders. Epilepsy Curr. 2013;13(2):62–8.
304. Park M, et al. Delayed diagnosis of SLE in a patient presenting with intractable status epilepticus. Lupus. 2009;18:474–5.
305. Fernandez-Torre JL, Sanchez JM, Gonzalez C, et al. Complex partial status epilepticus of extratemporal origin in a patient with systemic lupus erythematosus. Seizure. 2003;12(4):245–8.
306. Appenzeller S, Cendes F, Costallat LT. Epileptic seizures in systemic lupus erythematosus. Neurology. 2004;63(10):1808–12.
307. Benavente E, Paira S, Roverano S, et al. Encephalitis and status epilepticus in a patient with systemic lupus erythematosus. Reumatol Clín. 2013;9(2):123–7.
308. Tsuji M, Tanaka H, Yamakawa M, et al. A case of systemic lupus erythematosus with complex partial status epilepticus. Epileptic Disord. 2005;7(3):249–51.
309. Koppel BS. Connective tissue diseases. In: Engel J, Pedley TA, editors. Epilepsy: a comprehensive textbook. Philadelphia: Lippincott-Raven; 1997. p. 2597–604.
310. Urbach H, Soeder BM, Jeub M, et al. Serial MRI of limbic encephalitis. Neuroradiology. 2006;48(6):380–6.
311. Kruer MC, Hoeftberger R, Lim KY, et al. Aggressive course in encephalitis with opsoclonus, ataxia, chorea, and seizures: the first pediatric case of γ-aminobutyric acid type B receptor autoimmunity. JAMA Neurol. 2014;71(5):620–3.
312. Dhamija R, Renaud DL, Pittock SJ, et al. Neuronal voltage-gated potassium channel complex autoimmunity in children. Pediatr Neurol. 2011;44(4):275–81.
313. Vincent A. Stiff, twitchy or wobbly—are GAD antibodies pathogenic? Brain. 2008;131(10):2536–7.
314. Reznik ME, Berger K, Claassen J. Comparison of intravenous anesthetic agents for the treatment of refractory status epilepticus. J Clin Med. 2016;5(5).
315. Sutter R, Kaplan PW, Rüegg S. Outcome predictors for status epilepticus—what really counts[J]. Nat Rev Neurol. 2013;9(9):525–34.
316. Trinka E, Höfler J, Zerbs A. Causes of status epilepticus. Epilepsia. 2012;53(s4):127–38.
317. Shorvon S. Guidelines for status epilepticus: are we there yet? Neurocrit Care. 2012:1–2.
318. Kirkpatrick MNP, Clarke CD, Sonmezturk HH, et al. Rhythmic delta activity represents a form of nonconvulsive status epilepticus in anti-NMDA receptor antibody encephalitis. Epilepsy Behav. 2011;20(2):392–4.
319. Chang HR, Kuo CC. Molecular determinants of the anticonvulsant felbamate binding site in the N-methyl-D-aspartate receptor. J Med Chem. 2008;51(6):1534–45.
320. Harty TP, Rogawski MA. Felbamate block of recombinant N-methyl-D-aspartate receptors:

selectivity for the NR2B subunit. Epilepsy Res. 2000;39(1):47–55.
321. Atwater BD, Ai Z, Wolff MR. Fulminant myopericarditis from phenytoin-induced systemic lupus erythematosus. WMJ. 2008;107(6):298–300.
322. Gunther A, Schubert J, Bramer D, Witte OW. Autoimmune encephalitis. Dtsch Med Wochenschr. 2016;141(17):1244–9.
323. Sabin TD, Jednacz JA, Staats PN. Case 26-2008: a 26-year-old woman with headache and behavioral changes. N Engl J Med. 2008;359(8):842–53.
324. Ramanathan S, Mohammad SS, Brilot F, et al. Autoimmune encephalitis: recent updates and emerging challenges. J Clin Neurosci. 2014;21(5):722–30.
325. Ishiura H, Matsuda S, Higashihara M, et al. Response of anti-NMDA receptor encephalitis without tumor to immunotherapy including rituximab. Neurology. 2008;71:1921–3.
326. Martinez-Hernandez E, Horvath J, Shiloh-Malawsky Y, et al. Analysis of complement and plasma cells in the brain of patients with anti-NMDARencephalitis. Neurology. 2011;77:589–93.
327. Titulaer MJ, McCracken L, Gabilondo I, et al. Treatment and prognositc factorsfor long-term outcome in patients with anti-NMDA receptor encephalitis: an observational cohort study. Lancet Neurol. 2013;12:157–65.
328. Weimer T, Boling W, Pryputniewicz D, et al. Temporal lobectomy for refractory status epilepticus in a case of limbic encephalitis. J Neurosurg. 2008;109(4):742–5.
329. Costello DJ, Simon MV, Eskandar EN, et al. Efficacy of surgical treatment of de novo, adult-onset, cryptogenic, refractory focal status epilepticus. Arch Neurol. 2006;63(6):895–901.
330. Mohamed IS, Otsubo H, Donner E, et al. Magnetoencephalography for surgical treatment of refractory status epilepticus. Acta Neurol Scand. 2007;115(s186):29–36.
331. Ng Y, Kerrigan JF, Rekate HL. Neurosurgical treatment of status epilepticus. J Neurosurg Pediatr. 2006;105(5):378–81.
332. Ng Y, Kim HL, Wheless JW. Successful neurosurgical treatment of childhood complex partial status epilepticus with focal resection. Epilepsia. 2003;44(3):468–71.
333. Correa-Lima AR, de Barros M-FD, Valenca MM, Andrade-Valenca L. Risk factors for acute symptomatic seizure in bacterial meningitis in children. J Child Neurol. 2015;30(9):1182–5.
334. Annegers JF, Hauser WA, Beghi E, Nicolosi A, Kurland LT. The risk of unprovoked seizures after encephalitis and meningitis. Neurology. 1988;38(9):1407–10.
335. Prasanth S, Shaji VC, Lyla C, Jayalakshmi V. Refractory status epilepticus due to pneumococcal meningitis in an infant with congenital immunodeficiency. J Pediatr Neurosci. 2016;11(2):125–7.
336. Singhi SC, Khetarpal R, Baranwal AK, Singhi PD. Intensive care needs of children with acute bacterial meningitis: a developing country perspective. Ann Trop Paediatr. 2004;24(2):133–40.
337. Wang KW, Chang WN, Chang HW, Chuang YC, Tsai NW, Wang HC, Lu CH. The significance of seizures and other predictive factors during the acute illness for the long-term outcome after bacterial meningitis. Seizure. 2005;14(8):586–92.
338. Zoons E, Weisfelt M, de Gans J, Spanjaard L, Koelman JH, Reitsma JB, van de Beek D. Seizures in adults with bacterial meningitis. Neurology. 2008;70(22 Pt 2):2109–15.
339. Maegaki Y, Kurozawa Y, Tamasaki A, Togawa M, Tamura A, Hirao M, Nagao A, Kouda T, Okada T, Hayashibara H, et al. Early predictors of status epilepticus-associated mortality and morbidity in children. Brain Dev. 2015;37(5):478–86.
340. Chang CJ, Chang HW, Chang WN, Huang LT, Huang SC, Chang YC, Hung PL, Chang CS, Chuang YC, Huang CR, et al. Seizures complicating infantile and childhood bacterial meningitis. Pediatr Neurol. 2004;31(3):165–71.
341. Wall EC, Cartwright K, Scarborough M, Ajdukiewicz KM, Goodson P, Mwambene J, Zijlstra EE, Gordon SB, French N, Faragher B, et al. High mortality amongst adolescents and adults with bacterial meningitis in sub-Saharan Africa: an analysis of 715 cases from Malawi. PLoS One. 2013;8(7):e69783.
342. Kim MA, Park KM, Kim SE, Oh MK. Acute symptomatic seizures in CNS infection. Eur J Neurol. 2008;15(1):38–41.
343. Casado-Flores J, Rodrigo C, Aristegui J, Martinon JM, Fenoll A, Mendez C. Decline in pneumococcal meningitis in Spain after introduction of the heptavalent pneumococcal conjugate vaccine. Pediatr Infect Dis J. 2008;27(11):1020–2.
344. Inoue S, Nakazawa T, Takahashi H, Kaneko K. Seizures in the acute phase of aseptic and bacterial meningitis. No To Hattatsu. 1998;30(6):494–9.
345. Phillips SA, Shanahan RJ. Etiology and mortality of status epilepticus in children. A recent update. Arch Neurol. 1989;46(1):74–6.
346. Frenkel AL, Bour F, Plouin P, Jalin C. Prognostic value of EEG in pneumococcal meningitis in children. Rev Electroencephalogr Neurophysiol Clin. 1983;13(1):83–7.
347. Tuncer O, Caksen H, Arslan S, Atas B, Uner A, Oner AF, Odabas D. Cranial computed tomography in purulent meningitis of childhood. Int J Neurosci. 2004;114(2):167–74.
348. Lambrechtsen FA, Buchhalter JR. Aborted and refractory status epilepticus in children: a comparative analysis. Epilepsia. 2008;49(4):615–25.
349. Chaptal J, Passouant P, Brunel D, Latour H, Jean R, Cadilhac J, Carli G. Temporal epilepsy of tuberculous meningitis. Arch Fr Pediatr. 1953;10(4):350–7.
350. Carletti B, Guareschi A. Aspects of convulsions in sequels of treated tuberculous meningitis. Minerva Pediatr. 1957;9(40):1022–38.
351. Hacquard M, Henry J, Poire R, Colmart C. Modifications in epilepsy following tuberculous

meningitis: electro-clinical & radiological study. Revue Medicale de Nancy. 1958;83:688–95.
352. Bahemuka M, Murungi JH. Tuberculosis of the nervous system. A clinical, radiological and pathological study of 39 consecutive cases in Riyadh, Saudi Arabia. J Neurol Sci. 1989;90(1):67–76.
353. Ulvi H, Yoldas T, Mungen B, Yigiter R. Continuous infusion of midazolam in the treatment of refractory generalized convulsive status epilepticus. Neurol Sci. 2002;23(4):177–82.
354. Barzegar M, Mahdavi M, Galegolab Behbehani A, Tabrizi A. Refractory convulsive status epilepticus in children: etiology, associated risk factors and outcome. Iran J Child Neurol. 2015;9(4):24–31.
355. Sinha M, Shafiulla M, Trupti K, Namrata NR, Nadimul H, Sabitha KS, Kumar RV, Jayshree RS. No evidence of association of xenotropic murine leukemia virus-related virus with oral cancers: experience from a tertiary care center in South India. Indian J Cancer. 2015;52(1):61–4.
356. Pandian JD, Thomas SV, Santoshkumar B, Radhakrishnan K, Sarma PS, Joseph S, Kesavadas C. Epilepsia partialis continua—a clinical and electroencephalography study. Seizure. 2002;11(7):437–41.
357. Zorn-Olexa C, Laugel V, Martin Ade S, Donato L, Fischbach M. Multiple intracranial tuberculomas associated with partial status epilepticus and refractory infantile spasms. J Child Neurol. 2008;23(4):459–62.
358. Raut T, Garg RK, Jain A, Verma R, Singh MK, Malhotra HS, Kohli N, Parihar A. Hydrocephalus in tuberculous meningitis: incidence, its predictive factors and impact on the prognosis. J Infect. 2013;66(4):330–7.
359. Patwari AK, Aneja S, Ravi RN, Singhal PK, Arora SK. Convulsions in tuberculous meningitis. J Trop Pediatr. 1996;42(2):91–7.
360. Saitoh A, Pong A, Waecker NJ Jr, Leake JA, Nespeca MP, Bradley JS. Prediction of neurologic sequelae in childhood tuberculous meningitis: a review of 20 cases and proposal of a novel scoring system. Pediatr Infect Dis J. 2005;24(3):207–12.
361. Yaramis A, Gurkan F, Elevli M, Soker M, Haspolat K, Kirbas G, Tas MA. Central nervous system tuberculosis in children: a review of 214 cases. Pediatrics. 1998;102(5):E49.
362. Sutlas PN, Unal A, Forta H, Senol S, Kirbas D. Tuberculous meningitis in adults: review of 61 cases. Infection. 2003;31(6):387–91.
363. Arman F, Kaya D, Akgun Y, Kocagoz S. Tuberculous meningitis presenting with nonconvulsive status epilepticus. Epilepsy Behav. 2011;20(1):111–5.
364. Ranjan P, Kalita J, Misra UK. Serial study of clinical and CT changes in tuberculous meningitis. Neuroradiology. 2003;45(5):277–82.
365. Rossetti AO, Bromfield EB. Determinants of success in the use of oral levetiracetam in status epilepticus. Epilepsy Behav. 2006;8(3):651–4.
366. Kalita J, Misra UK, Ranjan P. Predictors of long-term neurological sequelae of tuberculous meningitis: a multivariate analysis. Eur J Neurol. 2007;14(1):33–7.
367. Mazigo HD, Morona D, Kweka EJ, Waihenya R, Mnyone LL, Heukelbach J. Epilepsy and tropical parasitic infections in sub-Saharan Africa: a review. Tanzan J Health Res. 2013;15(2):102–19.
368. Crawley J, Smith S, Kirkham F, Muthinji P, Waruiru C, Marsh K. Seizures and status epilepticus in childhood cerebral malaria. QJM. 1996;89(8):591–7.
369. Newton CR, Kariuki SM. Status epilepticus in sub-Saharan Africa: new findings. Epilepsia. 2013;54(Suppl 6):50–3.
370. Kariuki SM, Kakooza-Mwesige A, Wagner RG, Chengo E, White S, Kamuyu G, Ngugi AK, Sander JW, Neville BG, Newton CR, et al. Prevalence and factors associated with convulsive status epilepticus in Africans with epilepsy. Neurology. 2015;84(18):1838–45.
371. Crawley J, Waruiru C, Mithwani S, Mwangi I, Watkins W, Ouma D, Winstanley P, Peto T, Marsh K. Effect of phenobarbital on seizure frequency and mortality in childhood cerebral malaria: a randomised, controlled intervention study. Lancet. 2000;355(9205):701–6.
372. Ikumi ML, Muchohi SN, Ohuma EO, Kokwaro GO, Newton CR. Response to diazepam in children with malaria-induced seizures. Epilepsy Res. 2008;82(2–3):215–8.
373. Singh G, Prabhakar S. The effects of antimicrobial and antiepileptic treatment on the outcome of epilepsy associated with central nervous system (CNS) infections. Epilepsia. 2008;49(Suppl 6):42–6.
374. Medina MT, Aguilar-Estrada RL, Alvarez A, Duron RM, Martinez L, Dubon S, Estrada AL, Zuniga C, Cartagena D, Thompson A, et al. Reduction in rate of epilepsy from neurocysticercosis by community interventions: the Salama, Honduras study. Epilepsia. 2011;52(6):1177–85.
375. Chuang MJ, Chang WN, Chang HW, Lin WC, Tsai NW, Hsieh MJ, Wang HC, Lu CH. Predictors and long-term outcome of seizures after bacterial brain abscess. J Neurol Neurosurg Psychiatry. 2010;81(8):913–7.
376. Koszewski W. Epilepsy following brain abscess. The evaluation of possible risk factors with emphasis on new concept of epileptic focus formation. Acta Neurochir. 1991;113(3–4):110–7.
377. Patel NH, Jain AR, Iyer VK, Shah AG, Jain DA, Shah AA. Clinico—diagnostic and therapeutic relevance of computed tomography scan of brain in children with partial seizures. Ann Indian Acad Neurol. 2013;16(3):352–6.
378. Intan HI, Zubaidah CD, Norazah A, Norlijah O. Subdural collections due to non-typhi salmonella infections in two Malaysian children. Singap Med J. 2008;49(7):e186–9.
379. Shimohata M, Naruse S, Kawasaki S, Watanabe Y, Koyama M, Ito Y, Tanaka H. Brain abscess due to fusobacterium necrophorum in a patient with convulsion and no signs of meningitis. Rinsho Shinkeigaku. 2012;52(6):429–32.

380. Carrasco-Moro R, Garcia-Navarrete E, Pedrosa-Sanchez M, Pascual-Garvi JM, Minervini-Marin M, Sola RG. Refractory epilepsy as the presenting symptom of a brucellar brain abscess. Rev Neurol. 2006;43(12):729–32.
381. Pitkanen A, Roivainen R, Lukasiuk K. Development of epilepsy after ischaemic stroke. Lancet Neurol. 2015.
382. Armstrong-Wells J, Ferriero DM. Diagnosis and acute management of perinatal arterial ischemic stroke. Neurol Clin Pract. 2014;4(5):378–85.
383. Ozdemir HH, Mungen B, Ilhan S. Evaluation of the efficacy of sodium valproate in convulsive status epilepticus following to ischemic stroke. Arq Neuropsiquiatr. 2015;73(4):293–7.
384. Lowenstein DH, Alldredge BK. Status epilepticus at an urban public hospital in the 1980s. Neurology. 1993;43(3 Pt 1):483–8.
385. Sung CY, Chu NS. Status epilepticus in the elderly: etiology, seizure type and outcome. Acta Neurol Scand. 1989;80(1):51–6.
386. Koubeissi MZ, Mayor CL, Estephan B, Rashid S, Azar NJ. Efficacy and safety of intravenous lacosamide in refractory nonconvulsive status epilepticus. Acta Neurol Scand. 2011;123(2):142–6.
387. Kirton A, Armstrong-Wells J, Chang T, Deveber G, Rivkin MJ, Hernandez M, Carpenter J, Yager JY, Lynch JK, Ferriero DM, et al. Symptomatic neonatal arterial ischemic stroke: the International Pediatric Stroke Study. Pediatrics. 2011;128(6):e1402–10.
388. Hofler J, Unterberger I, Dobesberger J, Kuchukhidze G, Walser G, Trinka E. Intravenous lacosamide in status epilepticus and seizure clusters. Epilepsia. 2011;52(10):e148–52.
389. Goodwin H, Hinson HE, Shermock KM, Karanjia N, Lewin JJ 3rd. The use of lacosamide in refractory status epilepticus. Neurocrit Care. 2011;14(3):348–53.
390. Rosati A, Ilvento L, L'Erario M, De Masi S, Biggeri A, Fabbro G, Bianchi R, Stoppa F, Fusco L, Pulitano S, et al. Efficacy of ketamine in refractory convulsive status epilepticus in children: a protocol for a sequential design, multicentre, randomised, controlled, open-label, non-profit trial (KETASER01). BMJ Open. 2016;6(6):e011565.
391. Miras Veiga A, Moreno DC, Menendez AI, Siscart IM, Fernandez MD, Sanchez EG, Gonzalez MG, Saez FG. Effectiveness of electroconvulsive therapy for refractory status epilepticus in febrile infection-related epilepsy syndrome. Neuropediatrics. 2017;48(1):45–8.
392. Appavu B, Vanatta L, Condie J, Kerrigan JF, Jarrar R. Ketogenic diet treatment for pediatric super-refractory status epilepticus. Seizure. 2016;41:62–5.
393. Thakur KT, Probasco JC, Hocker SE, Roehl K, Henry B, Kossoff EH, Kaplan PW, Geocadin RG, Hartman AL, Venkatesan A, et al. Ketogenic diet for adults in super-refractory status epilepticus. Neurology. 2014;82(8):665–70.
394. Yoshimura H, Matsumoto R, Ueda H, Ariyoshi K, Kawamoto M, Ishii J, Ikeda A, Takahashi R, Kohara N. Status epilepticus in the elderly: prognostic implications of rhythmic and periodic patterns in electroencephalography and hyperintensities on diffusion-weighted imaging. J Neurol Sci. 2016;370:284–9.
395. Canoui-Poitrine F, Bastuji-Garin S, Alonso E, Darcel G, Verstichel P, Caillet P, Paillaud E. Risk and prognostic factors of status epilepticus in the elderly: a case-control study. Epilepsia. 2011;52(10):1849–56.
396. Kalita J, Nair PP, Misra UK. A clinical, radiological and outcome study of status epilepticus from India. J Neurol. 2010;257(2):224–9.
397. Nanau RM, Neuman MG. Adverse drug reactions induced by valproic acid. Clin Biochem. 2013;46(15):1323–38.
398. Labovitz DL, Hauser WA, Sacco RL. Prevalence and predictors of early seizure and status epilepticus after first stroke. Neurology. 2001;57(2):200–6.
399. Makihara N, Arimura K, Ago T, Tachibana M, Nishimura A, Nakamura K, Matsuo R, Wakisaka Y, Kuroda J, Sugimori H, et al. Involvement of platelet-derived growth factor receptor Beta in fibrosis through extracellular matrix protein production after ischemic stroke. Exp Neurol. 2015;264:127–34.
400. Bell RD, Winkler EA, Sagare AP, Singh I, LaRue B, Deane R, Zlokovic BV. Pericytes control key neurovascular functions and neuronal phenotype in the adult brain and during brain aging. Neuron. 2010;68(3):409–27.
401. So EL, Annegers JF, Hauser WA, O'Brien PC, Whisnant JP. Population-based study of seizure disorders after cerebral infarction. Neurology. 1996;46(2):350–5.
402. Koubeissi M, Alshekhlee A. In-hospital mortality of generalized convulsive status epilepticus: a large US sample. Neurology. 2007;69(9):886–93.
403. Sinha S, Satishchandra P, Mahadevan A, Bhimani BC, Kovur JM, Shankar SK. Fatal status epilepticus: a clinico-pathological analysis among 100 patients: from a developing country perspective. Epilepsy Res. 2010;91(2–3):193–204.
404. Jeon SB, Parikh G, Choi HA, Lee K, Lee JH, Schmidt JM, Badjatia N, Mayer SA, Claassen J. Acute cerebral microbleeds in refractory status epilepticus. Epilepsia. 2013;54(5):e66–8.
405. Liberalesso PB, Garzon E, Yacubian EM, Sakamoto AC. Higher mortality rate is associated with advanced age and periodic lateralized epileptiform discharges in patients with refractory status epilepticus. Arq Neuropsiquiatr. 2013;71(3):153–8.
406. Albers JM, Moddel G, Dittrich R, Steidl C, Suntrup S, Ringelstein EB, Dziewas R. Intravenous lacosamide—an effective add-on treatment of refractory status epilepticus. Seizure. 2011;20(5):428–30.
407. Kang X, Jiang H, Wu C, Liu X, Qiang J, Liu F, Guo Y, Xiao D, Liu J, Yu J, et al. Application of continuous video-electroencephalographic monitoring in patients with consciousness disorders in intensive care unit. Zhonghua Yi Xue Za Zhi. 2015;95(21):1663–6.

408. Kennel C, Michas-Martin A, Berman BD, Poisson S. Non convulsive status epilepticus masquerading as stroke. Am J Emerg Med. 2015;33(3):482.e1–2.
409. Synowiec AS, Yandora KA, Yenugadhati V, Valeriano JP, Schramke CJ, Kelly KM. The efficacy of topiramate in adult refractory status epilepticus: experience of a tertiary care center. Epilepsy Res. 2012;98(2–3):232–7.
410. Drislane FW, Blum AS, Lopez MR, Gautam S, Schomer DL. Duration of refractory status epilepticus and outcome: loss of prognostic utility after several hours. Epilepsia. 2009;50(6):1566–71.
411. Privitera M, Hoffman M, Moore JL, Jester D. EEG detection of nontonic-clonic status epilepticus in patients with altered consciousness. Epilepsy Res. 1994;18(2):155–66.
412. Tasker RC, Goodkin HP, Sanchez Fernandez I, Chapman KE, Abend NS, Arya R, Brenton JN, Carpenter JL, Gaillard WD, Glauser TA, et al. Refractory status epilepticus in children: intention to treat with continuous infusions of midazolam and pentobarbital. Pediatr Crit Care Med. 2016;17(10):968–75.
413. Fernandez-Torre JL, Burgueno P, Ballesteros MA, Hernandez-Hernandez MA, Villagra-Teran N, de Lucas EM. Super-refractory nonconvulsive status epilepticus secondary to fat embolism: a clinical, electrophysiological, and pathological study. Epilepsy Behav. 2015;49:184–8.
414. Legros B, Depondt C, Levy-Nogueira M, Ligot N, Mavroudakis N, Naeije G, Gaspard N. Intravenous lacosamide in refractory seizure clusters and status epilepticus: comparison of 200 and 400 mg loading doses. Neurocrit Care. 2014;20(3):484–8.
415. Belcastro V, Vidale S, Pierguidi L, Sironi L, Tancredi L, Striano P, Taborelli A, Arnaboldi M. Intravenous lacosamide as treatment option in post-stroke non convulsive status epilepticus in the elderly: a proof-of-concept, observational study. Seizure. 2013;22(10):905–7.
416. Alexopoulos A, Lachhwani DK, Gupta A, Kotagal P, Harrison AM, Bingaman W, Wyllie E. Resective surgery to treat refractory status epilepticus in children with focal epileptogenesis. Neurology. 2005;64(3):567–70.
417. Atkinson M, Atkinson B, Norris G, Shah A. Refractory status epilepticus secondary to CNS vasculitis, a role for epilepsy surgery. J Neurol Sci. 2012;315(1–2):156–9.
418. Miras Veiga A, Moreno DC, Menendez AI, Siscart IM, Fernandez MD, Sanchez EG, Gonzalez MG, Saez FG. Effectiveness of electroconvulsive therapy for refractory status epilepticus in febrile infection-related epilepsy syndrome. Neuropediatrics. 2016.
419. Chiusolo F, Diamanti A, Bianchi R, Fusco L, Elia M, Capriati T, Vigevano F, Picardo S. From intravenous to enteral ketogenic diet in PICU: a potential treatment strategy for refractory status epilepticus. Eur J Paediatr Neurol. 2016;20(6):843–7.
420. Farias-Moeller R, Bartolini L, Pasupuleti A, Brittany Cines RD, Kao A, Carpenter JL. A practical approach to ketogenic diet in the pediatric intensive care unit for super-refractory status epilepticus. Neurocrit Care. 2017;26(2):267–72.
421. Rossetti AO, Alvarez V, Januel JM, Burnand B. Treatment deviating from guidelines does not influence status epilepticus prognosis. J Neurol. 2013;260(2):421–8.
422. Khoujah D, Abraham MK. Status epilepticus: what's new? Emerg Med Clin North Am. 2016;34(4):759–76.
423. Capizzi G, Vittorini R, Torta F, Davico C, Raino E, Conio A, Longobardo A, Briatore E, Podesta B, Calzolari S. Lidocaine treatment in refractory status epilepticus resulting from febrile infection-related epilepsy syndrome: a case report and follow-up. Neuropediatrics. 2015;46(1):65–8.
424. Tunkel AR, Glaser CA, Bloch KC, Sejvar JJ, Marra CM, Roos KL, et al. The management of encephalitis: clinical practice guidelines by the Infectious Diseases Society of America. Clin Infect Dis. 2008;47(3):303–27. doi:10.1086/589747.
425. Venkatesan A, Tunkel AR, Bloch KC, Lauring AS, Sejvar J, Bitnun A, et al. Case definitions, diagnostic algorithms, and priorities in encephalitis: consensus statement of the international encephalitis consortium. Clin Infect Dis. 2013;57(8):1114–28. doi:10.1093/cid/cit458.
426. Janz D, Kautz G. Etiology and therapy of status epilepticus. Dtsch Med Wochenschr. 1963;88:2189–94. doi:10.1055/s-0028-1112345.
427. Resnick J. Pre-eruptive varicella encephalitis presenting as status epilepticus. Minn Med. 1970;53(1):65–7.
428. Hayakawa T, Sato J, Hara H, Murakami F, Goto T, Fukuyama Y. Therapy and prognosis of status convulsivus in childhood. Folia Psychiatr Neurol Jpn. 1979;33(3):445–56.
429. Uldry PA, Bernasconi A, Despland PA. Fatal status epilepticus in the course of HIV encephalitis. Presse Med. 1991;20(43):2216–8.
430. Vooturi S, Jayalakshmi S, Sahu S, Mohandas S. Prognosis and predictors of outcome of refractory generalized convulsive status epilepticus in adults treated in neurointensive care unit. Clin Neurol Neurosurg. 2014;126:7–10. doi:10.1016/j.clineuro.2014.07.038.
431. Misra UK, Kalita J, Nair PP. Status epilepticus in central nervous system infections: an experience from a developing country. Am J Med. 2008;121(7):618–23. doi:10.1016/j.amjmed.2008.02.012.
432. Kalita J, Nair PP, Misra UK. Status epilepticus in encephalitis: a study of clinical findings, magnetic resonance imaging, and response to antiepileptic drugs. J Neurovirol. 2008;14(5):412–7. doi:10.1080/13550280802266523.
433. Sonneville R, Mariotte E, Neuville M, Minaud S, Magalhaes E, Ruckly S, et al. Early-onset sta-

tus epilepticus in patients with acute encephalitis. Medicine. 2016;95(30):e4092. doi:10.1097/MD.0000000000004092.
434. Glaser CA, Gilliam S, Honarmand S, Tureen JH, Lowenstein DH, Anderson LJ, et al. Refractory status epilepticus in suspect encephalitis. Neurocrit Care. 2008;9(1):74–82. doi:10.1007/s12028-007-9042-y. Epub 2007/12/22.
435. Lin JJ, Lin KL, Wang HS, Hsia SH, Wu CT. Analysis of status epilepticus related presumed encephalitis in children. Eur J Paediatr Neurol. 2008;12(1):32–7. doi:10.1016/j.ejpn.2007.05.007. Epub 2007/06/23.
436. Lin JJ, Lin KL, Hsia SH, Wu CT, Chou IJ, Wang HS. Analysis of status epilepticus with Mycoplasma pneumoniae encephalitis. Pediatr Neurol. 2010;43(1):41–5. doi:10.1016/j.pediatrneurol.2010.02.017.
437. Vehapoglu A, Turel O, Uygur Sahin T, Kutlu NO, Iscan A. Clinical significance of human metapneumovirus in refractory status epilepticus and encephalitis: case report and review of the literature. Case Rep Neurol Med. 2015;2015:131780. doi: 10.1155/2015/131780. Epub 2015/12/15.
438. Greco F, Cocuzza MD, Smilari P, Sorge G, Pavone L. Nonconvulsive status epilepticus complicating epstein-barr virus encephalitis in a child. Case Rep Pediatrics. 2014;2014:547396. doi:10.1155/2014/547396.
439. Bick SK, Izzy S, Rubin DB, Zafar SF, Rosenthal ES, Eskandar EN. Anterior temporal lobectomy for refractory status epilepticus in herpes simplex encephalitis. Neurocrit Care. 2016. doi: 10.1007/s12028-016-0302-6. Epub 2016/07/31.
440. Kramer AH, Jette N, Pillay N, Federico P, Zygun DA. Epileptiform activity in neurocritical care patients. Can J Neurol Sci. 2012;39(3):328–37.
441. Carrera E, Claassen J, Oddo M, Emerson RG, Mayer SA, Hirsch LJ. Continuous electroencephalographic monitoring in critically ill patients with central nervous system infections. Arch Neurol. 2008;65(12):1612–8. doi:10.1001/archneur.65.12.1612.
442. Rautonen J, Koskiniemi M, Vaheri A. Prognostic factors in childhood acute encephalitis. Pediatr Infect Dis J. 1991;10(6):441–6.
443. Panagariya A, Jain RS, Gupta S, Garg A, Sureka RK, Mathur V. Herpes simplex encephalitis in North West India. Neurol India. 2001;49(4):360–5.
444. Misra UK, Kalita J. Seizures in encephalitis: predictors and outcome. Seizure. 2009;18(8):583–7. doi:10.1016/j.seizure.2009.06.003.
445. Armangue T, Moris G, Cantarin-Extremera V, Conde CE, Rostasy K, Erro ME, et al. Autoimmune postherpes simplex encephalitis of adults and teenagers. Neurology. 2015;85(20):1736–43. doi:10.1212/WNL.0000000000002125.
446. Gunduz A, Beskardes AF, Kutlu A, Ozkara C, Karaagac N, Yeni SN. Herpes encephalitis as a cause of nonconvulsive status epilepticus. Epileptic Disord. 2006;8(1):57–60.
447. Lee JH, Nam DH, Oh SY, Shin BS, Seo MW, Jeong SK, et al. Nonconvulsive status epilepticus presenting as epileptic nystagmus in a patient with herpes encephalitis. J Neuroophthalmol. 2012;32(3):249–51. doi:10.1097/WNO.0b013e3182413679.
448. Sutter R, Kaplan PW, Cervenka MC, Thakur KT, Asemota AO, Venkatesan A, et al. Electroencephalography for diagnosis and prognosis of acute encephalitis. Clin Neurophysiol. 2015;126(8):1524–31. doi:10.1016/j.clinph.2014.11.006.
449. Ch'ien LT, Boehm RM, Robinson H, Liu C, Frenkel LD. Characteristic early electroencephalographic changes in herpes simplex encephalitis. Arch Neurol. 1977;34(6):361–4.
450. Bradshaw MJ, Venkatesan A. Herpes simplex virus-1 encephalitis in adults: pathophysiology, diagnosis, and management. Neurotherapeutics. 2016;13(3):493–508. doi:10.1007/s13311-016-0433-7.
451. Misra UK, Kalita J. Seizures in Japanese encephalitis. J Neurol Sci. 2001;190(1–2):57–60.
452. van den Hoogen BG, de Jong JC, Groen J, Kuiken T, de Groot R, Fouchier RA, et al. A newly discovered human pneumovirus isolated from young children with respiratory tract disease. Nat Med. 2001;7(6):719–24. doi:10.1038/89098.
453. Arnold JC, Singh KK, Milder E, Spector SA, Sawyer MH, Gavali S, et al. Human metapneumovirus associated with central nervous system infection in children. Pediatr Infect Dis J. 2009;28(12):1057–60. doi:10.1097/INF.0b013e3181acd221.
454. Sanchez Fernandez I, Rebollo Polo M, Munoz-Almagro C, Monfort Carretero L, Fernandez Urena S, Rueda Munoz A, et al. Human metapneumovirus in the cerebrospinal fluid of a patient with acute encephalitis. Arch Neurol. 2012;69(5):649–52. doi:10.1001/archneurol.2011.1094.
455. Webster DL, Gardner AH, Dye TJ, Chima RS. Status epilepticus: a possible association with human metapneumovirus infection. Pediatrics. 2014;133(3):e747–50. doi:10.1542/peds.2013-0929.
456. Niizuma T, Okumura A, Kinoshita K, Shimizu T. Acute encephalopathy associated with human metapneumovirus infection. Jpn J Infect Dis. 2014;67(3):213–5.
457. Schildgen O, Glatzel T, Geikowski T, Scheibner B, Matz B, Bindl L, et al. Human metapneumovirus RNA in encephalitis patient. Emerg Infect Dis. 2005;11(3):467–70.
458. Kaida A, Iritani N, Kubo H, Shiomi M, Kohdera U, Murakami T. Seasonal distribution and phylogenetic analysis of human metapneumovirus among children in Osaka City, Japan. J Clin Virol. 2006;35(4):394–9. doi:10.1016/j.jcv.2005.12.009.
459. Hata M, Ito M, Kiyosawa S, Kimpara Y, Tanaka S, Yamashita T, et al. A fatal case of encephalopathy possibly associated with human metapneumovirus infection. Jpn J Infect Dis. 2007;60(5): 328–9.

460. Klein C, Kimiagar I, Pollak L, Gandelman-Marton R, Itzhaki A, Milo R, et al. Neurological features of West Nile virus infection during the 2000 outbreak in a regional hospital in Israel. J Neurol Sci. 2002;200(1–2):63–6.
461. Nash D, Mostashari F, Fine A, Miller J, O'Leary D, Murray K, et al. The outbreak of West Nile virus infection in the New York City area in 1999. N Engl J Med. 2001;344(24):1807–14. doi:10.1056/NEJM200106143442401.
462. Chowers MY, Lang R, Nassar F, Ben-David D, Giladi M, Rubinshtein E, et al. Clinical characteristics of the West Nile fever outbreak, Israel, 2000. Emerg Infect Dis. 2001;7(4):675–8. doi:10.3201/eid0704.010414.
463. Gandelman-Marton R, Kimiagar I, Itzhaki A, Klein C, Theitler J, Rabey JM. Electroencephalography findings in adult patients with West Nile virus-associated meningitis and meningoencephalitis. Clin Infect Dis. 2003;37(11):1573–8. doi:10.1086/379516.
464. Feki I, Marrakchi C, Ben Hmida M, Belahsen F, Ben Jemaa M, Maaloul I, et al. Epidemic West Nile virus encephalitis in Tunisia. Neuroepidemiology. 2005;24(1–2):1–7. doi:10.1159/000081042.
465. Bagic A, Boudreau EA, Greenfield J, Sato S. Electroclinical evolution of refractory non-convulsive status epilepticus caused by West Nile virus encephalitis. Epileptic Disord. 2007;9(1):98–103. doi:10.1684/epd.2007.0056. Epub 2007/02/20.
466. Barah F, Vallely PJ, Chiswick ML, Cleator GM, Kerr JR. Association of human parvovirus B19 infection with acute meningoencephalitis. Lancet. 2001;358(9283):729–30. doi:10.1016/S0140-6736(01)05905-0.
467. Palermo CI, Costanzo CM, Franchina C, Castiglione G, Giuliano L, Russo R, et al. Focal epilepsy as a long term sequela of parvovirus B19 encephalitis. J Clin Virol. 2016;80:20–3. doi:10.1016/j.jcv.2016.04.007.
468. Skaff PT, Labiner DM. Status epilepticus due to human parvovirus B19 encephalitis in an immunocompetent adult. Neurology. 2001;57(7):1336–7.
469. Erol I, Alehan F, Yalcin K. Refractory status epilepticus owing to human parvovirus B19 encephalitis in a child. J Child Neurol. 2006;21(9):820–2. Epub 2006/09/15.
470. Mazur-Melewska K, Brenska I, Jonczyk-Potoczna K, Kemnitz P, Pieczonka-Ruszkowska I, Mania A, et al. Neurologic complications caused by Epstein-Barr virus in pediatric patients. J Child Neurol. 2016;31(6):700–8.doi:10.1177/0883073815613563.
471. Majid A, Galetta SL, Sweeney CJ, Robinson C, Mahalingam R, Smith J, et al. Epstein-Barr virus myeloradiculitis and encephalomyeloradiculitis. Brain. 2002;125(Pt 1):159–65.
472. Johkura K, Momoo T, Kuroiwa Y. Thalamic involvement of Epstein-Barr virus encephalitis demonstrated by MRI. J Neurol. 2003;250(3):357–8.
473. Delgado S, Duran MI. Encephalitis in a renal transplantation patient. Nefrologia. 2004;24(Suppl 3):21–5.
474. Nishie M, Ogawa M, Kurahashi K. Epstein-Barr virus-associated encephalitis presenting as refractory status epilepticus that persisted for nearly 2 months with excellent recovery. Rinsho Shinkeigaku. 2003;43(7):422–6. Epub 2003/10/30.
475. Armengol CE, Hendley JO. Cat-scratch disease encephalopathy: a cause of status epilepticus in school-aged children. J Pediatr. 1999;134(5):635–8.
476. Lewis DW, Tucker SH. Central nervous system involvement in cat scratch disease. Pediatrics. 1986;77(5):714–21.
477. Singhal AB, Newstein MC, Budzik R, Cha JH, Rordorf G, Buonanno FS, et al. Diffusion-weighted magnetic resonance imaging abnormalities in Bartonella encephalopathy. J Neuroimaging. 2003;13(1):79–82. Epub 2003/02/21.
478. Laswell EM, Chambers KD, Whitsel DR, Poudel K. New-onset refractory status epilepticus in an adult with an atypical presentation of cat-scratch disease: successful treatment with high-dose corticosteroids. Pharmacotherapy. 2015;35(6):e106–10. doi:10.1002/phar.1595.
479. Hildebrand J, Lecaille C, Perennes J, Delattre JY. Epileptic seizures during follow-up of patients treated for primary brain tumors. Neurology. 2005;65(2):212–5.
480. Michelucci R, Pasini E, Meletti S, Fallica E, Rizzi R, Florindo I, Chiari A, Monetti C, Cremonini AM, Forlivesi S, et al. Epilepsy in primary cerebral tumors: the characteristics of epilepsy at the onset (results from the PERNO study—project of Emilia Romagna region on neuro-oncology). Epilepsia. 2013;54(Suppl 7):86–91.
481. Cowie CJ, Cunningham MO. Peritumoral epilepsy: relating form and function for surgical success. Epilepsy Behav. 2014;38:53–61.
482. Nowell M, Miserocchi A, McEvoy AW. Tumors in epilepsy. Semin Neurol. 2015;35(3):209–17.
483. Lhatoo SD, Moghimi N, Schuele S. Tumor-related epilepsy and epilepsy surgery. Epilepsia. 2013;54(Suppl 9):1–4.
484. Japp A, Gielen GH, Becker AJ. Recent aspects of classification and epidemiology of epilepsy-associated tumors. Epilepsia. 2013;54(Suppl 9):5–11.
485. Lynam LM, Lyons MK, Drazkowski JF, Sirven JI, Noe KH, Zimmerman RS, Wilkens JA. Frequency of seizures in patients with newly diagnosed brain tumors: a retrospective review. Clin Neurol Neurosurg. 2007;109(7):634–8.
486. Ullrich NJ, Pomeroy SL, Kapur K, Manley PE, Goumnerova LC, Loddenkemper T. Incidence, risk factors, and longitudinal outcome of seizures in long-term survivors of pediatric brain tumors. Epilepsia. 2015;56(10):1599–604.
487. van Breemen MSM, Wilms EB, Vecht CJ. Epilepsy in patients with brain tumors: epidemiology, mechanisms, and management. Lancet Neurol. 2007;6:421–30.

488. Maschio M. Brain tumor-related epilepsy. Curr Neuropharmacol. 2012;10:124–33.
489. Chang EF, Potts MB, Keles GE, Lamborn KR, Chang SM, Barbaro NM, Berger MS. Seizure characteristics and control following resection in 332 patients with low-grade gliomas. J Neurosurg. 2008;108:227–35.
490. Wojcik-Draczkowska H, Mazurkiewicz-Beldzinska M, Mankowska B, Dilling-Ostrowska E. Epileptic seizures as a manifestation of brain tumors: clinical and electroencephalographic correlations. Przegl Lek. 2003;60(Suppl 1):42–4.
491. Gottschalk J, Korves M, Skotzek-Konrad B, Goebel S, Cervos-Navarro J. Dysembryoplastic neuroepithelial micro-tumor in a 75-year-old patient with long-standing epilepsy. Clin Neuropathol. 1993;12(3):175–8.
492. Rheims S, Ducray F, Ryvlin P. Choosing the tumoral epilepsy surgery candidate. Epilepsia. 2013;54(Suppl 9):91–6.
493. van Breemen MS, Rijsman RM, Taphoorn MJ, Walchenbach R, Zwinkels H, Vecht CJ. Efficacy of anti-epileptic drugs in patients with gliomas and seizures. J Neurol. 2009;256(9):1519–26.
494. Weller M, Stupp R, Wick W. Epilepsy meets cancer: when, why, and what to do about it? Lancet Oncol. 2012;13(9):e375–82.
495. Weller M, Gorlia T, Cairncross JG, van den Bent MJ, Mason W, Belanger K, Brandes AA, Bogdahn U, Macdonald DR, Forsyth P, et al. Prolonged survival with valproic acid use in the EORTC/NCIC temozolomide trial for glioblastoma. Neurology. 2011;77(12):1156–64.
496. Singh G, Driever PH, Sander JW. Cancer risk in people with epilepsy: the role of antiepileptic drugs. Brain. 2005;128(Pt 1):7–17.
497. Glantz MJ, Cole BF, Forsyth PA, Recht LD, Wen PY, Chamberlain MC, Grossman SA, Cairncross JG. Practice parameter: anticonvulsant prophylaxis in patients with newly diagnosed brain tumors. Report of the quality standards Subcommittee of the American Academy of neurology. Neurology. 2000;54(10):1886–93.
498. Kong X, Guan J, Yang Y, Li Y, Ma W, Wang R. A meta-analysis: do prophylactic antiepileptic drugs in patients with brain tumors decrease the incidence of seizures? Clin Neurol Neurosurg. 2015;134:98–103.
499. Guerrini R, Rosati A, Giordano F, Genitori L, Barba C. The medical and surgical treatment of tumoral seizures: current and future perspectives. Epilepsia. 2013;54(Suppl 9):84–90.
500. Englot DJ, Berger MS, Barbaro NM, Chang EF. Predictors of seizure freedom after resection of supratentorial low-grade gliomas. A review. J Neurosurg. 2011;115(2):240–4.
501. Kim SK, Wang KC, Hwang YS, Kim KJ, Chae JH, Kim IO, Cho BK. Epilepsy surgery in children: outcomes and complications. J Neurosurg Pediatr. 2008;1(4):277–83.
502. Sherman JH, Moldovan K, Yeoh HK, Starke RM, Pouratian N, Shaffrey ME, Schiff D. Impact of temozolomide chemotherapy on seizure frequency in patients with low-grade gliomas. J Neurosurg. 2011;114(6):1617–21.
503. Ruda R, Magliola U, Bertero L, Trevisan E, Bosa C, Mantovani C, Ricardi U, Castiglione A, Monagheddu C, Soffietti R. Seizure control following radiotherapy in patients with diffuse gliomas: a retrospective study. Neuro-Oncology. 2013;15(12):1739–49.
504. Zaatreh MM, Spencer DD, Thompson JL, Blumenfeld H, Novotny EJ, Mattson RH, Spencer SS. Frontal lobe tumoral epilepsy: clinical, neurophysiologic features and predictors of surgical outcome. Epilepsia. 2002;43(7):727–33.
505. Tiamkao S, Suko P, Mayurasakorn N. Outcome of status epilepticus in Srinagarind hospital. J Med Assoc Thail. 2010;93(4):420–3.
506. Aladdin Y, Gross DW. Refractory status epilepticus during pregnancy secondary to cavernous angioma. Epilepsia. 2008;49(9):1627–9.
507. Kasai M, Aoki S, Kobayashi N, Hirahara F, Takahashi T. Status epilepticus due to brain tumor during pregnancy. Clin Case Rep. 2016;4(4):333–5.
508. Janz D. Status epilepticus and frontal lobe lesions. J Neurol Sci. 1964;1:446–57.
509. Goonawardena J, Marshman LA, Drummond KJ. Brain tumour-associated status epilepticus. J Clin Neurosci. 2015;22(1):29–34.
510. Moots PL, Maciunas RJ, Eisert DR, Parker RA, Laporte K, Abou-Khalil B. The course of seizure disorders in patients with malignant gliomas. Arch Neurol. 1995;52(7):717–24.
511. Swisher CB, Doreswamy M, Gingrich KJ, Vredenburgh JJ, Kolls BJ. Phenytoin, levetiracetam, and pregabalin in the acute management of refractory status epilepticus in patients with brain tumors. Neurocrit Care. 2012;16(1):109–13.
512. Chen JW, Wasterlain CG. Status epilepticus: pathophysiology and management in adults. Lancet Neurol. 2006;5(3):246–56.
513. Ng YT, Bristol RE, Schrader DV, Smith KA. The role of neurosurgery in status epilepticus. Neurocrit Care. 2007;7(1):86–91.
514. Yun C, Xuefeng W. Association between seizures and diabetes mellitus: a comprehensive review of literature. Curr Diabetes Rev. 2013;9(4):350–4.
515. Moloney TC, Idris I, Waters P, Howell S, Vincent A, Lang B, Maddison P. Autoantibodies to glutamic acid decarboxylase in patients with epilepsy and their relationship with type 1 diabetes: a pilot study. J Neurol Neurosurg Psychiatry. 2016;87(6):676–7.
516. Stagg CJ, Lang B, Best JG, McKnight K, Cavey A, Johansen-Berg H, Vincent A, Palace J. Autoantibodies to glutamic acid decarboxylase in patients with epilepsy are associated with low cortical GABA levels. Epilepsia. 2010;51(9):1898–901.

517. Vulliemoz S, Seeck M. An association between type 1 diabetes and idiopathic generalized epilepsy. Ann Neurol. 2006;59(4):728.
518. Kashihara K, Shohmori T, Otsuki S. Noninsulin-dependent diabetes mellitus-related encephalopathy presenting with amnesia, personality change, and autonomic seizure. Intern Med. 1997;36(9):633–6.
519. Yew TW, McCreight L, Colclough K, Ellard S, Pearson ER. tRNA methyltransferase homologue gene TRMT10A mutation in young adult-onset diabetes with intellectual disability, microcephaly and epilepsy. Diabet Med. 2016;33(9):e21–5.
520. Zwaveling-Soonawala N, Hagebeuk EE, Slingerland AS, Ris-Stalpers C, Vulsma T, van Trotsenburg AS. Successful transfer to sulfonylurea therapy in an infant with developmental delay, epilepsy and neonatal diabetes (DEND) syndrome and a novel ABCC8 gene mutation. Diabetologia. 2011;54(2):469–71.
521. Sanyoura M, Woudstra C, Halaby G, Baz P, Senee V, Guillausseau PJ, Zalloua P, Julier C. A novel ALMS1 splice mutation in a non-obese juvenile-onset insulin-dependent syndromic diabetic patient. Eur J Hum Genet. 2014;22(1):140–3.
522. Poulton CJ, Schot R, Kia SK, Jones M, Verheijen FW, Venselaar H, de Wit MC, de Graaff E, Bertoli-Avella AM, Mancini GM. Microcephaly with simplified gyration, epilepsy, and infantile diabetes linked to inappropriate apoptosis of neural progenitors. Am J Hum Genet. 2011;89(2):265–76.
523. Huang CW, Tsai JJ, Ou HY, Wang ST, Cheng JT, Wu SN, Huang CC. Diabetic hyperglycemia is associated with the severity of epileptic seizures in adults. Epilepsy Res. 2008;79(1):71–7.
524. Tsalikian E, Becker DJ, Crumrine PK, Daneman D, Drash AL. Electroencephalographic changes in diabetic ketosis in children with newly and previously diagnosed insulin-dependent diabetes mellitus. J Pediatr. 1981;99(3):355–9.
525. Burns CM, Rutherford MA, Boardman JP, Cowan FM. Patterns of cerebral injury and neurodevelopmental outcomes after symptomatic neonatal hypoglycemia. Pediatrics. 2008;122(1):65–74.
526. Cochin JP, Hannequin D, Delangre T, Guegan-Massardier E, Augustin P. Continuous partial epilepsy disclosing diabetes mellitus. Rev Neurol. 1994;150(3):239–41.
527. Schomer DL. Focal status epilepticus and epilepsia partialis continua in adults and children. Epilepsia. 1993;34(Suppl 1):S29–36.
528. Makimattila S, Malmberg-Ceder K, Hakkinen AM, Vuori K, Salonen O, Summanen P, Yki-Jarvinen H, Kaste M, Heikkinen S, Lundbom N, et al. Brain metabolic alterations in patients with type 1 diabetes-hyperglycemia-induced injury. J Cereb Blood Flow Metab. 2004;24(12):1393–9.
529. Tedrus GM, Albertin MC, Odashima NS, Fonseca LC. Partial motor seizures induced by movement in diabetic patients. Arq Neuropsiquiatr. 1991;49(4):442–6.
530. Caietta E, Halbert C, Lepine A, Khammar A, Cano A, Gavaret M, Mancini J, Villeneuve N, Chabrol B, Simonin G, et al. Association of type 1 diabetes mellitus and epilepsy in children. A cohort of 10 cases. Arch Pediatr. 2012;19(1):9–16.
531. Fisher BM, Frier BM. Nocturnal convulsions and insulin-induced hypoglycaemia in diabetic patients. Postgrad Med J. 1987;63(742):673–6.
532. Hennis A, Corbin D, Fraser H. Focal seizures and non-ketotic hyperglycaemia. J Neurol Neurosurg Psychiatry. 1992;55(3):195–7.
533. El-Hattab AW, Adesina AM, Jones J, Scaglia F. MELAS syndrome: clinical manifestations, pathogenesis, and treatment options. Mol Genet Metab. 2015.
534. Kim TH, Petrou S, Reid CA. Low glycaemic index diet reduces seizure susceptibility in a syndrome-specific mouse model of generalized epilepsy. Epilepsy Res. 2014;108(1):139–43.
535. Aylward NM, Shah N, Sellers EA. The ketogenic diet for the treatment of myoclonic astatic epilepsy in a child with type 1 diabetes mellitus. Can J Diabetes. 2014;38(4):223–4.
536. Roze E, Oubary P, Chedru F. Status-like recurrent pilomotor seizures: case report and review of the literature. J Neurol Neurosurg Psychiatry. 2000;68(5):647–9.
537. Batista MS, Silva DF, Ferraz HB, de Andrade LA. Complex partial seizures and aphasia as initial manifestations of non-ketotic hyperglycemia. Case report. Arq Neuropsiquiatr. 1998;56(2):296–9.
538. Eliasson B, Gudbjornsdottir S, Cederholm J, Liang Y, Vercruysse F, Smith U. Weight loss and metabolic effects of topiramate in overweight and obese type 2 diabetic patients: randomized double-blind placebo-controlled trial. Int J Obes. 2007;31(7):1140–7.
539. Baglietto MG, Mancardi MM, Giannattasio A, Minuto N, Rossi A, Capovilla G, Veneselli E, Lorini R, d'Annunzio G. Epilepsia partialis continua in type 1 diabetes: evolution into epileptic encephalopathy with continuous spike-waves during slow sleep. Neurol Sci. 2009;30(6):509–12.
540. Paiboonpol S. Epilepsia partialis continua as a manifestation of hyperglycemia. J Med Assoc Thail. 2005;88(6):759–62.
541. Mukherjee V, Mukherjee A, Mukherjee A, Halder A. Type I diabetes mellitus in a child presenting with epilepsy partialis continua. J Indian Med Assoc. 2007;105(6):340. 342
542. Mikdashi J, Krumholz A, Handwerger B. Factors at diagnosis predict subsequent occurrence of seizures in systemic lupus erythematosus. Neurology. 2005;64(12):2102–7.
543. Ramsey-Goldman R, Alarcon GS, McGwin G, Petri M, Vila LM, Edberg JC, et al. Time to seizure occurrence and damage in PROFILE, a multiethnic systemic lupus erythematosus cohort. Lupus. 2008;17(3):177–84.

544. Tsai JD, Lin CL, Lin CC, Sung FC, Lue KH. Risk of epilepsy in patients with systemic lupus erythematosus—a retrospective cohort study. Neuropsychiatr Dis Treat. 2014;10:1635–43.
545. Brey RL, Holliday SL, Saklad AR, Navarrete MG, Hermosillo-Romo D, Stallworth CL, Valdez CR, Escalante A, del Rincon I, Gronseth G, et al. Neuropsychiatric syndromes in lupus: prevalence using standardized definitions. Neurology. 2002;58(8):1214–20.
546. Nasri A, Bedoui I, Mrissa R, Riahi A, Derbali H, Zaouali J, Messelmani M. Mansour M:recurrent status epilepticus in posterior reversible encephalopathy syndrome as initial feature of pediatric lupus: a newly diagnosed case and literature review. Brain Dev. 2016;38:835–41.
547. Gonzalez-Duarte A, Cantu-Brito CG, Ruano-Calderon L, Garcia-Ramos G. Clinical description of seizures in patients with systemic lupus erythematosus. Eur Neurol. 2008;59(6):320–3.
548. Mackworth-Young CG, Hughes GR. Epilepsy: an early symptom of systemic lupus erythematosus. J Neurol Neurosurg Psychiatry. 1985;48(2):185.
549. Degirmencioglu H, Sari FN, Alyamac Dizdar E, Say B, Altug N, Uras N, Canpolat FE, Oguz SS. Coexistence of fetal cardiac malformation and maternal drug-induced lupus: is lamotrigine safe? Am J Ther. 2016;23(5):e1263–65.
550. Leroux G, et al. Posterior reversible encephalopathy syndrome during systemic lupus erythematosus: four new cases and review of the literature. Lupus. 2008:139–47.
551. Lin SC, Shyur SD, Li Hsin H, Wu JY, Ma YC. Focal seizures as an unusual presentation of neonatal lupus erythematosus. Asian Pac J Allergy Immunol. 2005;23(1):61–4.
552. Vincent A, Crino PB. Systemic and neurologic autoimmune disorders associated with seizures or epilepsy. Epilepsia. 2011;52(Suppl 3):12–7.
553. Ainiala H, Dastidar P, Loukkola J, Lehtimaki T, Korpela M, Peltola J, Hietaharju A. Cerebral MRI abnormalities and their association with neuropsychiatric manifestations in SLE: a population-based study. Scand J Rheumatol. 2005;34(5):376–82.
554. Jeong HW, Her M, Bae JS, Kim SK, Lee SW, Kim HK, Kim D, Park N, Chung WT, Lee SY, et al. Brain MRI in neuropsychiatric lupus: associations with the 1999 ACR case definitions. Rheumatol Int. 2015;35(5):861–9.
555. Hawro T, Bogucki A, Krupinska-Kun M, Maurer M, Wozniacka A. Intractable headaches, ischemic stroke, and seizures are linked to the presence of anti-beta2GPI antibodies in patients with systemic lupus erythematosus. PLoS One. 2015;10(3):e0119911.
556. Barile-Fabris L, Ariza-Andraca R, Olguin-Ortega L, Jara LJ, Fraga-Mouret A, Miranda-Limon JM, Fuentes de la Mata J, Clark P, Vargas F, Alocer-Varela J. Controlled clinical trial of IV cyclophosphamide versus IV methylprednisolone in severe neurological manifestations in systemic lupus erythematosus. Ann Rheum Dis. 2005;64(4):620–5.
557. Popescu A, Kao AH. Neuropsychiatric systemic lupus erythematosus. Curr Neuropharmacol. 2011;9(3):449–57.
558. Bertsias GK, Ioannidis JP, Aringer M, Bollen E, Bombardieri S, Bruce IN, Cervera R, Dalakas M, Doria A, Hanly JG, et al. EULAR recommendations for the management of systemic lupus erythematosus with neuropsychiatric manifestations: report of a task force of the EULAR standing committee for clinical affairs. Ann Rheum Dis. 2010;69(12):2074–82.
559. Chang RS, Cole AJ. Lamotrigine-induced lupus-like syndrome: a case report and literature review. Am J Ther. 2014;21(3):e85–7.
560. Pelizza L, De Luca P, La Pesa M, Minervino A. Drug-induced systemic lupus erythematosus after 7 years of treatment with carbamazepine. Acta Biomed. 2006;77(1):17–9.
561. Hanly JG, Urowitz MB, Su L, Gordon C, Bae SC, Sanchez-Guerrero J, Romero-Diaz J, Wallace DJ, Clarke AE, Ginzler E, et al. Seizure disorders in systemic lupus erythematosus results from an international, prospective, inception cohort study. Ann Rheum Dis. 2012;71(9):1502–9.
562. Cimaz R, Meroni PL, Shoenfeld Y. Epilepsy as part of systemic lupus erythematosus and systemic antiphospholipid syndrome (Hughes syndrome). Lupus. 2006;15(4):191–7.
563. Polychronopoulos P, Giannopoulos G, Litsardopoulos P, Soldatos P, Chroni E. Systemic lupus erythematosus manifested as drug-resistant mesial temporal lobe epilepsy. Neurol Sci. 2016.
564. Gieron MA, Khoromi S, Campos A. MRI changes in the central nervous system in a child with lupus erythematosus. Pediatr Radiol. 1995;25(3):184–5.
565. Prabhakar S, Bhatia R. Management of agitation and convulsions in hepatic encephalopathy. Indian J Gastroenterol. 2003;22(Suppl 2):S54–8.
566. Ardizzone G, Arrigo A, Schellino MM, Stratta C, Valzan S, Skurzak S, Andruetto P, Panio A, Ballaris MA, Lavezzo B, et al. Neurological complications of liver cirrhosis and orthotopic liver transplant. Transplant Proc. 2006;38(3):789–92.
567. Tanaka H, Ueda H, Kida Y, Hamagami H, Tsuji T, Ichinose M. Hepatic encephalopathy with status epileptics: a case report. World J Gastroenterol. 2006;12(11):1793–4.
568. Kumar R, Shalimar, Sharma H, Prakash S, Panda SK, Khanal S, Acharya SK. Persistent hyperammonemia is associated with complications and poor outcomes in patients with acute liver failure. Clin Gastroenterol Hepatol. 2012;10(8):925–31.
569. Rama Rao KV, Jayakumar AR, Norenberg MD. Glutamine in the pathogenesis of acute hepatic encephalopathy. Neurochem Int. 2012;61(4):575–80.

570. Derle E, Kibaroglu S, Ocal R, Kirnap M, Kilinc M, Benli S, Haberal M. Seizure as a neurologic complication after liver transplant. Exp Clin Transplant. 2015;13(Suppl 1):323–6.
571. Ghosh PS, Hupertz V, Ghosh D. Neurological complications following pediatric liver transplant. J Pediatr Gastroenterol Nutr. 2012;54(4):540–6.
572. Thabah MM, Singh KK, Madhavan SM, Gupta R. Adult onset Still's disease as a cause of acute liver failure. Trop Gastroenterol. 2008;29(1):35–6.
573. Ferro JM, Viana P, Santos P. Management of neurologic manifestations in patients with liver disease. Curr Treat Options Neurol. 2016;18(8):37.
574. Lacerda G, Krummel T, Sabourdy C, Ryvlin P, Hirsch E. Optimizing therapy of seizures in patients with renal or hepatic dysfunction. Neurology. 2006;67(12 Suppl 4):S28–33.
575. Asconape JJ. Use of antiepileptic drugs in hepatic and renal disease. Handb Clin Neurol. 2014;119:417–32.
576. Bhatia V, Batra Y, Acharya SK. Prophylactic phenytoin does not improve cerebral edema or survival in acute liver failure—a controlled clinical trial. J Hepatol. 2004;41(1):89–96.
577. Eleftheriadis N, Fourla E, Eleftheriadis D, Karlovasitou A. Status epilepticus as a manifestation of hepatic encephalopathy. Acta Neurol Scand. 2003;107(2):142–4.
578. Jo YM, Lee SW, Han SY, Baek YH, Ahn JH, Choi WJ, Lee JY, Kim SH, Yoon BA. Nonconvulsive status epilepticus disguising as hepatic encephalopathy. World J Gastroenterol. 2015;21(16):5105–9.
579. Scorza FA, Albuquerque M, Arida RM, et al. Seizure occurrence in patients with chronic renal insufficiency in regular hemodialysis program. Arq Neuropsiquiatr. 2005;63:757–60.
580. Rufo Campos M, Vazquez Florido AM, Madruga Garrido M, Fijo J, Sanchez Moreno A, Martin Govantes J. Renal failure as a factor leading to epileptic seizures. An Esp Pediatr. 2002;56(3):212–8.
581. Cassinotto C, Mejdoubi M, Signate A, Herbland A, Olindo S, Deramond H. MRI findings in star-fruit intoxication. J Neuroradiol. 2008;35(4):217–23.
582. Soliman AR, Helmy S. Status epilepticus induced by putrid salted gray mullet fish intoxication in patients with chronic kidney disease. Hemodial Int. 2010;14(4):523–5.
583. Kao LW, Nanagas KA. Carbon monoxide poisoning. Emerg Med Clin North Am. 2004;22(4):985–1018.
584. Abdulaziz S, Dabbagh O, Arabi Y, Kojan S, Hassan I. Status epilepticus and cardiopulmonary arrest in a patient with carbon monoxide poisoning with full recovery after using a neuroprotective strategy: a case report. J Med Case Rep. 2012;6:421.
585. Wong M, Mallory GB Jr, Goldstein J, Goyal M, Yamada KA. Neurologic complications of pediatric lung transplantation. Neurology. 1999;53(7):1542–9.
586. Laaban JP, Marsal L, Waked M, Vuong TK, Rochemaure J. Seizures related to severe hypophosphataemia induced by mechanical ventilation. Intensive Care Med. 1990;16(2):135–6.
587. Zhang YX, Liu JR, Jiang B, Liu HQ, Ding MP, Song SJ, Zhang BR, Zhang H, Xu B, Chen HH, et al. Lance-Adams syndrome: a report of two cases. J Zhejiang Univ Sci B. 2007;8(10):715–20.

Applications of Electroencephalography in Status Epilepticus

5

Yida Hu and Shichuo Li

Abstract

Status epilepticus (SE) is a critical neurological condition that may appear alone or during the course of a variety of neurological disorders, such as encephalitis, cerebrovascular disease, or toxic metabolic or ischemic hypoxic encephalopathy. Although the onset of prominent motor symptoms is usually noticed by medical staff and family members, patients who lack prominent motor symptoms are often not treated in time because of their atypical symptomology. Such patients are usually diagnosed with nonconvulsive status epilepticus (NCSE), which is difficult to identify without an electroencephalogram (EEG). Moreover, an EEG provides guidance for determining the prognosis and treatment options in patients with SE. In this chapter, we briefly introduce the history of EEG, its technical parameters, the principles used in interpreting abnormal EEGs, the association between EEG results and prevalent types of SE, the role of EEG in the treatment and prognosis of various pathologies, and the additional uses of EEG.

5.1 Introduction: the Basic Characteristics of the Electroencephalogram

5.1.1 The Development and Evolution of the Electroencephalogram

The first human EEG was recorded in 1924 by Hans Berger, the German engineer and psychiatrist, in Jena. This important finding has contributed to the rapid development of clinical neuroscience and neuroelectrophysiology. The earliest EEG recordings relied on a machine-driven marker to

Y. Hu, Ph.D. (✉)
Chongqing Key Laboratory of Neurology, Department of Neurology, The First Affiliated Hospital of Chongqing Medical University, 1 YouYi Road, Chongqing 400016, China
e-mail: hyd1112@126.com

S. Li
China Association Against Epilepsy (CAAE), Rm. 5102, Building 2, Beijing Exhibition Center Hotel, 135 Xizhimenwai Avenue, Xicheng District, Beijing 100044, People's Republic of China

X. Wang, S. Li (eds.), *Refractory Status Epilepticus*, DOI 10.1007/978-981-10-5125-8_5

depict the electrical activity of the human brain on blank sheets of paper, but these were inconvenient to read and resulted in massive paper waste. With the rapid development of computer technology, the EEG evolved into analog signal EEG and digital signal EEG, the former simply simulating the traditional recording on the paper, while the latter was truly a milestone that marked a new era in technology. Due to improvements in recording modes, output modes, and analysis algorithms, such as compressed spectral array technology, digital EEG enables real-time, noninvasive economic monitoring, analysis, and evaluation of patients via storage of large amounts of data, adjustment of analysis parameters, playback, automatic analysis, and other functions. Currently, in addition to the common EEG instruments, the following types of EEG are available: video EEG for synchronous monitoring of EEG and the behavior of patients; continuous EEG (cEEG) for long-term, noninvasive monitoring and assessment of drug efficacy and prognosis; intracranial EEG to locate epileptic foci; index EEG to evaluate coma depth; high-frequency EEG to detect the origin of epilepsy; and nuclear magnetic EEG, which can be obtained in the MRI room and fused with MR images.

5.1.2 Structure of the EEG Recorder

The traditional EEG recorder consists of several parts: power, input, amplification, regulation, and recording. Signal acquisition and input components include electrodes, input box, lead selection, standard voltage, resistance measurement, and other devices; the amplifying component consists of a preamplifier and a postamplifier; the adjustment components include gain, filter, running speed of paper, and damping; and the recording portion is composed of a marker and paper sheets. The core components of the EEG recorder are the amplifiers. Because the EEG signal is weak, in the range of millivolts or microvolts, and is further attenuated on its way through the skull, meninges, and scalp, it must be amplified millions of times. However, this produces environmental noise and interference that overwhelms the EEG signal; thus, amplifiers with high sensitivity and strong anti-interferent properties are necessary. In modern digital EEG systems, the amplifiers, as the core components, also contain adjustment and recording functions in addition to the traditional amplification function. Since there is no mechanical damping during the recording and display of the digital EEG, the term "damping" has disappeared from the vocabulary of modern clinical EEG. Therefore, the EEG systems commonly observed in many hospitals consist of the following parts: (1) electrodes or electrode cap, (2) amplifier, (3) video monitor, (4) computer (monitor and recorder), and (5) printer (Fig. 5.1).

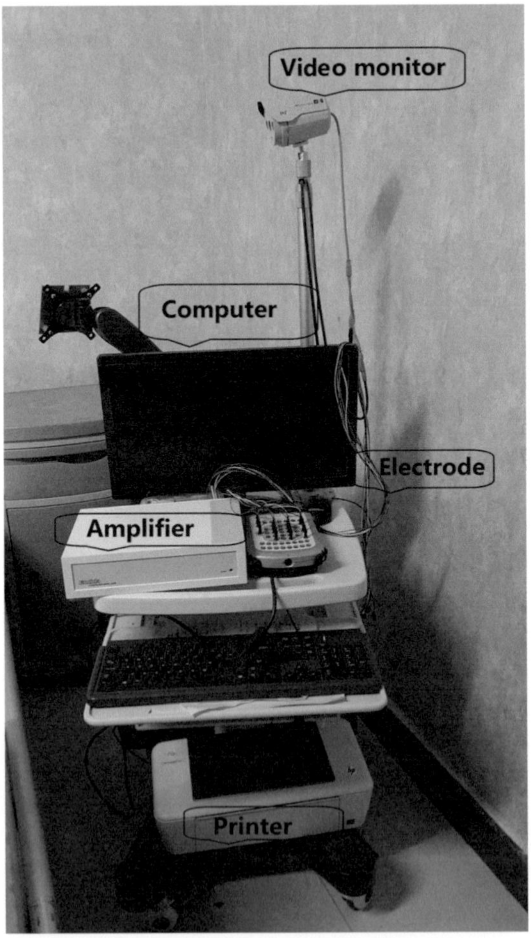

Fig. 5.1 The structure of an EEG recorder

5.1.3 Basic Knowledge of the EEG Wave

To interpret an EEG, the EEG frequency, amplitude, and waveform, as well as the distribution, form, and changes of abnormal waves, must be analyzed.

5.1.3.1 Frequency

Frequency equals the number of repetitions per second of EEG waves that share the same period. The frequency of EEG waves encountered in clinical analysis ranges from 0.1 to 100 Hz and is mainly within the 0.3–70 Hz interval. Internationally, the range of EEG wave frequency is divided into five bands represented by five Greek letters, of which delta and theta are slow wave bands, and beta and gamma are fast wave bands.

Alpha wave: 8–13 Hz (Fig. 5.2)
Beta wave: 14–30 Hz (Figs. 5.2 and 5.3)
Theta wave: 4–7.5 Hz (Fig. 5.3)
Delta wave: 0.3–3.5 Hz (Figs. 5.3 and 5.4)
Gamma wave: >30 Hz

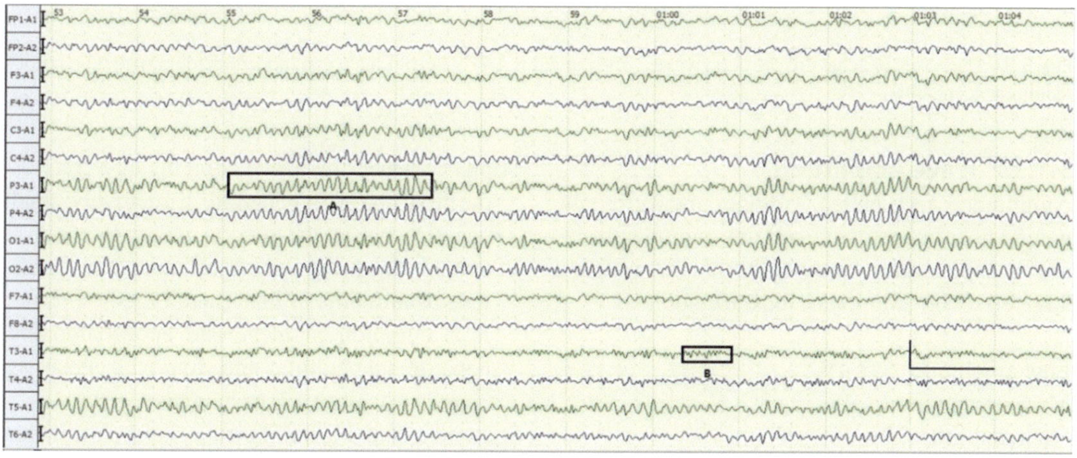

Fig. 5.2 Box A shows an alpha wave, and Box B shows a beta wave. The subject is a 53-year-old male who is awake with closed eyes

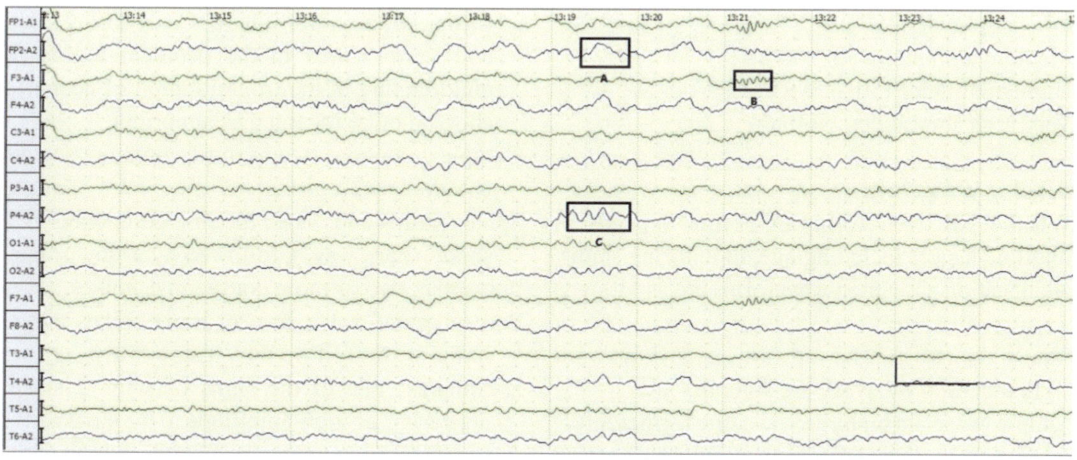

Fig. 5.3 Box A shows a delta wave, Box B shows a spindle wave in the beta band, and Box C shows a theta wave. The patient is a 69-year-old male in coma who is believed to have an intracranial infection

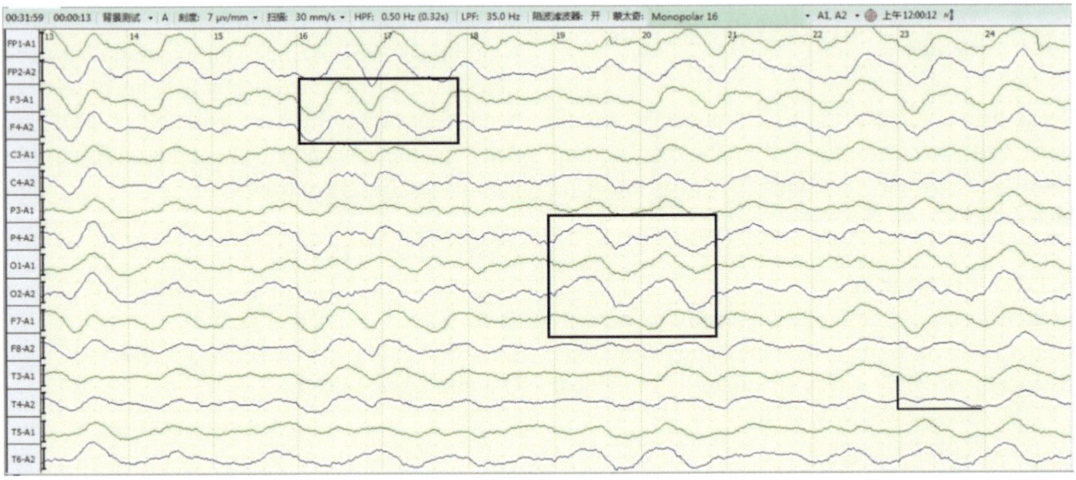

Fig. 5.4 The boxes indicate diffuse delta waves. The patient is a 47-year-old male in a moderate coma with tuberculous meningoencephalitis

5.1.3.2 Wave Amplitude

Amplitude, also called voltage, measures the potential difference between any two electrodes and is expressed in microvolts (μV). Age has a large effect on amplitude; thus, for adults:

Low amplitude: <25 μV
Medium amplitude: 25–75 μV
High amplitude: 75–150 μV
Very high amplitude: >150 μV

For children:

Low amplitude: <50 μV
Medium amplitude: 50–150 μV
High amplitude: 150–300 μV
Very high amplitude: >300 μV

5.1.3.3 Waveform

Whether EEG waveforms are normal depends on multiple factors including age, monitoring status, and location. Common waveforms are as follows:

Sinusoidal wave: the upward and downward branches of the wave are smooth.

Simple wave and biphasic wave: the former refers to a wave that deflects in a single direction from the baseline (up or down), whereas the latter contains one segment above the baseline and the other segment below the baseline.

Triphasic wave: this wave contains three phases; the first phase is generally a relatively small negative wave, the second phase is positive, and the third phase is negative with an amplitude usually higher than that of the first phase. It is common in metabolic encephalopathy, hepatorenal failure, and hypoxia. Positive-negative-positive triphasic waves exist.

Spike: the shape is similar to a sharp nail, with a time limit of 20–70 ms.

Sharp wave: this waveform is similar to those of spikes, with a time limit of 70–200 ms; spikes and sharp waves are usually abnormal waveforms, but the vertex sharp waves during sleep and sharp waves in the occipital region of children and in the frontal region of neonates should not be regarded as abnormal.

Complex: contains two or more continuous wave components.

Spike (sharp) and wave: the first component is a spike (sharp wave), followed by a slow wave.

Polyspike: two or more consecutive spikes.

Polyspike and wave: two or more spikes as the initial wave, followed by a slow wave.

K-complex: one of the signs of stage 2 sleep, appearing as high-amplitude 1 Hz slow activity of the brain hemisphere; under sound stimulation, short-range 12–14 Hz fast activity will appear.

5.1.3.4 EEG of Normal Adults

Alpha and beta waves are the basic waves in the awakened state (Fig. 5.2), and a few fast waves and slow waves are scattered during this state. The primary brain wave is the alpha wave, which is distributed in the back of the head and is symmetrical on both sides. On symmetrical sites of both hemispheres, the frequency difference of alpha waves should not exceed 20%, and the amplitude difference should be no more than 50% in the occipital region and no more than 20% in other regions. The average amplitude of alpha waves is less than 100 μV and that of beta waves less than 50 μV. During the opening and closing of the eyes, mental activity, or sensation of a stimulus, alpha waves should be attenuated. Slow waves of normal adults are random, low-amplitude waves, mostly theta waves, and continuous high-amplitude beta or delta waves should not be observed at any site. During sleep, brain waves should be symmetrical. Abnormal electrical activity should not be detected. There should not be spikes or spike and waves during waking or sleep.

5.1.3.5 Distribution of Abnormal Waves

According to the location of the abnormal waves identified by the electrodes, the distribution of abnormal waves is usually classified as follows:

Generalized: appearing in regions of both hemispheres, basically symmetrical (Fig. 5.5).

Diffuse: appearing in regions of both hemispheres, similar to the generalized type but with less symmetry.

Symmetrical: the waveform, amplitude, phase, and frequency of electrical activities are essentially the same in both hemispheres (Fig. 5.6).

Asymmetrical: the waveform, amplitude, phase, and frequency of electrical activities differ from one hemisphere to the other (Fig. 5.7).

Lateralized: abnormal electrical activity occurs in one hemisphere or mainly in one hemisphere.

Localized: abnormal electrical activity is limited in certain regions (Fig. 5.8).

Migratory: characteristic EEG activity gradually shifts from one region to another on the same or opposite side of the brain, often manifested as a weakening waveform in one region gradually emerging in another region.

5.1.3.6 Patterns of Abnormal Waves

The following terms are commonly used to describe abnormal waves according to the time and number of their occurrence:

Wave: wave in a single form.

Activity: several consecutive waves similar in form and prevalent within a certain range of time and space.

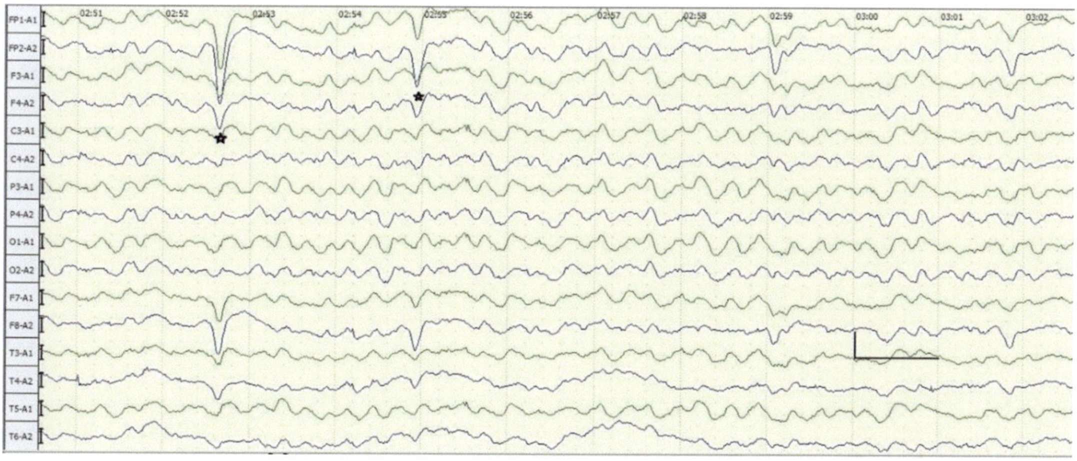

Fig. 5.5 Demonstrates generalized delta activity. The patient is 27 years old with autoimmune encephalitis and is in the lowest state of consciousness. The stars indicate eye-blink artifacts

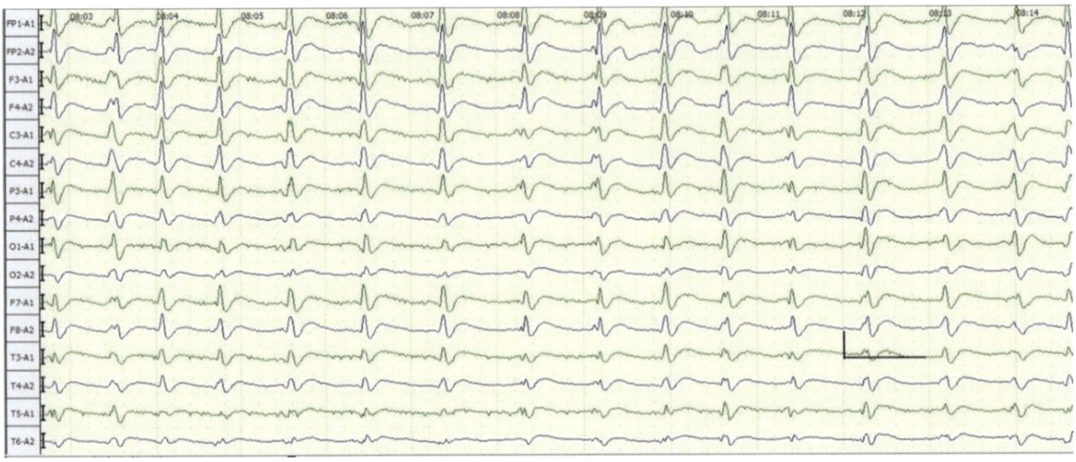

Fig. 5.6 Demonstrates discharges of symmetrical bilateral synchronous periodic spikes. The patient is 74 years old and in a deep coma after cardiopulmonary resuscitation

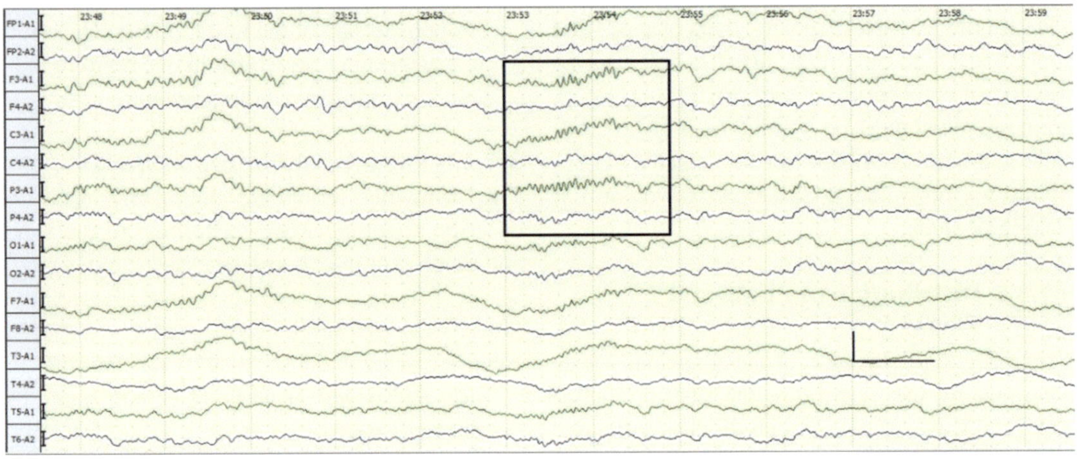

Fig. 5.7 Demonstrates asymmetrical electrical activity, in which the spindle wave is well developed on the left side of the brain (indicated by the box) but nonexistent on the right side. The patient, a 59-year-old male, is in a stupor after massive infarction of the right hemisphere

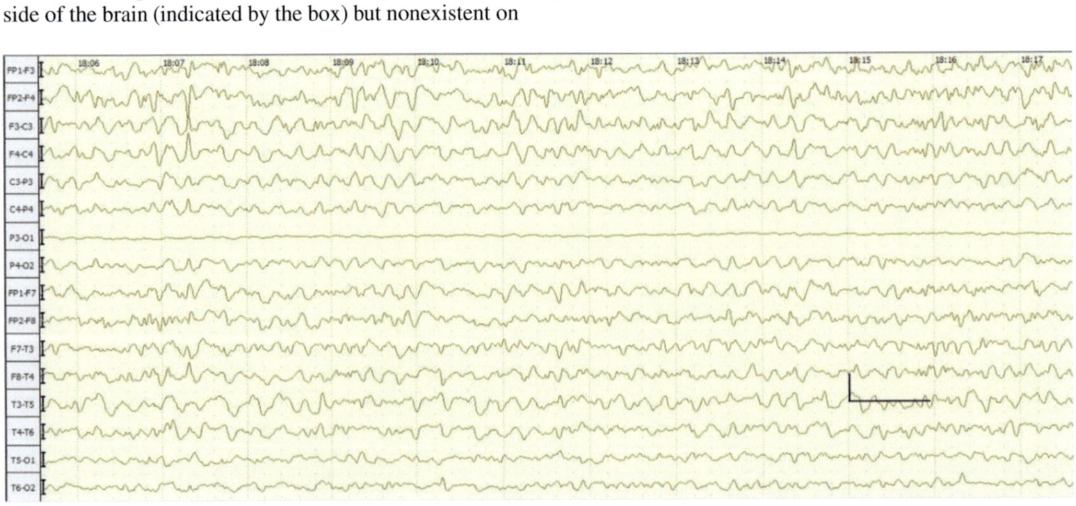

Fig. 5.8 Demonstrates localized discharge of spikes under the F4 electrode. This 49-year-old female patient with epilepsy is in a state of somnolence

Rhythm: the consecutive appearance of more than three identical waves. According to the time limit of occurrence, rhythms are classified into short-range (shorter than 1 s), medium-range (longer than 1 s but shorter than 3 s), and long-range (longer than 3 s).

Random: a single wave appearing at irregular intervals in the same lead or different leads.

Episode: only one or two occurrences of a particular waveform during one period of recording.

Transient: a certain waveform stands out from the background activity, with irregularity, a short range, and infrequent occurrence.

Periodicity: waves or wave groups of similar forms and phases that stand out from the background activity and recur at similar intervals (Fig. 5.6).

Synchronous: bilateral EEG changes with a fixed relationship of phase and the same frequency (Fig. 5.6). Bilateral EEG changes may have a time difference less than 25 ms; otherwise, they are regarded as secondary synchronization.

Asynchronous: bilateral EEG changes occur in a non-fixed relationship of phase and nonidentical frequencies.

Burst: brain waves prominent against the background activity with abrupt onset and termination (Fig. 5.9).

Paroxysm: brain waves prominent against the background activity with milder prominent components compared to bursts.

Hypsarrhythmia: asymmetry of amplitude, frequency, and waveform plus asynchronicity.

5.1.4 Electrode Placement and Montages

The principle of electrode placement is to record the abnormal potential as much as possible. Currently, the most internationally used method of electrode placement is the 10/20 system. The electrodes on both ears are usually designated reference electrodes, or the average potential of all electrodes is taken as the reference. Montages can be either referential or bipolar. The advantages and disadvantages of common lead settings are summarized as follows:

5.1.4.1 Ear Electrode Referential Montage

Advantages:

It helps to analyze abnormal waves and generalized waveforms.

The amplitude is higher and more stable than with bipolar montage.

The potential difference is close to the absolute value.

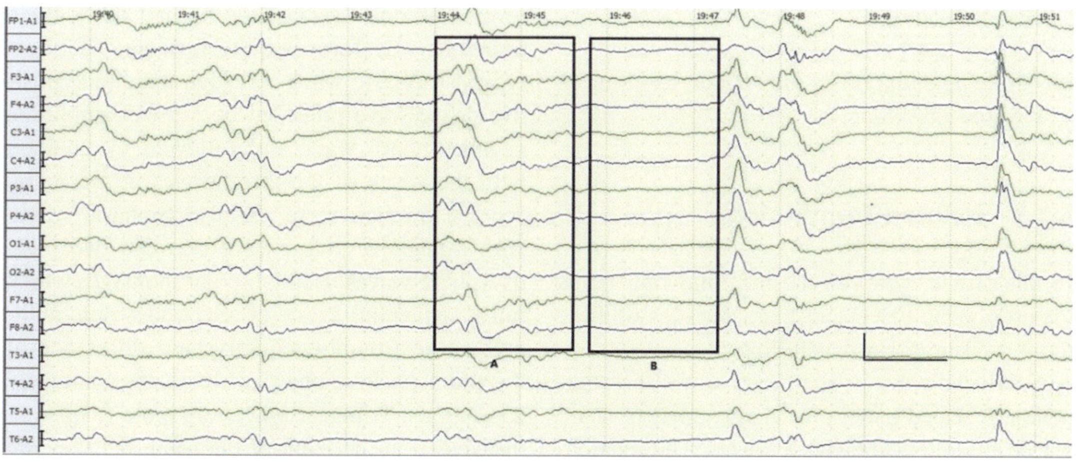

Fig. 5.9 Shows the typical pattern of burst suppression, with abrupt onset and termination. Box A indicates the burst phase, and Box B indicates the suppression phase. The patient is a 78-year-old male in a deep coma after cardiopulmonary resuscitation

It can be used to analyze the symmetry of bilateral normal phenomena.

Disadvantages:

It is difficult to locate small-scale lesions.
ECG artifacts may be obvious.
The activation of ear reference often leads to misunderstandings.

5.1.4.2 Average Referential Montage

Advantages:

The detection during a limited period of time is ideal.
It can be used to locate polyspike foci not distinct in the bipolar method.

Disadvantages:

Some generalized events may cause "referential montage activation," resulting in difficulty detecting focal lesions or the detection of pseudo-diffuse foci.

5.1.4.3 Bipolar Montage

Advantages:

Most electrical activities of the brain can be located by hemisphere and region.
The influence of unrelated electrodes is relatively small.

Disadvantages:

Electrode potential offset may occur, resulting in lowered amplitude.

5.1.5 Related Terminology

In this article, we will use the following terms to describe the EEG. The characteristics of these terms are summarized as follows:

Spike and wave or sharp and wave: the alternating, repeated pattern in which spikes or sharp waves are followed by slow waves. The relationship between the spikes (or sharp waves) and the slow waves is constant; there is no time interval between a spike and wave and the next (if intervals are present, the waveform should be described as a periodic waveform to be discussed below).

Periodic waveforms: repeated, relatively uniform, and continuous waveforms with approximately the same discharge interval. Periodic waveforms typically include periodic epileptiform discharges (PEDs) and burst suppression.

According to the focus of epileptic discharge, periodic epileptiform discharges in the EEG manifestation are divided into two types: generalized and lateralized.

EEG features of generalized periodic epileptiform discharges (GPDs): epileptiform discharges, such as spikes, sharp waves, spike and waves, and polyspikes, can be observed on EEG, and they are bilateral, synchronous, and generalized, with a similar discharge interval which is often observed with low-voltage slow activity or no activity. Periodic lateralized epileptiform discharges (PLEDs) are characterized by occurrence in mainly one hemisphere, involving the entire hemisphere or primarily a certain location.

EEG features of burst suppression: the alternation of explosive activity greater than 20 μV and electrical suppression. The bursts can be high-amplitude delta waves or theta waves with or without spikes or sharp waves. Between these bursts is low-voltage activity, whose amplitude should be less than 10 μV.

Characteristics of triphasic waves: as the name suggests, triphasic waves are waves that reverse around the baseline up and down three times. Its waveform is quite variable. The most typical triphasic wave is a high-amplitude positive-phase wave preceded by a lower-amplitude negative-phase wave and followed by another, with the width of the three waves in ascending order. However, there are also triphasic waves with a negative-phase wave between two positive-phase waves. Using bipolar montages which links sequential pairs of electrodes longitudinally, the frontal-occipital phase difference of the main positive-phase wave is approximately 25–140 ms. Triphasic waves are more frequently distributed at the front of the head, but they are not uncommon at the back of the head.

Rhythmic delta activity: its graphical characteristics include paroxysmal 2–3 Hz delta activity with a sinusoidal or zigzag waveform. When it appears intermittently, it is called intermittent rhythmic delta activity, which usually lasts for 2–5 s; when there is no time interval between successive waveforms, it is called continuous rhythmic delta activity. Rhythmic delta activity can be unilateral or bilateral.

5.2 Electroencephalographic Manifestations of SE

5.2.1 Introduction

As most recently defined by the International League Against Epilepsy (ILAE) in 2015, SE is a condition resulting either from the failure of the mechanisms responsible for seizure termination or from the initiation of mechanisms that lead to abnormally prolonged seizures [1]. The classification of SE by the ILAE in 2015 is based on semiology, etiology, EEG correlates, and age [1].

EEG to SE is what pathological examination is to tumors: they both play an irreplaceable role in the diagnosis, classification, and treatment monitoring of disease. There are many types of EEG manifestations of SE. Different types of SE can manifest in the same EEG, whereas the type of EEG in the same patient with SE can change over time. Therefore, physician and EEG technician must know how to explain these uncertainties when discussing electroencephalograms of SE.

5.2.2 EEG of SE with Prominent Motor Symptoms

5.2.2.1 Generalized Tonic-Clonic SE

Generalized tonic-clonic SE is a clinical emergency with extremely high mortality and morbidity. The EEG of idiopathic generalized tonic-clonic SE is similar to that of self-limiting generalized tonic-clonic seizure. At the beginning of the attack, the background amplitude is decreased in all electrodes, followed by the appearance of all-electrode low-amplitude fast rhythm (20–40 Hz) or low-amplitude polyspikes, gradually forming recruiting rhythms. The spike amplitude gradually increases, while the frequency gradually decreases (10–15 Hz), followed by the insertion of irregular slow theta waves; regular spike and waves have not yet been formed. In this period, the EEG signals may be overwhelmed by large amounts of electromyogram (EMG) artifacts due to tonic muscle contractions. In the clonic phase, the alternation of spikes or polyspikes and slow waves is gradually regularized. Simultaneously, spikes/polyspikes correspond to the contraction phase of the muscle, and slow waves correspond to the relaxation phase of the muscle, which forms the so-called checkerboard-like EEG [2]. After the last spike and wave disappears, the EEG signal goes into diffuse depression; during this period, the patient enters the postictal state when the disturbance of consciousness is usually present (see Fig. 5.10).

The diagnosis of generalized tonic-clonic SE is straightforward due to the clear and typical clinical symptoms. However, disturbance of consciousness usually follows the attack, and clinicians are often confused regarding how to explain the disturbance of consciousness and whether it is necessary to take measures. In this scenario, an EEG can help classify the disturbance of consciousness.

The first type of disturbance of consciousness is postictal suppression. This type of EEG features a generalized voltage suppression that continues for several tens of seconds to several minutes, followed by the gradual emergence of diffuse high-amplitude delta waves, which last for several minutes to more than 10 min. The delta waves are succeeded by the gradual appearance of the K-complex and/or sleep spindle. For this postictal suppression, intravenous antiepileptics are not necessary.

The second type of consciousness disturbance is an anticonvulsant drug-induced sleep state. The EEG of this type is similar to the first type, as there is no significant epileptic discharge, but there is a 15–20 Hz spindle-like fast rhythm mainly present in the front of the head. This type of rhythm must not be misinterpreted as epileptic

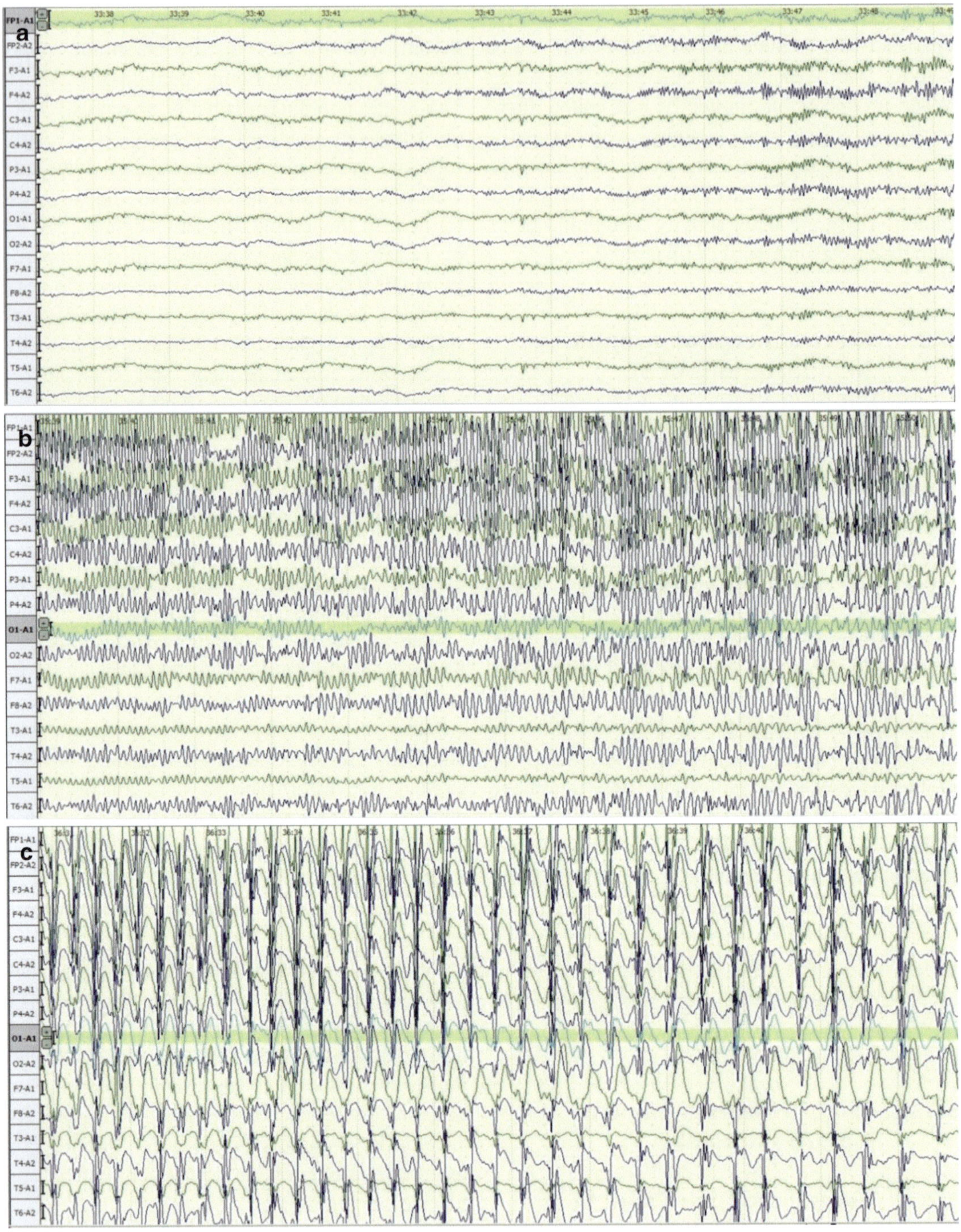

Fig. 5.10 Shows recurrent generalized tonic-clonic SE in a 28-year-old female patient. (**a**) Low-amplitude fast rhythm at the beginning of the attack. (**b**) Recruiting rhythm formed by spikes, with gradually increasing amplitude and gradually decreasing frequency. (**c**) Regular spike and waves, with spikes corresponding to muscle contraction and slow waves corresponding to muscle relaxation, forming a checkerboard-like appearance. (**d**) Termination of the attack and generalized low-voltage suppression observed after the disappearance of the last spike and wave

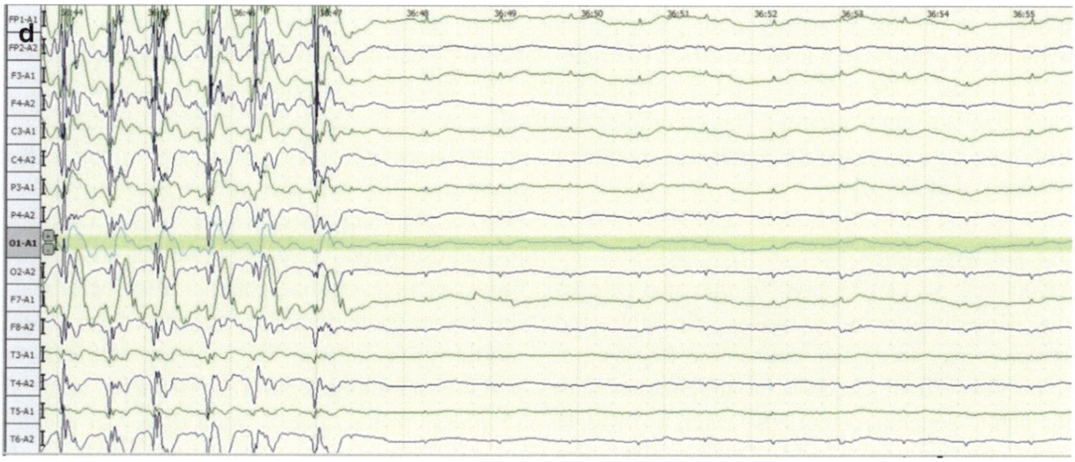

Fig. 5.10 (continued)

low-amplitude asynchronous discharge because this rhythm is fast wave and is induced by drugs, such as benzodiazepines and phenobarbital.

The third type of consciousness disturbance is subtle SE secondary to generalized tonic-clonic SE. Subtle SE is a type of nonconvulsive SE, which often follows convulsive SE. However, the literature notes that subtle SE secondary to idiopathic generalized tonic-clonic SE is rare, and most cases are eventually diagnosed as secondary generalized tonic-clonic SE [3]. This type of patient has no visible clinical attack or has only slight local twitching, but the EEG shows intermittent or continuous epileptiform discharge. For this type, it is necessary to actively follow the principle of antiepileptic drug treatment against convulsive SE.

The fourth type is coma caused by serious primary cerebral disorders. The EEG of this type shows sustained diffuse slow waves that are accompanied by varying amounts of spikes, sharp waves, spike and waves, sharp and waves, and other epileptiform discharges; however, it lacks sleep waveforms, such as K-complexes, sleep spindles, and other sleep waves. Even in patients with intravenous antiepileptics, sleep waveforms or drug-induced fast rhythms are not present, and the epileptic discharges and state of consciousness are not significantly improved. For this type, treatment should be based mainly on the primary disorder, assisted by antiepileptic drug therapy.

Another disorder that is easily confused with generalized tonic-clonic SE is pseudostatus epilepticus (PSE). The clinical manifestations of PSE can be tonic-clonic-like twitches similar to those of generalized tonic-clonic SE, but the EEG shows no epileptic discharge; instead, significant EMG artifacts are present. Patients may experience a coma after the onset, but good alpha rhythms can be demonstrated by EEG instead of generalized postictal electrical suppression. At this time, if the patient is given light stimulation with their eyes open, an alpha block can be observed.

DeLorenzo, R. J. et al. used 24-h continuous electroencephalogram (cEEG) monitoring and found that 52% of patients did not have after-SE ictal discharges (ASIDs) after convulsive SE was controlled; rather, they showed diffuse slow waves, wave amplitude attenuation, focal slow waves, periodic discharges, or burst suppression. Furthermore, nonconvulsive seizures and non-convulsion status appeared in 48% and 14% of patients, respectively [4]. After cEEG monitoring in the emergency rooms of 198 patients with disorders of consciousness, Privitera, M. et al. found that 74 (37%) patients were extremely likely to have NCSE [5]. Therefore, EEG, particularly cEEG, is very important for monitoring comatose patients, particularly after status convulsivus.

Because it can help identify potential patients with nonconvulsive seizures, the 2012 American Neurocritical Care Society Status Epilepticus Guideline Writing Committee has recommended EEG monitoring for the diagnosis and treatment of all types of SE [6].

5.2.2.2 Myoclonic SE

Myoclonic SE can be divided into two categories according to the etiology: idiopathic and symptomatic. Idiopathic myoclonic SE is rare. It is observed in children or adolescents with idiopathic generalized epilepsy, such as juvenile myoclonic epilepsy [7, 8]. These patients are often clinically manifested with bilateral, irregular continuous fast myoclonic manual movements. EEG shows all-electrode 2.5–5 Hz spike and waves, which are generalized outbreaks of polyspike and waves, with durations of a few seconds and intervals of 4–10 s. The corresponding EMG of contracting muscles shows muscle contraction that is synchronized with epileptic wave outbreaks or not. This discharge is increased when the eyes are closed or the patient is woken.

Symptomatic myoclonic SE usually occurs in patients with secondary generalized epilepsy and in patients with non-epileptic acute or subacute encephalopathy, such as early infant severe myoclonic encephalopathy, progressive myoclonic epilepsy, Lennox-Gastaut syndrome, and neurological diseases caused by infection, metabolic disorders, or intoxication. Various EEG patterns can be observed in this type of SE, such as outbreaks of spike and waves or polyspike and waves [8], triphasic waves with polyspikes (Fig. 5.11), and burst suppression waveforms [9–11]. Sustained myoclonic SE can usually be observed in comatose patients after cardiopulmonary resuscitation. These patients have a high mortality rate, and the EEG can show outbreaks of periodic pseudoepileptiform discharges or burst suppression that occur several times per second to once every few seconds. Ribeiro A. R. et al. monitored the EEG of 36 patients with cardiac arrest accompanied by myoclonic SE and found that 24 patients (66.7%) showed generalized epileptiform discharges (GEDs), and 12 patients (33.3%) had bilateral independent periodic discharges. Only ten patients (27.8%) survived, and the patients with an EEG response to sound, light, and pain during first-time EEG monitoring had a better prognosis than the patients with no response [12].

5.2.2.3 Tonic Status

Tonic status is a rare type of SE that occurs primarily in children or adolescents diagnosed with Lennox-Gastaut syndrome, some patients with

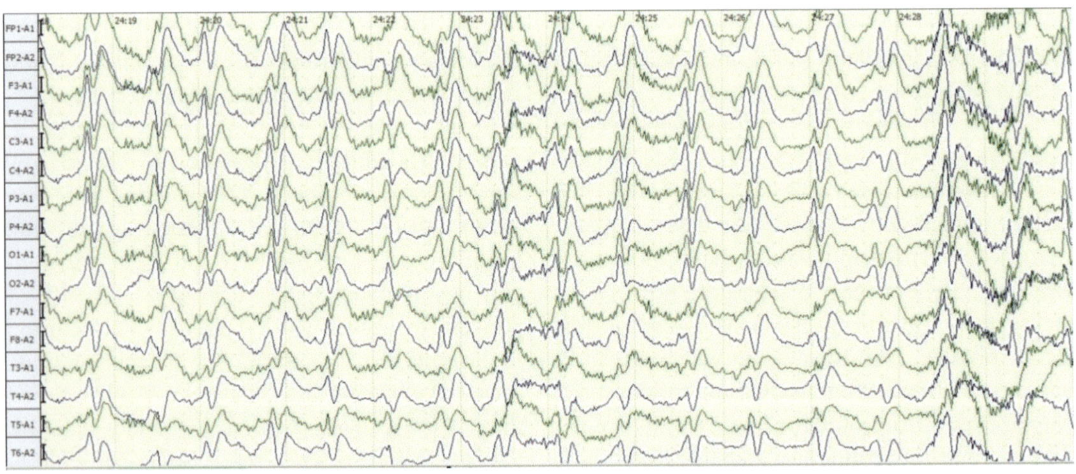

Fig. 5.11 Shows frequent episodes of generalized myoclonus of a 68-year-old male with rapid progressive cognitive impairment and mental and behavioral abnormalities. Cortical ribboning is observed on MRI, and the patient is suspected of Creutzfeldt-Jakob disease (CJD)

idiopathic generalized epilepsy and patients with drug-derived factors or specific infectious diseases [13–15]. Clinical manifestations are short-time axial muscle tonus, such as rigidity of the neck and trunk muscles and lower limb straightening, which is often accompanied by upward staring eyes and facial muscle twitching. Clinical manifestations of these patients are milder than in generalized tonic-clonic SE and can be difficult to detect. EEG upon onset shows a continuous low-amplitude fast activity of up to 20–30 Hz of frequency on the background of voltage attenuation in all electrodes, followed by a recruiting rhythm and the gradual slowing of spike frequency to 10–20 Hz with gradually increasing amplitude. Tonic status can occur as frequently as hundreds of times in a single night and can be sustained for several days. It may be exacerbated by a reduced level of awakening due to the use of benzodiazepines.

5.2.2.4 Clonic Status

Overall, 50–80% of patients with clonic status are children. Clinical manifestations are asymmetrical bilateral, rhythmic clonic tics. EEG shows a synchronous bilateral discharge of spikes or slow waves or the discharge of spike and waves following the recruiting rhythm formed by bursts of spikes. This disorder can be cryptogenic or caused by an acute brain injury or chronic encephalopathy. Cryptogenic clonic SE in children is usually accompanied by fever. The prognosis of cases with acute brain injury is relatively poor.

5.2.2.5 Secondary Generalized Tonic-Clonic SE

Treiman [16] and his colleagues summarized the EEG characteristics of secondary generalized tonic-clonic SE and the order of its development: (1) EEG changes of discrete seizures accompanied by episodic slow waves; (2) merging seizures with waxing and waning of the episodic discharge; (3) continuous epileptic discharge, such as spikes and spike and waves; (4) continuous ictal activity punctuated by low-voltage "flat periods"; and (5) periodic epileptiform discharges on a "flat" background. However, Lowenstein D. H. and Nei M. and other scholars have different views. They believe that not all cases of secondary generalized tonic-clonic SE develop in this order of EEG change, and some can be manifested with focal low-amplitude fast rhythms at first and EEG changes similar to primary generalized tonic-clonic SE during the late course of the attack [17, 18]. Therefore, although secondary generalized tonic-clonic SE often begins as focal seizures, it is difficult to distinguish between idiopathic and secondary generalized tonic-clonic SE purely by EEG if the patient's family and doctors failed to observe the onset [2]. It also requires attention to the differentiation with PSE. Professor Richard P. Brenner noted that in patients with PSE, generalized tonic-clonic symptoms are obvious; however, EMG artifacts rather than actual EEG changes are displayed on the EEG. In addition, PSE patients are usually in a state of "coma" but show a significant alpha rhythm in the back of the head, which can be suppressed by the passive opening of the eyes [2].

5.2.2.6 Epilepsia Partialis Continua (EPC)

First reported in 1895 by Koshenikov, EPC is a subtype of the former simple partial SE. At present, common clinical causes are thought to be infection, tumor, drug intoxication, cortical dysplasia, vascular malformation, genetics, and others [19–24]. The main presentation is focal myoclonus or clonus of the face and upper limbs. The typical EEG characteristics are slow waves, spikes, or sharp waves in the Rolandic region contralateral to motor symptoms [2, 3, 25], but in other cases, the following is observed: (1) bilateral discharge of spikes and spike and waves, with or without frequency differences between the two sides; (2) approximately 10% of patients have a normal EEG despite the typical clinical symptoms, which may be observed when the discharges originate from a very small region in the brain sulcus, and the direction of the electrode recording is tangent to the direction of discharge; thus, the electrodes fail to detect the discharge. In this case, detection by intracranial electrodes, magnetoencephalography, electric dipole, or SPECT [3] is necessary; (3) approximately 8–15% of patients can be detected with periodic lateralized epileptiform discharges, which mainly appears in cases with metastatic brain tumors and brain contusion. Injury of the spinal cord, the cerebellum, or the basal ganglia can also cause subcortical myoclonic-like twitches, whose clinical manifestations are very similar to epileptic myoclonus; thus, clinical differentiation is difficult, particularly when the EEG signals are masked by EMG artifacts produced by myoclonus. However, these two types of myoclonic status are significantly different regarding their clinical treatment and must, therefore, be clearly differentiated. First, appropriate amounts of muscle relaxants can be administered to patients with secured respiratory conditions to remove EMG artifacts and determine whether there is epileptiform discharge. Then, the median nerve or posterior tibial nerve can be stimulated to determine whether EMG shows myoclonus 50–90 ms after cortical somatosensory evoked potential (SEP) is induced. Another method is jerk-locked back averaging, which assumes the outburst of myoclonic EMG signals as the trigger point, extracts the precedent EEG signals, and then superimposes those to acquire the average, thus highlighting the originally unclear spikes. If the EMG signal outburst appears 15–50 ms later than the spikes and a fixed relationship can be established between the former and the latter, then the myoclonus should be of epileptic origin. In patients with partial SE, unilateral limb jerking is usually located contralateral to the epileptic discharges [26, 27], but there are also reports in which seizures and discharges are located ipsilaterally. Young G. B. and W. T. Blume studied a 47-year-old patient with a severely damaged right hemisphere and found that the patient's right upper and lower extremity convulsions were associated with lateralized periodic discharges beside the sagittal sinus in the right frontal lobe, but these periodic discharges were associated with ipsilateral convulsions with a delay of 100 ms in each episode. The clonic jerks were abolished after sectioning of the subcortical callosal and projection connections of the frontal lobe. Young, G. B. and W. T. Blume also indicated that ipsilateral convulsions may be associated with the presence of fibers from the ipsilateral auxiliary motor area to the medullary reticular formation, and this projection also explains the delay between discharge and seizure onset [28].

5.2.3 EEG of NCSE

5.2.3.1 Overview

NCSE refers to SE with no significant motor symptoms. NCSE patients usually have abnormalities in consciousness, cognitive status, mental state, and behavior, with or without minor facial and limb tics, nystagmus, and involuntary blinking [29]. Because these symptoms are mild and atypical, they are easily overlooked by family members and medical workers; thus, EEG is essential for the diagnosis of NCSE [30]. However, there are various EEG waveforms of NCSE. Although there have been many studies attempting to define the EEG characteristics of NCSE, a lack of consensus on the criteria remains [31–35]. In the Salzburg Consensus Criteria for Non-Convulsive Status Epilepticus, the new EEG diagnostic criteria for the NCSE were defined as follows:

Part 1: In patients without epileptic encephalopathy: if there is a repeat of >2.5 Hz of epileptiform discharges, regarded here as spikes, sharp waves, polyspikes, or spike and waves, then NCSE must be considered based on the clinical and time criteria. In patients with epileptiform discharges ≤2.5 Hz or slow waves >0.5 Hz AND at least one of the additional criteria, EEG of NCSE should be considered: (1) clinical and EEG improvements with IV antiepileptic drugs (AEDs): note that if there is only EEG improvement without clinical improvement or fluctuation without decisive improvement of clinical symptoms, "possible NCSE" should be diagnosed, (2) subtle clinical phenomena, and (3) typical spatiotemporal evolution. In fact, all EEG specialists understand that to diagnose epilepsy from an EEG, EEG evolutions must be identified, especially those in the following three categories: (A) incrementing onset (in voltage and frequency), (B) evolution of pattern (change in frequency >1 Hz or change in location), or (C) decreasing termination (in voltage and frequency).

PART 2: In patients with preexisting encephalopathy, NCSE should be considered in case of observable changes of the clinical presentation compared to baseline, increased amplitude or frequency of epileptiform discharges, or improvement of clinical and EEG features with IV AEDs [30]. According to the latest criteria, in all patients with clinical and EEG improvement after the administration of IV AEDs, a diagnosis of NCSE must be considered. The procedures of the auxiliary test for the diagnosis of NCSE with IV benzodiazepines are as follows [29]:

Patient selection: patients with rhythmic or periodic focal or generalized epileptic discharge on EEG accompanied by impaired neurological function.

Patient preparation: accompanied by nursing professionals under EEG, pulse, ECG, blood oxygen, and blood pressure monitoring.

Testing

Test implementation:

1. Sequential injection of small doses of rapid-onset and short-acting benzodiazepine, e.g., midazolam (1 mg per time).
2. Evaluate clinical and EEG performance during each injection.
3. Stop injection when:

(a) EEG continues to improve.
(b) Clinical improvement is affirmative.
(c) Respiratory depression, dropping blood pressure, or other adverse events occurs.
(d) Maximum dose of injection is achieved (midazolam 0.2 mg/kg).

Interpretation of the end result: NCSE should be confirmed with the disappearance of abnormal EEG discharges with clinical improvement or the emergence of a normal EEG rhythm, e.g., alpha waves in the back of the head. If the EEG abnormalities disappear without clinical improvement, NCSE should be neither confirmed nor excluded.

In 2007, Shorvon studied and summarized the etiology and clinical characteristics of each type of SE and proposed the classification of NCSE based on age and clinical subtypes [36]. According to the above classification, Sutter and Kaplan proposed the corresponding EEG features and criteria of each type of NCSE in 2012 [37]. To view EEGs of each type of NCSE, please refer to the corresponding literature. In 2015, the ILAE updated the criteria of the classification for NCSE [1]. According to the presence or absence of coma symptoms, NCSE is divided into NCSE with coma and NCSE without coma. Typical absence status, atypical absence status, aura continua, myoclonic absence status, focal NCSE with impaired consciousness, and aphasic status are types of NCSE without coma.

5.2.3.2 EEG of NCSE Without Coma

Typical Absence Status

Typical absence status can be observed at any age [38] and is not limited to children or adolescents. Patients may or may not be diagnosed with epilepsy prior to this diagnosis. Unlike the transient typical absence seizures, patients with typical absent status rarely show complete loss of consciousness or stoppage of movement but are usually in continuous confusion or a twilight state. Although they can communicate with people, go to work, or attend school, their work efficiency and responsiveness are significantly compromised. Such an episode can last for hours or even days. EEG during an episode shows outbursts of continuous generalized 3–6 Hz spike and waves [39, 40] or discontinuous spike and waves [38]. The discharges of spike and waves are discontinuous but still frequent during sleep and regain continuity after the patient wakes. Intravenous benzodiazepines can terminate the discharge of spike and waves, and the consciousness of the patient recovers immediately.

Atypical Absence Status

Atypical absence status is common in children or adolescents with symptomatic epilepsy accompanied by psychomotor developmental disorders, such as Lennox-Gastaut syndrome (LGS) [41, 42]. Compared to the baseline non-attack state, patients are confused during the attacks and may have mild myoclonus jerks. In some patients, a slight tonus or atonia can also be observed [3]. Ictal

EEG shows continuous generalized discharge of a 1–2.5 Hz wave-spike-wave complex [43], with varying amounts of spikes or epileptic recruiting rhythm occasionally observed [3, 44].

Myoclonic Absence Status

Myoclonus absence status is often observed in children with idiopathic generalized epilepsy, such as myoclonus absence epilepsy. The patient shows frequent episodes of myoclonic absence, which is rhythmic myoclonic jitters of both shoulders and the upper and lower extremities during the course of absence, often accompanied by a disturbance of consciousness. The myoclonus component is more obvious than the absence component. Ictal EEG is similar to the 3 Hz spike and wave outbreaks typical of absence seizures. If EMG is monitored simultaneously, the synchronous myoclonic-like jerks and the discharge of spike and waves on EEG are time-locked.

Aura Continua

The clinical manifestations of aura continua are continuous sensory episodes. During the attacks, the patient's consciousness is complete, and there are persistent superficial sensory, deep sensory, visionary, auditory, gustatory and autonomic symptoms, and emotional or experiential sensations. Most ictal EEGs can be normal because approximately 6 cm^2 of cortical discharges is necessary for detection by scalp EEG, whereas the range of the epileptogenic focus of aura continua is smaller. Special electrodes, such as sphenoid or intracranial electrodes, can increase positive findings. The few patients with ictal EEG findings show discharge of focal spikes, polyspikes, spike and waves, and rhythmic slow waves [34, 45].

Focal NCSE with Impaired Consciousness

This type was formerly known as complex partial status epilepticus (CPSE) or psychomotor status. Patients are in varying degrees of a fluctuating disturbance of consciousness or a dream-like state. Some patients are associated with automatism. Ictal EEG can often be detected by scalp EEG, but it has various forms, such as the continuous discharge of spikes, spike and waves, 0.5–1 Hz delta rhythm, or 5–7 Hz theta rhythm, depending on the depth of the epileptogenic foci. The discharges of epileptogenic foci near the scalp are mostly fast rhythms, whereas the deep discharges demonstrate a slow frequency. Although the origin of the discharge is unilateral, the discharge in some patients may extend to both cerebral hemispheres [3, 43].

Aphasic Status

Aphasic status is usually secondary to the sustained discharge of the dominant hemisphere, and the duration of aphasia is associated with the site involved. Aphasia may persist for 1 h after continuous temporal lobe epileptic discharges [46, 47], and mixed aphasia induced by frontal lobe epileptic discharges can last for 48 h [48]. EEG of aphasic status mainly shows PLEDs or lateralized rhythmic slow wave of the dominant hemisphere [49, 50].

5.2.3.3 EEG of NCSE with Coma

Among patients with NCSE, the comatose patients deserve more attention. Because of the lack of clinical symptoms for chronological comparison in these patients, EEG becomes the only basis for the diagnosis of NCSE with coma [51–53]. According to the scope of the regions involved in the discharge, the EEG of NCSE with coma is divided into the generalized type (coma-GED) and the lateralized type (coma-LED), between which the only distinction is the EEG. The EEG changes in coma-GED usually include bilateral periodic epileptiform discharge (Fig. 5.12), burst suppression waveforms (Fig. 5.13), and bilateral triphasic waves (Fig. 5.11). The EEG of coma-LED mainly displays persistent focal spikes, PLEDs (Fig. 5.14), bilateral independent periodic epileptiform discharges (BiPEDs), and lateralized burst suppression. Notably, the presence of NCSE cannot be determined by the presence of these types of EEGs, and the diagnosis of NCSE from EEG changes must conform to the previously discussed diagnostic criteria of EEG changes in NCSE.

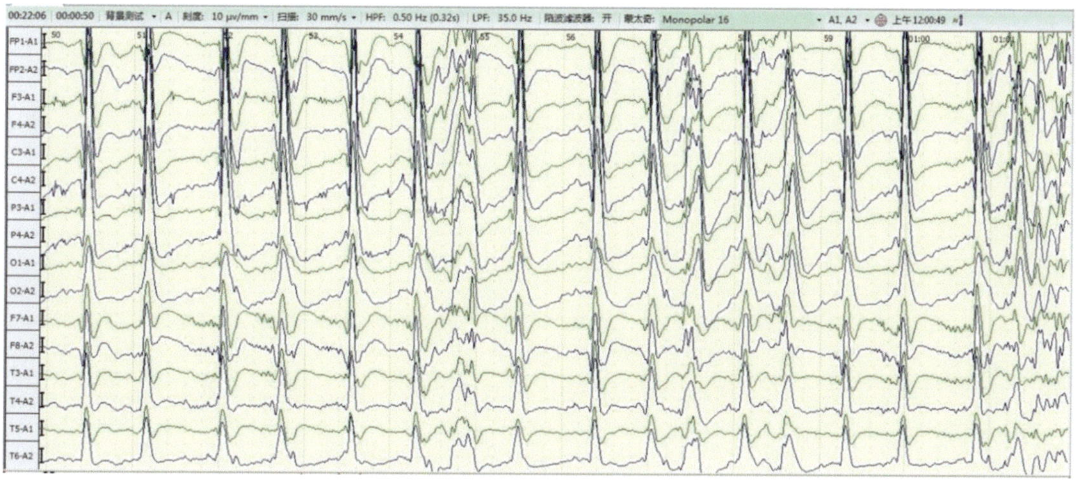

Fig. 5.12 A 66-year-old male with ischemic anoxic encephalopathy and in a moderate coma with NCSE, showing bilateral periodic epileptiform discharge with intervals of 0.8–1 s

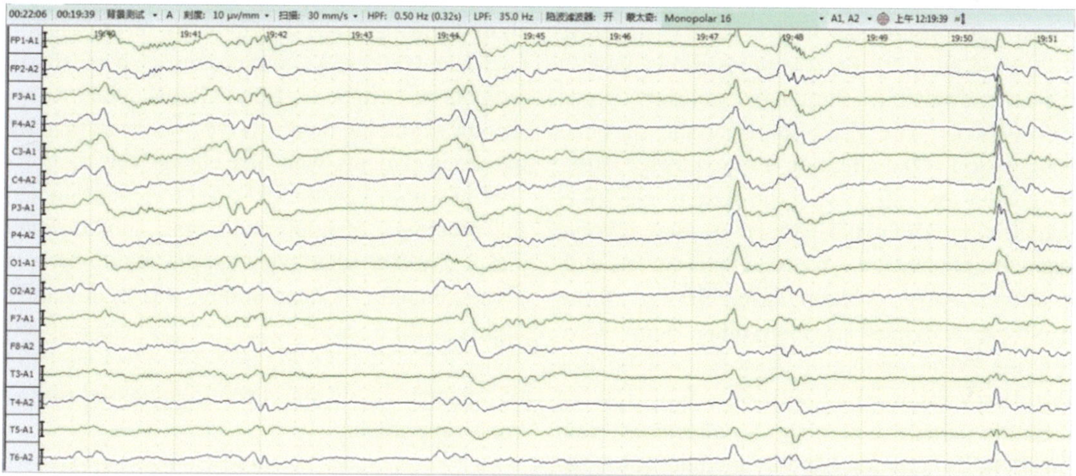

Fig. 5.13 A 78-year-old male with cardiac arrest after cardiopulmonary resuscitation and in a moderate coma with NCSE; the right side of his face was involuntarily twitching. Sharp waves, delta waves, and theta waves were observed during the burst period. The amplitude in the suppression period was less than 10 μV

Generalized Epileptiform Discharges

GEDs are often observed in intensive care units (ICU) [33]. In a follow-up study of over 3000 cEEG monitoring results in the ICU, NCSE was found in 27% of patients with generalized discharges [54]. The study found that cerebral hypoxia, metabolism disorders, infection, intoxication of central nervous system (CNS)-inhibiting drugs, and traumatic brain injury may all lead to generalized epileptiform discharges (GEDs), but the prognosis differs depending on the etiology. The prognosis is poor in patients with ischemic hypoxia and severe craniocerebral trauma or infection, but the prognosis is better in patients with metabolism disorders or intoxication with CNS-inhibiting drugs [43, 53, 55]. Although most types of GEDs do not determine prognosis [29], Pederson and colleagues noted that for patients with acute brain injury, mortality and morbidity are high in patients with generalized periodic

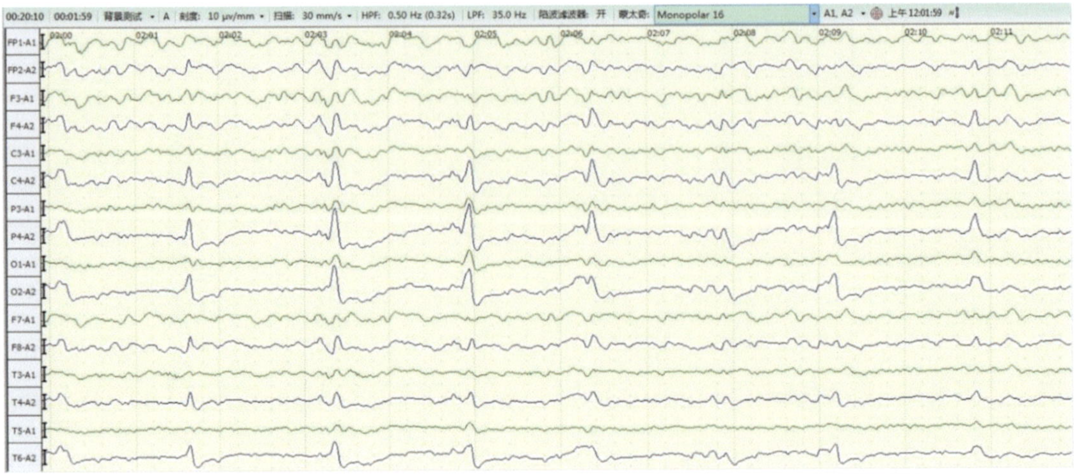

Fig. 5.14 A 71-year-old male in a deep coma with massive cerebral hemorrhage of the right basal ganglia region broken into cerebral ventricles, showing periodic epileptiform discharges on the right side with intervals of approximately 1.5 s

pseudoepileptiform discharges (OR = 2.5, 95% CI 1.43–4.40) [56]. Burst suppression is another EEG waveform that is thought to be closely related to prognosis. The EEG characteristic of burst suppression is the alternation of explosive activity greater than 20 μV and the state of electrical suppression. The explosive activity may involve high-amplitude delta waves and theta waves, with or without spikes or sharp waves. Between those explosive activities are low-voltage slow-wave activities. The inhibition phase should be less than 10 μV for at least 1 s. Burst suppression is a common pattern in severely compromised brain function. Its common etiology includes intoxication with CNS-inhibiting drugs, severe hypoxic encephalopathy, hypothermia, and anesthesia. Burst suppression after hypoxia often indicates poor prognosis; most drug intoxication-induced burst suppression allows recovery, but sequelae are common. Bursts with a single feature and increased rate of burst suppression usually indicate exacerbation of the patient's condition and a poor prognosis. Here, the features of bursts refer to the burst duration, burst interval, maximum peak-to-peak voltage, and energy ratio of high/low frequency. After extraction and an all-electrode correlation coefficient analysis of the features of bursts, we found that patients with significantly skewed distributions of correlation coefficients showed a poor prognosis, particularly patients with hypoxic-ischemic encephalopathy, among whom the mortality rate was significantly higher in patients who had bursts with a single feature within 12–36 h [57]. Yang et al. evaluated the prognosis of adults with post-anoxic coma and found that when burst suppression ratio was greater than 0.239, the mortality was significantly higher, with a sensitivity of 97.1% and a specificity of 73.3% [58]. Figure 5.15 shows the EEG of a patient with a significantly increased rate of burst suppression.

Lateralized Epileptiform Discharges

The most common waveforms of lateralized epileptiform discharges are PLEDs and BiPEDs. EEG features of PLED are spikes, sharp waves, sharp and waves, polyspikes, and other epileptiform discharges in local or unilateral hemispheric electrodes. The epileptiform discharges have similar intervals that are often manifested as no activity or low-voltage slow activity. There has been controversy over whether PLEDs suggest epilepsy or SE [59, 60]. Because PLED often occurs in cerebrovascular disease, infection, metabolism disorders, head injury, or tumors, there is currently no consensus as to whether

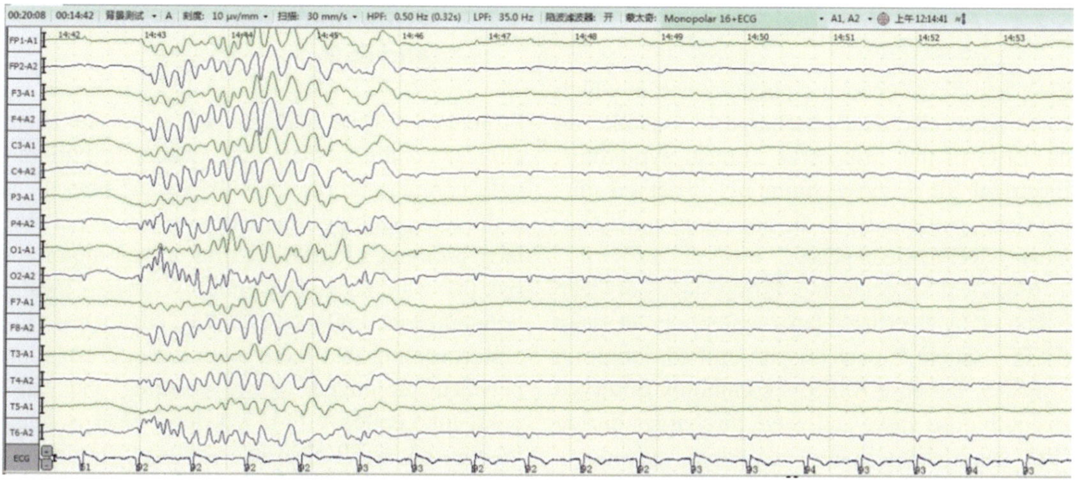

Fig. 5.15 A 51-year-old male in a deep coma after a car accident injury, with left upper limb involuntary twitches, showing the new type of burst suppression waveform with significantly prolonged periods of suppression

PLED is associated with epilepsy or caused by a primary disorder. However, if post-PLED discharge is prolonged, followed by a burst of low-amplitude electrical activity more frequent than 4 Hz, it is called PLED plus (PLED+). PLED+ often indicates nonconvulsive seizures or NCSE in comatose patients [2, 3, 61, 62]. BiPEDs have the same waveforms as PLED, but bilateral hemispheric discharges are not synchronized in amplitude, frequency, or distribution. These patients often have positive symptoms, including minor limb or facial twitching, hallucinations, and negative symptoms, including aphasia or cortical blindness, resulting in a higher mortality rate compared to PLED patients [62–64].

5.2.3.4 Duration of EEG Monitoring for NCSE Patients

The incidence of NCSE is 32–85 cases per ten million person-years. In the United States, 30,000–170,000 NCSE patients are newly diagnosed every year. Of all patients treated in the ICU, 8% have NCSE, 5% have epileptic status, 8–15% of comatose patients have NCSE, and more than 14% of patients with tonic-clonic seizures experience NCSE afterward. Although these data suggest that the occurrence of NCSE is considerably high, the authors conclude that these numbers are still below the true incidence because numerous patients remain undiagnosed. Misdiagnosis occurs largely because of the inability to perform EEG monitoring in a timely manner or for a sufficient duration [53, 65, 66]. The current study suggests that EEG should be monitored after the patient enters the ICU [6]. The literature has slightly different points of view regarding the duration of monitoring. One document stated that approximately 50% of patients with a final diagnosis of NCSE develop epileptiform discharges within 1 h of admission to the ICU [67]; 88% of patients will have seizures recorded by EEG within 24 h, but the other 12% of patients require 48 h or more for their EEG to display evidence of seizures. Another document showed that the likelihood of monitored NCSE seizures during hospitalization was extremely low if no seizure discharges were observed within the first 4 h of admission to the ICU [68]. The authors believe that the EEG of NICU patients should be continuously monitored for 48 h after routine admission; for those patients who have periodic discharges or burst suppression during recording, the recording time should be extended appropriately. The detection rate of NCSE is increased when patients with tonic-clonic SE continue to be monitored 24 h after onset.

5.2.4 EEG of Electrical SE

Electrical SE is a peculiar phenomenon in which continuous electrical discharge is visible on the EEG in the absence of clinical symptoms. Electrical SE is most commonly observed during sleep, particularly in the non-rapid eye movement (NREM) sleep phase.

Electrical SE occurring during stages of sleep is known as electrical status epilepticus in sleep (ESES). There is currently no unified definition of ESES. Because ESES is commonly observed as continuous spike and wave discharges during slow wave sleep, some researchers consider a spike and wave index greater than 85% as one of the diagnostic criteria of ESES [69]; that is, ESES is considered when the spike and wave discharge comprises more than 85% of the total duration of the NREM stage of sleep. There are also reports that ESES can be considered when this rate exceeds 50%. As a special clinical phenomenon, ESES is not an independent epilepsy syndrome. ESES can be hereditary, symptomatic, or cryptogenic. ESES is often observed in Landau-Kleffner syndrome (LKS), benign epilepsy in childhood with central temporal spikes plus its variants, epilepsy with continuous spike and waves during slow wave sleep and LGS.

Before the onset of ESES, the EEG of waking patients mostly shows focal or random multifocal spike and waves, which are increased and often generalized during sleep; during ESES, the spike and waves of waking patients are more diffuse than before the onset, and slow-wave sleep is the emergence of continuous spike and wave discharge. The spike and wave is usually 1.5–3.5 Hz in frequency and more generalized, but in some children, the site with the maximum amplitude can differ [70]. However, differences in the spike and wave index and the site of peak amplitude are not associated with the responsiveness of children to antiepileptics. Mental and psychological trauma of childhood patients is usually alleviated by the disappearance of ESES, but it is difficult for most patients to return to normal levels. The duration, severity and cumulative site of ESES discharges are usually associated with the patient's prognosis and must be adequately addressed by the medical staff [69, 71].

5.2.5 Prolonged Febrile Seizures and EEG

Prolonged febrile seizures are a severe acute clinical condition that often occurs in children with complex febrile convulsions. At present, it is thought that long-time febrile seizures, particularly prolonged febrile seizures, are an important risk factor for secondary epilepsy, such as mesial temporal lobe epilepsy [72, 73], but there is literature stating that there is no direct correlation between prolonged febrile seizures and temporal lobe epilepsy [74, 75]. Ictal EEG is often manifested as all-electrode or focal continuous bursts of spikes and spike and waves. The EEG wave patterns have a low value in predicting the future possibility of epilepsy. A prospective blind study evaluating the prognosis of children with prolonged febrile seizures (The Consequences of Prolonged Febrile Seizures, FEBSTAT) [76] showed that nearly half of the patients (45.2%) had EEG abnormalities after prolonged febrile seizures, with 36.2% showing focal slow wave or voltage attenuation. When a focal slow wave or voltage attenuation occurs within 72 h after prolonged febrile seizures, it is considered to be a biomarker of neuron damage; this result was supported by MRI findings [76, 77]. Studies have also shown that the predictive value of epileptiform discharges is very low and appears only in a small number of patients. This is likely because prolonged febrile seizures are not a type of epilepsy but merely represent acute brain injury, which is one of the risk factors of epilepsy. Previous studies have found that hippocampal sclerosis induced by prolonged febrile seizures is significantly more frequent in the right hemisphere than in the left; thus, patients with postictal EEG abnormalities in the right hemisphere are more likely to develop epilepsy in the future [72, 78].

5.2.6 Refractory Status Epilepticus (RSE) and EEG

Refractory status epilepticus refers to prolonged seizures that remain clinically uncontrollable, even with sufficient doses of at least two categories of the first-line antiepileptic drugs, particularly benzodiazepines, and often requires special treatment. The morbidity and mortality of RSE are high [79, 80]. There is evidence that the longer the seizures last, the more difficult they are to control [81, 82]. At least 14% of NCSE cases occur after the clinical signs of convulsions disappear [4]. At this time, the failure to detect and control continuous discharges is the greatest potential risk for the clinical recurrence of convulsions [83, 84]. Once the SE relapses, termination is more difficult, and it will very likely develop into RSE [85, 86]. A survey of NICU construction in China showed that the number of devices used for EEG monitoring is insufficient: less than 2/3 of NICUs are equipped with EEG monitoring devices, only half of which are video-EEG monitors, whereas the rate at which EEG was considered for monitoring SE or RSE was even lower [87]. Another study showed that in the absence of EEG monitoring, 62% of patients with a prior history of epilepsy were immediately diagnosed in the presence of SE, whereas only 22% of patients without a previous history were diagnosed with SE after its emergence; the median delay of diagnosis for these two types of patients was 48 and 72 h, respectively [81]. Although the overall prognosis of patients with SE is most closely related to the etiology, longer attacks lead to more severe neuron damage. Thus, the duration of the attack also affects the prognosis [88]. Therefore, an increased rate of cEEG monitoring and prolonged monitoring time is important to reduce the incidence of refractory epilepsy [81, 89, 90]. Meanwhile, for the treatment of RSE, the termination of clinical convulsion is not the only criterion; no epileptic discharges or burst suppression waveforms should be observed on the EEG. When burst suppression occurs after drug use, it is only sufficient for the criteria recommended in current guidelines with intervals of at least 10 s. Although there is a large body of literature supporting burst suppression on EEG as a marker for a sufficient dose of narcotics to control RSE [91–94], some patients may still have epileptic episodes during burst suppression sustained by narcotics [95, 96]. Others believe that neither the length of intervals between bursts nor the rate of burst suppression (the ratio of time of suppression to total time) predicts whether refractory epilepsy will be terminated [97]. Some studies even suggest that prolonged burst suppression by narcotics cannot reduce patient mortality or improve prognosis, and it even prolongs hospital stays [98]. In 2016, one article indicated that the number of epileptiform discharges during bursts is associated with seizure control, and a maximum burst amplitude less than 125 μV is a fairly good predictor of whether a seizure will be satisfactorily controlled (sensitivity: 84.6%, specificity: 61.1%) [97]. The suggested time of burst suppression maintained by drugs ranges from 24 to 48 h in different studies [90, 95, 96]. Our own experience is that in the absence of significant epileptiform discharges and clinical attacks during cEEG monitoring, narcotic drugs used to maintain burst suppression can be carefully reduced or withdrawn after 24 h; in the case of recurrence, burst suppression should be maintained.

5.3 The Role of EEG in Predicting the Prognosis of SE

The general view is that the prognosis of SE is closely related to the etiology, age, duration of seizures, necessity to use mechanical ventilation, and other clinical factors [99–101]. Although EEG can be used to predict the likelihood of SE recurrence [102], it is controversial whether it can predict the prognosis. The literature suggests that periodic epileptiform discharges may indicate poor prognosis [59, 61, 63–64], and the presence of PLEDs is associated with high mortality and high morbidity [103], regardless of etiology. However, some scholars do not support this claim, believing that the phenomenon of periodic discharges, particularly PLEDs and GEDs, mainly occurs in hypoxic-ischemic encephalopathy and severe intracranial infection, which have poor prognoses, and that statistical correction indicates that the prognosis should be related to age or etiology rather than periodic discharges [104, 105]. Another view is that etiology and EEG types should be integrated into the evaluation of prognosis. For example, Orta and colleagues found that compared to PLEDs of acute causes, PLEDs of chronic causes result in a lower mortality rate [106]. Burst suppression is another EEG waveform considered to be representative of a poor prognosis. Hofmeijer and colleagues collected the EEGs of 101 comatose patients with cardiac arrest after cardiopulmonary resuscitation from 2005 and showed that if burst suppression waveforms with identical bursts occurred within 12–36 h after cardiac arrest, the mortality was 100% compared to 36% for burst suppression without identical bursts; however, the accuracy of the results was reduced beyond 36 h after cardiac arrest [57]. In another study, Neligan, A. and Shorvon, S. D. reviewed all prospective studies between 1990 and 2009 that enrolled more than 30 patients with tonic-clonic SE; the longer the duration of epileptic seizures, which was found to be 1–2 h overall, the poorer the prognosis, but this association disappeared 10 h after onset. Moreover, only periodic epileptiform discharge was found to be associated with a poor prognosis, whereas the other types of abnormal discharges were not closely related to prognosis [107]. Recently, more articles have focused on the relationship between the EEG background and prognosis. Many studies have shown that in addition to particular abnormal discharge waveforms that may be valuable for the prediction of prognosis, the EEG background rhythm, sleep-related waveforms, and drug-induced EEGs may also be useful as tools to predict the prognosis of SE. In a prospective observational study designed by Alvarez et al., 120 adult patients with SE were enrolled. During the first 24 h of cEEG monitoring, 49 patients (40.8%) had no periodic or rhythmic abnormalities, 45 patients (37.5%) developed periodic discharges, 20 patients (16.7%) had rhythmic slow wave activity, and the other 6 patients (5%) developed spike and wave discharges. However, after rectifying the Status Epilepticus Severity Score (STESS), age, etiology, and other risk factors, no statistical correlation was found between any of these EEG abnormalities and prognosis, except that risk of death was significantly higher in patients in whom EEG rhythmicity disappeared within the first 24 h (OR 9.8; $p = 0.033$) or who had spindle loss in stage 2 of NREM sleep (OR 2.59; $p = 0.002$) [105]. Another study with a small sample size found that after an injection of ketamine, a narcotic commonly used to treat refractory epilepsy, better curative effects and prognosis of refractory epilepsy were shown in patients with the emergence of a generalized 7–20 Hz arcuate theta or beta rhythm [108]. In a study of 62 patients with cardiac arrest, Milani, P. and colleagues found that within 48 h after cardiac arrest, 26 patients showed an initial background rhythm, of whom 16 patients (61%) survived, and all 36 cases without an initial background rhythm died. They noted that the prognosis was poor for those patients with continuous inhibition of background rhythms, even if they had received mild hypothermia therapy after cardiac arrest [109].

Conclusion

EEG patterns, such as continuous spikes, spike and waves, polyspike and waves, or rhythmic slow waves and periodic waveforms, can vary in SE. Diagnosis of SE is not difficult when clinical symptoms are significant and EEG manifestations are typical. However, when clinical symptoms are atypical, particularly when patients in the ICU display alterations of consciousness, cognitive functions, mental state, or behavior that are difficult to explain, cEEG monitoring often helps to detect occult NCSE. Continuous or intermittent EEG monitoring is critical in the treatment and evaluation of ESES prognosis, prolonged febrile seizures, and SE. This article introduces the applications of burst suppression, which may be an important marker for drug use in the treatment of RSE. Finally, it should be emphasized that explanations of EEG changes and EEG responses to sound, light, pain, or drug therapy are central when interpreting EEGs of SE.

References

1. Trinka E, Cock H, Hesdorffer D, et al. A definition and classification of status epilepticus—report of the ILAE Task Force on Classification of Status Epilepticus. Epilepsia. 2015;56:1515–23.

2. Brenner RP. EEG in convulsive and nonconvulsive status epilepticus. J Clin Neurophysiol. 2004;21:319–31.
3. Kaplan PW. The EEG of status epilepticus. J Clin Neurophysiol. 2006;23:221–9.
4. DeLorenzo RJ, Waterhouse EJ, Towne AR, et al. Persistent nonconvulsive status epilepticus after the control of convulsive status epilepticus. Epilepsia. 1998;39:833–40.
5. Privitera M, Hoffman M, Moore JL, Jester D. EEG detection of nontonic-clonic status epilepticus in patients with altered consciousness. Epilepsy Res. 1994;18:155–66.
6. Brophy GM, Bell R, Claassen J, et al. Guidelines for the evaluation and management of status epilepticus. Neurocrit Care. 2012;17:3–23.
7. Gelisse P, Crespel A. Mixed myoclonic-absence status epilepticus in juvenile myoclonic epilepsy. Epileptic Disord. 2015;17:95–6.
8. Larch J, Unterberger I, Bauer G, Reichsoellner J, Kuchukhidze G, Trinka E. Myoclonic status epilepticus in juvenile myoclonic epilepsy. Epileptic Disord. 2009;11:309–14.
9. Fernandez-Torre JL, Calleja J, Infante J. Periodic eye opening and swallowing movements associated with post-anoxic burst-suppression EEG pattern. Epileptic Disord. 2008;10:19–21.
10. Ohtahara S, Yamatogi Y. Epileptic encephalopathies in early infancy with suppression-burst. J Clin Neurophysiol. 2003;20:398–407.
11. Knezevic-Pogancev M. Ohtahara syndrome—early infantile epileptic encephalopathy. Med Pregl. 2008;61:581–5.
12. Ribeiro A, Singh R, Brunnhuber F. Clinical outcome of generalized periodic epileptiform discharges on first EEG in patients with hypoxic encephalopathy postcardiac arrest. Epilepsy Behav. 2015;49:268–72.
13. Kobayashi E, Thomas P, Andermann F. Tonic status epilepticus in patients with idiopathic generalized epilepsy. Epileptic Disord. 2005;7:327–31.
14. Grande-Martin A, Pardal-Fernandez JM, Carrascosa-Romero MC, De Cabo C. Tonic seizure status epilepticus triggered by valproate in a child with Doose syndrome. Neuropediatrics. 2016;47:187–9.
15. Karatas H, Dericioglu N, Kursun O, Saygi S. Creutzfeldt-Jakob disease presenting as hyperparathyroidism and generalized tonic status epilepticus. Clin EEG Neurosci. 2007;38:203–6.
16. Treiman DM, Walton NY, Kendrick C. A progressive sequence of electroencephalographic changes during generalized convulsive status epilepticus. Epilepsy Res. 1990;5:49–60.
17. Lowenstein DH, Aminoff MJ. Clinical and EEG features of status epilepticus in comatose patients. Neurology. 1992;42:100–4.
18. Nei M, Lee JM, Shanker VL, Sperling MR. The EEG and prognosis in status epilepticus. Epilepsia. 1999;40:157–63.
19. Hwang KJ, Yoon S, Park KC. Non-ketotic hyperglycaemia presenting as epilepsia partialis continua. Epileptic Disord. 2016;18(2):201–3.
20. Ribeiro JJ, Sousa M, Teotonio R, Bento C, Sales F. Epilepsia partialis continua of the abdominal muscles due to cerebrovascular disease. Epileptic Disord. 2015;17:72–6. quiz 6.
21. Steve TA, Gross DW. Alcohol-responsive epilepsia partialis continua. Epileptic Disord. 2014;16:107–11.
22. Shrivastava V, Burji NP, Basumatary LJ, Das M, Goswami M, Kayal AK. Etiological profile of epilepsia partialis continua among adults in a tertiary care hospital. Neurol India. 2013;61:156–60.
23. Krysl D, Zamecnik J, Senolt L, Marusic P. Chronic repetitive nonprogressive epilepsia partialis continua due to rheumatoid meningitis. Seizure. 2013;22:80–2.
24. Kravljanac R, Djuric M, Jovic N, Djordjevic M, Zamurovic D, Pekmezovic T. Etiology, clinical features and outcome of epilepsia partialis continua in cohort of 51 children. Epilepsy Res. 2013;104:112–7.
25. Capovilla G, Paladin F, Bernardina BD. Rasmussen's syndrome: longitudinal EEG study from the first seizure to epilepsia partialis continua. Epilepsia. 1997;38:483–8.
26. Guerrini R. Physiology of epilepsia partialis continua and subcortical mechanisms of status epilepticus. Epilepsia. 2009;50(Suppl 12):7–9.
27. Espay AJ, Schmithorst VJ, Szaflarski JP. Chronic isolated hemifacial spasm as a manifestation of epilepsia partialis continua. Epilepsy Behav. 2008;12:332–6.
28. Young GB, Blume WT. Periodic lateralized frontal epileptiform discharges with ipsilateral epilepsia partialis continua. Epilepsia. 2007;48:597–8.
29. Jirsch J, Hirsch LJ. Nonconvulsive seizures: developing a rational approach to the diagnosis and management in the critically ill population. Clin Neurophysiol. 2007;118:1660–70.
30. Beniczky S, Hirsch LJ, Kaplan PW, et al. Unified EEG terminology and criteria for nonconvulsive status epilepticus. Epilepsia. 2013;54(Suppl 6):28–9.
31. Hirsch LJ, Brenner RP, Drislane FW, et al. The ACNS subcommittee on research terminology for continuous EEG monitoring: proposed standardized terminology for rhythmic and periodic EEG patterns encountered in critically ill patients. J Clin Neurophysiol. 2005;22:128–35.
32. Kaplan PW. EEG criteria for nonconvulsive status epilepticus. Epilepsia. 2007;48(Suppl 8):39–41.
33. Leitinger M, Beniczky S, Rohracher A, et al. Salzburg consensus criteria for non-convulsive status epilepticus—approach to clinical application. Epilepsy Behav. 2015;49:158–63.
34. Sutter R, Kaplan PW. Electroencephalographic criteria for nonconvulsive status epilepticus: synopsis and comprehensive survey. Epilepsia. 2012;53(Suppl 3):1–51.
35. Zandi AS, Dumont GA, Javidan M, Tafreshi R. Detection of epileptic seizures in scalp electroencephalogram: an automated real-time wavelet-based approach. J Clin Neurophysiol. 2012;29:1–16.
36. Shorvon S. What is nonconvulsive status epilepticus, and what are its subtypes? Epilepsia. 2007;48(Suppl 8):35–8.

37. Sutter R, Kaplan PW. The neurophysiologic types of nonconvulsive status epilepticus: EEG patterns of different phenotypes. Epilepsia. 2013;54(Suppl 6):23–7.
38. Fernandez-Torre JL, Rebollo M. Typical absence status epilepticus as late presentation of idiopathic generalised epilepsy in an elderly patient. Seizure. 2009;18:82–3.
39. Bilo L, Meo R, de Leva MF, Vicidomini C, Salvatore M, Pappata S. Thalamic activation and cortical deactivation during typical absence status monitored using [18F]FDG-PET: a case report. Seizure. 2010;19:198–201.
40. Baykan B, Gokyigit A, Gurses C, Eraksoy M. Recurrent absence status epilepticus: clinical and EEG characteristics. Seizure. 2002;11:310–9.
41. Arzimanoglou A, Resnick T. Diagnosing and treating epileptic drop attacks, atypical absences and episodes of nonconvulsive status epilepticus. Epileptic Disord. 2011;13(Suppl 1):S1–2.
42. Yang Z, Liu X, Qin J, Zhang Y, Bao X, Xiong H. Partial seizures and atypical absence seizures as a single ictal event in a patient with Lennox-Gastaut syndrome. J Child Neurol. 2008;23:1319–23.
43. Trinka E, Leitinger M. Which EEG patterns in coma are nonconvulsive status epilepticus? Epilepsy Behav. 2015;49:203–22.
44. Kaplan PW. Intravenous valproate treatment of generalized nonconvulsive status epilepticus. Clin Electroencephalogr. 1999;30:1–4.
45. Manford M, Shorvon SD. Prolonged sensory or visceral symptoms: an under-diagnosed form of nonconvulsive focal (simple partial) status epilepticus. J Neurol Neurosurg Psychiatry. 1992;55:714–6.
46. Adam C, Rouleau I, Saint-Hilaire JM. Postictal aphasia and paresis: a clinical and intracerebral EEG study. Can J Neurol Sci. 2000;27:49–54.
47. Goldberg-Stern H, Gadoth N, Cahill W, Privitera M. Language dysfunction after frontal lobe partial seizures. Neurology. 2004;62:1637–8.
48. Yankovsky AE, Treves TA. Postictal mixed transcortical aphasia. Seizure. 2002;11:278–9.
49. Ericson EJ, Gerard EE, Macken MP, Schuele SU. Aphasic status epilepticus: electroclinical correlation. Epilepsia. 2011;52:1452–8.
50. Rosche J, Schley A, Schwesinger A, et al. Recurrent aphasic status epilepticus after prolonged generalized tonic-clonic seizures versus a special feature of Todd's paralysis. Epilepsy Behav. 2011;20:132–7.
51. Vespa PM, O'Phelan K, Shah M, et al. Acute seizures after intracerebral hemorrhage: a factor in progressive midline shift and outcome. Neurology. 2003;60:1441–6.
52. McCoy B, Hahn CD. Continuous EEG monitoring in the neonatal intensive care unit. J Clin Neurophysiol. 2013;30:106–14.
53. Bauer G, Trinka E. Nonconvulsive status epilepticus and coma. Epilepsia. 2010;51:177–90.
54. Foreman B, Claassen J, Abou Khaled K, et al. Generalized periodic discharges in the critically ill: a case-control study of 200 patients. Neurology. 2012;79:1951–60.
55. Boulanger JM, Deacon C, Lecuyer D, Gosselin S, Reiher J. Triphasic waves versus nonconvulsive status epilepticus: EEG distinction. Can J Neurol Sci. 2006;33:175–80.
56. Pedersen GL, Rasmussen SB, Gyllenborg J, Benedek K, Lauritzen M. Prognostic value of periodic electroencephalographic discharges for neurological patients with profound disturbances of consciousness. Clin Neurophysiol. 2013;124:44–51.
57. Hofmeijer J, Tjepkema-Cloostermans MC, van Putten MJ. Burst-suppression with identical bursts: a distinct EEG pattern with poor outcome in postanoxic coma. Clin Neurophysiol. 2014;125:947–54.
58. Yang Q, Su Y, Hussain M, Chen W, Ye H, Gao D, Tian F. Poor outcome prediction by burst suppression ratio in adults with post-anoxic coma without hypothermia. Neurol Res. 2014;36(5):453–60.
59. Sen-Gupta I, Bernstein RA, Macken MP, Schuele SU, Gerard EE. Ictal sensory periodic lateralized epileptiform discharges. Epilepsy Behav. 2011;22:796–8.
60. Pohlmann-Eden B, Hoch DB, Cochius JI, Chiappa KH. Periodic lateralized epileptiform discharges—a critical review. J Clin Neurophysiol. 1996;13:519–30.
61. Chong DJ, Hirsch LJ. Which EEG patterns warrant treatment in the critically ill? Reviewing the evidence for treatment of periodic epileptiform discharges and related patterns. J Clin Neurophysiol. 2005;22:79–91.
62. Fitzpatrick W, Lowry N. PLEDs: clinical correlates. Can J Neurol Sci. 2007;34:443–50.
63. Hirsch LJ, LaRoche SM, Gaspard N, et al. American Clinical Neurophysiology Society's Standardized Critical Care EEG Terminology: 2012 version. J Clin Neurophysiol. 2013;30:1–27.
64. Husain AM, Mebust KA, Radtke RA. Generalized periodic epileptiform discharges: etiologies, relationship to status epilepticus, and prognosis. J Clin Neurophysiol. 1999;16:51–8.
65. Meierkord H, Holtkamp M. Non-convulsive status epilepticus in adults: clinical forms and treatment. Lancet Neurol. 2007;6:329–39.
66. Bearden S, Eisenschenk S, Uthman B. Diagnosis of nonconvulsive status epilepticus (NCSE) in adults with altered mental status: clinico-electroencephalographic considerations. Am J Electroneurodiagnostic Technol. 2008;48:11–37.
67. Claassen J, Mayer SA, Kowalski RG, Emerson RG, Hirsch LJ. Detection of electrographic seizures with continuous EEG monitoring in critically ill patients. Neurology. 2004;62:1743–8.
68. Shafi MM, Westover MB, Cole AJ, Kilbride RD, Hoch DB, Cash SS. Absence of early epileptiform abnormalities predicts lack of seizures on continuous EEG. Neurology. 2012;79:1796–801.
69. Scheltens-de BM. Guidelines for EEG in encephalopathy related to ESES/CSWS in children. Epilepsia. 2009;50(Suppl 7):13–7.
70. Gencpinar P, Dundar NO, Tekgul H. Electrical status epilepticus in sleep (ESES)/continuous spikes and waves during slow sleep (CSWS) syndrome in children: an electroclinical evaluation according to the EEG patterns. Epilepsy Behav. 2016;61:107–11.

71. Fernandez IS, Chapman KE, Peters JM, et al. The tower of Babel: survey on concepts and terminology in electrical status epilepticus in sleep and continuous spikes and waves during sleep in North America. Epilepsia. 2013;54:741–50.
72. Janszky J, Woermann FG, Barsi P, Schulz R, Halasz P, Ebner A. Right hippocampal sclerosis is more common than left after febrile seizures. Neurology. 2003;60:1209–10.
73. Spooner CG, Berkovic SF, Mitchell LA, Wrennall JA, Harvey AS. New-onset temporal lobe epilepsy in children: lesion on MRI predicts poor seizure outcome. Neurology. 2006;67:2147–53.
74. Shinnar S. Febrile seizures and mesial temporal sclerosis. Epilepsy Curr. 2003;3:115–8.
75. Sanchez J, Centanaro M, Solis J, Delgado F, Yepez L. Factors predicting the outcome following medical treatment of mesial temporal epilepsy with hippocampal sclerosis. Seizure. 2014;23: 448–53.
76. Nordli DR Jr, Moshe SL, Shinnar S, et al. Acute EEG findings in children with febrile status epilepticus: results of the FEBSTAT study. Neurology. 2012;79:2180–6.
77. Shinnar S, Bello JA, Chan S, et al. MRI abnormalities following febrile status epilepticus in children: the FEBSTAT study. Neurology. 2012;79:871–7.
78. Dube CM, Ravizza T, Hamamura M, et al. Epileptogenesis provoked by prolonged experimental febrile seizures: mechanisms and biomarkers. J Neurosci. 2010;30:7484–94.
79. Shorvon S, Ferlisi M. The treatment of super-refractory status epilepticus: a critical review of available therapies and a clinical treatment protocol. Brain. 2011;134:2802–18.
80. Mayer SA, Claassen J, Lokin J, Mendelsohn F, Dennis LJ, Fitzsimmons BF. Refractory status epilepticus: frequency, risk factors, and impact on outcome. Arch Neurol. 2002;59:205–10.
81. Drislane FW, Lopez MR, Blum AS, Schomer DL. Detection and treatment of refractory status epilepticus in the intensive care unit. J Clin Neurophysiol. 2008;25:181–6.
82. Kapur J, Macdonald RL. Rapid seizure-induced reduction of benzodiazepine and Zn2+ sensitivity of hippocampal dentate granule cell GABAA receptors. J Neurosci. 1997;17:7532–40.
83. Alroughani R, Javidan M, Qasem A, Alotaibi N. Nonconvulsive status epilepticus; the rate of occurrence in a general hospital. Seizure. 2009;18:38–42.
84. Thomke F, Weilemann SL. Poor prognosis despite successful treatment of postanoxic generalized myoclonus. Neurology. 2010;74:1392–4.
85. Holtkamp M, Othman J, Buchheim K, Meierkord H. Predictors and prognosis of refractory status epilepticus treated in a neurological intensive care unit. J Neurol Neurosurg Psychiatry. 2005;76: 534–9.
86. Rossetti AO, Logroscino G, Bromfield EB. Refractory status epilepticus: effect of treatment aggressiveness on prognosis. Arch Neurol. 2005;62:1698–702.
87. Su YY, Wang M, Feng HH, et al. An overview of neurocritical care in China: a nationwide survey. Chin Med J. 2013;126:3422–6.
88. Meldrum BS. Anatomy, physiology, and pathology of epilepsy. Lancet. 1990;336:231–4.
89. Kalviainen R, Eriksson K, Parviainen I. Refractory generalised convulsive status epilepticus : a guide to treatment. CNS Drugs. 2005;19:759–68.
90. Hocker S, Tatum WO, LaRoche S, Freeman WD. Refractory and super-refractory status epilepticus—an update. Curr Neurol Neurosci Rep. 2014;14:452.
91. Jordan KG, Hirsch LJ. In nonconvulsive status epilepticus (NCSE), treat to burst-suppression: pro and con. Epilepsia. 2006;47(Suppl 1):41–5.
92. Musialowicz T, Mervaala E, Kalviainen R, Uusaro A, Ruokonen E, Parviainen I. Can BIS monitoring be used to assess the depth of propofol anesthesia in the treatment of refractory status epilepticus? Epilepsia. 2010;51:1580–6.
93. Parviainen I, Uusaro A, Kalviainen R, Mervaala E, Ruokonen E. Propofol in the treatment of refractory status epilepticus. Intensive Care Med. 2006;32:1075–9.
94. Claassen J, Hirsch LJ, Emerson RG, Bates JE, Thompson TB, Mayer SA. Continuous EEG monitoring and midazolam infusion for refractory nonconvulsive status epilepticus. Neurology. 2001;57:1036–42.
95. Thompson SA, Hantus S. Highly epileptiform bursts are associated with seizure recurrence. J Clin Neurophysiol. 2016;33:66–71.
96. Rossetti AO, Milligan TA, Vulliemoz S, Michaelides C, Bertschi M, Lee JW. A randomized trial for the treatment of refractory status epilepticus. Neurocrit Care. 2011;14:4–10.
97. Johnson EL, Martinez NC, Ritzl EK. EEG characteristics of successful burst suppression for refractory status epilepticus. Neurocrit Care. 2016;25(3):407–14.
98. Kang BS, Jung KH, Shin JW, et al. Induction of burst suppression or coma using intravenous anesthetics in refractory status epilepticus. J Clin Neurosci. 2015;22:854–8.
99. Lowenstein DH, Alldredge BK. Status epilepticus at an urban public hospital in the 1980s. Neurology. 1993;43:483–8.
100. Koubeissi M, Alshekhlee A. In-hospital mortality of generalized convulsive status epilepticus: a large US sample. Neurology. 2007;69:886–93.
101. Leitinger M, Kalss G, Rohracher A, et al. Predicting outcome of status epilepticus. Epilepsy Behav. 2015;49:126–30.
102. Kalita J, Misra UK, Patel R. Initial EEG in status epilepticus is helpful in predicting seizure recurrence. Electromyogr Clin Neurophysiol. 2006;46: 139–44.
103. Jaitly R, Sgro JA, Towne AR, Ko D, DeLorenzo RJ. Prognostic value of EEG monitoring after status epilepticus: a prospective adult study. J Clin Neurophysiol. 1997;14:326–34.

104. Garzon E, Fernandes RM, Sakamoto AC. Serial EEG during human status epilepticus: evidence for PLED as an ictal pattern. Neurology. 2001;57:1175–83.
105. Alvarez V, Drislane FW, Westover MB, Dworetzky BA, Lee JW. Characteristics and role in outcome prediction of continuous EEG after status epilepticus: a prospective observational cohort. Epilepsia. 2015;56:933–41.
106. Orta DS, Chiappa KH, Quiroz AZ, Costello DJ, Cole AJ. Prognostic implications of periodic epileptiform discharges. Arch Neurol. 2009;66:985–91.
107. Neligan A, Shorvon SD. Prognostic factors, morbidity and mortality in tonic-clonic status epilepticus: a review. Epilepsy Res. 2011;93:1–10.
108. Basha MM, Alqallaf A, Shah AK. Drug-induced EEG pattern predicts effectiveness of ketamine in treating refractory status epilepticus. Epilepsia. 2015;56:e44–8.
109. Milani P, Malissin I, Tran-Dinh YR, et al. Prognostic EEG patterns in patients resuscitated from cardiac arrest with particular focus on Generalized Periodic Epileptiform Discharges (GPEDs). Neurophysiol Clin. 2014;44:153–64.

Drugs Commonly Used to Treat Refractory Status Epilepticus in Clinical Practice

6

Xuefeng Wang and Shichuo Li

Abstract

Status epilepticus (SE) is an emergency condition that requires immediate treatment. Some cases of SE are resistant to traditional first-line antiepileptic drugs (AEDs), a condition that is commonly known as refractory status epilepticus (RSE). In RSE, long-duration and uninterrupted seizures can cause irreversible brain damage and have been associated with a variety of serious complications. Thus, it is vital to select rapid-onset, safe, and effective AEDs to control seizures while treating RSE. In this section, we describe seven drugs that are commonly used to treat RSE. These drugs are principally discussed with respect to their clinical pharmacokinetics and pharmacodynamics and their use in clinical practice, including routes of administration, time of onset, adverse reactions, and precautions. RSE is also known to result from a variety of causes, and alterations have been observed in neurotransmitters during its different stages. Polytherapy may therefore be considered a feasible choice for treating RSE when single-drug treatment for SE fails.

X. Wang (✉)
Chongqing Key Laboratory of Neurology, Department of Neurology, The First Affiliated Hospital of Chongqing Medical University, 1 YouYi Road, Chongqing 400016, China
e-mail: xfyp@163.com

S. Li
China Association Against Epilepsy (CAAE), Rm. 5102, Building 2, Beijing Exhibition Center Hotel, 135 Xizhimenwai Avenue, Xicheng District, Beijing 100044, People's Republic of China

6.1 Midazolam

6.1.1 Clinical Pharmacokinetics and Pharmacodynamics

Midazolam (MDZ) is a water-soluble benzodiazepine which will open its imidazole ring to become hydrophilic in low-pH environment. While, in the physiological environment, it closes its imidazole ring to become lipophilic and acts quickly on the central nervous system [1, 2], MDZ is metabolized by cytochrome P450 3A (CYP3A) in the liver and intestine [3], and approximately 60–70% of them are excreted by

X. Wang, S. Li (eds.), *Refractory Status Epilepticus*, DOI 10.1007/978-981-10-5125-8_6

the kidneys. MDZ is a positive allosteric modulator of GABA-A synaptic receptors in the brain, which enhances the GABAergic inhibition, reduces the release of neurotransmitters, opens up chloride ion channels to induce chloride influx, and depolarizes the cell membrane to inhibit excessive excitement and seizures.

6.1.2 Clinical Practice

In 1983, Kaneko et al. [4] reported the clinical use of MDZ in the treatment of SE for the first time: a 14-year-old female SE patient experienced successful control of her seizures by intravenous MDZ at the dose of 15 mg after the previous failure by diazepam.

Currently, MDZ, as a clinical guideline-recommended drug for anti-SE in many countries, is known to work rapidly, potently, and safely and has been widely used as a first-line therapy for SE and for RSE after the failure of other first-line drugs [5–7]. A retrospective study of continuous intravenous MDZ (cIV-MDZ) which has been used on 33 patients with refractory nonconvulsive status epilepticus (NCSE) (17 patients had generalized convulsive status epilepticus (GCSE), 16 had NCSE, and all patients were in NCSE at the time cIV-MDZ started) showed that the mean duration of cIV-MDZ therapy was 4.2 ± 3.3 days, the mean loading dose was 0.19 ± 0.09 mg/kg, and the mean infusion rate was 0.08–0.22 mg/kg/h. Eighty-two percent (27/33) of episodes were terminated within 60 min, 57.6% (19/33) recurred within 48 h after withdrawal, and 6% ultimately were failed [8]. In an open prospective study, Ulvi et al. [9] reported that 19 patients (mean age: 40.4 years) with refractory generalized convulsive status epilepticus (RGCSE) whose episodes were not controlled by diazepam, phenytoin, or phenobarbital (PB) were administered with intravenous MDZ. In 94.7% (18/19) of patients, seizures were completely controlled; and 21% (4/19) had a slightly increase in pharyngeal secretions. No patient experienced significant change in heart rate, blood pressure, or oxygen saturation. The mean time to full consciousness after stopping MDZ was 1.6 h (range: 2.0–8.5 h) for all patients. In 2012, Ferlisi et al. [10] conducted a review about therapy outcome in refractory and super-refractory status epilepticus (SRSE). In the report, 585 patients were treated with MDZ infusions (with the doses varying from 0.02 to 1.8 mg/kg/h). The rate of initial control was 78%, and only 0.3% of patients experienced withdrawal seizures. Ninety-three percent of patients reported regaining control among those patients whose episodes occurred upon tapering or withdrawal and who accepted MDZ re-treatment.

Due to the elevated efficacy and safety, MDZ might be a better choice compared to other anti-SE drugs. In a retrospective review, 20 RSE patients treated with MDZ or propofol were included [11]. Similar efficiency was observed between the two drugs (MDZ vs. propofol, 67% vs. 64%, $p \geq 0.61$). However, the mortality of the patients with APACHE II scores higher than 20 was lower in the MDZ group than that in the propofol group ($p = 0.05$). A prospective randomized study reviewed the efficacy of MDZ ($n = 54$), propofol ($n = 33$), and pentobarbital ($n = 106$) in 193 patients with RSE [12]. The rate of failed seizure suppression in the MDZ group was higher than that in pentobarbital (20% vs. 8%, $p < 0.01$, 6 h after administration), but hypotension was lower (30% vs. 77%, $p < 0.001$). Singhi et al. [13] evaluated the efficacy and prognosis of MDZ and diazepam in a clinical randomized controlled trial (RCT). Forty RSE patients were enrolled with ages ranging 2–12 years including 21 patients who received MDZ and 19 who received diazepam. There was no significant difference between the two drugs regarding the response rate (85.7% vs. 89.5%), time from therapy to seizure suppression (both means: 16 min), and recurrence rate after withdrawal (19% vs. 16%). The proportion of intubation or mechanical ventilation was similar; however, there was a shorter time of required mechanical ventilation in the MDZ group: 19.7 ± 15.9 h vs. 93.5 ± 78.1 h, $p < 0.005$.

The clinical and experimental data show that seizures may bring immediate and long-term adverse effects to immature brains and brains in development, and the mortality and incidence rate of children's SE are very high [14]. Therefore, children's SE requires timely and rational treatment. MDZ is also applicable in the treatment of children with RSE. Ozdemir et al. [15] included 27 patients (ages 5.1 ± 3.5 years) in a study wherein he gave each a bolus of 0.2 mg/kg MDZ intravenously followed by cIV-MDZ at 1–5 μg/kg/min (average: 3.1 μg/kg/min). Ninety-six percent (26/27) of the children returned to normal, without respiratory depression, hypotension, bradycardia, or other adverse events. In the course of medical treatment, serum electrolytes and blood glucose stayed within a normal range. Only one patient's SE failed to be controlled, which was considered to be related to etiology (acute meningoencephalitis). In another study including 17 children with RSE (mean age: 3.5 years), intravenous MDZ was administered after first-line treatment (including MDZ and other drugs) failed to control seizures. Fifteen episodes were terminated at an average time of 0.3 h (0.1–1.5 h), and the median of the peak infusion rates was 4 μg/kg/min (mean: 8.7 μg/kg/min, 2–32 μg/kg/min). No patient experienced significant adverse event [16].

In addition to treating RSE secondary to infection, trauma, or unexplained etiologies, MDZ still has a therapeutic effect for some other etiologies of RSE. Bello-Espinosa et al. [17] reported on a child with Sturge-Weber syndrome with infraslow SE. Fosphenytoin, PB, lorazepam (LZP), and valproate were ineffective for 48 h; then, MDZ was administered intravenously at 240 μg/kg/h. The seizure was quickly controlled, and no significant sequelae remained. Another 18-year-old patient was suffering from SE caused by carbamazepine overdose. A bolus of 14 mg of MDZ followed by 2 mg/h continuous intravenous maintenance was given after PB, phenytoin, diazepam, and other ineffective treatments. Seizures gradually decreased and then stopped [18].

6.1.3 Administration and Time of Onset

MDZ can be administered via intravenous, oral, buccal, intranasal, and intramuscular routes. Among them, continuous intravenous infusion is often used to treat RSE. In Status Epilepticus Guideline Writing (2012) [19], the Neurocritical Care Society recommended intravenous MDZ with an initial loading dose of 0.2 mg/kg via injection (at a speed of 2 mg/min), followed by 0.05–2 mg/kg/h continuous intravenous infusion, gradually adjusting the dosage according to its success at controlling symptoms. To test the efficacy of MDZ as an anticonvulsant drug, Galcin et al. [20] treated 12 tonic–clonic SE patients with intravenous MDZ 3.0–15.0 mg which rapidly terminated all seizures in 1 min without obvious cardiopulmonary inhibition. In a systematic review, a total of nine studies were included, involving 521 RSE patients with two or three types of anticonvulsant drugs to which they were resistant. The patients received intravenous MDZ therapy (an initial dose of 0.15–0.5 mg/kg injection, then a 1–2 μg/kg/min continuous infusion, adjusted according to the symptoms, with a maximum rate of up to 5–24 μg/kg/min), and the efficacy was 76% (396/521) [21]. In response to the recommended dose, some scholars have advocated a higher one. Fernandez et al. [22] found that higher doses of MDZ (0.4 mg/kg/h or more) compared to smaller doses (0.2 mg/kg/h) yielded lower recurrence (15% vs. 64%) at 48 h after discontinuation, lower mortality (40% vs. 62%), and lower rate of tracheotomy (48% vs. 59%), but a higher proportion of cases relying on pharmacotherapeutic blood pressure support (53% vs. 32%).

Intravenous MDZ acts quickly, usually in seconds to 45 min. Parent et al. [23] reported a 64-year-old patient with SE secondary to hyperosmosis. After ineffective PB, phenytoin, and LZP treatment, injection of MDZ 17 mg (220 μg/kg) was given and continued with a rate of 1.0 μg/kg/min infusion. The seizures stopped within 90 s. In a study by Singhi et al. [13], 21 patients with RSE (2–12 years of age) underwent MDZ treatment (viz., a loading dose of 0.2 mg/kg, sustained 2.0 μg/kg/min infusion, gradually increased, with the highest of 10.0 μg/kg/min). The effective rate was 85.7%, and the average time from administration to termination was 16 min. Ulvi et al. [9] gave the RGCSE patients a 0.2 mg/kg MDZ injection, followed by continuous infusion, starting at 1 μg/kg/min and gradually increasing to an average of 8 μg/kg/min (3–21 μg/kg/min). The episodes of 18 patients were controlled within 45 min (5–120 min), on average.

6.1.4 Adverse Reaction and Precaution

The most common adverse effects of MDZ are short-term dizziness and drowsiness [24] and, more rarely, euphoria, diplopia, and blurred vision [25]. Furthermore, a larger dose of intravenous MDZ may lead to a decrease in consciousness, hypotension, respiratory depression, or acute, even life-threatening, respiratory distress syndrome [8, 26]. In addition, there was a case of metabolic acidosis induced by intravenous MDZ. A 9-year-old SE girl was given continuous infusion of MDZ from 15 μg/kg/min, gradually increasing to 200 μg/kg/min. Forty-eight hours later, intense hyperchloremic and non-anion gap metabolic acidosis occurred, which was minimally corrected by carbonate. Moreover, arterial blood pH reached as low as 7.16, and serum osmotic pressure, level of lactate, serum creatinine, and urea nitrogen were abnormal. Then, MDZ was discontinued after 81 h of treatment. Less than 5 h later, the patient's metabolic acidosis was corrected, and the administration of vasopressor drugs and positive inotropic agents was also been ceased [27].

Tachyphylaxis was observed in cIV-MDZ after treatment for 24–48 h, and its rate of occurrence approached 38% [26, 28]. This forced a constant increase in dose over the course of controlling seizures. At the same time, there was a cumulative effect of the drug, especially in critically ill patients and those with liver or kidney dysfunction; thus, monitoring of vital signs was necessary.

After the seizures have been controlled for 12 h, withdrawal should be considered. MDZ should be reduced slowly until discontinuation over the next 12 h [29]. If the seizure recurs, another 12-h medication cycle should be given, and the reduction be repeated then. Acute or rapid withdrawal may lead to a withdrawal response. According to some reports in the literature, 17% of children in ICUs experienced withdrawal reactions due upon stopping MDZ treatment too rapidly after long-term sedation [30]. Common symptoms of withdrawal responses include anxiety, irritability, diaphoresis, fasciculation, tremor, and so on. Epstein et al. [31] reported on a 4-year-old NCSE child who was administered with large doses of MDZ (cumulative dose: 26 mg/kg), fentanyl, and morphine. After the drugs were discontinued over 12 h, she experienced a sustained mania, disordered periods of sleep, intermittent visual hallucinations, orofacial dyskinesia, and somatic myoclonic jerks. Electroencephalogram (EEG) suggested diffused slow and triphasic waves, while the magnetic resonance and cerebrospinal fluid examination results revealed negative. Without any specific interventions, the patient recovered gradually in 4–5 days after the onset of reactions, leaving no neurological sequelae.

6.2 Propofol

6.2.1 Clinical Pharmacokinetics and Pharmacodynamics

Propofol, having the chemical name 2,6-diisopropylphenol, is an alkyl acid used as a short-acting intravenous anesthetic; the agent is lipophilic at room temperature and is insoluble in water. Its half-life is 1.8–8.3 min. It can be distributed throughout the body quickly after intravenous injection; it induces anesthesia within 40 s and produces a rapid and steady anesthetic effect. It is mainly combined with glucuronic acid during liver metabolism, and its metabolites are excreted in the urine. Recovery from propofol is also rapid, at approximately 8 min, even in the case of extended use. Propofol, as an inhibitor of the central nervous system, can directly activate GABA-A receptors and inhibit the expression of *N*-methyl-D-aspartic acid receptors (NMDARs) [32], as well as adjust the influx of calcium ions through slow calcium channels.

6.2.2 Clinical Practice

Since Wood et al. [33] reported the first intravenous injection of propofol in SE treatment in 1988, propofol has been widely used in clinical practice.

Propofol is a reasonable choice when first-line AEDs are ineffective. Langer et al. [34] conducted a study on the treatment of GCSE and observed seizure termination, intubation rate, and mortality rate after drug therapy. It was found that among the 177 GCSE seizures, the most commonly used first-line, second-line, and third-line therapies were benzodiazepines, phenytoin, and propofol, respectively. The therapeutic effective rate of the first-line drug is 56%. Three quarters of the patients who were irresponsive to the first-line drug were responsive to the third-line drugs such as propofol. Melloni et al. [35] reported three cases of SE who were nonresponsive to the first-line anti-SE drug, but their SE seizures and EEG abnormal activities were rapidly controlled after continuous intravenous injection of propofol [3–6 mg/(kg·h)]. After 7 days of intravenous propofol injection, the patient woke up rapidly without sequelae. Rossetti et al. [36] believes that it is necessary to use intravenous anesthesia drugs such as propofol, thiopental, and MDZ, among other AEDs, to treat SE resistant to diazepam and other AEDs, and these drugs can control SE effectively.

Propofol is a commonly used drug for the treatment of RSE [28, 37–39]. Rossetti et al. [36] have retrospectively analyzed therapy in 27 adult patients with RSE (31 seizures) in the intensive care unit of an internal medicine section of the hospital during years 1997 to 2002. After the use of propofol, 21 (67%) seizures were controlled successfully; another three (10%) were also controlled after the subsequent usage of thiopental. From the author's point of view, propofol may be a valuable drug under this condition. In recent years, different views on the efficacy and safety of propofol in treating RSE have been revealed. Power et al. [40] retrospectively analyzed the status of 18 patients with RSE (27 seizures) who accepted propofol treatment in the intensive care unit during 2001 to 2010. The average dose of propofol used for those patients was 7885.1 mg, and the average duration was 34.4 h. Complications occurred in 17 episodes of RSE. The most common complication was pneumonia (9/27), and one patient presented propofol infusion syndrome (PRIS). Eight patients exhibited no sequelae after 14 episodes of RSE, minor sequelae were observed in 7 seizures, severe sequelae were observed in four seizures, and two patients died. The study supports the use of propofol as an effective drug for the treatment of RSE, but it should be noted that PRIS may occur if propofol usage lasts for more than 48 h. Rossetti et al. [36] found that in 20 seizures of the surviving RSE patients treated with propofol, chills, short-term dystonia, and hyperlipidemia occurred after ten dosage iterations, and mild neuropsychological impairment occurred in five cases after seizure termination. Seven cases of death were not directly related to propofol usage. Niermeijer et al. [41] also reported that several guidelines recommended the use of propofol in the treatment of RSE, but after the large-dose and extended course coupled with the use of propofol, the patient's mortality increased. Subsequently, the authors assessed the relevant literature on the efficacy and safety of propofol in the treatment of RSE. Through a Medline search, 22 reports about the use of propofol for RSE treatment were found, and there was no randomized clinical trial. Two nonrandomized studies were conducted to compare the effects of propofol with those of barbiturates and MDZ. Both of these two studies reported high risk of death from propofol. In addition, several fatal cases were reported in case reports, and a case analysis of the use of propofol as an anesthetic or sedative drug for children and adults was developed, which indicated the need to reevaluate the safety of propofol in the treatment of RSE.

The European Federation of Neurological Societies (EFNS) emphasized that achieving a burst suppression pattern for at least 24 h on EEG is the important indicator of therapeutic success in RSE treatment. Parviainen et al. [42] reported on the results of a prospective study of ten RSE cases treated with propofol and found that the drug's usage could rapidly terminate clinical seizures as well as electrophysiological seizures; however, it was necessary to increase the propofol dosage to maintain the burst suppression EEG pattern. It was considered that it was not easy to maintain a burst suppression EEG pattern without the use of a large dosage of propofol; as such, it is emphasized that the gradual increase of a propofol dosage should be conducted under continuous EEG monitoring. However, Kang et al. [43] retrospectively analyzed the effect of EEG burst suppression (induced by intravenous injection of anesthetic drugs) on the prognosis of 22 cases with RSE, among whom three were treated with MDZ and propofol, one was treated with MDZ and phenobarbital, and the others were treated with MDZ. It was found that burst suppression induced by treating RSE with intravenous anesthesia could not alter the mortality and prognosis of RSE but could increase the duration of hospitalization.

Propofol can also be used in the treatment of SRSE. Sabharwal et al. [44] retrospectively analyzed 67 cases with SRSE, who were treated with propofol and ketamine (KE) used in combination for 1–28 days (mean: 3.6 days) with a dosage up to 145 and 175 mg/kg/min. Fifty-three patients used hypertensor, 48 of which were administered within 5 days after being admitted into the ICU. The overall remission rate of SRSE was 91%, and the total mortality rate was 39% (including patients with hypoxic brain injury). Of these, 13 patients with SRSE had hypoxic brain damage, and five cases of SRSE were controlled. A study by Höfler et al. [45] found similar results overall. In their retrospective study, 40% (17/42) of patients with SRSE received propofol treatment, among whom 65% (11/17) used propofol in the 12–72 h prior to KE usage (seizures were controlled for all these patients), and 35% (6/17) used propofol and KE simultaneously (SE ceased in 4/6 of patients, and propofol dosage was 2–6 mg/kg/h.)

In SE treatment guidelines, EFNS noted that anesthesia drugs should not be used in refractory complex partial SE [46]. Rossetti [36] noted that intravenous anesthetics had poor therapeutic effects on complex partial SE or absence SE. However, Begemann et al. [47] reported one case with refractory complex partial SE: a 65-year-old female patient with subarachnoid and intracerebral hemorrhage secondary to ruptured anterior communicating artery aneurysm; moreover, she had phenytoin, phenobarbital, valproate, and LZP resistance. Her EEG pattern showed burst suppression after continuous propofol injection for 7 days: seizures ceased, and the patient regained consciousness. Despite some complications, the patient gradually returned to normal and was discharged 4 months after surgery. The authors believed that this was the first case of a successful therapeutic usage of propofol in the treatment of a NCSE.

The Italian Association Against Epilepsy recommended that continuous intravenous injection of thiopental, MDZ, and propofol could be used for children with RSE to suppress EEG burst and epileptic seizures [48]. Van Gestel et al. [49] evaluated the efficacy and safety of propofol and thiopental in the treatment of children with RSE and found that thiopental was effective for most patients (34 seizures), but with serious side effects; propofol was also effective, and its side effects were unusual—and very light and reversible. The author suggested a preferable use of propofol prior to thiopental usage. However, a survey on experts of SE treatment found that physicians often used MDZ and propofol for adults with RSE, while they were less likely to choose propofol for children patients [50]. Hubert et al. [14] found that in the treatment of infants and children with convulsive status epilepticus (CSE), the efficacy/risk ratio does not support the use of propofol in children for RSE resistant to benzodiazepines, phenytoin, or phenobarbital. Many pediatricians tend to use large doses of MDZ instead of propofol; however, Tully et al. [51] reported that thiopental was commonly used in children with RSE in the PICU (65.6%), whereas propofol was only used in 4% of patients. The study was supported by research from Moreno-Medinilla et al. [52], who retrospectively analyzed 39 children with SE with an average age of 4.8 years and a total of 51 seizures. Among the patients, ten patients needed third-line drugs, and

MDZ was the most commonly used drug in this center, followed by thiopental and propofol.

Compared with other AEDs, the efficacy of propofol is controversial. Propofol and thiopental are two drugs commonly used in the treatment of RSE, and Prabhakar et al. [53] conducted a literature review of the two drugs in the treatment of RSE. The search of multiple databases found only one small-scale, single-blind, multicenter trial [54, 55]. The trial ended 3 years after starting and enrolled 24 patients, 14 of whom were treated with propofol and nine with phenobarbital (including thiopental sodium and phenobarbital). The trial compared the efficacy and side effects, as well as short-term and long-term prognoses of these two types of drugs for RSE treatment, and found that the mechanical ventilation time in patients treated with barbiturates was longer than patients treated with propofol and that there was no significant difference in a 3-month prognosis (such as seizure control and functional prognosis). The side effects of the drugs were infection, hypotension, and intestinal ischemia. The authors noted that there was still a lack of a strong RCT comparing the efficacy of both drugs in the treatment of RSE, and as such, a large-scale RCT was needed to verify efficacy. In a literature review, Parviainen et al. [56] discussed the state of propofol and barbiturate usage in RSE treatment. Their team found that the use of propofol in the treatment of RSE had increased because it could quickly terminate the clinical seizures and EEG epileptic discharges in patients with epilepsy. However, 19–33% of the patients had SE recurrence, especially when the drug dose was reduced. The advantage of barbiturate treatment was that the frequency of short-term treatment failure was very low, but its long-term use could lead to prolonged mechanical ventilation, intensive care, and hospital stay. The use of large doses of propofol infusion should be limited to 48 h, and relevant personnel should always pay attention to the risk of intravenous propofol syndrome; high doses of barbiturates can effectively terminate seizures, but recovery to consciousness needs some time after anesthesia, which has led to prolonged ventilation and intensive care. Prasad et al. [11] explored the differences in efficacy between propofol and MDZ in RSE treatment. By reviewing the chart documentation of patients with RSE treated between 1995 and 1999, it was found that in the initial treatment, 14 patients were treated with propofol and 6 patients were treated with MDZ. Propofol and MDZ, respectively, controlled 64% and 67% of the clinical seizures and 78% and 67% of the EEG seizures. There was no significant difference, but the overall mortality rate (57%) of propofol was higher than that of MDZ (17%) ($P = 0.16$). According to the APACHE II (Acute Physiology and Chronic Health Evaluation II) score evaluation, except for the fact that APACHE scores of patients treated with propofol were greater than or equal to 20, a comparison of mortality between the propofol and MDZ subgroups showed no significant difference. It was noted that in the small sample study of RSE patients, there was no difference between the use of propofol and MDZ for clinical and EEG seizure control. In RSE patients with APACHE II scores greater than or equal to 20, the survival rate of RSE patients using MDZ may be higher than those using propofol.

6.2.3 Administration and Time of Onset

The treatment of RSE requires continuous intravenous injection of propofol. It was advocated that the first dosage should be 2 mg/kg IV bolus and then 3–6 mg/(kg·h) for intravenous maintenance therapy [35]. The median of propofol injection rate should be 4.8 mg/(kg·h) [2.1–13 mg/(kg·h)] [36], and the average duration for propofol usage was 34.4 h–7 days [35, 40]. Studies have also shown that the median of usage time is 63 h (2–391 h) or 3 days (1–9 days) [36, 57]. The maximum accumulated dose for the treatment process was 7885.1–12,750 mg [40, 57], and the time required for propofol usage from the start of treatment to RSE being controlled was 2.6 min [58]. The effective rate for seizure control of propofol was 63–100% [35, 36, 58].

Combination therapy of propofol and KE could be used to treat SRSE. Combined administration should last for 1–28 days (3.6 days at average), and the infusion rates should be 145 and 175 μg/kg/min, yielding a total remission rate of SRSE of 91% [44]. Studies have also shown that [45] the use of propofol 12–72 h prior to the use of KE could control all seizures of SRSE patients, whereas the SRSE remission rate for the simultaneous use of propofol and KE (the median of administration duration at 4 days) was approximately 66%.

There is a case report on the successful treatment of refractory NCSE by propofol. Propofol 1 mg/kg was administered by intravenous injection and continued with infusion at 5 μg/kg/min. Continuous electroencephalogram (cEEG) monitoring was provided, and the speed of infusion increased to 110 μg/kg/min until burst suppression. Drug withdrawal was carried out after continuous intravenous injection of propofol for 7 days [47].

The onset time of propofol is rapid. In the study of propofol in the treatment of 16 patients with RSE, Stecker et al. [58] found that seizures in 63% of patients were controlled after propofol usage, and therapeutic effect of propofol was slightly worse than that of barbiturates (at 82%), but with no significant difference. From the start of the treatment until RSE was controlled, the time required for a large-dose intravenous injection of barbiturate (123 min) was longer than that for propofol (2.6 min). The authors believed that propofol could terminate the attack quickly and effectively if used appropriately. However, it was not effective for all RSE patients, and patients who were irresponsive to propofol still needed other drugs to control their seizures.

6.2.4 Adverse Reaction and Precaution

Propofol has the advantages of rapid onset, short duration, rapid and stable awakening, and fewer adverse reactions, but it has a marked impact on the central nervous system, cardiovascular system, and respiratory system. Mäkelä et al. [59] reported five cases of epileptic seizure induced by propofol and noted that although propofol can be used to treat SE, a possible sudden onset of epilepsy in the implementation of anesthesia should be considered, especially in patients with epilepsy. Marik et al. [60] reported that dose-dependent hypotension often occurred in treatment with propofol, especially in patients with low capacity failure. In addition, Ku et al. [61] found that in a rare case, the urine of a patient with refractory epilepsy turned dark green after propofol treatment. The shade of the urine's color depended on the propofol infusion dose. Reducing the dose of propofol could lighten the urine's color and return it to normal. This phenomenon was benign and reversible.

PRIS, a fatal complication, may occur when the dosage of propofol exceeds 4 mg/kg/h and the usage lasts for more than 48 h. PRIS accompanied with high-dose injection of propofol is a potentially fatal complication, with characteristics such as metabolic acidosis and severe circulatory failure. PRIS has 30% mortality [62] and over a 1% incidence rate [63]; its deduced risk factors include the use of high doses of propofol (>83 μg/kg/min), treatment time > 48 h, and simultaneous blood vessel pressure-raising therapy. Walli et al. [64] searched five databases and found 21 cases with PRIS: all patients had arrhythmias (100%), nine cases with rhabdomyolysis (42%), 13 (62%) cases with lactic acidosis, eight cases with renal failure (38%), seven cases with hyperlipidemia (33%), six cases with liver enzyme elevation (28%), and 13 cases with death (66%). Some scholars reported that a 17-year-old woman with RSE treated with propofol (8.8 mg/kg/h lasting for 58 h) had PRIS, and its manifestations were renal failure, severe metabolic acidosis, and rhabdomyolysis [65]. In addition, Da-Silva et al. [66] described a 4-year-old boy with malignant SE treated with propofol as the dose increased from 0.6 to 15.6 mg/kg/h, where EEG burst suppression occurred. PRIS occurred after 48 h of propofol use. In another retrospective analysis by another scholar on the prognosis of RSE when being treated by propofol, three patients in a propofol treatment group (3/31, 10%) experienced the occurrence of cardiac pulmonary sudden arrest, two of which were fatal, and 11 patients (11/31, 35%) had non-life-threatening PRIS [57].

Baumeister et al. [67] reported fatal PRIS associated with the ketogenic diet. PRIS is caused by abnormal fatty acid oxidation; therefore, a ketogenic diet and a high-fat, low-carbohydrate diet with appropriate protein diet, in addition to AEDs, can effectively reduce the seizures of RSE, but the literature has described a case of a 10-year-old boy with severe epilepsy who died from PRIS when he was on a ketogenic diet. Because the class of propofol drugs could hinder fatty acid oxidation, using it together with a ketogenic diet increases that risk.

Kumar et al. [68] found that irreversible acidosis occurred after extended injection of propofol. The authors retrospectively analyzed three cases of patients admitted to the NICU at Massachusetts General Hospital from October 2001 to September 2004: case 1 was a 27-year-old female patient with epilepsy secondary to arteriovenous malformation hemorrhage accompanied by metabolic acidosis, hypotension, and bradycardia after propofol usage, who ultimately died; case 2 was a 64-year-old male with SE who had metabolic acidosis, hypotension, and rhabdomyolysis after long-term injection of propofol, who died eventually; and case 3 was a 24-year-old female with SE secondary to encephalitis who was given propofol to control seizures; whose presentation was characterized by hypotension, metabolic acidosis, and chronic arrhythmia; and who eventually died despite transvenous pacing. These data suggest that in adult and pediatric patients, the long-term use of propofol is related to metabolic acidosis, rhabdomyolysis, and death.

Biochemical indicators should be closely monitored in the case of long-term propofol usage to quickly identify PRIS, at which point administration of the drug should be stopped immediately, and appropriate therapeutic measures should be taken. Fang et al. [69] reported that extracorporeal membrane oxygenation and sustained hemodialysis filtration could lead to successful recovery from PRIS in RSE treatment. Guitton et al. [65] used blood filtration and extracorporeal membrane oxygenation to treat PRIS, which resulted in the gradual improvement of symptoms; their patient improved in an ICU ward over 36 days and was discharge from hospital after 2 months. Some scholars have used partial exchange of blood therapy (PEBT) to treat PRIS, which improves the metabolic abnormalities and cardiac insufficiency [66]. Moreover, Mayette [70] described the occurrence of PRIS in a young female SE patient after propofol treatment, which progressed to refractory cardiac arrest. Extracorporeal pulmonary membrane oxygenation was enabled during cardiopulmonary resuscitation, and her heartbeat recovered after cardiac arrest for more than 8 h. The patient was finally discharged with improved prognosis. Similarly, Levin et al. [71] also reported a 16-year-old patient with SE accompanied by head injury who had PRIS manifestations such as severe lactic acidosis, rhabdomyolysis, and hemodynamic disorder and who recovered completely after plasma exchange treatment. In conclusion, renal replacement therapy, blood exchange, and extracorporeal pulmonary membrane oxygenation appear to be promising approaches for the treatment of PRIS.

In patients treated with propofol, withdrawal-related "seizures" should be noted. Zubair et al. [72] reported a case in which an SE patient who was successfully treated with propofol experienced convulsive seizures upon each drug withdrawal, despite EEG monitoring finding no abnormal discharge. Therefore, propofol treatment was ceased; seizure occurrence gradually reduced and disappeared. The author noted that seizure EEGs related to propofol withdrawal were in essence not seizures, so there would be no need for further propofol treatment. However, Bhatt et al. [73] found that five patients receiving phenobarbital and propofol to treat intracranial hypertension, encephalopathy, and RSE showed generalized periodic discharges related to anesthetic withdrawal (GRAW). The anesthetic withdrawal was carried out 24–48 h after EEG burst suppression, and all patients showed generalized periodic discharges at 1–4 Hz after drug withdrawal. Different from their previous EEG pattern, this EEG performance could remit spontaneously after 12–120 h. Because this did not constitute seizure recurrence, no treatment was needed.

6.3 Ketamine

6.3.1 Clinical Pharmacokinetics and Pharmacodynamics

KE is a water-soluble drug with a low plasma protein binding rate of approximately 10–30% [74]. The peak concentration of a single dose is reached in 20–30 min [75]. The elimination half-life period is 2–3 h, which is sooner in children by approximately 100 min [76]. KE is metabolized through a microsomal enzyme system. It is mainly oxidized into norketamine, a component with pharmacological action, and KE is primarily excreted via bile and urine.

KE has both anticonvulsant and neuroprotective effects. The possible mechanism of KE on anticonvulsion is as follows. As a noncompetitive antagonist of NMDAR, KE can reduce the epileptiform discharges and afterpotentials by combining with the phencyclidine site that is located in the inner side of the cation channel, thus inhibiting transmission of excitatory nerve impulses and playing an antiepileptic role [77]. The neuroprotective effect of KE may be achieved through multiple approaches. The NMDAR antagonist KE not only can block the influx of Ca^{2+} but also alleviate neuroinflammation, neuronal oxidative stress, and the decrease of brain-derived neurotrophic factor (BDNF) [78–80]. Therefore, KE plays a neuroprotective role in RSE. Fujikawa [81] induced 12 rat SE models with lithium and pilocarpine; then, they were injected with saline ($n = 5$) or 100 mg/kg KE ($n = 7$) intraperitoneally after 10 min of SE onset. Three hours later, intraperitoneal injections with atropine, phenobarbital, and diazepam were initiated to terminate seizures. Then, they performed perfusion-fixation to the rat brain slices on the next day, with subsequent processing of these slices for microscopic examination. The researchers observed that 24 of 25 brain regions had suffered from neuronal injury in the saline group, whereas in the KE group, none of the brain regions were damaged in the three rats whose SEs were terminated within 30 min after KE administration. In the remaining four rats, KE also provides neuroprotection in 21 of the 24 damaged brain regions despite the pronged SE that had persisted over 90 min. Moreover, the neuroprotective effect of this drug was still present regardless of whether SE had ultimately ceased or not.

6.3.2 Clinical Practice

In 1962, KE was developed by a pharmaceutical company in the USA. Three years later, while researching electrically or chemically generated animal models of epilepsy, McCarthy [82] first discovered that KE exerts anticonvulsant effects, which was soon confirmed in patients [83], raising the possibility of treating SE using KE. However, this possibility was later questioned by Kayama et al. [84]. Through their animal experiments using cat models, they revealed that KE could induce epileptiform discharges in EEG recordings. However, a similar study of human volunteers carried out by Corssen et al. [85] rejected this conclusion; instead, these researchers argued that KE caused epileptic changes neither in epilepsy patients nor in normal subjects and that there was no evidence indicating that KE could exacerbate or induce convulsions.

Recently KE has been commonly used in RSE. Gaspard [86] conducted a multicenter retrospective study that included 58 RSE patients receiving intravenous KE treatment between 1999 and 2012, among whom were 46 adult patients and 12 child patients. The results indicated that among the 60 episodes of RSE that were identified, among which approximately 57% (34/60) of the seizures were ultimately resolved, 32% (19/60) considered KE to be the "likely" (7/19) or "possible" (12/19) agent responsible for gaining permanent control over the RSE. Similarly, the results of a prospective study published in 2015 [87] also approved of the possible efficacy and safety of KE in RSE treatment. This research included 13 children (0.16–11.4 years old) who experienced a total of 19 episodes of RSE from 2009 to 2015, most of which (14/19) manifested as CSE. The results indicated that the RSE resolution rate achieved 73.6% (14/19) after intravenous KE administration and that KE treatment was accompanied by no severe side effects except mildly increased saliva secretion. Additionally, KE was selected as the first anesthetic in five children when the first-line and second-line AEDs failed, and four out of the five patients avoided endotracheal intubation, which was due to KE's minimal influence on cardiopulmonary function.

In 2003, Mewasingh [88] reported six cases of RSE in children manifesting NCSE; oral KE administration was initiated after the seizures had continued for approximately 4.4 weeks (2–10 weeks) despite the use of many anticonvulsants, and the results showed that all of the seizures were controlled within 24–48 h after KE initiation, no matter their clinical manifestations or epileptiform discharges. Although one of the patients suffered a relapse a few months later, oral KE was still effective in NCSE treatment, and no significant adverse reactions were recorded during KE administration.

In addition, in Tables 6.1 and 6.2, we have summarized the studies of KE in RSE treatment over the most recent 2 years, and more reports that were published from 1996 to 2014 about this topic were also summarized in a review [89]. From the results of all the published reports stated above, we can draw a conclusion that KE treatment is primarily suitable for RSE and SRSE. This conclusion is also supported by the animal experiment ($n = 4$) of Borris [90], who found that if KE was initiated after 15 min of SE, none of the seizures could be resolved, but when KE administration was selected 1 h after stimulation, the seizure resolution rate was 100%; thereafter, correspondingly increasing the dosages of KE continued to be effective within a certain period despite a prolonged SE.

KE is primarily suitable for the treatment of RSE and SRSE during prolonged seizures, but the specific timing of KE administration is still controversial. According to the results of some past successful studies [45, 86, 91–93], we concluded that KE might be suitable for RSEs that have been resistant to five to six AEDs, which is coincident with the gradual downregulation of GABA-A receptors and upregulation of NMDARs [94–98]. However, some scholars have recommended that KE should be considered even earlier—just after the failure of those commonly used first-line and second-line AEDs, including sodium-channel inhibitors and γ-aminobutyric acid (GABA) receptor antagonists [44, 87, 99], for the purpose of achieving earlier control of seizures to relieve the neuronal injuries and endotracheal intubation ratios that would occur during prolonged SE; however, this view still needs further confirmation.

A systematic evaluation of NMDAR antagonists for the treatment of RSE published in 2014 [101] ultimately included 23 original studies that consisted of 52 children (range: 2 months–18 years old) and 110 adults (range: 19–88 years old), all of whom were RSE patients treated with KE. Finally, this evaluation revealed that KE was responsible for 56.5% (59/110) of the resolutions in adults and 63.5% (33/52) in children and that the accompanying untoward effects consisted of arrhythmia in adults (1.8%, $n = 2$) and increased saliva secretion in children (17.3%, $n = 17$). As a result, the authors deemed that there was evidence to support the relative efficacy and safety of KE for the treatment of RSE in both adults and children. However, some limitations also existed in this review, such as the small sample size of the included studies, the heterogeneous nature of the retrospective studies, the diversity of medications prior to KE, the timing of KE initiation, and the dosages and durations of this drug. Therefore, more prospective studies with larger sample sizes are warranted to further confirm the efficacy and safety of KE for the treatment of RSE.

6.3.3 Administration and Time of Onset

Intravenous administration: (a) Intravenous bolus followed by infusion: When KE is selected for adult RSE patients, the recommended average loading dose is 1.5 mg/kg, followed by continuous infusion at a median rate of 2.75 mg/kg/h, maintained for approximately 4 days (0–24 days) [86], and Gaspard [86] also summarized that the peak loading dose could reach 5 mg/kg, with a maximum infusion rate as high as 10 mg/kg/h.

Table 6.1 Demographics and clinical data of ketamine treatment in RSE

Year	Number of patients	Age (Y)	Sex	History of epilepsy	Study type	Etiologies	SE types	SE duration prior to KE	Medications prior to KE	References
2016	2	57,56	Female (2)	No	Case report	Autoimmune encephalitis, cardiac arrest	My, NC	>5d, unknown	5 (PRO, VPA, LEV, PHT, PB), 4 (MDZ, LEV, PB, VPA)	[91]
2016[a]	42	68 (59.3–72)	Male (22) Female (20)	Yes (7) No (35)	Retrospective	CNS tumor (3), CNS infection (4), cerebrovascular disease (7), epilepsy relapse (7), unknown (7), postanoxic encephalopathy (14)	My (6), NC (28), tonic–clonic (6), focal motor (20)	3d (2–6.8d)	5 (4–7) (unknown)	[45]
2015	67	58 (8–85)	Male (18) Female (49)	Unknown	Retrospective	Gene mutation (2), autoimmune disease (3), tumor (3), systemic infection (5), CNS infection (5), stroke (7), unknown (11), anoxic encephalopathy (13), metabolic/toxic encephalopathy (18)	Convulsive	1-2d	Unknown	[44]
2015	2	23, 30	Male (18)	Yes (1) No (1)	Case report	Unknown	Convulsive	1-2d	6 (DZP, PHT, MDZ, VPA,LEV, PB), 5(MDZ, PHT, VPA, LEV, CLZ)	[92]
2015	11	54 (33–68)	Male (5) Female (6)	Yes (4) No (7)	Retrospective	Cerebral hemorrhage (1), mucous cyst (1), anoxic encephalopathy (1), brain abscess (1), drugs (1), intracranial metastases (1), epidural and subdural hematoma(1, mesial temporal sclerosis (1), unknown (2), autoimmune disease (3)	NC (1), SPS (2), CPSl + SG (5), CPS (1), SG (2)	0.7-11d	1–5 (unknown)	[100]
2015	13	5 (0.17–11.5)	Male (6) Female (7)	Yes (11) No (2)	Prospective	Hemimegalencephaly (1), mitochondrial diseases (1), focal cortical dysplasia (2), Rett syndrome (1), MELAS (1), congenital malformation (1), unknown (6)	Focal (1), focal, My (3), focal, My, GC (2); focal ± SG (7)	7d (5 h-26d)	Unknown	[87]

AED antiepileptic drug, *CLB* clobazam, *CPS* complex partial seizure, *CNS* central nervous system, *d* days, *DZP* diazepam, *GC* generalized convulsive, *h* hours, *KE* ketamine, *LEV* levetiracetam, *MDZ* midazolam, *MELAS* mitochondrial encephalomyopathy, lactic acidosis, and stroke-like episodes, *My* myoclonus, *NC* nonconvulsive, *PB* phenobarbital, *PHT* phenytoin, *PRO* propofol, *SE* status epilepticus, *SG* secondary generalization, *SPS* simple partial seizure, *VPA* valproate, *w* weeks, *Y* years

[a]The drug selected was (S)-ketamine

Table 6.2 Ketamine treatment regime and efficacy

Year	Number of patients	Administration	Dosages			Duration of treatment (d)	Onset time	Time from ketamine initiation to seizure cessation	Resolution rate of seizures	Outcome	References
			Bolus (mg/kg)	Infusion (mg/kg/h)	Oral						
2016	2	IV	0, 0	0.1, 0.5	0,0	2–3, 19	12 h, Unknown	Unknown	100%	Died (1), need nursing (1)	[91]
2016[a]	42	IV	200 mg (200–250 mg) (only 7 patients)	2.39 (1.52–3.02) (all)	0	4 (2.0–6.8)	Unknown	Unknown	64%	Died (45.2%)	[45]
2015	67	IV	0	1.5–10.5	0	3.6 (1–28)	Unknown	Unknown	91%	Died (39%)	[44]
2015	2	IV	1	2,	0,0	2–3	1-2d	1-2d	100%	Died (1), rehabilitation (1)	[92]
2015	11	IV	1.1–4 (only 4 patients)	3.5 (1–5)	0	2–27	5–10 min (2),10–15 min (1),35 min (1),2.75 h (1), unknown (6)	Unknown	36%	Died (3), rehabilitation (3), recurred (2), need nursing (3)	[100]
2015	13	IV	(2–3) × 2	1.8 (0.42–3.6)	0	3 (1–17)	Unknown	Unknown	73.7%	Unknown	[87]

d day(s), *h* hour(s), *kg* kilogram, *mg* milligram, *min* minutes, *IV* intravenous
[a]The drug selected was (S)-ketamine

Additionally, Synowiec [102] revealed that if a bolus of 1–2 mg/kg KE was injected first, followed by a median infusion rate of 1.3 mg/kg/h (0.45–2.1 mg/kg/h) for approximately 9.8 days (4–28 days), all of the RSE patients (11/11) could have their seizures completely resolved. When KE is used in pediatric RSE patients, a bolus of 2–3 mg/kg KE is administered every 5 min followed by an initial infusion rate of 5–10 μg/kg/min, with a gradual increase of the infusion rate at a magnitude of 2–10 μg/kg/min every 10 min according to the changes on manifestation and EEG, and the average infusion rate is 30 μg/kg/min (7–60 μg/kg/min) [87, 93]. (b) Continuous infusion: Zelier [103] selected continuous infusion of KE at a rate of 10–40 μg/kg/min for RSE treatment, and all of the seizures (2/2) were ultimately terminated. Moreover, Basha [100] reported that when KE was initiated from 1 mg/kg/h, then gradually increased its infusion rate to 3.5 mg/kg/h (1–5 mg/kg/h), and was maintained for 2–14 days, the complete response rate could reach 57% (4/7), and in the remaining three patients who did not respond, one of them was previously controlled by KE but relapsed and was ultimately resolved through neurosurgery, and the other two died separately of sudden cardiac arrest and giving up of treatment. If infusion administration of KE is used in pediatric patients, the recommended dosage is 32.5 μg/kg/min (10–60 μg/kg/min) [104].

Until now, reports of oral KE for the treatment of RSE have been few in number and only used in NCSE, so we can only limitedly describe that the effective dosage of oral KE is 1500–2000 mg/d in adults [105]; in children, it is 1.5 mg/kg/d, administered in two divided doses [88].

From a pharmacological point of view, KE manifests the property of short onset time, which could be due to its low binding rate with plasma protein, high lipid solubility, and high permeability through the blood–brain barrier (BBB) [106]. A report by Kramer [107] supports this view insofar as the researchers immediately observed decreased seizure frequency and duration and reduced epileptiform discharge amplitude after a loading dose of 50 mg of KE followed by an initial infusion rate of 0.6 mg/kg/h, indicating a possible rapid-onset time of KE in the application of RSE treatment. Similarly, Sheth [108] also described that when KE was administered intravenously to a girl, improvement of manifestations and epileptiform discharges was observed approximately 90 s after KE administration had initiated, thereby supporting the rapid-onset property of KE in the treatment of RSE. Additionally, it was reported that most seizures were terminated within 2–3 days of KE initiation [101]. At present, cEEG is a critical tool for us to recognize whether anticonvulsants work. Basha [100] used KE to treat 11 RSE patients, among whom only four patients' seizures were ultimately terminated; coincidentally, 5–35 min after KE administration, all of the four resolved patients exhibited specific diffused θ-β rhythms (7–20 Hz) on cEEG. Therefore, the authors deemed that this specific KE-induced EEG change might be a "marker" that could help us predict the success of this drug in RSE treatment.

6.3.4 Adverse Reaction and Precaution

A systematic review conducted by Zeiler [101] indicated that the side effects related to KE use in RSE were rare, but concerns remain warranted. Herein, we have described the major adverse reactions.

Increased intracranial pressure (ICP): 40 years ago, researchers knew that KE could increase intracranial pressure through improving the brain's metabolic rate and increasing the brain blood flow [109]. However, further opinions have been prompted regarding the effect of KE on intracranial pressure, and recent studies have revealed that when RSE patients breathe spontaneously, KE increases ICP due to an elevation of $PaCO_2$ in the arteries, but when patients are sedated and breathe in the form of mechanical ventilation, the effects of KE on ICP are actually quite small [110]. Additionally, a systematic review published in 2014 indicated that when KE was administered in RSE patients without traumatic brain injuries, it would not increase ICP and might even decrease ICP under proper conditions

[111]. As a result, mechanical ventilation should be warranted during KE use, to minimize the risk of KE-induced intracranial hypertension and respiratory depression, and head CT should be performed previously to exclude the intracranial lesions that might aggravate the intracranial pressure [112, 113]. Moreover, if KE use is combined with GABA-A receptor activators for RSE treatment, its adverse effects on ICP could be diminished [114].

Psychiatric symptoms: The major psychiatric symptoms related to KE use for RSE treatment include delirium, hallucinations, and blurred vision, and the incidence rate ranges from 5 to 30%, with children being at the lowest risk [115]. These adverse reactions are easier to occur in female patients, in patients above 16 years old, or when the KE dosage or administration rate is too high [116]. A relaxing and quiet environment, slower administration rate, and gradual titration of the dose are helpful for reducing the incidence of psychiatric symptoms [110, 112]. Additionally, prophylactic administration of MDZ (3.75–7.5 mg) could reduce the severity and probability of these side effects [110].

Increased saliva secretion: The KE-induced increase of saliva secretion is common in children, and this hypersecretion of saliva, accompanied by increased secretion of bronchial mucus, might cause transient respiratory depression or apnea. Therefore, attention should be paid to monitoring respiratory status during KE administration. A slower administration rate and a gradual titration of the KE dosage can reduce the incidence of respiratory depression related to this drug [112], and prophylactic use of anticholinergic drugs, such as atropine or scopolamine, can help us to prevent this side effect [106].

Tachyarrhythmia: This adverse reaction is thought to be associated with KE-induced excitation of the sympathetic nervous system and shortening of the atrial conduction [117, 118]. Gaspard [86] and his colleagues studied the adverse reactions of 58 RSE patients who had undergone KE administration. They found that only three patients exhibited tachyarrhythmia, among whom one patient manifested as atrial fibrillation, and the other two exhibited supraventricular tachycardia; moreover, all of these arrhythmias were relieved after KE was withdrawn or after using amiodarone.

Increased intraocular pressure (IOP): The effect of KE on IOP is still controversial [115]: some researchers deem that it could increase IOP [119], but others believe that it does not affect IOP [120] or even believe that it reduces IOP [121]. This controversy may be ascribed to the multiple factors that affect IOP, such as the dynamic equilibrium of aqueous humor, blood flow of choroid, tension of extraocular muscle, and volume of vitreous body [78]. Actually, KE exerts only a trifling impact on IOP and is even weaker than the influence experienced during laryngoscopy [78]. Consequently, KE has little influence on IOP when it is administered for RSE, and when it is combined with benzodiazepines, the effect of KE on IOP could be alleviated [115].

Neurotoxicity: The influence of KE on CNS for human beings remains controversial. Twenty-five years ago, it was reported that KE exerted neurotoxic effects that could induce neuronal degeneration and even necrosis on the pallium of rats. Since then, clinicians have become more cautious when considering this drug. However, KE-induced neurotoxicity has not been fully identified in human beings [122]. Most researchers have suggested that the neurotoxicity of KE is often mild and might only be limited to children during its clinical applications, and this mild effect is thought to be associated with the short half-life of KE and the low affinity of this drug for NMDARs [123, 124]. In recent years, animal studies have implicated the neuroprotective effect of KE combined with atropine, thus reversing KE-induced neurotoxicity [125, 126].

6.4 Levetiracetam

6.4.1 Clinical Pharmacokinetics and Pharmacodynamics

Levetiracetam (LEV), a pyrrolidone derivative and piracetam analog with the trade name Keppra, is a novel broad-spectrum AED [127]. LEV is highly permeable and readily dissolvable and can reach its peak plasma concentration within 1 h. The bioavailability of LEV is 95%, which is not affected by food [128, 129]. Animal experiments show that LEV can rapidly penetrate the blood–brain barrier and is distributed into the brain tissue and cerebrospinal fluid, where its concentrations are similar to its blood drug concentration [130]. LEV has a linear pharmacokinetic profile [131, 132] and is not metabolized in the liver [133]. In addition, its hydrolytic metabolism does not rely on the hepatic cytochrome P450 enzyme system; therefore, interactions of LEV with other AEDs are rare [134]. Furthermore, the drug plasma protein binding rate is low (only 10%), 66% of LEV is renally metabolized, and the duration of action is twice the plasma half-life (6–8 h) [135]. The pharmacokinetics of the intravenous formulation are similar to those of the oral formulations [136], indicating that oral and intravenous uses of LEV are almost equivalent.

LEV can effectively reduce seizures in pilocarpine-induced and kainate-induced epileptic models, but it was devoid of anticonvulsant activity in acute maximal electroshock-kindled and pentylenetetrazole (PTZ)-kindled epileptic mice, suggesting that its mechanism may be different from traditional AEDs [137]. At present, studies suggest that LEV may exert antiepileptic effects via binding to the synaptic vesicle protein 2A (SV2A) and affecting neurotransmitter release, particularly the release of excitatory amino acids [138]. In addition, Rigo et al. [139] have found that LEV can also block the downregulation of GABA receptors in the cerebral cortex and selectively inhibit N-type high-voltage activated calcium channels in hippocampal pyramidal cells, thereby reducing the influx of calcium ions induced by excessive activation of the NMDAR. This inhibition consequently reduces conduction of excitatory nerve impulses, which exerts the antiepileptic effects. Animal experimentation has shown that during the maintenance phase of SE, LEV can reduce or terminate seizures, exhibit potent neuroprotective effects, and decrease the incidence of epilepsy after seizure [140]. Besides, the animal experiment results of Zheng et al. [141], which also support the above conclusion, further found that compared with a placebo, LEV can significantly reduce the intensity of seizure and neuronal injury induced by the episode in pilocarpine-induced animal models of SE. However, others have found that the prophylactic use of LEV after SE had no effect on epileptogenesis, neuronal damage, and behavioral changes induced by SE [142].

6.4.2 Clinical Practice

The potential anticonvulsant effect of LEV was originally discovered in animal experiments [143]. Furthermore, Klitgaard et al. [144] have found that LEV not only controls seizures but also has few effects on the normal behavior of animals even upon large doses in drug-induced epileptic models, indicating its safe and effective antiepileptic effects. In 1999, LEV was approved for the treatment of adults with partial seizures by the US Food and Drug Administration (FDA). In 2005, this drug began to be broadly used as an add-on therapy for children aged 4 years or older with partial seizures. One year later, LEV was recommended for the treatment of SE. Since then, researchers [39, 145] have also found that intravenous LEV can be a useful alternative to traditional first-line AEDs for RSE. This conclusion was supported by the European Society for Neuroscience and the Italian League Against Epilepsy [48, 146].

Oral administration of LEV is a new method of treatment for SE. Unfortunately, the majority of these studies have been retrospective. Especially rare prospective controlled trials have been conducted to evaluate the feasibility and safety of oral LEV for the treatment of RSE. Patel et al. [147] reported six patients (five adults and one adolescent) who were administered LEV via a nasogastric tube at a dosage of 500–3000 mg/day. Seizures of all patients were under control, and no significant adverse reactions were observed. Rossetti et al. [148] used nasogastric LEV at an average dose of 2000 mg (range of 750–9000 mg) to treat 23 adult patients with SE (including nine patients with RSE). Finally, remission was observed in 43% (10/23) of the patients after the treatment. Trabacca et al.

[149] reported that one 9-year-old child with refractory NCSE was given oral LEV at a dosage of 10–40 mg/(kg d) for 2 weeks, resulting in the improvement of symptoms. However, with such a long period of drug administration, seizure termination may not be an effect of drug action.

Currently, there are many reports about intravenous LEV therapy for RSE. Knake et al. [150] used intravenous LEV to treat 18 patients with benzodiazepine-resistant SE, with an average dose of 944 mg/30 min (range of 250–1500 mg/30 min) and a mean maintenance dose of 2166 mg/day. Seizure termination was observed in 16 patients. Möddel et al. [151] reported 36 RSE patients with intravenous injection or continuous infusion of LEV, at the loading dose of 500–2000 mg/30–60 min. Seizure termination was observed in 69% (25/36) of the patients, and no obvious adverse reactions occurred. Eue et al. [152] used intravenous LEV to treat 43 SE patients after ineffective treatment with benzodiazepines. Patients with NCSE and subtle SE were administered LEV as a short infusion at a dose of 1000 or 2000 mg, and in cases of CSE, a fractionated injection of 1000 or 2000 mg was used. Eventually, 44% (19/43) of the patients showed cessation of SE. Tripathi et al. [153] administered intravenous sodium valproate and LEV to treat 82 patients diagnosed with RSE. Effective control of RSE was achieved in approximately 68% of the patients in the sodium valproate group (28/41) and in 73% of those in LEV group (30/41). No severe adverse reactions occurred during the course of administration.

LEV for the treatment of RSE has been studied in specific populations. In 2009, a study of pediatric patients with RSE, NCSE, or acute recurrent seizures showed that LEV can completely abolish seizures and reduce epileptiform discharges on EEG and no significant adverse reactions were observed [154]. Kim et al. [155] retrospectively analyzed 14 pediatric patients (eight boys and six girls) with a mean age of 4.4 ± 5.5 years (range: 4 days to 14.6 years) who received intravenous LEV for the treatment of RSE. The average loading dose of LEV for intravenous infusion was 26 ± 4.6 mg/kg. Ultimately, they found that the clinical symptoms were under control in 43% (6/14) of these children. In particular, remission was observed in 57% (4/7) of the patients younger than 2 years of age, with no obvious side effects. Isguder et al. [156] used intravenous LEV to treat 46 pediatric patients with RSE, at the loading dose of 20 mg/kg; the response rate was 78.3% (36/46), and no adverse effects were observed during or after the course of the treatments. In addition, some studies have reported that LEV is also effective and safe for the treatment of electrical status epilepticus in sleep (ESES) in pediatric patients [157, 158]. Taken together, these studies demonstrate that intravenous LEV is also effective and tolerable in pediatric patients with RSE. In light of the good pharmacokinetic characteristics of LEV, the drug becomes a better option to control seizures in elderly and critically ill patients with SE, but the use of LEV for the treatment of RSE in these specific populations has rarely been reported. Bevenburg et al. [159] reported on 14 elderly patients with repeated complex partial seizures, CSE, or NCSE who were treated with intravenous LEV. The mean age of the patients was 73.9 years (range: 61–97). The average dosage of LEV was 1643 mg/d (range: 500–4000 mg/d). Treatment failure was observed in only three patients. Berning et al. [160] examined the use of LEV to treat 30 SE patients with comorbid conditions with an average age of 71 years. The average bolus dose was 2000 mg, and the median total dose was 3500 mg per day. Ultimately, the seizures were controlled in 76.7% (23/30) of the patients. Fattouch et al. [161] treated nine elderly SE patients with LEV at a loading dose of 1500 mg/100 mL/15 min and an average maintenance dose of 2500 mg/d. All of the patients presented with comorbid medical conditions (arrhythmia/respiratory distress/hepatic disease). LEV therapy resulted in control of the clinical symptoms in eight patients (including seizure termination in seven cases) and was ineffective in only one patient. In 2008, Rüegg et al. [162] administered intravenous LEV to treat 50 critically ill patients, and nearly half of these patients' conditions were characterized by myoclonic SE induced by anoxia. The initial dose was 20 mg/kg in 15 min, and the maintenance dose was 15 mg/kg. The seizure ended in

67% (16/24) of the patients. Additionally, LEV does not affect liver metabolism and has no significant interactions with other AEDs. Thus, one liver transplant patient with NCSE [163] and one patient with acute intermittent porphyria [164] achieved good results after the administration of LEV.

Yasiry et al. [165] performed a meta-analysis on the efficacy of five AEDs—LEV, phenobarbital, phenytoin, valproate, and lacosamide—for the treatment of convulsive benzodiazepine-resistant SE. Twenty-seven studies were identified, and 22 were included in the meta-analysis. Ultimately, they found that the efficacy of LEV was 68.5% (95% CI: 56.2–78.7%). Meanwhile, those of phenobarbital, phenytoin, and sodium valproate were 73.6% (95% CI: 58.3–84.8%), 50.2% (95% CI: 34.2–66.1%), and 75.7% (95% CI: 63.7–84.8%), respectively. There is not enough evidence to support the routine use of lacosamide due to insufficient data. Thus, from the above results, the author drew the conclusion that LEV could be used as an effective therapy in benzodiazepine-resistant SE. However, this study has certain limitations, such as the limited number of included prospective studies, lack of randomized double-blind controlled trials, insufficient homogeneity of the findings, and interference of benzodiazepine administration prior to LEV treatment. Therefore, additional RCTs are urgently needed to further confirm the efficacy of LEV for the treatment of RSE.

6.4.3 Administration and Time of Onset

For the treatment of RSE in adults, the initial dose is considered to be 1000–1500 mg IV at a rate of 2–5 mg/(kg min). If seizures do not stop, additional doses can be used according to EEG findings, but sustainable infusion is limited to 0.05–2 mg/(kg h), and the recommended daily dose of LEV is 1500–3000 mg [150, 166, 167]. Attention is called to the need for further investigations to confirm the regimes of LEV to treat RSE because the patient numbers of most studies are quite low. The effective dosage of RSE in the treatment of children and adolescents has not yet been unified. However, one scholar has recommended that the loading dose of intravenous LEV should be set at 20–30 mg/kg and administered over 15 min [168].

From the pharmacology point of view, LEV has high solubility and permeability, a short time to peak, and the property of penetrating the BBB rapidly. Thus, LEV can be used to treat seizures in RSE and exhibits short onset time. Patel et al. [147] successfully controlled seizures in six patients through the use of a nasogastric tube injection of LEV. The termination time of the seizure was 12–96 h. Rossetti et al. [148] reported on 23 adult patients with SE treated with nasogastric LEV. Seizure termination was observed within 72 h after the start of the treatment. Möddel et al. [151] analyzed 25 patients whose seizures were successfully controlled among 36 patients with RSE treated by intravenous LEV and found that seizure termination was observed within 3 days. Gallentine et al. [169] performed the study of 11 pediatric RSE patients who received intravenous LEV. The median time to cessation of seizures was 1.5 days after the start of the treatment. Thus, the duration from oral LEV administration to achieving seizure control was 12–96 h, and the intravenous use time of LEV for the treatment of RSE was 1–3 days.

6.4.4 Adverse Reaction and Precaution

There are rare reports of SE patients receiving LEV having had significant side effects. Some patients have drowsiness, weakness, and dizziness, especially when the initial dose is high [169]. Rare adverse reactions are behavioral and psychiatric side effects (PSEs), such as depression, nervousness, hostility, mood swings, and anxiety; these reactions are not clearly associated with dose but can be reversed after withdrawal [170]. Möddel et al. [151] reported on only two patients with nausea and vomiting after having examined 36 patients treated with intravenous LEV therapy for RSE. Berning et al. [161] examined 32 RSE patients treated with LEV, observing only one patient who had nausea and vomiting and one case of elevated liver enzymes during intravenous administration of LEV. McTague et al. [171] reported that among 45 pediatric patients with acute seizures or RSE, only three children exhibited aggressive response after LEV treatment. It is necessary to note that Atefy et al. [172] reported on two patients with astrocytoma following LEV treatment for the complex partial seizures caused by radiotherapy and central temporal lobe sclerosis. NCSE was observed during the course of the LEV treatments and was presumably associated with LEV. This may be the only report on LEV-induced SE, although it was difficult to determine whether this was caused by LEV.

PSEs may be caused by LEV, and patients with underlying psychiatric disorders may exhibit pejorative behavioral changes after treatment with LEV, which is concerning [173]. For patients with severe hepatic impairment, their renal function should be examined first to establish the dose adjustment requirements corresponding with the creatinine clearance rates of patients [174]. Due to differences in individual sensitivity, drowsiness or other central nervous system symptoms may occur at the initial stage of treatment or after an increased dose, which is concerning. In addition, patients who are allergic to LEV, pyrrolidone derivatives, or any of the ingredients in the drug should not use LEV.

6.5 Valproic Acid

6.5.1 Clinical Pharmacokinetics and Pharmacodynamics

Valproic acid (VPA) is a type of short-chain fatty acid and has a chemical structure different from that of other clinical AEDs [175]. It can be widely combined with plasma proteins, especially albumin. With the increase of VPA dosages, the degree to which it can be combined with plasma proteins is reduced [176]. A nonlinear shape exists between the total plasma drug concentration and the drug dose [177]. VPA concentration ratios in the brain and plasma depend on the ratio of total and uncombined plasma protein [178]. The apparent volume of distribution is 0.13–0.19 L/kg [175]. The half-life of VPA is approximately 9–18 h; when paired with enzyme-inducing co-medication, its half-life will be reduced to 5–12 h [179–181]. In newborns, its elimination is slower, particularly in premature neonates. Its clearance rate will also increase in children [175]. Although the total plasma concentrations of VPA in elderly and young people are the same, unbound VPA concentrations in elderly are increased because of their reduced plasma protein binding and reduced clearance [182]. Pregnant women, because of changes in the pharmacokinetics of VPA, experience reduced drug total concentrations of VPA in their blood, but free VPA concentrations are basically unchanged [183], so the dose should be adjusted depending on the patient. VPA is primarily metabolized in the liver though mitochondrial β-oxidation, microsomal glucuronide conjugation, and cytochrome P450 (CYP)-dependent ω-, (ω-1)-, and (ω-2)-oxidation. Plasma clearance of VPA in healthy people ranges from 0.4 to 0.6 L/h [175, 178, 179, 184], whereas only a small portion of VPA is excreted unchanged in the urine.

VPA possesses broad-spectrum antiepileptic effects. The characteristics by which it can be safe and effective to treat various types of epilepsy, which determine its antiepileptic mechanism, may be varied. Currently, the antiepileptic mechanism of VPA is still being explored.

Increasing GABA concentrations in the brain: VPA can increase the synthesis of GABA and reduce the degradation of GABA. Taberner et al. [185] confirmed that VPA can increase the synthesis of GABA in a similar experiment with mice, especially with respect to the substantia nigra of the brain. The synthesis of GABA by VPA is mainly via increasing the activity of glutamic acid decarboxylase (GAD), but high dose of VPA will decrease the activity of GAD. Recent studies have shown that VPA increases GABA which potassium ion induced in the cerebral cortex of rats. Similarly, VPA in clinical doses can increase the release of GABA, which showed potassium ion induction in cultured cortical neurons. At present, however, the antiepileptic mechanism of VPA by increasing the GABA concentrations of the brain is not fully elucidated.

Inhibiting release of γ-hydroxybutyrate (GHB): Whittle et al. [186] studied the changes made by VPA in the brain homogenate of mice and found that VPA can inhibit the release of GHB, and Snead [187] confirmed that GHB has an epileptogenic effect in a variety of species.

Potentiating neuronal responses to GABA: Macdonald et al. [188] was the first to find that VPA can enhance the neuronal reaction to GABA via the postsynaptic effect, thereby increasing the depolarization reaction of IPSPs. However, subsequent in vitro research suggested that only at high concentrations of VPA can neuronal responses to GABA be potentiated. Olpe et al. [189] proved that VPA in therapeutic doses also potentiates neuronal responses to GABA and summarized how different research results may reflect how VPA increases GABA in specific areas of the brain.

Reducing the excitability of NMDAR: Zeise [190] studied that VPA can effectively inhibit NMDAR-evoked transient depolarization in the rat neocortex. zeise assert that VPA can reduce the excitability of NMDAR-mediated, which is the important antiepileptic mechanism of VPA. Recently, many studies have also confirmed that VPA can inhibit transient depolarization of the rat hippocampus and the amygdala and that NMDAR activation triggers the transient depolarization; such research has also confirmed that VPA can antagonize the excitability of neurons that the NMDAR serves to stimulate.

Influencing neuronal membrane: McLean [191] posited that VPA can inhibit the high-frequency repetitive firing of action potentials of central neurons (the effect might be involved in antiepileptic action of valproate on generalized tonic–clonic seizures (GTCS)), the most probable explanation behind which is that VPA produces a use-dependent inhibition of inward sodium current. Yet the study of the effects of VPA on the sodium channel is indirectly inferred from changes in the increased maximum rate that sodium-dependent action potentials produce. Research data show that VPA increases potassium outflow, which causes neuronal hyperpolarization and increases the conductance of the potassium ion across the membrane. Although the concentrations of VPA used in these studies were high, this may yet represent the antiepileptic mechanism of VPA [192, 193].

Influencing calcium ions: Ethosuximide treats absence epilepsy by preventing the use-dependent activation of T-type Ca^{+} channels of thalamic neurons (which are associated with a spike wave produced in absence epilepsy). VPA can also treat absence epilepsy as effectively as ethosuximide, but in contrast to ethosuximide's antiepileptic mechanism, VPA may play a role through blocking low-threshold T-type calcium ion channels of the peripheral nerve [192, 194].

Reducing the cGMP of the cerebellum: In the experimental model of induced epilepsy seizures, at the beginning of the seizure, the cGMP of the cerebellum and cortex increases rapidly [192]. Lust [195] and McCandless [196] proposed that at the beginning or during the maintenance of seizures, the cerebellum's cGMP level increases are regulated by Purkinje cell activity, and VPA has been proven to reduce the levels of cGMP in the cerebellum during epileptic seizures.

6.5.2 Clinical Practice

VPA was synthesized having a history dating back more than 100 years as a derivative of pentanoic acid. Prior to 1963, it was a solvent of organic compounds; a novel systematic screening of a series of derivatives of kellin dissolved in VPA has permitted scientists to find out the antiepileptic effects of VPA [197]. Then, Honack et al. [198] found that VPA has anti-SE effects in a mouse GCSE model and proposed that intravenous injection of VPA may be used to treat diazepam-resistant SE.

Neurological intensive care guidelines (2012) recommend that VPA can be used as a choice for controlling RSE in emergencies [199]. A number of studies and reports show that intravenous injection of VPA can be safe and effective to control RSE in children [200–204]. Mehta [202] conducted an RCT to compare the efficacy and safety of intravenous VPA and diazepam in the treatment of RSE. The test was carried out according to strict standards of diagnosis and inclusion/exclusion criteria. The researchers brought in 40 5-month- to 12-year-old children with RSE who were randomly divided into a VPA group and a diazepam group; the two groups were given intravenous VPA or diazepam intravenously. First, the loading dose of the VPA group is 30 mg/kg (diluted 1: 1 with normal saline), which should be intravenously injected within 2–5 min; should SE not be controlled after approximately 10 min, a bolus dose of 10 mg/kg is repeated, followed by intravenous infusion of VPA at the rate of 5 mg/kg/h. The diazepam group began to intravenously infused at 10 μg/kg/min and then every 5 min, with the rate increased by 10 μg/kg/min, until the SE was controlled or diazepam achieved the maximum dose of 100 μg/kg/min. Experimental results show that within 30 min of treatment, the effectiveness of valproate and diazepam for controlling RSE is 80% and 85%, respectively. Moreover, Uberall et al. [200], in a retrospective study of control children with RSE, found that the efficiency of VPA treatment for RSE was 78% (32/41). In a number of related reports on VPA treatment for RSE in adults, the effective treatment rate of VPA is 63–91% [205–207]. To understand how different drugs provide treatment for SE when patients do not respond to benzodiazepine drug treatment, Yasiry et al. [208] systematically analyzed 798 patients from 27 studies and found that the therapeutic response rate for RSE that benzodiazepine drugs failed to treat but VPA successfully treated was 75.7%. Chen et al. [209] studied intravenous valproate to treat refractory CSE for which benzodiazepine drugs were ineffective for treatment in Mainland China; their study included a total of 48 patients who came from the neurology department at West China Hospital in China's Sichuan province between January 1996 and December 2007, with all patients according with the inclusion and exclusion criteria of the research objectives. After the initial failure of diazepam and phenobarbital treatment, VPA was begun via intravenous injection, at a first loading dose of 15 mg/kg (diluted 1:1 with normal saline or dextrose 5%) over 5 min (repeated after 10–15 min, if necessary), then continuous valproate at 30 mg/kg, infused at the rate of 6 mg/kg/h to maintain. Ultimately, 42 patients with RSE (87.5%) were effectively controlled. SE in all 42 patients had been relieved within 1 h, neurologic function returned to baseline at the same time, and CSE did not recur within the next 12 h. The Italian League Against Epilepsy (2006) established guidelines for the treatment of adult SE and recommended the use of phenytoin and then to try phenobarbital to treat SE patients who do not respond to benzodiazepine drugs in the initial treatment for SE. If there are contraindications with both, it is recommended to use VPA to treat RSE (Level 3, Rating B).

VPA can be used in the treatment of various types of epilepsy. A systemic evaluation [207], which included 166 generalized tonic–clonic SE patients from ten studies, found that VPA effectively treated the majority of the research subjects (119/166), and the overall efficiency is 71.7% [200, 205, 206, 210–215]. A systemic evaluation [207] that analyzed 107 simple or complex focal SE patients from nine studies established an effective rate of treatment of 83/107; the overall efficiency of VPA is 77.6% [200, 203, 205, 206, 211–216]. Intravenous VPA administered alone for the absence SE is rare. A systemic evaluation [207] included a total of 16 patients with the absence SE from six studies. The results showed that the absence SE can quickly be eliminated by VPA. The overall efficiency of VPA is 75.0% [200, 205, 210, 211, 217, 218]. Giroud [211] and Jha [205] studied VPA treatment for myoclonus SE. The total effective rate was 71.0%. Uberall et al. [200] reported that VPA treated two cases of infant patients with spastic SE successfully.

Some studies have compared the efficacy of VPA with other AEDs. Tripthi (2010) and colleagues [153] chose 209 patients older than 14 years with RSE in neurology and neurosurgery at AIIMS hospitalized in December 2006–June 2008 as the research objects, in which 82 patients with RSE were randomly divided into an IV valproate group (41 patients) and an IV lamotrigine group (41 patients). The two groups received 30 mg/kg of valproate or lamotrigine intravenously at a rate of 5 mg/kg/min; the treatment effectiveness of RSE in the valproate group was 68.3%, whereas in the lamotrigine group, it was 73.2% ($p = 0.696$). The differences in treatment efficiency for RSE were not statistically significant, and liver function damage, low blood pressure, respiratory depression, and thrombocytopenia in the two groups were not found in the process of treatment. Agarwal [219] (2007) and others, in RCTs that compared the efficiency of valproate and phenytoin sodium for the treatment of RSE, ultimately found that the treatment effectiveness of valproate was 88%, and the treatment effectiveness of phenytoin sodium was 84%, thereby suggesting that VPA treatment for RSE might be effective by targeting those individuals who do not respond to benzodiazepine drugs. Malamiri [220] compared the treatments of intravenous VPA and phenobarbital for children with SE against diazepam and other benzodiazepine drugs that had failed to be effective in children; the results showed that both types of drugs effectively control SE. In 24 h, VPA showed less recurrence of RSE (37% vs. 77%).

6.5.3 Administration and Time of Onset

VPA can be administered intravenously, orally, and rectally. VPA is used to treat RSE mainly via intravenous administration. In 1996, the US FDA approved intravenous administration of VPA and later approved it for the treatment of SE. The most commonly used effective doses of VPA were intravenous injection with 15–40 mg/kg (<6 mg/kg/min), followed by 1–2 mg/kg/h infusion. Ueberall et al. [200] used intravenous VPA to treat 41 pediatric patients with SE who did not respond to benzodiazepines, phenytoin sodium, or phenobarbital. All were given IV VPA at first loading doses of 20–40 mg/kg (diluted 1:1 with normal saline or dextrose 5%) over 1–5 min (and repeated after 10–15 min, if necessary) and then infusion at a rate of 5 mg/kg/h for maintenance. Ultimately, the RSE of 78% of the children was effectively controlled, and the majority of patients (65.9%) responded immediately after 2–6 min of VPA administration in bolus. Several studies show that intravenous injection of VPA to treat RSE in children is effective and has almost no obvious side effects [200–204]. Intravenous administration of VPA works quickly; for instance, its maximum serum levels are achieved with minutes after the start of infusion. An open-label, multicenter, parallel-group, randomized, prospective epileptic treatment trial involving 112 patients (37 were randomized to 1.5 mg/kg/min valproate injection, other 75 were randomized to 3.0 mg/kg/min valproate injection) determined that intravenous valproate is well tolerated when the dose is up to 15 mg/kg per infusion at a rate of 3 mg/kg/min [221]. Only two patients had significant hypotension. Thus, in an emergency, the intravenous application of VPA can feasibly occur quickly and in a large quantity to treat RSE.

Varieties of oral VPA include syrup, capsules, and ordinary, enteric-coated, and sustained-release tablets. Enteric-coated tablets increase gastrointestinal tolerance; sustained-release tablets reduce the plasma wave of drug concentration, extending the dosing intervals, to improve the patients' compliance [179, 222–224]. Oral VPA absorbs quickly and completely; the traditional common tablets and syrup reach peak concentrations after oral medication for 1–2 h. Enteric-coated tablets and sustained-release tablets reach peak concentrations in the blood after 3–6 h and 10–12 h, respectively, although absorption occurs more slowly with oral medication after a meal [225].

VPA can be absorbed quickly with rectal administration, and the drug concentration in the blood that results from anal suppositories or solutions is roughly similar to the blood drug concentration following oral administration [225].

6.5.4 Adverse Reaction and Precaution

VPA is a broad-spectrum, non-sedating drug for the treatment of RSE. Intravenous VPA has a low incidence of adverse events: the overall incidence of adverse events is <10% [207]. Devinsky et al.

[226] studied 318 children and adults who had been hospitalized with epilepsy and administered a first dose of VPA at 15 mg/kg/day in four divided doses, and the subsequent doses were adjusted by the researchers based on VPA functional blood drug concentrations. Among them, 54 patients reported transient adverse reactions mainly dizziness, headache, drowsiness, injection reaction, nausea, and other symptoms. Limdi [227] reported an open-label, prospective clinical study about securing prompt intravenous injection of valproate. Forty patients with epilepsy received an intravenous valproate loading dose of 20 or 30 mg/kg (undiluted), and each dose group was divided into ten individuals to infuse at the rate of 6 or 10 mg/kg/min; the results show that rapid intravenous injection of VPA is well tolerated. Only 60.5% of patients complained of pain ,burning and sensation in the injection site which last not for more than 3 min, moreover the injection site did not appear red, swollen. Although sodium valproate was not diluted, there was no significant stimulation in the injection site. Only 7.5% of the patients complained of sedation; moreover, patients complained about somnolence. Thus, rapid intravenous administration of undiluted valproate in the treatment of epilepsy at infusion rate of 10 mg/kg/min and doses up to 30 mg/kg is safe and well tolerated. Ramsay et al. (2003) [221] compared intravenous infusion of VPA at the rate of 1.5 and 3 mg/kg/min to treat 112 patients with epilepsy in a hospital; the maximum doses per infusion in the two groups were both 15 mg/kg. The results show that two patients had temporary low blood pressure initially, but the overall patients' average blood pressure did not change with intravenous infusion at the rate of 3 mg/kg/min. Moreover one patient who was infused at the rate of 3mg/kg/min experienced encephalopathy that resolved within 3 days upon discontinued use of oval VPA. Other most common adverse reactions are vomiting, nausea, drowsiness, and dizziness.

VPA may lead to hyperammonemia, with or without encephalopathy. Sousa C et al. reported that valproate-induced hyperammonemic encephalopathy in one diagnosed patient. This patient manifested altered consciousness after 10 days of VPA treatment. Blood ammonia level significantly increased, but hepatic function and VPA serum level were within normal ranges. The classic manifestations of valproate-induced hyperammonemic encephalopathy are disturbances of consciousness, somnolence, focal or bilateral signs, and increased seizure frequency [228]. DeWolfe et al. (2009) [229] prospectively studied intravenous injection of VPA with loading dose (20 or 30 mg/kg) at 6 or 10 mg/kg/min for the treatment of 40 epileptic patients and found that 30/40 of the patients after treatment for 1 h experienced high blood ammonia without symptoms, but the incidence of high blood ammonia without symptoms decreased after infusion for 24 h. Consequently, no patients' consciousness changed or transaminase levels rose. Some scholars believe that reducing the dose of VPA is effective for those non-symptomatic hyperammonemia [230].

Using VPA during pregnancy is related to major fetal malformation. Hernández-Díaz et al. reported that 9.3% (30/323) of patients who used VPA during pregnancy had major malformation of fetuses. They believed that compared with using other AEDs such as lamotrigine or LEV, using VPA is more likely to cause major malformation [231]. Jentink et al. found that the use of VPA monotherapy during early pregnancy is more likely to cause major congenital malformations compared with not using AEDs or using other AEDs [232]. Thus, avoiding the use of VPA in pregnant women is reasonable.

6.6 Phenobarbital

6.6.1 Clinical Pharmacokinetics and Pharmacodynamics

This drug is easy to absorb, and its bioavailability is above 95%. Its peak plasma concentration is usually reached in 0.5–4 h [233, 234]. In adults, its plasma half-life period is approximately 50–120 h, whereas in children, it is approximately 60–180 h. The drug is a liver enzyme inducer and can improve the activity of liver enzymes, which means that it not only accelerates its own metabolism but also accelerates the metabolism of other drugs [235]. Most of this drug combines with glucuronic acid or sulfate and is excreted by the kidneys into the urine. Twenty-five percent of the drug is excreted via the kidneys into the urine in its original form [236].

The exact antiepileptic mechanism of phenobarbital remains unknown. Phenobarbital increases GABA receptor activity by increasing their mean open time without altering channel-opening frequency or burst frequency [237]. In conditions characterized by a lack of GABA, Phenobarbital can also directly activate GABA-A receptors [238].

6.6.2 Clinical Practice

Phenobarbital was first synthesized by German organic chemist Emil Fischer in 1911 and subsequently used as a hypnotic agent for epilepsy patients by Alfred Hauptmann, who found phenobarbital to have anticonvulsant properties. The World Health Organization now recommends phenobarbital as a first-line drug for treatment of partial and generalized tonic–clonic seizures [239].

Thus far, a few studies have confirmed that phenobarbital can be an effective treatment for RSE. In 1998, Treiman et al. [240] conducted a 5-year randomized, double-blind study. Patients were randomized to one of the following four regimens: diazepam (0.15 mg/kg) followed by phenytoin (18 mg/kg), LZP (0.1 mg/kg), phenobarbital (15 mg/kg), or phenytoin (18 mg/kg). Successful treatment was considered when seizure activity ceased within 20 min without the return of seizure activity during the next 40 min. For overt GCSE (384 patients), the success rate of phenobarbital was 58.2%, which was comparable to the other three regimens. For subtle GCSE (134 patients), the success rate of GCSE was 24.2%, showing that phenobarbital had a better trend that did not reach statistical significance for the other regimens. Kravljanac et al. [26] retrospectively studied 602 episodes of CSE in 395 children. Among these SE cases, 50.57% were RSE, and 7.1% were SRSE. Treatment was judged to be effective when seizures clinically ceased within 20 min and when there was no return to seizure activity within the next 6 h. In total, 135 patients received phenobarbital (20 mg/kg) treatment, with an effectiveness rate of 67.4% (91/135). In a meta-analysis including two studies, an efficacy of 73.6% (95% CI: 58.3–84.8%) of phenobarbital in benzodiazepine-resistant CSE was observed [208]. These studies suggest that phenobarbital is an effective drug for the treatment of SE and RSE.

Phenobarbital is not the first choice for the treatment of SE. In 2013, the Italian League Against Epilepsy's treatment guidelines for SE in children noted that phenobarbital or phenytoin is considered when the treatment of benzodiazepine fails. For adults, the efficacy of phenobarbital is better than that of phenytoin. For children, phenobarbital can be used as a second-line therapy for SE treatment [241]. Muramoto et al. [242] observed 43 cases of SE patients who received phenobarbital treatment. Thirty-nine cases identified potential etiologies. Eighteen patients had been treated with AEDs prior to SE. Before receiving phenobarbital treatment, 39 patients received intravenous benzodiazepine therapy, 17 patients received intravenous phenytoin treatment, and 15 cases received lidocaine treatment. The first dose of phenobarbital was 125–1250 mg (1.9–20.0 mg/kg), and 24 of the 43 patients experienced the end of SE after the first dose of phenobarbital. Twelve patients used additional phenobarbital, leading to the end of seizures for 11 of the 12. Three patients experienced respiratory depression, one patient experienced drug eruption, and no patient experienced any other serious adverse reaction. In addition, in a retrospective cohort study, Mayer et al. [243] observed 74 patients manifesting 83 consecutive SE episodes. The average patient age was 63 years. The patients were first administered with benzodiazepine drugs, but 69% of SE cases could not be effectively controlled. When phenytoin was used, SE went uncontrolled 26 times, which became RSE. Finally, upon being treated with phenobarbital, 15 of the 26 patients achieved control of SE.

Some studies reported phenobarbital in the treatment of SRSE. Byun et al. [244] observed the administration of megadose of phenobarbital (MDPB) to treat ten patients with SRSE who were viral encephalitis patients without previous histories of epilepsy. The six patients were experiencing CSE and NCSE, whereas four patients were experiencing CSE. Before MDPB treatment, the median duration of SE was 17.5 days (range: 6–60 days). The median treatment time of anesthesia was 14 days (range: 2–54 days). The patients had taken at least two AEDs. For these SRSE patients, the median duration of MDPB treatment was 45.5 days (range: 11–84 days), the median of the maximum 24-h drug concentrations was 38.6 mg/kg/day (range: 18–95.7), and the median of the maximum plasma concentrations was 151.5 mg/mL (82.2–353.7 mg/mL). SE was under control for eight of the patients after their initial treatments, including five cases of MDPB without recurrence after withdrawal from the drug. One case died of septic shock during the treatment, two cases recurred upon withdrawal from phenobarbital, and two cases failed to respond to initial MDPB treatment and thus did not continue MDPB treatment. All patients had systemic infections, with five cases presenting with pneumonia, four cases presenting with urinary tract infection, two cases presenting with fungal infection, and two cases presenting with central line infection. Other adverse reactions included seven cases of hypotension, four cases of intestinal obstruction, three cases of elevated liver enzymes, one case of pseudomembranous peritonitis, one case of atelectasis, and one case of rhabdomyolysis. In addition, Pugin et al. [245] conducted a retrospective cohort study and observed the effects of continuous intravenous phenobarbital treatment for SRSE. The study included 31 patients treated with phenobarbital. The patients also received other treatments. Twenty-five of the 31 patients also received combined benzodiazepine and phenytoin treatment. Twenty-nine of the 31 patients received MDZ treatment. Depending on the nature of how the SE was controlled, the dose of phenobarbital was maintained at 0.5–3.7 mg/kg/h, with 6 days as the median duration of phenobarbital treatment. Eventually, SE was controlled in 28 cases (90%), but recurrence after phenobarbital withdrawal occurred in 15 cases (48%). Complications of the 31 patients included ten cases of pneumonia, nine cases of hypotension and the need for boost therapy, four cases of urinary tract infection, and one case of cardiac arrest.

VPA is a commonly used drug for benzodiazepine-resistant SE. The efficacies of phenobarbital and VPA have been compared with inconsistent conclusions. Malamiri et al. [220] conducted a study comparing phenobarbital and VPA in children with SE and acute prolonged seizures. Thirty patients in each group were recruited. The efficacies were observed within 20 min of anticonvulsant drug administration. The seizure termination rate was 77% (23/30) for the phenobarbital group, which was comparable to that for the VPA group (90%, 27/30). In a recent prospective RCT, 73 adult Chinese GSCE patients who had failed diazepam treatment were randomly assigned to receive either phenobarbital or VPA therapy. The success rate of the phenobarbital group was 81.1%, which was better than that of VPA group (44.4%). The relapse rate of SE within 24 h for the phenobarbital group was 6.7%, which was lower than that for the VPA group (31.3%). These inconsistent results may be primarily due to the patients included in the two studies: the former study included newly treated patients, whereas the latter included refractory patients who had failed diazepam treatment [246]. This demonstrates the superiority of phenobarbital in the treatment of benzodiazepine-resistant SE.

In recent years, LEV, a new type of AED, has become widely used in the treatment of epilepsy. Intravenous LEV is gradually administered in SE. In a retrospective study, Lee et al. [247] reviewed 88 children with benzodiazepine RSE or acute repetitive seizure. Fifty patients received phenobarbital, and 38 patients received LEV. The median initial loading dose of PB was 20 mg/kg (range: 10–20 mg/kg) and that of LEV was 30 mg/kg (range: 20–30 mg/kg). The success rate was 74.0% (37/50) in the phenobarbital group and 57.9% (22/38) in the LEV group, showing a superior trend of phenobarbital to LEV, but the therapeutic effect was not statistically significant.

6.6.3 Administration and Time of Onset

Routine intravenous administration: The most common administration route is intravenous administration. Several treatment guidelines and expert opinions have offered recommendations for intravenous administration. In 2005, Finnish scholars recommended that in children, intravenous administration starts with a loading dose of 15–20 mg/kg with a maximum infusion rate of 100 mg/min. The 24-h maintenance doses should be 2.5 mg/kg. Maintaining administration for 48 h is sufficient to ensure the serum concentration is within the therapeutic range for 72 h [241]. In 2012, the Neurocritical Care Society recommended intravenous administration with an initial dose of 20 mg/kg and an administration rate of 50–100 mg/min for critically ill adults and children. If efficacy is poor, an additional 5–10 mg/kg in 10 min may be considered [199]. In 2013, the Italian League Against Epilepsy recommended a dose of 15–20 mg/kg with a maximum dose of no more than 1 g, and an administration rate of no more than 1 mg/kg/min be used for children. Usually, the administration time is no less than 20 min, and the drug concentration is no higher than 10 mg/mL [48].

High-dose intravenous administration: An increase in the drug's dosage may increase its adverse effects. However, studies have indicated that high-dose intravenous administration for RSE, especially multidrug-resistant SRSE, shows good effects and safety. In 1988, Crawford et al. [248] reported on 50 patients with RSE who were treated with very-high-dose phenobarbital, which yielded maximum serum levels ranging from 70 to 344 mg/mL (median: 114 mg/mL). The results showed that the seizures of all 50 patients were effectively controlled. In terms of safety, 40 patients were intubated prior to the very-high-dose phenobarbital administration and successfully removed from their ventilators. Hypotension was uncommon and easily treated. This study showed that, in the treatment of RSE, high-dose phenobarbital had marked effectiveness and acceptable safety. Lee et al. [249] reported on three children (7–9 years of age) with RSE that likely was the result of viral encephalitis. The conventional doses of phenobarbital, phenytoin, and MDZ intravenous infusions were unable to effectively control SE. When their daily doses of phenobarbital reached 80 mg/kg (i.e., serum concentrations exceeding 1000 μmol/L), the seizures were effectively controlled. The Italian League Against Epilepsy has recommended in its treatment guidelines that in children with refractory CSE, high-dose phenobarbital can be used for the induction of coma when the use of sodium thiopental and propofol are contraindicated. The recommended dosage is a bolus of 20 mg/kg, with a maximum daily maintenance dose of 80–120 mg/kg, to achieve serum levels greater than 100 μg/mL. The patient should be intubated and ventilated.

Non-intravenous administration: Non-intravenous administration, including intramuscular and rectal administration, is rarely reported for the treatment of multiple drug-resistant SE. Sudoh et al. [250] observed three patients with long-term RSE whose seizures were not controlled by continuous MDZ and/or pentobarbital. The authors used non-intravenous high-dose phenobarbital treatment. Phenobarbital was initially administered intramuscularly or rectally followed by orally to achieve a phenobarbital serum concentration of 50–58 mg/mL, completely controlling the seizures. The patients did not develop significant hypotension or respiratory depression.

In addition, Tiamkao et al. [251] observed the efficacy of adjunctive rectal phenobarbital in six patients with RSE, including five patients with CSE and one patient with NCSE. All patients first received 10 mg diazepam treatment and other intravenous anticonvulsants, but SE was not effectively controlled. Finally, rectal administration of phenobarbital was initiated with loading doses of 900 mg, with a repeated 900 mg if needed. The SE of three patients was completely controlled; however, for two patients, complete control yielded to relapse within 24 h, and one patient did not respond to this treatment. After the initial dose, the dose was gradually reduced to 180 mg/day for maintenance treatment. No severe adverse reaction was observed in any patient.

In 1987, Simon et al. [252] observed the brain uptake of phenobarbital during SE in sheep. In the first 30 min of SE, hypertension, increased cerebral blood flow, and decreased brain pH were observed. Phenobarbital administered during this time produced a higher phenobarbital concentration in the brain compared with nonseizure sheep. The highest brain concentration was achieved 5 min after infusion, and elevated brain phenobarbital concentration persisted for 3 h. During the established phase of SE, blood pressure and cerebral blood flow returned to pre-seizure levels. Phenobarbital administered during this phase did not produced different brain phenobarbital concentrations between the sheep with SE and those in the non-seizure group.

The SE termination time was consistent with the peak time of drug concentration. In 1988, Shaner et al. [253] carried out a randomized, nonblinded clinical trial. In 36 cases of GCSE patients, phenobarbital monotherapy was compared to combination diazepam and phenytoin (DZ/DPH) therapy. For the phenobarbital condition, the dose was 10 mg/kg, the rate of administration was 100 mg/min, and the results showed that the median time of cumulative convulsion in the phenobarbital group was 5 min, shorter than that of the DZ/DPH group (9 min). The response latency of the phenobarbital group was 5.5 min, less than that of the DZ/DPH group (15 min), but there were no differences in the rates of endotracheal intubation, hypotension, or arrhythmia. Moreover, because administration of phenobarbital occurs rapidly, a time of 20 or 30 min to SE control has been used as the therapeutic index in several clinical studies. For example, Malamiri et al. [220] reported seizure termination at 20 min as the outcome. Treiman et al. [240] recommended that seizures were completely controlled once the effects were delivered within 20 min and when no recurrence had occurred after 40 min. Kravljanac et al. [26] recommended that seizures be judged to be terminated once the effects were delivered within 20 min and when no recurrence had occurred within 6 h. In a retrospective study, Lee et al. [247] used termination within 30 min and no recurrence within 24 h to judge successful outcomes.

6.6.4 Adverse Reaction and Precaution

The Italian League Against Epilepsy has clearly stated that [48] phenobarbital can lead to adverse effects such as sedation, respiratory depression, and decreased blood pressure. Respiratory depression is the most dangerous adverse reaction. The Italian League Against Epilepsy recommends that patients who are spontaneously breathing should be assisted by professionals with cardiopulmonary resuscitation training when using phenobarbital treatment for the purpose of providing high-level ventilator support (mask or nasal intubation) [48]. Ultra-high-dose phenobarbital has more obvious inhibitory effects on respiration. Therefore, putting this into practice, Byun et al. [244] reported that MDPB treatment for ten cases of SRSE patients, all of whom underwent tracheotomies for respiratory support, resulted in eight smoothly going offline of said support, with a median phenobarbital concentration of 81.3 μg/mL (range: 24.0–124.6). The incidence of hypotension is not high, and low blood pressure can be treated with vasoconstrictors. After high-dose treatment, blood pressure decreases significantly. Byun et al. [244] used MDPB to treat ten cases of SRSE, seven of whom had low blood pressure, which was maintained by one to two vasoconstrictors.

6.7 Clonazepam

6.7.1 Clinical Pharmacokinetics and Pharmacodynamics

Clonazepam (CZP) belongs to the class of benzodiazepines (BZDs). CZP can be administered orally, intravenously, or rectally. When CZP is taken orally, it is absorbed quickly via the gastrointestinal tract. Via intravenous injection, CZP can rapidly pass through the BBB and diffuse into the central nervous system [254]. Seventy percent of CZP is eliminated through the urine, with an elimination half-life of approximately 40 h. To control most epileptic seizures, the CZP blood concentration must be 15–50 μg/L [255]. CZP is an agonist of γ-aminobutyric acid A receptors (GABAARs) and binds to the BZD recognition site of GABAARs [256], which consists of alpha and gamma subunits. This binding induces a conformation chance in the GABAARs. Consequently, the GABAAR chloride channel also undergoes a conformation change that leads to hyperpolarization of the cell. Thus, the inhibitory action of GABA in the central nervous system is imitated. CZP is a long-acting GABAAR agonist with high efficiency [257].

6.7.2 Clinical Practice

The use of CZP for the treatment of SE was first reported in 1971 [258]. Gaustaut et al. conducted a study that included 37 patients who had 39 episodes of SE and were administered with CZP. These patients with SE included unilateral SE, partial SE, absence SE, and generalized SE. All but one patient was able to control their SE. The authors believed that CZP had a short onset time, mild side effects, and a low effective dose.

CZP can be used to treat generalized or partial SE. Sorel et al. [259] compared the efficacy of 4–10 mg of intravenously injected LZP and/or 1 mg of CZP for the treatment of SE in 61 cases. LZP was administered in 22 cases, CZP was administered in 9 cases, and both drugs were administered at different times in 30 cases. In the cases treated with LZP, the EEG improvements were better compared with cases treated with CZP. Meanwhile, the clinical symptoms were more improved in the cases that were administered with CZP compared with cases treated with LZP. CZP and LZP both showed effectiveness in treating secondary generalized epilepsy with mild side effects. Moreover, Alvarez et al. [260] utilized CZP, LZP, or MDZ as first-line drugs to treat SE in a prospective observational study. To compare the relative efficacies of these drugs, they estimated the risk of developing RSE and the number of drugs required to control SE. They found that when MDZ and LZP were not appropriate, CZP was a reasonable alternative. A group of scholars [261] conducted a retrospective study that included 167 seizure episodes of 118 patients with SE from 2000 to 2009 in the neurology department of Rostock University. Forty-eight episodes of GCSE were treated with CZP (efficacy rate of 63%), and CZP was used in 73 episodes of NCSE or partial SE (efficacy rate of 42%). Compared with diazepam, MDZ, LEV, and sodium valproate, CZP seems to be more effective in terminating GCSE. Nevertheless, no significant differences were observed among these AEDs regarding the efficacy for terminating partial SE or NCSE. Singh et al. [262] examined 24 SE patients administered with CZP intravenously. After the administration, all (7/7) patients with absence seizures, half of the patients with GTCS (7/14), and two patients with complex partial seizures (2/3) were fully controlled. Moreover, these patients exhibited no obvious vital sign changes before and after the administration. Thus, intravenously administered CZP is a safe option with rapid onset and effectiveness in treating SE, and it is an alternative to diazepam. Furthermore, Fernández-Torre and colleagues [263] reported a patient with simple partial frontal lobe SE. After CZP was administered intravenously, this 44-year-old patient's seizures were fully controlled.

Navarro et al. [264] performed a double-blind, add-on, randomized, and placebo-controlled phase III clinical trial that concerned the prehospital treatment of patients with GCSEs. This study compared the efficacy of combination therapy of intravenous LEV and CZP with CZP alone in treating GCSE. The treatment group was administered with 1 mg of CZP and 2.5 g of LEV, and the control group was treated with 1 mg of CZP and a placebo. The patients were included in this study when they had episodes of GCSE lasting more than 5 min, and the outcome was primarily measured by the percentage of patients who showed seizure cessation within 15 min after the administration of these drugs. The study was terminated because there was no treatment difference. However, the researchers recently analyzed the modified intention-to-treat population. In this analysis, 68 patients were included in each group. The researchers found that convulsions ceased within 15 min after drug injection in 84% of patients (57/68) using CZP and placebo and in 74% of patients (50/68) using CZP and LEV. Therefore, LEV combined with CZP showed no advantage compared with CZP alone in the pre-hospital treatment of patients with GCSEs.

NCSE commonly occurs in children and the elderly. The manifestation of NCSE ranges from confusion to coma, which is caused by different etiologies. This range makes NCSE difficult to diagnose and treat [265, 266]. In addition, there are currently no unified treatment guidelines for NCSE [267]. Livingston and his colleagues [268] examined seven NCSE patients, ranging from 3 to 13 years of age (mean age: 7 years), who all had Lennox-Gastaut syndrome. Every patient had at least one seizure with NCSE and was intravenously administered with BZDs under cEEG monitoring. Diazepam at the dose of 0.2–0.3 mg/kg was injected in five cases, CZP at the dose of 0.02 mg/kg was injected in one case, and a combination of diazepam and CZP was administered in one case. After treatment, the seizures were completely controlled in only one patient, indicating that BZDs are probably not the most effective drugs for the treatment of NCSE in patients with Lennox-Gastaut syndrome. However, regarding the limitations in this study for treating this condition, the unresponsiveness to BZDs might not be generalizable to other subtypes of NCSE. Other scholars [261] retrospectively studied and compared the efficacies of diazepam, CZP, MDZ, VPA, and LEV for treating NCSE and observed no significant differences among these drugs. Additionally, other studies have found that CZP is effective in treating absence SE. Gaustaut et al. [258] found that all 12 patients with absence SE were rapidly controlled after the administration of CZP, and Singh et al. [262] used intravenous CZP to treat seven patients with absence SE, which ended in all seven patients.

Hubert et al. [14] suggested that CZP should be the first-line treatment for infants and children with CSE lasting longer than 5 min and that the intravenous administration of phenytoin/fosphenytoin or phenobarbital could be the second-line option. Congdon and colleagues [269] treated 17 patients with SE ranging from 2 weeks to 15 years old with intravenous administration of CZP. In all the patients, the SE was quickly controlled. However, seizures subsequently relapsed in six patients, and these seizures ultimately stopped after the administration of diazepam. The authors believed that CZP had a longer duration of action than that of diazepam, and neither drug exhibited severe side effects. Therefore, the authors suggested that CZP could be the primary choice for the treatment of SE, especially in children. Their opinions have been supported by several studies. Padma et al. [270] reported a case in which the electrophysiological and clinical manifestations of an 11-year-old child with focal SE were markedly improved after oral CZP administration.

6.7.3 Administration and Time of Onset

When CZP is used to treat SE in adults, the first dose should generally be a 1–2 mg intravenous injection [258, 259, 261, 262]. The injection rate should be within 0.25–0.5 mg/min [271], and the drug can be readministered after 20 min when necessary [259]. When the duration of GCSE is within 5–30 min, CZP monotherapy is reasonable. If the seizure duration exceeds 30 min before treatment, the initial treatment dose of CZP should be combined with phenobarbital or fosphenytoin [272, 273]. When intravenous CZP is used in pediatric patients ranging from 2 weeks to 15 years old, the dose should be adjusted to a total dose of 0.25–0.75 mg or 0.01 to 0.09 mg/kg based on the child's weight [269]. For recurrent cases, seizures ceased after the administration of diazepam at 0.25–0.75 mg/kg.

CZP can be used orally, and this route is commonly seen in treating partial SE and prolonged convulsive seizures (PCSs). For the treatment of partial SE, CZP could be administered orally at a dose of 1 mg three times per day [270]. For the urgent treatment of PCSs in pediatric patients, oral CZP wafers at a total dose of 0.25–2 mg were given, based on the child's weight [274].

Kosterskov and colleagues [275] examined the absorption of CZP when it is administered rectally. A dose of 0.02 mg/kg of CZP was given to ten non-epileptic adults, and blood samples were collected at various times to evaluate the concentration of CZP by gas chromatography.

CZP (1 mg) was intravenously administered to two additional volunteers, and the plasma concentrations were measured after intravenous administration. The peak plasma concentration was reached 10–30 min after rectal administration and approximately 10–15 min after intravenous administration. The peak concentrations were approximately equal for both rectal and intravenous administration, indicating that CZP can be well absorbed upon rectal administration. Consequently, the rectal administration of CZP is a choice for the treatment of SE.

SE can be controlled within 1–3 min by the administration of intravenous CZP [258, 262, 269]. The seizures of 50% of patients with PCS can be controlled within 1 min, 24% within 1–5 min, and 26% within 5–10 min after the administration of oral CZP wafers [274].

6.7.4 Adverse Reaction and Precaution

CZP is a BZD. Because sedation can be induced by BZDs, excitatory symptoms could also develop, such as excitement, emotional release, increased speech, and excessive movement. The incidence of these excitatory symptoms is relatively low, at less than 1% [276]. Patients using BZDs often show fatigue, drowsiness, and lethargy [257]. Additionally, dizziness, vertigo, blurred vision, slurred speech, motor coordination disorder, euphoria, and mood swings can appear in patients who have been administered higher doses of BZDs, and erratic or hostile behavior can occur in some patients. Major symptoms, such as confusion, disorientation, slurred speech, and impaired thinking, may occur in overmedicated patients. Hyperactivity, hypotonia, obvious ataxia, and dystonia have been observed in a few cases, and these side effects have disappeared if the administration was continued longer than 2–4 weeks. The primary reasons for treatment withdrawal are fatigue and lethargy, and bronchial hypersecretion and excessive salivation are the main side effects after administration in pediatric patients [277]. Some studies have found that BZDs are related to memory impairment [278]. Induced anterograde amnesia is less likely to occur in response to treatment with CZP when compared with other BZDs, given its low lipid solubility [257]. Upon applying CZP to treat SE, Sorel et al. [259] demonstrated that CZP had good safety and tolerability; drowsiness appeared following administration, and psychomotor agitation was identified in only 12% of cases. When Congdon et al. [269] administered CZP to treat SE, no obvious respiratory depression or serious side effects occurred. Moreover, some scholars have observed that heart rate, respiration, and blood pressure have no significant changes when CZP is administered intravenously for the treatment of SE [262], and only transient, mild to moderate somnolence was observed in 40% of patients [262]. Thus, intravenous CZP seems to be an effective and safe choice for the treatment of SE. Although CZP can be safely administered, it is necessary to pay attention to a rare but serious side effect of CZP, respiratory depression.

6.8 Polytherapy as a Treatment for Status Epilepticus

6.8.1 Introduction

SE is a common neurological emergency with high mortality and disability rates. Terminating SE early and effectively can improve the prognosis of patients. The traditional therapeutic regimen is ineffective in 30–40% of SE cases [38]. Considering the diverse etiology and complex pathogenesis of SE, polytherapy using anticonvulsants with diverse mechanisms might be more beneficial for SE patients than monotherapy for increasing curative effects and reducing side effects. This paper expounds upon the advantages of polytherapy by studying the combination drug therapies in clinical trials. The study of combination drug therapies for SE may be useful due to the recent date of which the advantage of polytherapy over monotherapy has been identified [279, 280].

6.8.2 Definition of Polytherapy

A treatment meeting any of following three criteria can be defined as polytherapy:

1. The simultaneous use of two or more anticonvulsants (including add-on therapeutic regimen)
2. Progressive sequential therapy, such that prior anticonvulsants interact with following ones to produce a combined effect
3. Anticonvulsants combined with immunomodulating drugs, non-pharmacological drugs, or neuromodulatory drugs

6.8.3 Polytherapy in Clinical Practice

Initial polytherapy may be effective to prevent the SE from progressed to RSE. Mundlamuri et al. [281] carried out a prospective RCT to study the efficacy of polytherapy of LZP along with phenytoin, VPA, and LEV separately for the SE treatment. The study enrolled 150 GCSE patients (33.71 ± 17.0 years; 88 males and 62 females). All patients meeting the inclusion criteria were treated with 0.1 mg/kg LZP (4–6 mg) within 5 min of arrival. Then, the patients were randomly divided into three groups. Within 10 min, the patients were treated with a predesigned progressive sequential protocol: Group 1 (n = 50), phenytoin (first AED) → VPA (second AED) → LEV (third AED); Group 2 (n = 50), VPA (first AED) → phenytoin (second AED) → LEV (third AED); and Group 3 (n = 50), LEV (first AED) → phenytoin (second AED) → VPA (third AED). The loading dose of the drugs was phenytoin 20 mg/kg (0.8–1.6 g), VPA 30 mg/kg (1.2–2.4 g), and LEV 25 mg/kg (1–2 g), followed by maintenance dose (in three divided doses): phenytoin 5 mg/kg/day, VPA 30 mg/kg/day, and LEV 25 mg/kg/day. According to the protocol, the next AED was given if seizure termination failed within 30 min after the last drug was used. The initial polytherapy using LZP and phenytoin controlled 68% (34) of GCSE cases. The polytherapy of LZP and valproate controlled 68% (34) of GCSE cases, and LZP + LEV controlled 78% (39) of GCSE cases. The efficacies of three combination therapies were not remarkably distinguished statistically. The polytherapy of LZP and the first AED controlled 71.3% (107/150) of total GCSE cases. By adding the second AED, the GCSE of 130/150 (86.7%) patients was controlled. By adding the third AED, the GCSE of 138/150 (92%) patients was controlled. In other words, SE was controlled in 92% of patients by AEDs, and anesthetic was avoided, thereby preventing admission to the ICU and the occurrence of ICU-related complications. This study demonstrated that the progressive sequential protocol of IV AEDs was quite beneficial for those SE patients who were nonresponsive to the initial monotherapy.

The polytherapy may be more effective if the patient recovers from SE upon administration of the first- or second-line anticonvulsants. In a retrospective study by Synowiec et al. [102], 11 SE patients used KE intravenously as an additional drug. All of the patients were resistant to benzodiazepines. The etiologies included infections (n = 7), metabolic disease (n = 1), and inadequate initial dose of AEDs (n = 3). The termination of RSE was defined as the complete arrest of SE in clinical and/or EEG evaluation after 24 h of KE discontinuation. The polytherapy of KE and other anticonvulsants such as LZP and phenytoin was effective in 11 (100%) patients. Patients in the study did not experience obvious adverse drug events. In a retrospective study [167], 11 RSE children using LEV as an additional drug were studied to understand the feasibility, safety, and efficacy of LEV. All of the patients with RSE had symptomatic etiologies. LEV added to the traditional AEDs showed definite efficiency in 45% (5/11) of cases and possible efficiency in 27% (3/11) of cases. The termination time of RSE was 1–8 (mean: 1.5) days after the administration of LEV. No LEV-related adverse reactions were observed in this study.

6.8.4 The Potential Advantages of Polytherapy

The above date of clinical trials proved the feasibility of polytherapy for SE and RSE. Cook et al. [282] found that polytherapy for SE and RSE is much more common in clinical practice than has been previously reported. In recent years, with further study of the mechanisms by which RSE develops, polytherapy has also received more attention. Why is polytherapy useful for SE and RSE? The answer is as follows:

Polytherapy may act on multiple mechanisms: As a multifactorial and heterogeneous disease, SE has both various causes and complicated pathogenic mechanisms [283–285]. Polytherapy with anticonvulsants having different pharmacological effects may be more effective in stopping SE than monotherapy with anticonvulsants of a single mechanism of action [279, 280, 286].

Polytherapy may act on different neurotransmitters: Some studies have proven that the pathogenesis is distinguished at disparate time points of the development process of SE [287, 288]. Complex brain alterations happen in the process of SE. As found by Wasterlain et al. [289], the number and activity of receptors on the postsynaptic membrane changed as seizures became more prolonged and epilepsy attacks iterated. Moreover, it was found that the GABA receptors decreased, and the NMDAR increased in the progress of SE, which might result in drug resistance and the formation of RSE [290]. Polytherapy might be more efficient because different anticonvulsants can act on different neurotransmitters to avoid drug resistance. It is worth noting that the addition of some novel anticonvulsants may be helpful for terminating SE [38, 279, 291].

Polytherapy may moderate brain insults: Persistent repeated attack of epileptic seizures can seriously damage the brain, leading to the death of brain neurons [289, 292]. The study by Vespa et al. [293, 294] found that the poor outcomes of traumatic brain injury patients were attributable to posttraumatic nonconvulsive electrographic seizures.

Polytherapy may shorten SE duration: The delayed treatment of SE may make SE difficult to control and further develop into RSE or SRSE or increase the incidence of poor prognosis or even death [38, 295, 296]. A review by Sutter et al. [297] studied the factors related to the outcomes of SE patients. The duration of SE is a crucial factor in the prognosis of SE patients. With the increased SE duration, both the hospital stays and fatality rate were distinctly increased as well.

6.8.5 Polytherapy of Different Anticonvulsants

6.8.5.1 KE

KE is a potent noncompetitive *N*-methyl-D-aspartic acid (NMDA) antagonist with properties such as not causing cardiac or respiratory depression and facilitating neuroprotection [298, 299]. The hemodynamic stabilization profile of KE along with aggressive fluid resuscitation makes it dependable for RSE patients. Numerous basic studies [208, 209, 292] have found that prolonged seizures are accompanied by the decline of GABA agonists and upregulation of NMDAR. Increasing attention has been directed to the polytherapy of KE with other anticonvulsants for the treatment of SE. It has been proven that KE has evident synergism to combine with diazepam in SE animal studies [102, 280, 300]. In case reports and small series [102, 301, 302], KE has been used as an add-on drug for the treatment of RSE in humans. KE is administered as an adjunctive anticonvulsant if SE is resistant to the standard first-line or second-line drug or administered together with other anticonvulsants [44, 102].

Polytherapy of KE with other anticonvulsants is indicated for children or adults with RSE or SRSE [44, 303]. Sabharwal et al. [44] retrospectively studied 67 SRSE patients (8–85 years; 18 males, 49 females) who were treated with polytherapy of intravenous propofol and KE from 2012 to 2015. The start time of KE occurred earlier in this study than in other previous clinical studies, and the initiation time of polytherapy of propofol and KE was within 24–48 h mostly. KE was the initial agent used in six patients and propofol in 61. The duration of KE combined with propofol ranged from 1 to 28 (mean: 3.6) days. SRSE had a higher resolution rate compared to previous clinical studies, and the study attributed this to the early administration of KE. The termination proportion of SRSE was 91% (n = 61). The final mortality rate was 39%, and patients with anoxic brain injuries were included. Among the 13 patients with anoxic brain injuries, SRSE was controlled in five (56%). Despite the mortality rate of the study being high, the main determining factor was the basic cause of the serious systemic or nervous diseases. According to the research, the combination scheme of KE and propofol is very effective for treating SRSE. Importantly, KE was thought to be quite effective in controlling SRSE whether with short-term or long-term use or whether used with or without propofol. A small retrospective series [102] analyzed 11 RSE adults who used KE intravenously as an add-on agent, and other anticonvulsants, such as LZP and phenytoin, were administered with KE. The time of KE use was 4–28 days. The study considered that, due to the use of KE, six of seven patients were able to be removed from vasopressors early in the treatment. Seizure termination was ultimately achieved in all 11 RSE patients.

Sabharwal et al. [44] treated SRSE with polytherapy of intravenous propofol and KE. The weights of the 67 patients (8–85 years; 18 males, 49 females) ranged from 20 to 176 (median: 82.5) kg. The initial dosage of KE was 25 μg/kg/min, and the maximum dose was 175 μg/kg/min. Propofol infusion rates ranged from 25 to 140 μg/kg/min. The SRSE of 91% of patients was terminated. Synowiec et al. [102] treated RSE with polytherapy of intravenous KE with other anticonvulsants such as LZP and phenytoin. The administration process was as follows: first step, a loading dose of 1–2 mg/kg and, second step, intravenous 0.45–2.1 mg/kg/h (mean: 1.3 mg/kg/h) continuously. The maximal dose was 1392–4200 mg/d. Seizure termination was finally achieved in all 11 RSE patients.

In the clinical trial by Synowiec et al. [102], the duration from KE administration to seizure termination (i.e., behavioral and/or electrographic seizure disappearing over 24 h after drug discontinuation) was 4–28 (mean: 9.8) days. In the clinical trial of Sabharwal et al. [44], the time of joint use of KE and propofol was 1–28 (mean: 3.6) days.

Zeiler et al. [101] found that KE was responsible for rare side effects such as arrhythmia, mental symptoms, and ICP. The study by Synowiec et al. [102] found no clinically significant treatment-limiting adverse events in patients using KE. In the study of Sabharwal et al. [44], SRSE patients were treated with polytherapy of propofol and KE, and 53 (79%) patients needed to use vasopressors. A variety of factors were considered, such as the hemodynamic/intravascular status of the patients upon presentation and the side effects of the anesthetic agent.

6.8.5.2 MDZ

MDZ is a water-soluble benzodiazepine that inhibits GABA neurons. Multiple existing formulations of MDZ exist: intravenous, intramuscular, buccal, and intranasal. Continuous IV MDZ is not a coma-inducing treatment, and mechanical ventilation is not conventionally used. MDZ possesses better results for SE children with rapid initial effects, no obvious side effects, high convenience, and no contraindications [304, 305]. Monotherapy effects are not as good in SE children, whereas the progressive sequential protocol of MDZ has lower mortality and a better prognosis [306, 307]. The rationally progressive sequential protocol of administering drugs by degrees could avoid arbitrary drug administration effects, such as improper medication times or drug alterations; as a result, sequential protocols will reduce the occurrence of adverse events [306, 308]. The polytherapy method of MDZ and other anticonvulsants is mainly via progressive sequential protocol [306, 308].

Polytherapy of MDZ is mostly applicable to CSE children [306, 308]. To know the efficacy of the progressive sequential protocol called the Ege Pediatric SE Protocol (EPSEP), Saz et al. [308] studied 27 SE (including nine RSE) patients. The etiology was meningitis or encephalitis in 11 (40%) children, cortical dysplasia in 5 (19%), hypoxic-ischemic encephalopathy in three (11%), trauma in one, and febrile seizures in seven (26%). Polytherapy of diazepam and MDZ was given to 22 children, and it was effective for 21 (95%) episodes (including nine RSE). Brevoord et al. [306] studied 122 SE children (ages 0.5–197.4 months) treated with the second progressive sequential protocol exhibited below. Idiopathic epilepsy was demonstrated in 37.7% of children. Febrile epilepsy was observed in 36.1% of children. Polytherapy of MDZ and phenytoin was effective for 89% of the SE children.

Some studies recommended the progressive sequential protocol. In a retrospective clinical trial [308] for pediatric SE, a four-step therapy protocol was assessed:

Step 1: In the first 10 min of the episode, rectal diazepam (0.5 mg/kg) was twice administered when the seizure was lasting over 5 min.
Step 2: After 15 min of the episode, there were two administration choices, 20 mg/kg of phenytoin intravenously or a bolus of 0.15 mg/kg IV of MDZ.
Step 3: If the arrest of SE was not achieved by the former two steps, a dosage of MDZ was added per 5 min (up to 0.6 μg/kg/min) until the seizure stopped, and this added dosage lasted for 24 h. Then, MDZ infusion was decreased by 0.05 μg/kg/min every 6 h. If the arrest of SE was not achieved over 1 h of 0.6 μg/kg/min IV MDZ, the dosage was increased to 1.2 μg/kg/min, and the monitoring of life sign parameters became necessary.
Step 4: If the seizures lasted for 1–1.5 h, 1 mg/kg/h IV of propofol was preferable.

The study included 27 SE children, and nine (33%) had RSE. Two children achieved complete arrest of SE in Step 1, six in Step 2, 18 in Step 3, and one in Step 4. The peak dose of MDZ is 1.2 μg/kg/min in this study. The polytherapy of diazepam and MDZ was given to 22 children (including nine RSE children) sequentially, and 21 of 22 episodes were halted completely. The protocol was valid with no severe treatment-limiting side effects. In a study of Brevoord et al. [306], another progressive sequential protocol for children with GCSE was recommend:

Step 1: An initial administration of MDZ was rectally (0.5 mg/kg) or intravenously (0.1 mg/kg) employed, and another administration of IV MDZ (0.1 mg/kg) was given 10 min later.
Step 2: If SE persisted, 10 min later, IV phenytoin (20 mg/kg) was given over 20 min.
Step 3: When SE continued, 0.2 mg/kg IV MDZ was given, followed by 0.1 mg/kg/h intravenously (increased by 0.1 mg/kg/h per 10 min, up to 1 mg/kg/h).
Step 4: Before MDZ reached the maximum 1 mg/kg/min in Step 3, the following treatment could start early based on the SE features: (1) phenobarbital (20 mg/kg) IV and (2) a load dose of pentobarbital (2–5 mg/kg) IV, followed by a 1–2 mg/kg/h infusion.

The study included 122 SE patients. Fifty-eight children achieved complete arrest of SE in Step 1, 19 in Step 2, 32 in Step 3, and 13 in Step 4. In Step 3, the dosage of MDZ was 0.05–0.8 mg/kg/h. In Step 4, the dosage of MDZ was 0.1–1.0 mg/kg/h. In conclusion, 89% of children achieved complete arrest of GCSE, treated sequentially with MDZ and phenytoin.

The reported side effects of MDZ were alteration of the cardiovascular system, the respiratory system, consciousness, and urinary retention [309]. In the EPSEP therapy [308] study, mild hypotension was observed in three children and transient desaturation in one. No patients died in the study. In the trial of Brevoords et al. [306], 52 children needed assisted ventilation. Respiratory dysfunction was observed in 39 children using MDZ. All of the patients who died in the study did not do so because of anticonvulsants or SE. MDZ should be given slowly and progressively; in the meantime, monitoring of vital signs is obligatory. Mechanical ventilation is a requisite to prevent the side effect of respiratory dysfunction.

6.8.5.3 LEV

LEV is a broad-spectrum AED that acts on the NMDAR, calcium channels, and GABA receptors [167, 291]. As a novel AED, LEV has a favorable pharmacological profile marked by rapid action, neuroprotective effects, and limited influence on other drugs, among other characteristics [138, 310], making it a favorable agent for use in patients with SE. Valid synergistic effects were found in the polytherapy of diazepam and LEV in SE animal models [138]. In clinical studies, polytherapy of LEV and other anticonvulsants for SE patients has been increasingly valued [167, 264, 291]. LEV is used either in conjunction with benzodiazepines or is added if the first- or second-line anticonvulsants fail [167, 264, 291]. LEV polytherapy is used to treat SE and RSE in adults and RSE and ESES syndromes in children [167, 264, 291, 311].

LEV and benzodiazepines are simultaneously used to treat SE and RSE in adults. The recommended dosage of LEV is 2.5 g, and LEV is administered by IV (>5 min) [291, 312, 313]. Earlier treatment with LEV may lead to a better control of SE than when treatment occurs later [148]. The 11 SE adults in a study by Uges et al. [291] all received 2.5 g LEV while being administered first-line and/or second-line anticonvulsants (benzodiazepines and phenytoin). The time from hospital admission to the administration of LEV was 15–90 (mean: 36) min. The simultaneous polytherapy of LEV and benzodiazepines was used in nine patients at the beginning of treatment; LEV was added later in the SE process for two patients when sufficient first-line and/or second-line anticonvulsants (e.g., benzodiazepines, phenytoin, VPA) were invalid. All patients had terminations of the SE within 24 h after the administration of LEV; the only fatality was attributed to multiple organ failure rather than as a side effect of LEV. However, a randomized, double-blind, phase III study by Navarro et al. [264] compared the curative effects of IV LEV (2.5 g) or placebo in combination with CZP (1 mg) for the pre-hospital treatment of adults (>18 years) with GCSE. The treatment was efficient if SE was terminated within 15 min from the first injection of drugs. CZP combined with LEV was efficient in 57 of 68 patients (84%). CZP combined with placebo was efficient in 50 of 68 patients (74%). The study proved that polytherapy of LEV and CZP for GCSE is not superior to CZP monotherapy. LEV is a safe drug, with no apparent side effects being observed in either study.

The recommended IV dosage of LEV is 15–70 mg/kg in RSE children [314]. In the retrospective study by Gallentine et al. [167], LEV was administered as an add-on drug for 11 RSE children. During the period of LEV use, other anticonvulsants (diazepam, MDZ, barbiturates, etc.) were simultaneously used or concomitantly added. LEV (15–60 mg/kg) was given by nasal feeding or orally in four patients. LEV (15–62.5 mg/kg) was given by intravenous administration in six patients. LEV was given rectally (70 mg/kg) and followed by nasal feeding (20 mg/kg) in one patient. The effective rate of this treatment proposal was 73% (8/11). The termination time of RSE from its initial use of LEV was 1–8 (mean: 1.5) days. No obvious side reactions were observed. The working dose of LEV was more than 30 mg/kg/d (median: 40 mg/kg/d) in this study. The recommended initial dose of LEV in polytherapy was 30 mg/kg/d for RSE children. The administration method of LEV was intravenously, orally, and via nasal feeding.

Polytherapy of LEV and CZP in children with ESES syndrome was studied by Su et al. [311]. The study consisted of 15 patients with ESES syndrome, in whom LEV monotherapy was useless for both the EEG and clinical symptoms. Later, LEV (20–40 mg/kg/d) together with CZP was used orally at bedtime for 2 months. The treatment method of CZP was 0.02–0.03 mg/kg once per day for the first month and once every other day for the second month. Clinical convulsions disappeared in 14/15 patients. Sleep EEGs of the 14 patients were normal or showed mild low-amplitude discharge. The neuropsychological functioning of all of the patients was apparently improved in terms of language expression and academic performance. The polytherapy of LEV and CZP was proven to be more effective than monotherapy in this study.

Within 24 h after being given LEV, adults' SE was controlled in the research of Uges et al. [291]. The mean time until children's RSE was controlled was 1.5 days after LEV use [167].

The reported side effects of LEV were allergic reactions and mental confusion [167, 291]. In the report by Uges et al. [291], transient allergic reactions were observed in one patient, and confusion of consciousness was observed in five patients after SE had been stopped for 24 h. The disorientation may have presented secondary to the seizures and had nothing to do with LEV. In the study by Navarro et al. [264], the polytherapy of CZP and LEV had no apparent side reactions.

6.8.5.4 Topiramate

As a broad-spectrum AED, topiramate works by blocking voltage-sensitive sodium channels, thereby enhancing the activity of GABA at GABA-A receptors and inhibiting excitatory transmission. The polytherapy of phenytoin or carbamazepine with topiramate could make topiramate metabolize more rapidly [315]. Absorption is rapid after the enteral or oral administration of topiramate. A small number of reports have described the use of topiramate as an adjunctive drug for adults or children with SE and RSE. The feasibility, safety profile, and efficacy of topiramate (enterally or orally) as an add-on drug were demonstrated [316–318]. Topiramate is used as an adjunctive drug if SE is resistant to the standard first- to fourth-line therapies [318–320].

The polytherapy of topiramate is mainly used in adult RSE. In a retrospective study [321], topiramate was administered enterally in 35 adults (19–84 years, mean: 60.5 years) with RSE. All of the patients were resistant to first- and second-line AEDs. Topiramate was used together with other anticonvulsants (LZP or LEV). Within 72 h of the administration of topiramate, 71% of patients experienced RSE termination, and 9% experienced RSE termination within 24 h. Mortality (31%) was attributed to the primary disease causing the RSE, rather than to RSE or topiramate administration. In another prospective open-label nonrandomized clinical trial [315], 20 RSE adults who were treated with enteral topiramate were studied. As an adjunctive drug, topiramate was successful in terminating SE in 5 (25%) patients, was possibly successful in 11 (55%), and was unsuccessful in 4 (20%).

The recommended initial dosage is 200–400 mg/day. The alternative subsequent dosage is 300–1600 mg/day orally (divided 2–4 times per day) [199]. Topiramate was enterally administered as an add-on drug in studies by Hottinger et al. [321] and Asadi-Pooya et al. [315]. In the study by Hottinger et al. [321], patients were divided based on the topiramate dosage (Group 1, 800 mg/day; Group 2, 400–799 mg/day; Group 3, <400 mg/day). In Group 1, topiramate was definitely successful in terminating SE in no patients and was possibly successful in three of six (50%) patients. In Group 2, topiramate was definitely successful in terminating SE in two of 23 (9%) patients and possibly successful in 14 of 23 (61%) patients. In Group 3, topiramate was definitely successful in terminating SE in one of nine (11%) patients and possibly successful in five of nine (56%) patients.

Hottinger et al. [321] and Asadi-Pooya et al. [315] observed no clinically significant adverse events directly related to topiramate treatment. Slight hyperammonemia and hyperchloremic acidosis were found in patients treated with topiramate combined with VPA.

6.8.5.5 Lacosamide

Lacosamide is a relatively novel AED that acts on slow sodium channels. It has the following functions: stabilizing hyperexcitable neuronal membranes, inhibiting repetitive firing, neuroprotecting, and acting synergistically with other AEDs [322, 323]. The existing formulations of lacosamide are oral and intravenous. A small number of reports [324–326] have described the use of lacosamide as an adjunctive drug for the treatment of SE and RSE. Lacosamide efficacy was thought to be dependent on synergism with other AEDs because of its unique mechanism [325]. Comparatively speaking, lacosamide combined with other AEDs for the treatment of SE is well tolerated and efficacious. Lacosamide is used as an adjunctive drug if SE is resistant to the standard first- or second-line drugs or used together with benzodiazepines [322, 325].

Polytherapy of lacosamide is mainly used in adults' SE whether it is convulsive or nonconvulsive [322, 327]. Moreno Morales et al. [325]

designed a prospective observational study to observe the role of lacosamide in the treatment of CSE and NCSE. Once the patient was confirmed to meet the inclusion criterion, lacosamide was given intravenously whether as the first-line drug or as a concomitant drug with other AEDs at SE onset. Of 53 patients (55.2 ± 16.78 years), 69.8% were male, and 43.4% (n = 23) had CSE. Polytherapy of lacosamide and other AEDs (LEV, MDZ, VPA, pentobarbital, phenytoin) was received by 79.2% of patients. Among the polytherapy variations, 34% received lacosamide with one concomitant AED, 22.6% with two, and 22.6% with three. The most common polytherapy agents in this study were lacosamide + MDZ (n = 9), lacosamide + MDZ + VPA (n = 8), and lacosamide +LEV +MDZ + VPA (n = 12), including MDZ (54.7%), VPA (52.8%), and an hour of LEV (30.2%). EEGs were recorded to judge the termination of SE. In summary, seizures were controlled in 90% of NCSE patients and 91.3% of CSE patients in both the clinical and EEG assessments. Although the efficiency of polytherapy was not assessed independently, the overall efficiency of lacosamide monotherapy and polytherapy was satisfactory.

In a retrospective study [322], 111 adult patients suffering from RSE were studied, and 53% of them received intravenous lacosamide. Lacosamide, as an adjunctive drug, was used together with other AEDs like LZP and LEV if the standard AED was useless. SE control was observed more commonly in patients who received lacosamide ($p = 0.252$). Twenty-three of the 45 RSE patients were administered with lacosamide as the last AED, and 21 (91%) of the 23 experienced successful termination of RSE. The persistent periods of SE in patients treated with or without lacosamide were 87.2 ± 159.4 h and 134.3 ± 188.7 h, respectively.

In a study by Sutter et al. [322], the agent of RSE treatment was IV lacosamide with concomitant AEDs, such as LZP and LEV. The normal dosage of lacosamide was 200 mg twice a day. The dosage of lacosamide was reduced if patients had renal failure: 150 mg twice daily if the creatinine clearance was 30–50 mL and 100 mg twice daily if the creatinine clearance was <30 mL. One obese patient of 110 kg weight received a total daily dosage of 600 mg. In a study by Moreno Morales [325], SE patients received IV lacosamide 400 mg/day (over 30 min) for 8 days.

No clinically significant adverse effects were directly observed in the reports relative to the adjunctive lacosamide treatment [324, 325]. Minor adverse events of lacosamide were noted in some trials, such as skin allergies, angioedema, hypotension, and pruritus [323].

6.8.5.6 Phenytoin, Fosphenytoin, and Barbiturates

Phenytoin, fosphenytoin, and barbiturates (including phenobarbital, thiopentone, and pentobarbital) are traditional second-line AEDs [328]. The antiepileptic properties of these drugs for SE have been recognized and used for decades. Physicians have long-term clinical experiences with these drugs for both children and adults. The drugs are inexpensive and have widespread availability, even in some resource-scarce areas. The synergistic effects of these drugs with benzodiazepines have been demonstrated by Bankstahl et al. via animal studies [329, 330]. In a clinical RCT [240] including 570 GCSE patients, the polytherapy of diazepam and phenytoin was compared with other monotherapies. Any of the following four treatments was given to the patients initially: diazepam + phenytoin, phenytoin, phenobarbital, or LZP. All of the drugs were used intravenously. The doses of diazepam, phenytoin, phenobarbital, and LZP were 0.15 mg/kg, 18 mg/kg, 15 mg/kg, and 0.1 mg/kg, respectively. The statistical data analysis proved that the treatment effects of diazepam + phenytoin, LZP, and phenobarbital did not differ, but they all performed better than phenytoin treatment alone. However, Chen et al. [279] noted that the study did not include the polytherapy of LZP and phenytoin in the comparison. Because LZP is much more effective than diazepam in seizure termination, more clinical research is needed at present to compare the effects of polytherapy and monotherapy in different phases of SE.

Outin et al. [272] speculated that the attack time of GCSE preceding the initial therapy should provide the guideline for drug chosen. First, if the

SE duration is 5–30 min, CZP alone is used; if the arrest of SE had failed, polytherapy of CZP with either fosphenytoin or phenobarbital is given 5 min later. Second, if the SE duration is 30 min, monotherapy is almost always unsuccessful, and the polytherapy of CZP with either fosphenytoin or phenobarbital should be performed immediately. Without a doubt, the feasibility, safety profile, and efficacy of this regimen for treating SE should be explored further.

6.8.5.7 Immunomodulating Therapy

Immunomodulating therapy consists of a corticosteroid, plasma exchange, and intravenous immunoglobulin (IVIG) [331]. In the last few years, doctors have gradually found that autoimmune encephalitis, new-onset refractory status epilepticus (NORSE) syndrome, and some epilepsy syndromes in children were special causes of SE [332, 333]. SE induced by these causes is always refractory to the first- and/or second-line anticonvulsants [331, 334]. Hence, the polytherapy of anticonvulsants and immunomodulating therapy can halt SE as well as improve outcomes. Immunomodulating therapy is used with anticonvulsants concurrently [331, 334].

The indications for immunomodulating therapy include autoimmune encephalitis, such as anti-GABAR encephalitis; epilepsy syndromes in children, such as ESES; and NORSE syndrome [331, 334–336]. A retrospective clinical research study [334] investigated five NORSE syndrome patients (22–34 years, male/female = 3:2) who were previously healthy people with no history of epilepsy. Premonitory symptoms were observed in these patients before seizure attack. Adequate AEDs and anesthetic were all useless for these five patients. Polytherapy of anticonvulsants and immunomodulating therapy (corticosteroid or IVIG) was used in three patients in the early stage. Complete arrest of RSE was achieved in all the three patients. According to the follow-up, serious neuropsychological defects were absent in them. To our delight, two of them resumed full-time work. One patient, the one who did not use immunomodulating therapy, ultimately died of complications. One patient lost communication during the follow-up. Sinclair et al. [335] studied ten children (2–11 years, male/female = 7:3) with Landau-Kleffner syndrome (LKS) (n = 8) and epilepsy with continuous spikes and waves during slow-wave sleep (CSWS) (n = 2); these children were treated with corticosteroids combined with anticonvulsants. All of the patients' EEGs were characterized by ESES. The dose of prednisone was 1 mg/kg/day for 6 months continuously. The follow-up period was 1–10 years. All of the patients experienced great improvement in language, cognition, and action after the treatment, except one. All of the patients' EEGs almost returned to normal in 3–6 months after the corticosteroid treatment. The patients' prognoses were good comparatively, and transient side effects were observed in four children. The study proved the effectiveness and safety of the polytherapy of corticosteroids and AEDs for CSWS and LKS children with ESES.

In a case report [334] of a 26-year-old patient with NORSE syndrome, polytherapy of anticonvulsants and corticosteroid was used. The patient had the following features: no previous history of epilepsy, no pathogenic factors of epilepsy, with a history of hyperthyroidism, with positive anti-TPO antibody, and with nonspecific symptoms (headache and vomit). In the course of the disease, different seizures appeared and gradually developed into GCSE, where upon the patient was admitted to the ICU for treatment with general anesthesia. The patient received both anesthesia (propofol, thiopental, and phenobarbital) and AEDs (phenytoin, VPA, LEV), but failed to stop their SEs. Etiologies considered to be immunological factors and infections were ruled out. On the 12th day following admission, corticosteroid treatment was used. The administration approaches of immunomodulating therapy were as follows: (1) on the first 3 days, methylprednisolone was given 1 g/d intravenously; (2) next, prednisone was given 60 mg/d orally; (3) finally, on the 18th day after admission, intravenous immunoglobulin was given intravenously for 5 days with an accumulated dose of 150 g. After 2 months of inhospital treatment, the patient recovered and returned home. The polytherapy of oral immunosuppressors and AEDs continued outside the hospital to prevent epilepsy. Dubey et al. [337] retrospectively analyzed three patients (33–55 years, male/female = 2:1) with focal NCSE caused by autoimmune encephalitis. The etiology was considered to be an immunological factor, whereas infection and tumor were ruled out. Some antibodies directed against the cell membrane or synaptic receptors were positive in all patients. The symptoms included dysmnesia and mental disorders. The polytherapy of AEDs (LEV, lacosamide, phenobarbital, lamotrigine, and VPA), immunomodulatory therapy (corticosteroid, plasma exchange, and IVIG), and rituximab was administered to the patients with no severe adverse events. In two patients, the following four-step therapies were used sequentially: 5 g of intravenous methylprednisolone over 5 days, five cycles of plasmapheresis, 2 g/kg IVIG over 5 days, and 0.5 or 1 g of intravenous rituximab. In the course of treatment, anticonvulsants were used simultaneously. Plasmapheresis and IVIG were given because symptoms were not completely relieved, and rituximab was used to achieve long-term immune suppression. In another patient, the 2 g/kg IVIG over 5 days and 0.5 g of intravenous rituximab were administered together with anticonvulsants. After 4–6 weeks of inhospital treatment, all of the patients with SE were discharged.

It is recommended that the polytherapy of anticonvulsants and immune inhibitors (azathioprine, mycophenolate mofetil, etc.) for longer than 1 year is needed after patients are discharged to prevent seizures and SE recurrence [331, 334].

6.8.5.8 Neuromodulatory Drugs and Non-Pharmacological Strategies

In recent years, neuromodulatory drugs and non-pharmacological strategies have been gradually combined with anticonvulsants for the treatment of RSE. Neuromodulatory drugs include steroids, melatonin, coenzymes, and neurosteroid metabolites. Non-pharmacological strategies include vagus nerve stimulation, surgical treatment, ketogenic diet, and transcranial magnetic stimulation, among others [305, 338–342]. Most of the strategies listed above are based on rare animal experiments or small amount of clinical research data. These interventions have little support from evidence-based medicine. These radical and novel therapies should be used as last resorts.

References

1. Fountain NB, Adams RE. Midazolam treatment of acute and refractory status epilepticus. Clin Neuropharmacol. 1999;22(5):261–7.
2. Ulgey A, Aksu R, Bicer C. Nasal and buccal treatment of midazolam in epileptic seizures in pediatrics. Clin Med Insights Pediatr. 2012;6:51–60.
3. Lee JI, Chaves-Gnecco D, Amico JA, Kroboth PD, Wilson JW, Frye RF. Application of semisimultaneous midazolam administration for hepatic and intestinal cytochrome P450 3A phenotyping. Clin Pharmacol Ther. 2002;72(6):718–28.
4. Kaneko S, Kurahashi K, Fujita S, Fukushima Y, Sato T, Hill RG. Potentiation of GABA by midazolam and its therapeutic effect against status epilepticus. Folia Psychiatr Neurol Jpn. 1983;37(3):307–9.
5. Sanchez Fernandez I, Loddenkemper T. Therapeutic choices in convulsive status epilepticus. Expert Opin Pharmacother. 2015;16(4):487–500.
6. Ferlisi M, Hocker S, Grade M, Trinka E, Shorvon S, A. International Steering Committee of the StEp. Preliminary results of the global audit of treatment of refractory status epilepticus. Epilepsy Behav. 2015;49:318–24.
7. Rossetti AO, Bleck TP. What's new in status epilepticus? Intensive Care Med. 2014;40(9):1359–62.
8. Claassen J, Hirsch LJ, Emerson RG, Bates JE, Thompson TB, Mayer SA. Continuous EEG monitoring and midazolam infusion for refractory nonconvulsive status epilepticus. Neurology. 2001;57(6):1036–42.
9. Ulvi H, Yoldas T, Mungen B, Yigiter R. Continuous infusion of midazolam in the treatment of refractory generalized convulsive status epilepticus. Neurol Sci. 2002;23(4):177–82.
10. Ferlisi M, Shorvon S. The outcome of therapies in refractory and super-refractory convulsive status epilepticus and recommendations for therapy. Brain. 2012;135(Pt 8):2314–28.
11. Prasad A, Worrall BB, Bertram EH, Bleck TP. Propofol and midazolam in the treatment of refractory status epilepticus. Epilepsia. 2001;42(3):380–6.
12. Claassen J, Hirsch LJ, Emerson RG, Mayer SA. Treatment of refractory status epilepticus with pentobarbital, propofol, or midazolam: a systematic review. Epilepsia. 2002;43(2):146–53.
13. Singhi S, Murthy A, Singhi P, Jayashree M. Continuous midazolam versus diazepam infusion for refractory convulsive status epilepticus. J Child Neurol. 2002;17(2):106–10.
14. Hubert P, Parain D, Vallée L. Management of convulsive status epilepticus in infants and children. Rev Neurol (Paris). 2009;165(4):390–7.
15. Ozdemir D, Gulez P, Uran N, Yendur G, Kavakli T, Aydin A. Efficacy of continuous midazolam infusion and mortality in childhood refractory generalized convulsive status epilepticus. Seizure. 2005;14(2):129–32.
16. Morrison G, Gibbons E, Whitehouse WP. High-dose midazolam therapy for refractory status

epilepticus in children. Intensive Care Med. 2006;32(12):2070–6.
17. Bello-Espinosa LE. Infraslow status epilepticus: a new form of subclinical status epilepticus recorded in a child with Sturge-Weber syndrome. Epilepsy Behav. 2015;49:193–7.
18. Spiller HA, Carlisle RD. Status epilepticus after massive carbamazepine overdose. J Toxicol Clin Toxicol. 2002;40(1):81–90.
19. Brophy GM, Bell R, Claassen J, Alldredge B, Bleck TP, Glauser T, Laroche SM, Riviello JJ Jr, Shutter L, Sperling MR, Treiman DM, Vespa PM, Neurocritical Care Society Status Epilepticus Guideline Writing. Guidelines for the evaluation and management of status epilepticus. Neurocrit Care. 2012;17(1):3–23.
20. Galvin GM, Jelinek GA. Midazolam: an effective intravenous agent for seizure control. Arch Emerg Med. 1987;4(3):169–72.
21. Wilkes R, Tasker RC. Intensive care treatment of uncontrolled status epilepticus in children: systematic literature search of midazolam and anesthetic therapies*. Pediatr Crit Care Med. 2014;15(7):632–9.
22. Fernandez A, Lantigua H, Lesch C, Shao B, Foreman B, Schmidt JM, Hirsch LJ, Mayer SA, Claassen J. High-dose midazolam infusion for refractory status epilepticus. Neurology. 2014;82(4):359–65.
23. Parent JM, Lowenstein DH. Treatment of refractory generalized status epilepticus with continuous infusion of midazolam. Neurology. 1994;44(10):1837–40.
24. Tomalik-Scharte D, Suleiman AA, Frechen S, et al. Population pharmacokinetic analysis of circadian rhythms in hepatic CYP3A activity using midazolam. J Clin Pharmacol. 2014;54(10):1162–9.
25. Veldhorst-Janssen NM, Fiddelers AA, Ph VDK, et al. Pharmacokinetics and tolerability of nasal versus intravenous midazolam in healthy Dutch volunteers: a single-dose, randomized-sequence, open-label, 2-period crossover pilot study. J Clinical Therapeutics. 2011;33(12):2022–8.
26. Kravljanac R, Djuric M, Jankovic B, Pekmezovic T. Etiology, clinical course and response to the treatment of status epilepticus in children: a 16-year single-center experience based on 602 episodes of status epilepticus. Eur J Paediatr Neurol. 2015;19(5):584–90.
27. Federman MD, Kelly R, Harrison RE. Refractory metabolic acidosis as a complication of high-dose midazolam infusion for pediatric status epilepticus. Clin Neuropharmacol. 2009;32(6):340–1.
28. Singh SP, Agarwal S, Faulkner M. Refractory status epilepticus. Ann Indian Acad Neurol. 2014;17(Suppl 1):S32–6.
29. Shorvon S. The treatment of status epilepticus. Curr Opin Neurol. 2011;24(2):165–70.
30. Hughes J, Gill A, Leach HJ, Nunn AJ, Billingham I, Ratcliffe J, Thornington R, Choonara I. A prospective study of the adverse effects of midazolam on withdrawal in critically ill children. Acta Paediatr. 1994;83(11):1194–9.
31. Epstein D, Difazio M. Orofacial automatisms induced by acute withdrawal from high-dose midazolam mimicking nonconvulsive status epilepticus in a child. Mov Disord. 2007;22(5):712–5.
32. Wang H, Wang Z, Mi W, Zhao C, Liu Y, Wang Y, Sun H. Propofol effectively inhibits lithium-pilocarpine-induced status epilepticus in rats via downregulation of N-methyl-D-aspartate receptor 2B subunit expression. Neural Regen Res. 2012;7(11):827–32.
33. Wood PR, Browne GP, Pugh S. Propofol infusion for the treatment of status epilepticus. Lancet. 1988;1(8583):480–1.
34. Langer JE, Fountain NB. A retrospective observational study of current treatment for generalized convulsive status epilepticus. Epilepsy Behav. 2014;37:95–9.
35. Melloni C, Fusari M, Scesi M, Franzoni E, Marchiani V, Mazzarino A, Candiani A, De Maria G. The use of propofol in status epilepticus. Minerva Anestesiol. 1992;58(9):553–6.
36. Rossetti AO, Santoli F. Drug treatment of refractory status epilepticus. Rev Neurol (Paris). 2009;165(4):373–9.
37. Yamanouchi H. Treatment of status epilepticus. Nihon Rinsho. 2014;72(5):895–901.
38. Rossetti AO, Lowenstein DH. Management of refractory statu s epilepticus in adults: still more questions than answers. Lancet Neurol. 2011;10(10):922–30.
39. Holtkamp M. Treatment strategies for refractory status epilepticus. Curr Opin Crit Care. 2011;17(2):94–100.
40. Power KN, Flaatten H, Gilhus NE, Engelsen BA. Propofol treatment in adult refractory status epilepticus. Mortality risk and outcome. Epilepsy Res. 2011;94(1–2):53–60.
41. Niermeijer JM, Uiterwaal CS, Van Donselaar CA. Propofol in status epilepticus: little evidence, many dangers? J Neurol. 2003;250(10):1237–40.
42. Parviainen I, Uusaro A, Kälviäinen R, Mervaala E, Ruokonen E. Propofol in the treatment of refractory status epilepticus. Intensive Care Med. 2006;32(7):1075–9.
43. Kang BS, Jung KH, Shin JW, Moon JS, Byun JI, Lim JA, Moon HJ, Kim YS, Lee ST, Chu K, Lee SK. Induction of burst suppression or coma using intravenous anesthetics in refractory status epilepticus. J Clin Neurosci. 2015;22(5):854–8.
44. Sabharwal V, Ramsay E, Martinez R, Shumate R, Khan F, Dave H, Iwuchukwu I, McGrade H. Propofol-ketamine combination therapy for effective control of super-refractory status epilepticus. Epilepsy Behav. 2015;52(Pt A):264–6.
45. Höfler J, Rohracher A, Kalss G, et al. (S)-Ketamine in refractory and super-refractory status epilepticus: a retrospective study. CNS Drugs. 2016;30(9):869–76.
46. Meierkord H, Boon P, Engelsen B, Göcke K, Shorvon S, Tinuper P, Holtkamp M. European Federation of Neurological Societies. EFNS guideline on the management of status epilepticus in adults. Eur J Neurol. 2010;17(3):348–55.
47. Begemann M, Rowan AJ, Tuhrim S. Treatment of refractory complex-partial status epilepticus with propofol: case report. Epilepsia. 2000;41(1):105–9.

48. Capovilla G, Beccaria F, Beghi E, Minicucci F, Sartori S, Vecchi M. Treatment of convulsive status epilepticus in childhood: recommendations of the Italian League Against Epilepsy. Epilepsia. 2013;54(Suppl 7):23–34.
49. van Gestel JP, Blussé van Oud-Alblas HJ, Malingré M, Ververs FF, Braun KP, van Nieuwenhuizen O. Propofol and thiopental for refractory status epilepticus in children. Neurology. 2005;65(4):591–2.
50. Riviello JJ Jr, Claassen J, LaRoche SM, Sperling MR, Alldredge B, Bleck TP, Glauser T, Shutter L, Treiman DM, Vespa PM, Bell R, Brophy GM, Neurocritical Care Society Status Epilepticus Guideline Writing Committee. Treatment of status epilepticus: an international survey of experts. Neurocrit Care. 2013;18(2):193–200.
51. Tully I, Draper ES, Lamming CR, Mattison D, Thomas C, Martland T, Appleton R. Admissions to paediatric intensive care units (PICU) with refractory convulsive status epilepticus (RCSE): a two-year Multi-Centre Study. Seizure. 2015;29:153–61.
52. Moreno-Medinilla EE, Negrillo-Ruano R, Calvo-Medina R, Mora-Ramírez MD, Martínez-Antón JL. Status epilepticus in paediatrics: a retrospective study and review of the literature. Rev Neurol. 2015;60(9):394–400.
53. Prabhakar H, Kalaivani M. Propofol versus thiopental sodium for the treatment of refractory status epilepticus. Cochrane Database Syst Rev. 2015;(6):CD009202.
54. Prabhakar H, Bindra A, Singh GP, Kalaivani M. Propofol versus thiopental sodium for the treatment of refractory status epilepticus (review). Evid Based Child Health. 2013;8(4):1488–508.
55. Rossetti AO, Milligan TA, Vulliémoz S, Michaelides C, Bertschi M, Lee JW. A randomized trial for the treatment of refractory status epilepticus. Neurocrit Care. 2011;14(1):4–10.
56. Parviainen I, Kälviäinen R, Ruokonen E. Propofol and barbiturates for the anesthesia of refractory convulsive status epilepticus: pros and cons. Neurol Res. 2007;29(7):667–71.
57. Iyer VN, Hoel R, Rabinstein AA. Propofol infusion syndrome in patients with refractory status epilepticus: an 11-year clinical experience. Crit Care Med. 2009;37(12):3024–30.
58. Stecker MM, Kramer TH, Raps EC, O'Meeghan R, Dulaney E, Skaar DJ. Treatment of refractory status epilepticus with propofol: clinical and pharmacokinetic findings. Epilepsia. 1998;39(1):18–26.
59. Mäkelä JP, Iivanainen M, Pieninkeroinen IP, Waltimo O, Lahdensuu M. Seizures associated with propofol anesthesia. Epilepsia. 1993;34(5):832–5.
60. Marik PE. Propofol: therapeutic indications and side-effects. Curr Pharm Des. 2004;10(29):3639–49. Review.
61. Ku BD, Park KC, Yoon SS. Dark green discoloration of the urine after prolonged propofol infusion: a case report. J Clin Pharm Ther. 2011;36(6):734–6.
62. Wong J. Propofol infusion syndrome. Am J Ther. 2010;17:487–91.
63. Roberts RJ, Barletta JF, Fong JJ, Schumaker G, Kuper PJ, Papadopoulos S, Yogaratnam D, Kendali E, Xamplas R, Gerlach AT, Szumita PM, Anger KE, Arpino PA, Voils SA, Grgurich P, Ruthazer R, Devlin JW. Incidence of propofol-related infusion syndrome in critically ill adults: a prospective, multicenter study. Crit Care. 2009;13:R169.
64. Walli A, Poulsen TD, Dam M, Børglum J. Propofol infusion syndrome in refractory status epilepticus: a case report and topical review. Case Rep Emerg Med. 2016;2016:3265929.
65. Guitton C, Gabillet L, Latour P, Rigal JC, Boutoille D, Al Habash O, Derkinderen P, Bretonniere C, Villers D. Propofol Infusion syndrome during refractory status epilepticus in a young adult: successful ECMO resuscitation. Neurocrit Care. 2011;15(1):139–45.
66. Da-Silva SS, Wong R, Coquillon P, Gavrilita C, Asuncion A. Partial-exchange blood transfusion: an effective method for preventing mortality in a child with propofol infusion syndrome. Pediatrics. 2010;125(6):e1493–9.
67. Baumeister FA, Oberhoffer R, Liebhaber GM, Kunkel J, Eberhardt J, Holthausen H, Peters J. Fatal propofol infusion syndrome in association with ketogenic diet. Neuropediatrics. 2004;35(4):250–2.
68. Kumar MA, Urrutia VC, Thomas CE, Abou-Khaled KJ, Schwartzman RJ. The syndrome of irreversible acidosis after prolonged propofol infusion. Neurocrit Care. 2005;3(3):257–9.
69. Fang YT, Wu VC, Tang SC, Yeh HM. Extracorporeal membrane oxygenation and sustained low-efficiency diafiltration successfully resuscitated propofol infusion syndrome during refractory status epilepticus. J Formos Med Assoc. 2015;114(11):1145–6.
70. Mayette M, Gonda J, Hsu JL, Mihm FG. Propofol infusion syndrome resuscitation with extracorporeal life support: a case report and review of the literature. Ann Intensive Care. 2013;3(1):32.
71. Levin PD, Levin V, Weissman C, Sprung CL, Rund D. Therapeutic plasma exchange as treatment for propofol infusion syndrome. J Clin Apher. 2015;30(5):311–3.
72. Zubair S, Patton T, Smithson K, Sonmezturk HH, Arain A, Abou-Khalil B. Propofol withdrawal seizures: non-epileptic nature of seizures in a patient with recently controlled status epilepticus. Epileptic Disord. 2011;13(1):107–10.
73. Bhatt AB, Popescu A, Waterhouse EJ, Abou-Khalil BW. De novo generalized periodic discharges related to anesthetic withdrawal resolve spontaneously. J Clin Neurophysiol. 2014;31(3):194–8.
74. Dayton PG, Stiller RL, Cook DR, Perel JM. The binding of ketamine to plasma proteins: Emphasis on human plasma. Eur J Clin Pharmacol. 1983;24:825–31.
75. Noppers I, Niesters M, Aarts L, Smith T, Sarton E, Dahan A. Ketamine for the treatment of chronic noncancer pain. Expert Opin Pharmacother. 2010; 11:2417–29.

76. Grant IS, Nimmo WS, McNicol LR, Clements JA. Ketamine disposition in children and adults. Br J Anaesth. 1983;55:1107–11.
77. Aram JA, Martin D, Tomczyk M, Zeman S, Millar J, Pohler G, et al. Neocortical epileptogenesis in vitro: studies with N-methyl-D-aspartate, phencyclidine, sigma and dextromethorphan receptorligands. J Pharmacol Exp Ther. 1989;248(1):320–8.
78. Aroni F, Iacovidou N, Dontas I, Pourzitaki C, Xanthos T. Pharmacological aspects and potential new clinical applications of ketamine: reevaluation of an old drug. J Clin Pharmacol. 2009;49(8):957–64.
79. Potter DE, Choudhury M. Ketamine: repurposing and redefining a multifaceted drug. Drug Discov Today. 2014;19(12):1848–54.
80. Peng S, Zhang Y, Wang H, Ren B, Zhang J. Anesthetic ketamine counteracts repetitive mechanical stress-induced learning and memory impairment in developing mice. Mol Biol Rep. 2011;38(7):4347–51.
81. Fujikawa DG. Neuroprotective effect of ketamine administered after status epilepticus onset. Epilepsia. 1995;36(2):186–95.
82. McCarthy D, Chen G, Kaump DH, Ensor C. General anesthetic and other pharmacological properties of 2-(O-chlorophenyl)-2-methylamino-cyclohexanone HCl (CI-58L). J New Drugs. 1965;5(1):21–33.
83. Corssen G, Miyasaka M, Domino EF. Changing concepts in pain control during surgery: dissociative anesthesia with CI-581. A progress report. Anesth Analg. 1968;47(6):746–59.
84. Kayama Y, Iwama K. The EEG, evoked potentials, and single-unit activity during ketamine anesthesia in cats. Anesthesiology. 1972;36(4):316–28.
85. Corssen G, Little SC, Tavakoli M. Ketamine and epilepsy. Anesth Analg. 1974;53(2):319–35.
86. Gaspard N, Foreman B, Judd LM, Brenton JN, Nathan BR, McCoy BM, et al. Intravenous ketamine for the treatment of refractory status epilepticus: a retrospective multicenter study. Epilepsia. 2013;54(8):1498–503.
87. Ilvento L, Rosati A, Marini C, L'Erario M, Mirabile L, Guerrini R. Ketamine in refractory convulsive status epilepticus in children avoids endotracheal intubation. Epilepsy Behav. 2015;49:3436.
88. Mewasingh LD, Skhara T, Aeby A, Christiaens FJ, Dan B. Oral ketamine in paediatric non-convulsive status epilepticus. Seizure. 2003;12(7):483–9.
89. Fang Y, Wang XF. Ketamine for the treatment of refractory status epilepticus. Seizure. 2015;30:14–20.
90. Borris DJ, Bertram EH, Kapur J. Ketamine controls prolonged status epilepticus. Epilepsy Res. 2000;42(2–3):117–22.
91. McGinn KA, Bishop L, Sarwal A. Use of ketamine in barbiturate coma for status epilepticus. Clin Neuropharmacol. 2016;39(1):62–5.
92. Shrestha GS, Joshi P, Chhetri S, Karn R, Acharya SP. Intravenous ketamine for treatment of super-refractory convulsive status epilepticus with septic shock: A report of two cases. Indian J Crit Care Med. 2015;19(5):283–5.
93. Rosati A, Erario LM, Ilvento L, Cecchi C, Pisano T, Mirabile L, et al. Efficacy and safety of ketamine in refractory status epilepticus in children. Neurology. 2012;79(24):2355–8.
94. Loscher W. Mechanisms of drug resistance in status epilepticus. Epilepsia. 2007;48(Suppl 8):74–7.
95. Deeb TZ, Maguire J, Moss SJ. Possible alterations in GABAA receptor signaling that underlie benzodiazepine-resistant seizures. Epilepsia. 2012;53(Suppl 9):79–88.
96. Feng HJ, Mathews GC, Kao C, Macdonald RL. Alterations of GABAA-receptor function and allosteric modulation during development of status epilepticus. J Neurophysiol. 2008;99(3):1285–93.
97. Dingledine R, Borges K, Bowie D, Traynelis SF. The glutamate receptor ion channels. Pharmacol Rev. 1999;51(1):7–61.
98. Fujikawa DG. Prolonged seizure and cellular injury: understanding the connection. Epilepsy Behav. 2005;7(Suppl 3):S3–11.
99. Zeiler FA. Early use of the NMDA receptor antagonist ketamine in refractory and superrefractory status epilepticus. Crit Care Res Pract. 2015;2015: 831260.
100. Basha MM, Alqallaf A, Shah AK. Drug-induced EEG pattern predicts effectiveness of ketamine in treating refractory status epilepticus. Epilepsia. 2015;56(4):e44–8.
101. Zeiler FA, Teitelbaum J, Gillman LM, West M. NMDA antagonists for refractory seizures. Neurocrit Care. 2014;20(3):502–13.
102. Synowiec AS, Singh DS, Yenugadhati V, Valeriano JP, Schramke CJ, Kelly KM. Ketamine use in the treatment of refractory status epilepticus. Epilepsy Res. 2013;105(1–2):183–8.
103. Zeiler FA, Kaufmann AM, Gillman LM, West M, Silvaggio J. Ketamine for medically refractory status epilepticus after elective aneurysm clipping. Neurocrit Care. 2013;19(1):119–24.
104. Rosati A, Erario LM, Ilvento L, Pisano T, Mirabile L, Guerrini R. An ongoing open-label uncontrolled study of the efficacy and safety of ketamine in children with refractory status epilepticus. Epilepsia. 2013;54(Suppl 3):17.
105. Yeh PS, Shen HN, Chen TY. Oral ketamine controlled refractory nonconvulsive status epilepticus in an elderly patient. Seizure. 2011;20(9):723–6.
106. Craven R. Ketamine. Anaesthesia. 2007;62(Suppl 1):48–53.
107. Kramer AH. Early ketamine to treat refractory status epilepticus. Neurocrit Care. 2012;16(2):299–305.
108. Sheth RD, Gidal BE. Refractory status epilepticus: response to ketamine. Neurology. 1998;51(6):1765–6.
109. Takeshita H, Okuda Y, Sari A. The effects of ketamine on cerebral circulation and metabolism in man. Anaesthesiology. 1972;36(1):69–75.
110. Himmelseher S, Durieux M. Ketamine for perioperative pain management. Anaesthesiology. 2005;102(1):211–20.

111. Zeiler FA, Teitelbaum J, West M, Gillman LM. The ketamine effect on intracranial pressure in nontraumatic neurological illness. J Crit Care. 2014;29(6):1096–106.
112. U.S. Food and Drug Administration. KETALAR-ketamine hydrochloride injection. 2013. https://www.fda.gov/safety/medwatch/safetyinformation/ucm299547.htm. Accessed 10 Dec 2014.
113. Roberts DJ, Hall RI, Kramer AH, Robertson HL, Gallagher CN, Zygun DA. Sedation for critically ill adults with severe traumatic brain injury: a systematic review of randomized controlled trials. Crit Care Med. 2011;39(12):2743–51.
114. Dorandeu F, Barbier L, Dhote F, Testylier G, Carpentier P. Ketamine combinations for the field treatment of soman-induced self-sustaining status epilepticus. Review of current data and perspectives. Chem Biol Interact. 2013;203(1):154–9.
115. Bergman SA. Ketamine: review of its pharmacology and its use in pediatric anesthesia. Anesth Prog. 1999;46(1):10–20.
116. Reich DL, Silvay G. Ketamine: an update on the first twenty five years of clinical experience. Can J Anaesth. 1989;36(2):186–97.
117. Wutzler A, Huemer M, Boldt LH, Parwani AS, Attanasio P, Tscholl V, et al. Effects of deep sedation on cardiac electrophysiology in patients undergoing radiofrequency ablation of supraventricular tachycardia: impact of propofol and ketamine. Europace. 2013;15(7):1019–24.
118. Haas DA, Harper DG. Ketamine: a review of its pharmacological properties and use in ambulatory anesthesia. Anesth Prog. 1992;39:61–8.
119. Antal M, Mucsi G, Faludi A. Ketamine anesthesia and intraocular pressure. Ann Ophthalmol. 1978;10(9):1281–4.
120. Blumberg D, Congdon N, Jampel H, Gilbert D, Elliott R, Rivers R, et al. The effects of sevoflurane and ketamine on intraocular pressure in children during examination under anesthesia. Am J Ophthalmol. 2007;143(3):494–9.
121. Chandorkar AG, Jain PK, Albal MV. Modulations in intraocular pressure under ketamine anaesthesia. Indian J Ophthalmol. 1975;23(1):22–4.
122. Olney JW, Labruyere J, Wang G, Wozniak DF, Price MT, Sesma MA. NMDA antagonist neurotoxicity: mechanism and prevention. Science. 1991;254(5037):1515–8.
123. Dorandeu F, Dhote F, Barbier L, Baccus B, Testylier G. Treatment of status epilepticus with ketamine, are we there yet? CNS Neurosci Ther. 2013;19(6):411–27.
124. Wang C, Liu F, Patterson T, Paule MG, Slikker W Jr. Preclinical assessment of ketamine. CNS Neurosci Ther. 2013;19(6):448–53.
125. Dhote F, Carpentier P, Barbier L, Peinnequin A, Baille V, Pernot F, et al. Combinations of ketamine and atropine are neuroprotective and reduce neuroinflammation after a toxic status epilepticus in mice. Toxicol Appl Pharmacol. 2012;259(2):195–209.
126. Fauvelle F, Carpentier P, Dorandeu F, Foquin A, Testylier G. Prediction of neuroprotective treatment efficiency using a HRMAS NMR-based statistical model of refractory status epilepticus on mouse: a metabolomic approach supported by histology. J Proteome Res. 2012;11(7):3782–95.
127. Zona C, Niespodziany I, Marchetti C, Klitgaard H, Bernardi G, Margineanu DG. Levetiracetam does not modulate neuronal voltage-gated Na+ and T-type Ca2+ currents. Seizure. 2001;10(4):279–86.
128. Patsalos PN. The pharmacokinetic characteristics of levetiracetam. Methods Find Exp Clin Pharmacol. 2003;25(2):123–9.
129. Perucca E, Johannessen SI. The ideal pharmacokinetic properties of an antiepileptic drug: how close does levetiracetam come? Epileptic Disord. 2003;5(Suppl 1):S17–26.
130. Tong X, Patsalos PN. A microdialysis study of the novel antiepileptic drug levetiracetam: extracellular pharmacokinetics and effect on taurine in rat brain. Br J Pharmacol. 2001;133(6):867–74.
131. Brodie MJ, Perucca E, Ryvlin P, Ben-Menachem E, Meencke HJ. Comparison of levetiracetam and controlled-release carbamazepine in newly diagnosed epilepsy. Neurology. 2007;68(6):402–8.
132. Doheny HC, Ratnaraj N, Whittington MA, Jefferys JG, Patsalos PN. Blood and cerebrospinal fluid pharmacokinetics of the novel anticonvulsant levetiracetam (ucb L059) in the rat. Epilepsy Res. 1999;34(2–3):161–8.
133. Radtke RA. Pharmacokinetics of levetiracetam. Epilepsia. 2001;42(Suppl 4):24–7.
134. Perucca E, Gidal BE, Baltes E. Effects of antiepileptic comedication on levetiracetam pharmacokinetics: a pooled analysis of data from randomized adjunctive therapy trials. Epilepsy Res. 2003;53(1–2):47–56.
135. Brockmoller J, Thomsen T, Wittstock M, Coupez R, Lochs H, Roots I. Pharmacokinetics of levetiracetam in patients with moderate to severe liver cirrhosis (Child-Pugh classes A, B, and C): characterization by dynamic liver function tests. Clin Pharmacol Ther. 2005;77(6):529–41.
136. Svalheim S, Tauboll E, Surdova K, Ormel L, Dahl E, Aleksandersen M, et al. Long-term levetiracetam treatment affects reproductive endocrine function in female Wistar rats. Seizure. 2008;17(2):203–9.
137. Klitgaard H. Levetiracetam: the preclinical profile of a new class of antiepileptic drugs? Epilepsia. 2001;42(Suppl 4):13–8.
138. Mazarati AM, Baldwin R, Klitgaard H, Matagne A, Wasterlain CG. Anticonvulsant effects of levetiracetam and levetiracetam-diazepam combinations in experimental status epilepticus. Epilepsy Res. 2004;58(2–3):167–74.
139. Rigo JM, Hans G, Nguyen L, Rocher V, Belachew S, Malgrange B, et al. The anti-epileptic drug levetiracetam reverses the inhibition by negative allosteric

modulators of neuronal GABA- and glycine-gated currents. Br J Pharmacol. 2002;136(5):659–72.
140. Gibbs JE, Walker MC, Cock HR. Levetiracetam: antiepileptic properties and protective effects on mitochondrial dysfunction in experimental status epilepticus. Epilepsia. 2006;47(3):469–78.
141. Zheng Y, Moussally J, Cash SS, Karnam HB, Cole AJ. Intravenous levetiracetam in the rat pilocarpine-induced status epilepticus model: behavioral, physiological and histological studies. Neuropharmacology. 2010;58(4–5):793–8.
142. Brandt C, Glien M, Gastens AM, Fedrowitz M, Bethmann K, Volk HA, et al. Prophylactic treatment with levetiracetam after status epilepticus: lack of effect on epileptogenesis, neuronal damage, and behavioral alterations in rats. Neuropharmacology. 2007;53(2):207–21.
143. Loscher W, Honack D, Rundfeldt C. Antiepileptogenic effects of the novel anticonvulsant levetiracetam (ucb L059) in the kindling model of temporal lobe epilepsy. J Pharmacol Exp Ther. 1998;284(2):474–9.
144. Klitgaard H, Matagne A, Gobert J, Wulfert E. Evidence for a unique profile of levetiracetam in rodent models of seizures and epilepsy. Eur J Pharmacol. 1998;353(2–3):191–206.
145. Rosenow F, Knake S, Hamer HM. Non-convulsive status epilepticus: temporary fad or reality in need of treatment? Der Nervenarzt. 2012;83(12):1551–8.
146. Meierkord H, Boon P, Engelsen B, Gocke K, Shorvon S, Tinuper P, et al. EFNS guideline on the management of status epilepticus in adults. Eur J Neurol. 2010;17(3):348–55.
147. Patel NC, Landan IR, Levin J, Szaflarski J, Wilner AN. The use of levetiracetam in refractory status epilepticus. Seizure. 2006;15(3):137–41.
148. Rossetti AO, Bromfield EB. Determinants of success in the use of oral levetiracetam in status epilepticus. Epilepsy Behav. 2006;8(3):651–4.
149. Trabacca A, Profice P, Costanza MC, Gesualdi M, De Rinaldis M. Levetiracetam in nonconvulsive status epilepticus in childhood: a case report. J Child Neurol. 2007;22(5):639–41.
150. Knake S, Gruener J, Hattemer K, Klein KM, Bauer S, Oertel WH, et al. Intravenous levetiracetam in the treatment of benzodiazepine refractory status epilepticus. J Neurol Neurosurg Psychiatry. 2008;79(5):588–9.
151. Moddel G, Bunten S, Dobis C, Kovac S, Dogan M, Fischera M, et al. Intravenous levetiracetam: a new treatment alternative for refractory status epilepticus. J Neurol Neurosurg Psychiatry. 2009;80(6):689–92.
152. Eue S, Grumbt M, Muller M, Schulze A. Two years of experience in the treatment of status epilepticus with intravenous levetiracetam. Epilepsy Behav. 2009;15(4):467–9.
153. Tripathi M, Vibha D, Choudhary N, Prasad K, Srivastava MV, Bhatia R, et al. Management of refractory status epilepticus at a tertiary care centre in a developing country. Seizure. 2010;19(2):109–11.
154. Abend NS, Monk HM, Licht DJ, Dlugos DJ. Intravenous levetiracetam in critically ill children with status epilepticus or acute repetitive seizures. Pediatr Crit Care Med. 2009;10(4):505–10.
155. Kim JS, Lee JH, Ryu HW, Lim BC, Hwang H, Chae JH, et al. Effectiveness of intravenous levetiracetam as an adjunctive treatment in pediatric refractory status epilepticus. Pediatr Emerg Care. 2014;30(8):525–8.
156. Isguder R, Guzel O, Ceylan G, Yilmaz U, Agin H. A comparison of intravenous levetiracetam and valproate for the treatment of refractory status epilepticus in children. J Child Neurol. 2016;31(9):1120–6.
157. Chen XQ, Zhang WN, Yang ZX, Zhao M, Cai FC, Huang SP, et al. Efficacy of levetiracetam in electrical status epilepticus during sleep of children: a multicenter experience. Pediatr Neurol. 2014;50(3):243–9.
158. Arhan E, Serdaroglu A, Aydin K, Hirfanoglu T, Soysal AS. Epileptic encephalopathy with electrical status epilepticus: an electroclinical study of 59 patients. Seizure. 2015;26:86–93.
159. Beyenburg S, Reuber M, Maraite N. Intravenous levetiracetam for epileptic seizure emergencies in older people. Gerontology. 2009;55(1):27–31.
160. Berning S, Boesebeck F, van Baalen A, Kellinghaus C. Intravenous levetiracetam as treatment for status epilepticus. J Neurol. 2009;256(10):1634–42.
161. Fattouch J, Di Bonaventura C, Casciato S, Bonini F, Petrucci S, Lapenta L, et al. Intravenous Levetiracetam as first-line treatment of status epilepticus in the elderly. Acta Neurol Scand. 2010;121(6):418–21.
162. Ruegg S, Naegelin Y, Hardmeier M, Winkler DT, Marsch S, Fuhr P. Intravenous levetiracetam: treatment experience with the first 50 critically ill patients. Epilepsy Behav. 2008;12(3):477–80.
163. Alehan F, Ozcay F, Haberal M. The use of levetiracetam in a child with nonconvulsive status epilepticus J Child Neurol 2008,23(3):331–3.
164. Zaatreh MM. Levetiracetam in porphyric status epilepticus: a case report. Clin Neuropharmacol. 2005;28(5):243–4.
165. Yasiry Z, Shorvon SD. The relative effectiveness of five antiepileptic drugs in treatment of benzodiazepine-resistant convulsive status epilepticus: a meta-analysis of published studies. Seizure. 2014;23(3):167–74.
166. Swisher CB, Doreswamy M, Gingrich KJ, Vredenburgh JJ, Kolls BJ. Phenytoin, levetiracetam, and pregabalin in the acute management of refractory status epilepticus in patients with brain tumors. Neurocrit Care. 2012;16(1):109–13.
167. Gallentine WB, Hunnicutt AS, Husain AM. Levetiracetam in children with refractory status epilepticus. Epilepsy Behav. 2009;14(1):215–8.
168. Betts T, Waegemans T, Crawford P. A multicentre, double-blind, randomized, parallel group study to evaluate the tolerability and efficacy of two oral doses of levetiracetam, 2000 mg daily and 4000 mg

daily, without titration in patients with refractory epilepsy. Seizure. 2000;9(2):80–7.
169. Weintraub D, Buchsbaum R, Resor SR Jr, Hirsch LJ. Psychiatric and behavioral side effects of the newer antiepileptic drugs in adults with epilepsy. Epilepsy Behav. 2007;10(1):105–10.
170. McTague A, Kneen R, Kumar R, Spinty S, Appleton R. Intravenous levetiracetam in acute repetitive seizures and status epilepticus in children: experience from a children's hospital. Seizure. 2012;21(7):529–34.
171. Atefy R, Tettenborn B. Nonconvulsive status epilepticus on treatment with levetiracetam. Epilepsy Behav. 2005;6(4):613–6.
172. Briggs DE, French JA. Levetiracetam safety profiles and tolerability in epilepsy patients. Expert Opin Drug Saf. 2004;3(5):415–24.
173. Yamamoto J, Toublanc N, Kumagai Y, Stockis A. Levetiracetam pharmacokinetics in Japanese subjects with renal impairment. Clin Drug Investig. 2014;34(11):819–28.
174. Bleck T, Cock H, Chamberlain J, Cloyd J, Connor J, Elm J, et al. The established status epilepticus trial 2013. Epilepsia. 2013;54(Suppl 6):89–92.
175. Perucca DE. Pharmacological and therapeutic properties of valproate. CNS Drugs. 2002;16(10): 695–714.
176. Cramer JA, Mattson RH. Valproic acid: in vitro plasma protein binding and interaction with phenytoin. Ther Drug Monit. 1979;1(1):105–16.
177. Gram L, Flachs H, Würtz-Jørgensen A, et al. Sodium valproate, serum level and clinical effect in epilepsy: a controlled study. Epilepsia. 1979;20(3): 303–11.
178. Shen DD, Ojemann GA, Rapport RL, et al. Low and variable presence of valproic acid in human brain. Neurology. 1992;42(3 Pt 1):582.
179. Davis R, Peters DH, Mctavish D. Valproic acid. A reappraisal of its pharmacological properties and clinical efficacy in epilepsy. Drugs. 1994;47(2):332–72.
180. Perucca E, Gatti G, Frigo GM, et al. Pharmacokinetics of valproic acid after oral and intravenous administration. Br J Clin Pharmacol. 1978;5(4):313–8.
181. Perucca E, Gatti G, Frigo G, et al. Disposition of sodium valproate in epileptic patients. Br J Clin Pharmacol. 1978;5(6):495.
182. Perucca E, Grimaldi R, Gatti G, et al. Pharmacokinetics of valproic acid in the elderly. Br J Clin Pharmacol. 1984;17(6):665–9.
183. Koerner M, Yerby M, Friel P, et al. Valproic acid disposition and protein binding in pregnancy. Ther Drug Monit. 1989;11(3):228–30.
184. Zaccara DG, Messori A, Moroni F. Clinical pharmacokinetics of valproic acid—1988. Clin Pharmacokinet. 1988;15(6):367–89.
185. Taberner PV, Charington CB, Unwin JW. Effects of GAD and GABA-T inhibitors on GABA metabolism in vivo. Brain Res Bull. 1980;5(80):621–5.
186. Whittle SR, Turner AJ. Effects of anticonvulsants on the formation of gamma-hydroxybutyrate from gamma-aminobutyrate in rat brain. J Neurochem. 1982;38(3):848–51.
187. Snead OC III. gamma-Hydroxybutyrate model of generalized absence seizures: further characterization and comparison with other absence models. Epilepsia. 1988;29(4):361.
188. Macdonald RL, Bergey GK. Valproic acid augments GABA-mediated postsynaptic inhibition in cultured mammalian neurons. Brain Res. 1979;170(3):558–62.
189. Olpe HR, Steinmann MW, Pozza MF, et al. Valproate enhances GABA-A mediated inhibition of locus coeruleus neurones in vitro. Naunyn Schmiedeberg's Arch Pharmacol. 1988;338(6):655–7.
190. Zeise ML, Kasparow S, Zieglgänsberger W. Valproate suppresses N -methyl-D-aspartate-evoked, transient depolarizations in the rat neocortex in vitro. Brain Res. 1991;544(2):345–8.
191. McLean MJ, MacDonald RL. Sodium valproate, but not ethosuximide, produces use- and voltage-dependent limitation of high frequency repetitive firing of action potentials of mouse central neurons in cell culture. J Pharmacol Exp Ther. 1986;237(3):1001–11.
192. Löscher W. Valproate: a reappraisal of its pharmacodynamic properties and mechanisms of action. Prog Neurobiol. 1999;58(1):31–59.
193. Schipp F. The action of valproate on spontaneous epileptiform activity in the absence of synaptic transmission and on evoked changes in [Ca2+] 0, and [K+] 0, in the hippocampal slice. Brain Res. 1986;386(1–2):1.
194. Coulter DA, Huguenard JR, Prince DA. Characterization of ethosuximide reduction of low-threshold calcium current in thalamic neurons. Ann Neurol. 1989;25(6):582–93.
195. Lust WD, Kupferberg HJ, Yonekawa WD, et al. Changes in brain metabolites induced by convulsants or electroshock: effects of anticonvulsant agents. Mol Pharmacol. 1978;14(2):347–56.
196. Mccandless DW, Feussner GK, Lust WD, et al. Metabolite levels in brain following experimental seizures: the effects of isoniazid and sodium valproate in cerebellar and cerebral cortical layers. J Neurochem. 1979;32(3):755–60.
197. Tomson T, Battino D, Perucca E. Valproic acid after five decades of use in epilepsy: time to reconsider the indications of a time-honoured drug. Lancet Neurol. 2016;15(2):210–8.
198. Hönack D, Löscher W. Intravenous valproate: onset and duration of anticonvulsant activity against a series of electroconvulsions in comparison with diazepam and phenytoin. Epilepsy Res. 1993;13(3):215–21.
199. Brophy GM, Bell R, Claassen J, et al. Guidelines for the evaluation and management of status epilepticus. Neurocrit Care. 2012;17(1):3–23.

200. Uberall MA, Trollmann R, Wunsiedler U, et al. Intravenous valproate in pediatric epilepsy patients with refractory status epilepticus. Neurology. 2000;54(11):2188–9.
201. Yu KT, Mills S, Thompson N, et al. Safety and efficacy of intravenous valproate in pediatric status epilepticus and acute repetitive seizures. Epilepsia. 2003;44(5):724–6.
202. Mehta V, Singhi P, Singhi S. Intravenous sodium valproate versus diazepam infusion for the control of refractory status epilepticus in children: a randomized controlled trial. J Child Neurol. 2007;22(10):1191–7.
203. Campistol J, Fernández A, Ortega J. Status epilepticus in children. Experience with intravenous valproate. Update of treatment guidelines. Rev Neurol. 1999;29(29):359–65.
204. Hovinga CA, Chicella MF, Rose DF, et al. Use of intravenous valproate in three pediatric patients with nonconvulsive or convulsive status epilepticus. Ann Pharmacother. 1999;33(5):579–84.
205. Jha S, Jose M, Patel R. Intravenous sodium valproate in status epilepticus. Neurol India. 2003;51(3):421–2.
206. Peters CN, Pohlmanneden B. Intravenous valproate as an innovative therapy in seizure emergency situations including status epilepticus—experience in 102 adult patients. Seizure. 2005;14(3):164–9.
207. Trinka E, Höfler J, Zerbs A, et al. Efficacy and safety of intravenous valproate for status epilepticus: a systematic review. CNS Drugs. 2014;28(7):623–39.
208. Yasiry Z, Shorvon SD. The relative effectiveness of five antiepileptic drugs in treatment of benzodiazepine-resistant convulsive status epilepticus: a meta-analysis of published studies. Seizure. 2014;23(3):167.
209. Chen L, Feng P, Wang J, et al. Intravenous sodium valproate in mainland China for the treatment of diazepam refractory convulsive status epilepticus. J Clin Neurosci. 2009;16(4):524–6.
210. Ajith C, Thomas SV. Status epilepticus. Ann Indian Acad Neurol. 2009;12(3):140–53.
211. Giroud M, Gras D, Escousse A, et al. Use of injectable valproic acid in status epilepticus. Clin Drug Investig. 1993;5(3):154–9.
212. Czapiński P, Terczyxski A. Intravenous valproic acid administration in status epilepticus. Neurol Neurochir Pol. 1998;32(32):11–22.
213. Naritoku DK. Outcome of status epileptcious treated with intravenous valproic acid. Adv Stud Med. 2011;1:279–80.
214. Olsen KB, Taubøll E, Gjerstad L. Valproate is an effective, well-tolerated drug for treatment of status epilepticus/serial attacks in adults. Acta Neurol Scand Suppl. 2007;187(s187):51–4.
215. Chen WB, Gao R, Su YY, et al. Valproate versus diazepam for generalized convulsive status epilepticus: a pilot study. Eur J Neurol. 2011;18(12):1391.
216. Peters C, Pohlman-Eden B. Efficacy and safety of intravenous valproate in status epilepticus. Epilepsia. 1999;40:149–50. (Abstract).
217. Katragadda S, Chand Aluri B, Burdette D. Intravenous administration of valproate for status epilepticus in 12 patients. Epilepsia. 2000;41:216. (Abstract).
218. Narayanan JT, Murthy JM. Nonconvulsive status epilepticus in a neurological intensive care unit: profile in a developing country. Epilepsia, 2007; 48(5):900.
219. Agarwal P, Kumar N, Chandra R, et al. Randomized study of intravenous valproate and phenytoin in status epilepticus. Seizure. 2007;16(6):527–32.
220. Malamiri RA, Ghaempanah M, Khosroshahi N, et al. Efficacy and safety of intravenous sodium valproate versus phenobarbital in controlling convulsive status epilepticus and acute prolonged convulsive seizures in children: a randomised trial. Eur J Paediatr Neurol. 2012;16(5):536–41.
221. Ramsay RE, Cantrell D, Collins SD, et al. Safety and tolerance of rapidly infused Depacon. A randomized trial in subjects with epilepsy. Epilepsy Res. 2003;52(3):189–201.
222. Bergmann A, Schmidt D, Hutt HJ. Epilepsietherapie mit retardierter Valproinsäure—Erfahrungen mit 1172 Patienten. Aktuelle Neurologie. 1999;26(3):121–6.
223. Brasfield KH. Pilot study of divalproex sodium versus valproic acid: drug acquisition costs versus all related costs. Curr Ther Res. 1999;60(3):138–44.
224. Cranor CW, Sawyer WT, Carson SW, et al. Clinical and economic impact of replacing divalproex sodium with valproic acid. Am J Health Syst Pharm. 1997;54(15):1716–22.
225. Johannessen CU, Johannessen SI. Valproate: past, present, and future. CNS Drug Rev. 2003;9(2):199–216.
226. Devinsky O, Leppik I, Willmore LJ, et al. Safety of intravenous valproate. Ann Neurol. 1995;38(4):670–4.
227. Limdi NA, Knowlton RK, Cofield SS, et al. Safety of rapid intravenous loading of valproate. Epilepsia. 2007;48(3):478–83.
228. Hamer HM, Knake S, Schomburg U, et al. Valproate induced hyperammonemic encephalopathy in the presence of topiramate. Neurology. 2000;54:230–2.
229. Dewolfe JL, Knowlton RCBeasley MT. Hyperammonemia following intravenous valproate loading. Epilepsy Res. 2009;85(1):65–71.
230. Raja M, Azzoni A. Valproate-induced hyperammonaemia. J Clin Psychopharmacol. 2002;22:631–3.
231. Hernándezdíaz S, Smith CR, Shen A, Mittendorf R, Hauser WA, Yerby M, et al. Comparative safety of antiepileptic drugs during pregnancy. Neurology. 2012;78(21):1692–9.
232. Jentink J, Loane MA, Dolk H, Barisic I, Garne E, Morris JK, et al. Valproic acid monotherapy in pregnancy and major congenital malformations. N Engl J Med. 2010;362(23):2185.
233. Nelson E, Powell JR, Conrad K, et al. Phenobarbital pharmacokinetics and bioavailability in adults. J Clin Pharmacol. 1982;22:141–8.

234. Wilensky AJ, Friel PN, Levy RH, et al. Kinetics of phenobarbital in normal subjects and epileptic patients. Eur J Clin Pharmacol. 1982;23:87–92.
235. Anderson GD. Phenobarbital and other barbiturates: chemistry, biotransformation, and pharmacokinetics. In: Levy RH, Mattson RH, Meldrum BS, Perucca E, editors. Antiepileptic drug. 5th ed. Philadelphia: Lippincott Williams & Wilkins; 2002. p. 596–603.
236. Bernus I, Dickinson RG, Hooper WD, et al. Urinary excretion of phenobarbitone and its metabolites in chronically treated patients. Eur J Clin Pharmacol. 1994;46:473–5.
237. Twyman RE, Rogers CJ, Macdonald RL. Differential regulation of gamma-aminobutyric acid receptor channels by diazepam and phenobarbital. Ann Neurol. 1989;25:213–20.
238. Rho JM, Donevan SD, Rogawski MA. Direct activation of GABAA receptors by barbiturates in cultured rat hippocampal neurons. J Physiol. 1996;497(Pt 2):509–22.
239. Kwan P, Brodie MJ. Phenobarbital for the treatment of epilepsy in the 21st century: a critical review. Epilepsia. 2004;45:1141–9.
240. Treiman DM, Meyers PD, Walton NY, Collins JF, Colling C, Rowan AJ, et al. A comparison of four treatments for generalized convulsive status epilepticus. Veterans Affairs Status Epilepticus Cooperative Study Group. N Engl J Med. 1998;339:792–8.
241. Kalviainen R, Eriksson K, Parviainen I. Refractory generalised convulsive status epilepticus: a guide to treatment. CNS Drugs. 2005;19:759–68.
242. Muramoto E, Mizobuchi M, Sumi Y, Sako K, Nihira A, Takeuchi A, et al. Efficacy of intravenous phenobarbital treatment for status epilepticus. Brain Nerve. 2013;65:983–7.
243. Mayer SA, Claassen J, Lokin J, Mendelsohn F, Dennis LJ, Fitzsimmons BF. Refractory status epilepticus: frequency, risk factors, and impact on outcome. Arch Neurol. 2002;59:205–10.
244. Byun JI, Chu K, Sunwoo JS, Moon J, Kim TJ, Lim JA, et al. Mega-dose phenobarbital therapy for super-refractory status epilepticus. Epileptic Disord. 2015;17:444–52.
245. Pugin D, Foreman B, De Marchis GM, Fernandez A, Schmidt JM, Czeisler BM, et al. Is pentobarbital safe and efficacious in the treatment of super-refractory status epilepticus: a cohort study. Crit Care. 2014;18:R103.
246. Su Y, Liu G, Tian F, Ren G, Jiang M, Chun B, et al. Phenobarbital versus valproate for generalized convulsive status epilepticus in adults: a prospective randomized controlled trial in China. CNS Drugs. 2016;30:1201–7.
247. Lee YJ, Yum MS, Kim EH, Ko TS. Intravenous levetiracetam versus phenobarbital in children with status epilepticus or acute repetitive seizures. Kor J Pediatrics. 2016;59:35–9.
248. Crawford TO, Mitchell WG, Fishman LS, Snodgrass SR. Very-high-dose phenobarbital for refractory status epilepticus in children. Neurology. 1988;38:1035–40.
249. Lee WK, Liu KT, Young BW. Very-high-dose phenobarbital for childhood refractory status epilepticus. Pediatr Neurol. 2006;34:63–5.
250. Sudoh A, Sugai K, Miyamoto T, Mimaki M, Fukumizu M, Hanaoka S, et al. Non-intravenous high-dose phenobarbital therapy for status epilepticus refractory to continuous infusion of midazolam or pentobarbital: report of three cases. No To Hattatsu. 2002;34:23–9.
251. Tiamkao S, Suttapan K, Pranbul S, Tiamkao S, Sawanyawisuth K, Integrated Epilepsy Research Group. Adjunctive enteral phenobarbital for adult status epilepticus: a brief report. Neuropsychiatr Dis Treat. 2013;9:1829–34.
252. Simon RP, Copeland JR, Benowitz NL, Jacob P III, Bronstein J. Brain phenobarbital uptake during prolonged status epilepticus. J Cereb Blood Flow Metab. 1987;7:783–8.
253. Shaner DM, McCurdy SA, Herring MO, Gabor AJ. Treatment of status epilepticus: a prospective comparison of diazepam and phenytoin versus phenobarbital and optional phenytoin. Neurology. 1988;38:202–7.
254. Riss J, Cloyd J, Gates J, Collins S. Benzodiazepines in epilepsy: pharmacology and pharmacokinetics. Acta Neurol Scand. 2008;118:69–86.
255. Debruyne D, Pailliet-Loilier M, Lelong-Boulouard V, et al. Therapeutic drug monitoring of clonazepam. Therapie. 2010;65(3):219–24.
256. Rundfeldt C, Löscher W. The pharmacology of imepitoin: the first partial benzodiazepine receptor agonist developed for the treatment of epilepsy. CNS Drugs. 2014;28(1):29–43.
257. Griffin CE 3rd, Kaye AM, Bueno FR, et al. Benzodiazepine pharmacology and central nervous system-mediated effects. Ochsner J. 2013;13(2): 214–23.
258. Gastaut H, Courjon J, Poiré R, Weber M. Treatment of status epilepticus with a new benzodiazepine more active than diazepam. Epilepsia. 1971;12(3):197–214.
259. Sorel L, Mechler L, Harmant J. Comparative trial of intravenous lorazepam and clonazepam in status epilepticus. ClinTher. 1981;4(4):326–36.
260. Alvarez V, Lee JW, Drislane FW, et al. Practice variability and efficacy of clonazepam, lorazepam, and midazolam in status epilepticus: a multicenter comparison. Epilepsia. 2015;56:1275–85.
261. Rantsch K, Walter U, Wittstock M, et al. Treatment and course of different subtypes of status epilepticus. Epilepsy Res. 2013;107(1–2):156–62.
262. Singh AN, Le Morvan P. Treatment of status epilepticus with intravenous clonazepam. Prog Neuro-Psychopharmacol Biol Psychiatry. 1982;6(4–6):539–42.
263. Fernández-Torre JL, Leno C. Teaching neuroimage: simple partial frontal status epilepticus with recurrent asymmetric tonic seizures. Neurology. 2008;70(7):e30–1.
264. Navarro V, Dagron C, Elie C, et al. Prehospital treatment with levetiracetam plus clonazepam

or placebo plus clonazepam in status epilepticus (SAMUKeppra): a randomised, double-blind, phase 3 trial. Lancet Neurol. 2016;15(1):47–55.
265. Akman CI. Nonconvulsive status epilepticus and continuous spike and slow wave of sleep In children. Semin Pediatr Neurol. 2010;17(3):155–62.
266. Cheng S. Non-convulsive status epilepticus in the elderly. Epileptic Disord. 2014;16(4): 385–94.
267. Pollak L, Gandelman-Marton R, Margolin N, et al. Clinical and electroencephalographic findings in acutely ill adults with non-convulsive vs convulsive status epilepticus. Acta Neurol Scand. 2014;129(6):405–11.
268. Livingston JH, Brown JK. Non-convulsive status epilepticus resistant to benzodiazepines. Arch Dis Child. 1987;62(1):41–4.
269. Congdon PJ, Forsythe WI. Intravenous clonazepam in the treatment of status epilepticus in children. Epilepsia. 1980;21(1):97–102.
270. Padma MV, Jain S, Maheshwari MC. Oral clonazepam sensitive focal status epilepticus (FSE). Indian J Pediatr. 1997;64(3):424–7.
271. Mazurkiewicz-Bełdzińska M, Szmuda M, Zawadzka M, Matheisel A. Current treatment of convulsive status epilepticus—a therapeutic protocol and review. Anaesthesiol Intensive Ther. 2014;46(4):293–300.
272. Outin H. Generalized convulsive status epilepticus in emergency situations in and out of hospital. Presse Med. 2009;38(12):1823–31.
273. Clair B, Demeret S, Dupont S, Tazarourte K. Management of convulsive status epilepticus: therapeutic strategies. Rev Neurol (Paris). 2009;165(4):366–72.
274. Troester MM, Hastriter EV, Ng YT. Dissolving oral clonazepam wafers in the acute treatment of prolonged seizures. J Child Neurol. 2010;25(12):1468–72.
275. Klosterskov Jensen P, Abild K, Nøhr PM. Serum concentration of clonazepam after rectal administration. Acta Neurol Scand. 1983;68(6):417–20.
276. Mancuso CE, Tanzi MG, Gabay M. Paradoxical reactions to benzodiazepines: literature review and treatment options. Pharmacotherapy. 2004;24(9):1177–85.
277. Pinder RM, Brogden RN, Speight TM, Avery GS. Clonazepam: a review of its pharmacological properties and therapeutic efficacy in epilepsy. Drugs. 1976;12(5):321–61.
278. Chavant F, Favrelière S, Lafay-Chebassier C, et al. Memory disorders associated with consumption of drugs: updating through a case/noncase study in the French PharmacoVigilance Database. Br J Clin Pharmacol. 2011;72(6):898–904.
279. Chen JW, Wasterlain CG. Status epilepticus: pathophysiology and management in adults. Lancet Neurol. 2006;5(3):246–56.
280. Wasterlain CG, Baldwin R, Naylor DE, Thompson KW, Suchomelova L, Niquet J. Rational polytherapy in the treatment of acute seizures and status epilepticus. Epilepsia. 2011;52(Suppl 8):70–1.
281. Mundlamuri RC, Sinha S, Subbakrishna DK, Prathyusha PV, Nagappa M, Bindu PS, et al. Management of generalised convulsive status epilepticus (SE): a prospective randomised controlled study of combined treatment with intravenous lorazepam with either phenytoin, sodium valproate or levetiracetam—Pilot study. Epilepsy Res. 2015;114:52–8.
282. Cook AM, Castle A, Green A, Lesch C, Morrison C, Rhoney D, et al. Practice variations in the management of status epilepticus. Neurocrit Care. 2012;17(1):24–30.
283. Abend NS, Dlugos DJ, Clancy RR. A review of long-term EEG monitoring in critically ill children with hypoxic-ischemic encephalopathy, congenital heart disease, ECMO, and stroke. J Clin Neurophysiol. 2013;30(2):134–42.
284. Arik Y, Leijten FS, Seute T, Robe PA, Snijders TJ. Prognosis and therapy of tumor-related versus non-tumor-related status epilepticus: a systematic review and meta-analysis. BMC Neurol. 2014;14:152.
285. Fernandez-Torre JL, Kaplan PW. Subacute encephalopathy with seizures in alcoholics (SESA syndrome) revisited. Seizure. 2014;23(5):393–6.
286. Kapur J, Macdonald RL. Rapid seizure-induced reduction of benzodiazepine and Zn2+ sensitivity of hippocampal dentate granule cell GABAA receptors. J Neurosci. 1997;17(19):7532–40.
287. Grohn O, Sierra A, Immonen R, Laitinen T, Lehtimaki K, Airaksinen A, et al. Multimodal MRI assessment of damage and plasticity caused by status epilepticus in the rat brain. Epilepsia. 2011;52(Suppl 8):57–60.
288. Rotheneichner P, Marschallinger J, Couillard-Despres S, Aigner L. Neurogenesis and neuronal regeneration in status epilepticus. Epilepsia. 2013;54(Suppl 6):40–2.
289. Wasterlain CG, Chen JW. Mechanistic and pharmacologic aspects of status epilepticus and its treatment with new antiepileptic drugs. Epilepsia. 2008;49(Suppl 9):63–73.
290. Avanzini G, Depaulis A, Tassinari A, de Curtis M. Do seizures and epileptic activity worsen epilepsy and deteriorate cognitive function? Epilepsia. 2013;54(Suppl 8):14–21.
291. Uges JW, van Huizen MD, Engelsman J, Wilms EB, Touw DJ, Peeters E, et al. Safety and pharmacokinetics of intravenous levetiracetam infusion as add-on in status epilepticus. Epilepsia. 2009;50(3): 415–21.
292. Winkler MK, Chassidim Y, Lublinsky S, Revankar GS, Major S, Kang EJ, et al. Impaired neurovascular coupling to ictal epileptic activity and spreading depolarization in a patient with subarachnoid hemorrhage: possible link to blood-brain barrier dysfunction. Epilepsia. 2012;53(Suppl 6):22–30.

293. Vespa PM, McArthur DL, Xu Y, Eliseo M, Etchepare M, Dinov I, et al. Nonconvulsive seizures after traumatic brain injury are associated with hippocampal atrophy. Neurology. 2010;75(9):792–8.
294. Vespa PM, Miller C, McArthur D, Eliseo M, Etchepare M, Hirt D, et al. Nonconvulsive electrographic seizures after traumatic brain injury result in a delayed, prolonged increase in intracranial pressure and metabolic crisis. Crit Care Med. 2007;35(12):2830–6.
295. Hocker S, Tatum WO, LaRoche S, Freeman WD. Refractory and super-refractory status epilepticus—an update. Curr Neurol Neurosci Rep. 2014;14(6):452.
296. Silbergleit R, Lowenstein D, Durkalski V, Conwit R. RAMPART (Rapid Anticonvulsant Medication Prior to Arrival Trial): a double-blind randomized clinical trial of the efficacy of intramuscular midazolam versus intravenous lorazepam in the prehospital treatment of status epilepticus by paramedics. Epilepsia. 2011;52(Suppl 8): 45–7.
297. Sutter R, Kaplan PW, Ruegg S. Outcome predictors for status epilepticus—what really counts. Nat Rev Neurol. 2013;9(9):525–34.
298. Hijazi Y, Bodonian C, Bolon M, Salord F, Boulieu R. Pharmacokinetics and haemodynamics of ketamine in intensive care patients with brain or spinal cord injury. Br J Anaesth. 2003;90(2):155–60.
299. Mazarati AM, Wasterlain CG. N-methyl-D-asparate receptor antagonists abolish the maintenance phase of self-sustaining status epilepticus in rat. Neurosci Lett. 1999;265(3):187–90.
300. Martin BS, Kapur J. A combination of ketamine and diazepam synergistically controls refractory status epilepticus induced by cholinergic stimulation. Epilepsia. 2008;49(2):248–55.
301. Gaspard N, Foreman B, Judd LM, Brenton JN, Nathan BR, McCoy BM, et al. Intravenous ketamine for the treatment of refractory status epilepticus: a retrospective multicenter study. Epilepsia. 2013;54(8):1498–503.
302. Esaian D, Joset D, Lazarovits C, Dugan PC, Fridman D. Ketamine continuous infusion for refractory status epilepticus in a patient with anticonvulsant hypersensitivity syndrome. Ann Pharmacother. 2013;47(11):1569–76.
303. Pruss H, Holtkamp M. Ketamine successfully terminates malignant status epilepticus. Epilepsy Res. 2008;82(2–3):219–22.
304. Inge A, Nasta F. New and old medications for croup and seizures in children. Oral dexamethasone and buccal midazolam may provide better treatment. Lakartidningen. 2013;110(48):2163.
305. Fallah R, Yadegari Y, Behdad S, Akhavan KS. Melatonin and intravenous midazolam administered orally in drug induced sleep electroencephalography of children: randomized clinical trial of efficacy. Arch Iran Med. 2014;17(11):741–5.
306. Brevoord JC, Joosten KF, Arts WF, van Rooij RW, de Hoog M. Status epilepticus: clinical analysis of a treatment protocol based on midazolam and phenytoin. J Child Neurol. 2005;20(6):476–81.
307. Hubert P, Parain D, Vallee L. Management of convulsive status epilepticus in infants and children. Rev Neurol. 2009;165(4):390–7.
308. Saz EU, Karapinar B, Ozcetin M, Polat M, Tosun A, Serdaroglu G, et al. Convulsive status epilepticus in children: etiology, treatment protocol and outcome. Seizure. 2011;20(2):115–8.
309. Tasker RC. Midazolam for refractory status epilepticus in children: higher dosing and more rapid and effective control. Intensive Care Med. 2006;32(12):1935–6.
310. Chen J, Cai F, Jiang L, Hu Y, Feng C. Levetiracetam efficacy in children with epilepsy with electrical status epilepticus in sleep. Epilepsy Behav. 2015;44:73–7.
311. Su TF, Xu SQ, Chen L. Efficacy of levetiracetam combined with short-term clonazepam in treatment of electrical status epilepticus during sleep in children with benign childhood epilepsy with centrotemporal spikes. Zhongguo dang dai er ke za zhi. 2014;16(8):829–33.
312. Navarro V, Dagron C, Demeret S, An K, Lamhaut L, Bolgert F, et al. A prehospital randomized trial in convulsive status epilepticus. Epilepsia. 2011;52(Suppl 8):48–9.
313. Ramael S, Daoust A, Otoul C, Toublanc N, Troenaru M, Lu ZS, et al. Levetiracetam intravenous infusion: a randomized, placebo-controlled safety and pharmacokinetic study. Epilepsia. 2006;47(7):1128–35.
314. Mastrangelo M, Celato A. Diagnostic work-up and therapeutic options in management of pediatric status epilepticus. World J Pediatrics. 2012;8(2):109–15.
315. Asadi-Pooya AA, Jahromi MJ, Izadi S, Emami Y. Treatment of refractory generalized convulsive status epilepticus with enteral topiramate in resource limited settings. Seizure. 2015;24:114–7.
316. Reuber M, Evans J, Bamford JM. Topiramate in drug-resistant complex partial status epilepticus. Eur J Neurol. 2002;9(1):111–2.
317. Towne AR, Garnett LK, Waterhouse EJ, Morton LD, DeLorenzo RJ. The use of topiramate in refractory status epilepticus. Neurology. 2003;60(2):332–4.
318. Akyildiz BN, Kumandas S. Treatment of pediatric refractory status epilepticus with topiramate. Childs Nerv Syst. 2011;27(9):1425–30.
319. Stojanova V, Rossetti AO. Oral topiramate as an add-on treatment for refractory status epilepticus. Acta Neurol Scand. 2012;125(2):e7–e11.
320. Synowiec AS, Yandora KA, Yenugadhati V, Valeriano JP, Schramke CJ, Kelly KM. The efficacy of topiramate in adult refractory status epilepticus: experience of a tertiary care center. Epilepsy Res. 2012;98(2–3):232–7.
321. Hottinger A, Sutter R, Marsch S, Ruegg S. Topiramate as an adjunctive treatment in patients

with refractory status epilepticus: an observational cohort study. CNS Drugs. 2012;26(9):761–72.
322. Sutter R, Marsch S, Ruegg S. Safety and efficacy of intravenous lacosamide for adjunctive treatment of refractory status epilepticus: a comparative cohort study. CNS Drugs. 2013;27(4):321–9.
323. Hofler J, Trinka E. Lacosamide as a new treatment option in status epilepticus. Epilepsia. 2013;54(3):393–404.
324. Kellinghaus C, Berning S, Immisch I, Larch J, Rosenow F, Rossetti AO, et al. Intravenous lacosamide for treatment of status epilepticus. Acta Neurol Scand. 2011;123(2):137–41.
325. Moreno Morales EY, Fernandez Peleteiro M, Bondy Pena EC, Dominguez Lorenzo JM, Pardellas Santiago E, Fernandez A. Observational study of intravenous lacosamide in patients with convulsive versus non-convulsive status epilepticus. Clin Drug Investig. 2015;35(7):463–9.
326. Papacostas SS. Status epilepticus developing during lacosamide monotherapy. BMJ Case Rep. 2015;27:2015.
327. Shiloh-Malawsky Y, Fan Z, Greenwood R, Tennison M. Successful treatment of childhood prolonged refractory status epilepticus with lacosamide. Seizure. 2011;20(7):586–8.
328. Abend NS, Dlugos DJ. Treatment of refractory status epilepticus: literature review and a proposed protocol. Pediatr Neurol. 2008;38(6):377–90.
329. Bankstahl JP, Loscher W. Resistance to antiepileptic drugs and expression of P-glycoprotein in two rat models of status epilepticus. Epilepsy Res. 2008;82(1):70–85.
330. Hasson H, Kim M, Moshe SL. Effective treatments of prolonged status epilepticus in developing rats. Epilepsy Behav. 2008;13(1):62–9.
331. Finne Lenoir X, Sindic C, van Pesch V, El Sankari S, de Tourtchaninoff M, Denays R, et al. Anti-N-methyl-D-aspartate receptor encephalitis with favorable outcome despite prolonged status epilepticus. Neurocrit Care. 2013;18(1):89–92.
332. Davis R, Dalmau J. Autoimmunity, seizures, and status epilepticus. Epilepsia. 2013;54(Suppl 6):46–9.
333. Hoftberger R, Titulaer MJ, Sabater L, Dome B, Rozsas A, Hegedus B, et al. Encephalitis and GABAB receptor antibodies: novel findings in a new case series of 20 patients. Neurology. 2013;81(17):1500–6.
334. Gall CR, Jumma O, Mohanraj R. Five cases of new onset refractory status epilepticus (NORSE) syndrome: outcomes with early immunotherapy. Seizure. 2013;22(3):217–20.
335. Sinclair DB, Snyder TJ. Corticosteroids for the treatment of Landau-kleffner syndrome and continuous spike-wave discharge during sleep. Pediatr Neurol. 2005;32(5):300–6.
336. Arts WF, Aarsen FK, Scheltens-de Boer M, Catsman-Berrevoets CE. Landau-Kleffner syndrome and CSWS syndrome: treatment with intravenous immunoglobulins. Epilepsia. 2009;50(Suppl 7): 55–8.
337. Dubey D, Konikkara J, Modur PN, Agostini M, Gupta P, Shu F, et al. Effectiveness of multimodality treatment for autoimmune limbic epilepsy. Epileptic Disord. 2014;16(4):494–9.
338. Rogawski MA, Loya CM, Reddy K, Zolkowska D, Lossin C. Neuroactive steroids for the treatment of status epilepticus. Epilepsia. 2013;54(Suppl 6): 93–8.
339. Tawfik MK. Coenzyme Q10 enhances the anticonvulsant effect of phenytoin in pilocarpine-induced seizures in rats and ameliorates phenytoin-induced cognitive impairment and oxidative stress. Epilepsy Behav. 2011;22(4):671–7.
340. Yis U, Topcu Y, Ozbal S, Tugyan K, Bayram E, Karakaya P, et al. Caffeic acid phenethyl ester prevents apoptotic cell death in the developing rat brain after pentylenetetrazole-induced status epilepticus. Epilepsy Behav. 2013;29(2):275–80.
341. Shahwan A, Bailey C, Maxiner W, Harvey AS. Vagus nerve stimulation for refractory epilepsy in children: more to VNS than seizure frequency reduction. Epilepsia. 2009;50(5):1220–8.
342. Alexopoulos A, Lachhwani DK, Gupta A, Kotagal P, Harrison AM, Bingaman W, et al. Resective surgery to treat refractory status epilepticus in children with focal epileptogenesis. Neurology. 2005;64(3):567–70.

Nondrug Treatment for Refractory Status Epilepticus

7

Guoming Luan and Xuefeng Wang

Abstract

Although various drugs, such as benzodiazepines, anesthetics, and intravenous antiepileptic drugs (AEDs), are used to control refractory status epilepticus (RSE), many cases of RSE are not effectively controlled. In such cases, efforts to control RSE may take the form of nonpharmacological measures, including therapeutic hypothermia, electroconvulsive therapy, neuromodulatory treatment, and the implementation of a ketogenic diet. These measures are not widely used in RSE, but studies have shown that they can play a role in controlling RSE. In this chapter, we summarize the efficacy, safety, and application of these treatments.

7.1 Therapeutic Hypothermia for Refractory Status Epilepticus

7.1.1 Historical Evolution

The beneficial effect of hypothermia has been indicated since ancient times. The Greek physician Hippocrates found that infants lived longer in the winter than in the summer when they were left exposed to the environment [1]. Later, a few researchers described the beneficial effects of hypothermia on the human body and on animals during hypoxic states [2]. Until the 1950s, Westin et al. [3] conducted a small uncontrolled study that found that immersing the participants' bodies in the cold water could be helpful for the recovery of the respiratory effort of infants who did not breathe for the first 5 min after birth. The primary understanding of hypothermia therapy

G. Luan
Beijing Key Laboratory of Epilepsy, Department of Neurology, Center of Epilepsy, Beijing Institute for Brain Disorders, Sanbo Brain Hospital Capital Medical University, 100093 Beijing, China

X. Wang (✉)
Chongqing Key Laboratory of Neurology, Department of Neurology, The First Affiliated Hospital of Chongqing Medical University, 1 YouYi Road, Chongqing 400016, China
e-mail: xfyp@163.com

X. Wang, S. Li (eds.), *Refractory Status Epilepticus*, DOI 10.1007/978-981-10-5125-8_7

stems from studies on hypoxic-ischemic brain injury that indicated that hypothermia was associated with alleviated cell death and improved clinical outcomes [2]. This sequence of studies suggested that hypothermia can affect the electrical activity of the cerebral cortex [4, 5].

The effect of hypothermia in treating status epilepticus (SE) originates from the implication that focal cooling of the cerebral cortex can lead to a good outcome for patients who experience a seizure. In 1963, Ommaya and colleagues were firstly reported to use direct focal cooling of the cerebral cortex at 20–25 °C for the effective cessation of SE [4]. In 1970, Sourek et al. [6] reported a series of 25 cases of refractory epilepsy who received a combination treatment of extravascular brain hypothermia (deep, general, and local) plus single dose of anticonvulsants (pentothal or diazepam). In most patients, the local temperature of the brain was below 24 °C, and the rectal temperature was 27–30 °C during surgery. The combination of hypothermia and anticonvulsants led to favorable outcomes. In 15 patients followed for at least 1 year after surgery, two patients had a 50% reduction of the frequency and the intensity of their seizures, five patients observed a reduction in activity to a single seizure, four patients had no seizures, and four patients had unaltered seizures. Not only had this therapy showed a good effect on the seizures, but it also showed an improvement in the behavior and the emotional stability in three patients. One patient died 6 weeks after surgery, and two patients had slight neurological deficits at 3 and 6 months postoperatively.

Hypothermia, which is used as a treatment measure for SE, originated in 1984, when Orlowski et al. [7] first reported three pediatric patients with SE that were unresponsive to conventional AEDs and who were successfully treated with a combination treatment of hypothermia (30–31 °C) and barbiturate coma. In 2008, Corry et al. [8] reported four patients with refractory tonic-clonic SE, who were controlled with hypothermia at 31–35 °C for 20–61 h using endovascular cooling, which demonstrated the effect of therapeutic hypothermia for super RSE. More recently, the multicenter randomized controlled trial HYBERNATUS was conducted to evaluate the effect of induced hypothermia on neurologic outcomes in patients with convulsive status epilepticus (CSE) [9].

7.1.2 Clinical Application and Efficacy in RSE

To date, there have been a handful of case reports that provide an experience of the application of hypothermia for SE [8, 10–12]. In 1984, Orlowski et al. [7] recorded the initial use of hypothermia for SE. Three patients with RSE were placed into moderate hypothermia (30–31 °C) by surface cooling for 48–120 h and then rewarmed to a normothermic state at a rate of 1 °C every 3–4 h. In combination with a thiopental barbiturate-induced coma, RSE in all three patients was controlled. Recently, there has been a recent resurgence of interest in the use of hypothermia as a treatment for RSE, which provides a growing experience of the use of hypothermia in general. The application parameters of 12 cases from 4 reports are summarized in Table 7.1.

Endovascular cooling systems and surface cooling are the most common methods for induced therapeutic hypothermia. Endovascular cooling systems have a balloon surrounding the catheter that is placed through the femoral vein into the inferior vena cava. When the core temperature reaches 36.5 °C after rewarming, the catheter needs to be removed as soon as possible to prevent venous thrombosis. The modern surface cooling system can modulate the patient's temperature with relative precision by circulating chilled water in pads that are directly adhered to the patient's skin [11].

The application parameters of therapeutic hypothermia for SE are not well established, but several case reports provided some references. The target temperature varied and, in most cases, was 31–35 °C [2–4, 8]. For pediatric cases, Guilliams et al. [11] used a mild hypothermia of 32–35 °C to treat RSE. No reports on target temperatures of less than 30 °C have been found to be useful for RSE. To achieve target temperature, the rate of cooling varied among cases but

Table 7.1 Cases about hypothermia for RSE

Study	Age/sex/etiology	Medication trails	Temperature management	Seizures controlled with hypothermia	Seizures controlled after rewarming	Outcome	Adverse effects during hypothermia
Corry et al. [8]	62-year-old/M/ cryptogenic	PHT, LEV, PRF, LZP, PB, MDZ	Endovascular cooling system. Targeted 34 °C over 4 h, maintained for 20 h; rewarming over 29 h	Yes	Yes	Survived	Acidosis, electrolyte abnormalities (↑K+), DVT
	66-year-old/M/ limbic encephalitis	OXZ, LEV, PHT, VPA, LZP, PB, TPM	Endovascular cooling system. Targeted 32 °C over 10 h, maintained for 61 h; rewarming over 50 h	Yes	Yes	Died	Acidosis, prolonged QT, elevated INR, DVT, infections
	54-year-old/M/ hepatic encephalopathy	PHT, LEV, LZP, MDZ	Endovascular cooling system. Targeted 35 °C over 1.5 h, maintained for 41 h; rewarming over 1.5 h	Yes	No	Died	Acidosis, elevated INR
	75-year-old/M/ limbic encephalitis	PHT, LEV, LZP, MDZ	Endovascular cooling system. Targeted 31 °C over 6.5 h, maintained for 25.5 h; rewarming over 45.5 h	Yes	No	Survived	Acidosis, elevated INR; ↓Ca/Mg/PO_4, DVT, PE, Tachy-Brady syndrome
Elting et al. [10]	3 days postpartum to 5 months old/M/ hemimegalencephaly	PB, VPA, VGB, LEV, CLZ, PHT, KTM, MDZ	Cooling blanket. Targeted 35.3–36 °C, maintained for 4 days	Yes	No	Hemispherectomy	N/A
Lin et al. [12]	10-year-old/M/viral encephalitis	LZP, DZP, PTH, PB, VPA, MDZ	External cooling mattress. Targeted 33 °C (bladder), maintained for 5 days; gradual rewarming (1 °C / day to 36 °C) over 3 days	Yes	Unclear	Survived	↓K+
	4.5-year-old/ F/viral encephalitis	ZP, DZP, PTH, PB, VPA, MDZ	External cooling mattress. Targeted 33 °C (bladder), maintained for 3 days; gradual rewarming (1 °C / day to 36 °C) over 4 days	Yes	Unclear	Survived	None

(continued)

Table 7.1 (continued)

Study	Age/sex/etiology	Medication trails	Temperature management	Seizures controlled with hypothermia	Seizures controlled after rewarming	Outcome	Adverse effects during hypothermia
Guilliams et al. [11]	10-year-old/F/ unknown	LZP, FPHT, LEV, PB, LZP, VPA, MDZ	Surface cooling. Targeted 34 °C (bladder) for 24 h; gradual rewarming by 0.5 °C/day to 36.5 °C	Yes	Yes	Survived	↓K+
	5-month-old/F/ hydrocephalus and perinatal injury	LZP, PB, FPHT, MZD (0.3 mg/kg/h), LEV	Cooling blanket. Targeted 32 °C (bladder) over 1 h, for 72 h; gradual rewarming by 1 °C every 6 h	Yes	Yes	Died	Abdominal hypertension, pneumatosis intestinalis, hypokalemia, elevated INR (2.48)
	11-month-old/M/ POLG-1 mutation	LZP, FPHT, PB, LVE, MDZ	Surface cooling (Arctic Sun). Targeted 34 °C (bladder) over 4 h, maintained for 4 days; rewarming by 0.5 °C every 12 h to 36 °C	Yes	No	Died	Unclear
	10-year-old/M/ epilepsy	LEV, LTG, DZP, CLZ, LZP, FPHT, PB, MDZ	Surface cooling (Arctic Sun). Targeted 33 °C (bladder) over 3 h, maintained for 5 days; rewarming by 0.5 °C every 12 h	Yes	Yes	Survived	Lactic acidosis, ↑Na + (155 mEq/L), ↓K+(2.0 mEq/L); hematuria; hypertension
	15-year-old/M/ anti-NMDAR encephalitis	ZNS, FPHT, OXC, PB, PRF, KTM, VPA, TPM, LEV, MDZ	Cooling blanket. Targeted 33–35 °C (esophageal) over 13 h, maintained for 5 days; rewarming 2 °C/8 h to 36 °C	Partly controlled	Yes	Survived	N/A

PB phenobarbital, *VPA* valproic acid, *VGB* vigabatrin, *LEV* levetiracetam, *CLZ* clonazepam, *MDZ* midazolam, *PHT* phenytoin, *KTM* ketamine, *LZP* lorazepam, *FPHT* fosphenytoin, *OXC* oxcarbazepine, *ZNS* zonisamide, *PRF* propofol, *INR* international normalized ratio, *DVT* deep venous thrombosis, *PE* pulmonary embolism ranged from 1 h for achieving 32 °C to 24 h for achieving 34 °C [8, 10–12]. After hypothermia was induced, the seizures ceased in most cases. In some cases, burst suppression was induced within several hours after hypothermia was induced. All cases reported a good control of seizures during the hypothermic state. The target temperature was usually maintained for 1–5 days, and then the patients were rewarmed. The rate of rewarming was often 0.5–1.0 °C/day. After rewarming, some cases remained in seizure remission with continuous AED treatment, but some cases had a recurrence of SE. The long-term outcome varied mainly by the etiology of the RSE [8, 10–12]. During the therapeutic hypothermia treatment, concomitant sedation was induced. Midazolam, thiopental, propofol, and ketamine were often used. However, some researchers suggested that barbiturates should be avoided and that midazolam and propofol were favorable [13].

7.1.3 Safety

Even mild hypothermia (30–35 °C) is not without its risks, and these adverse effects include acid-base and electrolyte disturbances, coagulation disorders, disseminated intravascular coagulation, cardiac arrhythmia, thrombosis, infection, bowel ischemia, and paralytic ileus [8, 10–12]. Most complications have a low incidence in other situations. In 41 clinical trials of mild hypothermia on postanoxic encephalopathy, only 29 (1%) adverse events related to a cooling device were reported. Adverse effects of hypothermia may be related to the cooling device or to the hypothermia itself [14].

The limited cases that used hypothermia for the treatment of RSE showed that adverse effects were not very common (Table 7.1). In the study conducted by Corry et al. [8], when the body temperature was lower than 30 °C, side effects occurred, including ventricular fibrillation, venous thromboses, and coagulation disorders. In the study by Cereda et al. [15], a patient with RSE received an appendectomy during the hypothermia treatment due to acute intestinal ischemia and necrosis. In the study by Lin et al. [12], a pediatric patient developed transient hypokalemia during hypothermia treatment. In the study by Guilliams et al. [11], the adverse events during therapeutic hypothermia included hypokalemia and hypernatremia, coagulation disorders, colonic necrosis, lactic acidosis, hematuria, and infection. These side effects suggest that the following situations may be contraindications for induced therapeutic hypothermia: immunosuppression, active infection, hemodynamic instability, pregnancy, and coagulopathy (INR > 2 or platelets < 75,000).

7.1.4 Potential Mechanisms

Animal studies have also shown the effect of hypothermia on epileptic activity. Micro-thermoelectric devices are useful tools to establish the antiseizure or antiepileptic effect of hypothermia in vivo. This effect is achieved by implanting micro-thermoelectric devices into the cerebral cortex of an animal model to manipulate the focal temperature [16]. Using thermoelectrically driven cooling devices and bipolar electrodes, the study of focal epileptic seizures that were established by penicillin G or cobalt powder in animal models also found that hypothermia reduced the seizure frequency and the neurological changes [17]. However, the mechanisms have been far from explained, but one potential mechanism pertains to neurotransmitter release and gated ion channels.

A study showed that presynaptic membrane excitatory neurotransmitter release was inhibited under low-temperature conditions [18]. Hypothermia can reduce cerebral metabolism, which regulates the release of the neurotransmitters and delays the onset of anoxic depolarization [19, 20]. It was suggested that hypothermia can lead to a loss of function of the voltage-gated sodium channels and can affect neuronal depolarization, which may be helpful for the suspension of epileptiform discharges [21, 22]. Motamedi et al. [23] found that low temperatures terminated epileptiform discharges, blocked action potentials, and interfered with neuronal firing rhythms. In addition, it was also suggested that low temperatures affected the expression change of excitatory glutamate receptors (GluRs), which further regulated the excitatory synaptic membrane current. Yu et al. [24] observed the decreased level of GluR1 and the increased level of GluR2 in the hippocampus of animal models with SE under hypothermic conditions. This study also observed the decreased neuronal excitability and seizure activity, which indicated that low-temperature-inhibited seizures may be related to the regulation of expression of the GluR.

7.1.5 Conclusion

For nearly half a century, hypothermia therapy has been gradually applied to RSE. Commonly used methods of inducing hypothermia include endovascular cooling systems and surface cooling. Hypothermia treatments have a positive effect on RSE. Therapeutic hypothermia could cause electrolyte imbalances, acid-base balance disorders, cardiovascular disorders, infections, and other adverse reactions, but their incidence is low.

7.2 Electroconvulsive Therapy for Refractory Status Epilepticus

7.2.1 Historical Evolution

In the 1930s, electroconvulsive therapy (ECT) was initially used to treat epilepsy [25, 26]. The first reported application of ECT for the treatment of SE was conducted by Viparelli and colleagues in 1992 [27]. The 19-year-old patient in that study had complex partial seizures that were not responsive to phenytoin and diazepam. Two sessions of ECT were provided over 3 days. The first session significantly reduced the frequency of the seizures, and the second session successfully led to the cessation of the seizures. From then on, a couple of cases were reported, but no well-designed trial has been conducted to confirm the effectiveness and safety of using ECT in the treatment of SE. Although psychiatric practice guidelines have mentioned the use of ECT for refractory epilepsy and SE, the use of ECT for epilepsy and SE is still rare in clinical practice [28].

7.2.2 Clinical Application and Efficacy in RSE

To date, ECT has been increasingly used in RSE but is still in its infancy in that there are only a handful of cases that have been reported [29, 30]. The clinical use of ECT for epilepsy is still lacking in the consensus of guidelines and in the expertise, and these case reports provide some referent experience.

In all reported cases, ECT was considered when a variety of AEDs were ineffective for SE. Meanwhile, ECT is mainly used for some psychiatric disorders. Therefore, when these diseases are present in a patient, there is a stronger indication for the use of ECT [31, 32]. Regenold et al. [31] reported a case of a 71-year-old man with major depression and RSE which was unresponsive to various AEDs (phenytoin, phenobarbital, diazepam, lorazepam, and carbamazepine). The patient received eight sessions of ECT over 16 days, which led to a cessation of SE. Subsequently, the patient's partial complex seizures and tonic-clonic seizures were well controlled by AEDs, and the depression did not relapse during the 6 months of follow-up.

ECT was usually administered using standard bifrontotemporal electrode placement. The stimulus parameters varied among practitioners and patients (Table 7.2). Usually, the duration of ECT treatment was no more than 1 week. The stimulus sessions ranged from three sessions per day to two sessions per week [33–36]. In one study, Koong et al. [36] used a relatively long-term treatment for 6 weeks that consisted of two sessions per week. This regimen led to a cessation of SE, and ECT was maintained weekly. The current was reported in four patients of either 800 or 900 mA [34, 35, 37, 38]. Stimulus is also largely varied. The lowest reported dose was 64 mC, which could also result in a motor seizure of 48 s [33].

Table 7.2 Cases about ECT for RSE

Study	Age (years)/sex/ etiology	Medication trails	Placement	Sessions	Parameters	Response	Outcome	Adverse effects during ECT
Carrasco Gonzalez et al. [39]	25/M/head injury	PHT, CBZ, PB, DZP	N/A	6 (3 per week)	N/A	N/A	Completely recovered within 1 month	N/A
Griesemer et al. [33]	15/M/ microgyria	PB, PHT, ACT, CLZ, VPA, GBP, LTG, FBM,	N/A	4 sessions over 9 days	Charge: 64–127 mC	Shortened seizure duration	Recurrence of SE	Lethargic
				3 sessions over 3 days	Charge: 201–302 mC	Cessation of SE	Recurrence of SE	N/A
				6 sessions over 2 days	Charge: 101–403 mC	Reduction of seizures	Recurrence of SE	N/A
				3 sessions over 1 day	Charge: 201–403 mC	Cessation of SE	N/A	N/A
	10/F/ microcephaly and osteoporosis	PB, PTH, CBZ, VPA, FBM, GBP	N/A	3 sessions over 2–5 days; 3 treatments for every other week	Charge: 180–576 mC	Reduction of seizures	Recurrence of SE	N/A
Regenold et al. [31]	71/M/primary epilepsy	PHT, PB, DZP, LZP, CBZ	Bilateral	8 sessions over 16 days	N/A	Cessation of SE	Continues to partial complex seizures and tonic-clonic seizures	None
Lisanby et al. [34]	36/M/bifrontal cortical dysplasia	VGB, PB, NTZ, PHT, MDZ, PTB	Right frontotemporal and left parietal	5 sessions over 5 days	Current: 0.8ACharge: 576–3379 mCPulse frequency: 90–120 HzPulse width: 1–1.4 ms	Cessation of SE	SE resolved	N/A
Cline et al. [35]	39/M/herpes viral encephalitis	FPHT, VPA, PTB, LEV, PHT, OXC, TPM, LZP, FBM	Bifrontotemporal	9 (3/day for consecutive 3 days)	Current: 800 mA Charge: 576 mC Pulse frequency: 90 Hz Pulse width: 1.0 s	Not seizure-free but improve mentally and physically	Seizure frequency reduced	N/A

(continued)

Table 7.2 (continued)

Study	Age (years)/sex/ etiology	Medication trails	Placement	Sessions	Parameters	Response	Outcome	Adverse effects during ECT
Viparelli et al. [27]	19/F/primary epilepsy	CLZ, DZP, PHT	N/A	2 sessions 48 h apart	Current: sinusoidalVoltage: 110 VDuration: 0.6 s	Cessation of SE	Seizure-free on CBZ	N/A
Wusthoff et al. [40]	29/F/ Rasmussen's encephalitis	PTB, PHT, LEV, PB, MDZ, VPA, PTM, PGB, FBM, DSF	N/A	10 sessions	N/A	No response	Continues to seizure	N/A
Kamel et al. [37]	32/F/viral encephalitis	VPA, PHT, PB, LEV, PTM, PB, KTM	Bifrontotemporal	4 sessions over 5 days	Current: 900 mA Charge: 504 mC Pulse frequency: 70 Hz Pulse width: 0.5 ms	Cessation of SE	Seizure resolved	Retrograde amnesia
	41/F/viral encephalitis	PHT, LEV, VPA, PB, KTM	Bifrontotemporal	4 sessions over 5 days	Current: 900 mA Charge: 504 mC Pulse frequency: 70 Hz Pulse width: 0.5 ms	No response	Died	N/A
	26/F/infectious cerebritis	PHT, VPA, PB, LEV, TPM, PB, ISF, KTM	Bifrontotemporal	4 sessions over 5 days	Current: 900 mA Charge: 504 mC Pulse frequency: 70 Hz Pulse width: 0.5 ms	Cessation of SE	Continues to have seizures	Retrograde amnesia
Koong et al. [36]	54/F/epilepsy with psychosis	N/A	N/A	2 sessions per week for 6 weeks	N/A	Cessation of SE	Recurrence of SE and ECT maintained weekly	Weight increased
Shin et al. [38]	7/F/primary epilepsy	VPA, TPM, LEV, CLZ, MDZ, KTM, PTB	Bilateral	2 sessions over 2 days, repeated 1 week later	Current: 0.8APulse frequency: 60–120 HzPulse width: 0.37–2 ms	Cessation of SE	Died	N/A

ACT acetazolamide, *CLZ* clonazepam, *FBM* felbamate, *ISF* isoflurane, *NTZ* nitrazepam, *PTB* pentobarbital, *DSF* desflurane, *PB* phenobarbital, *VPA* valproic acid, *VGB* vigabatrin, *LEV* levetiracetam, *MDZ* midazolam, *PHT* phenytoin, *KTM* ketamine, *LZP* lorazepam, *FPHT* fosphenytoin, *OXC* oxcarbazepine, *ZNS* zonisamide, *PRF* propofol, *GBP* gabapentin

The highest reported dose was 3379 mC [34]. The pulse frequency ranged from 40 to 120 Hz [34, 35, 37, 38]. The pulse width was 1.0–1.4 s [41–43], but lower pulse widths of 0.5 s were also used [37, 38].

Using these regimens, most patients achieved a cessation of SE during or after completion of the ECT treatment. Some patients reported shortened seizure durations or reduced seizure frequencies. In addition, some patients were unresponsive to ECT treatment (Table 7.2).

7.2.3 Safety

The biggest concern regarding the use of ECT was an impairment in cognitive function. Due to the lack of studies on treating RSE with ECT, safety was evaluated in studies that used ECT for the treatment of psychiatric disorders. The adverse cognitive effects usually included acute disorientation and anterograde amnesia, but the severity of cognitive impairment was usually low [41]. Brodaty et al. [42] investigated neuropsychological function in 81 elderly patients with major depressive disorder pre-ECT, immediately post-ECT and 1–3 years later. This study found that ECT did not lead to significant side effects or neuropsychological impairment in elderly patients. The safety of ECT using unilateral and bilateral approaches was assessed in 39 elderly patients with major depressive disorder. No serious adverse events were reported, and both groups showed an improvement in neuropsychological scores [43]. Sackeim et al. [44] assessed the depression severity and cognitive function before, during, immediately after, and 2 months after ECT in 80 depressed patients in a double-blind study. Bilateral ECT resulted in greater impairment than did unilateral ECT during short-term and long-term follow-up.

Some adverse events involving other systems were also common but were not severe. Cardiovascular complications, such as heart failure, cardiac arrhythmias, severe valvular heart disease, and other diseases, were common with the use of ECT [37]. These adverse events may be more severe [41]. Headaches, myalgias, and nausea were reported in most patients and were usually classified as minor. Other less common adverse events included prolonged seizures, prolonged apnea, mania, and postictal delirium [41].

7.2.4 Potential Mechanisms

The mechanism of ECT for SE is far from understood. Sackeim et al. [44] conducted a RCT on 52 depressed patients who received unilateral right and bilateral ECT treatments and observed that a 12-fold range of the minimum electrical intensity was necessary to produce a seizure and that bilateral ECT had a higher initial seizure threshold compared with unilateral ECT. GABAergic transmission plays a major inhibitory role in the central nervous system and in the γ-aminobutyric acid (GABA) dysfunction related to SE [45]. The increased seizure threshold may be involved in activating inhibitory mechanisms by enhancing GABAergic transmissions [30, 46]. This hypothesis was supported by the evidence from both animal and human studies. Clark [47] examined the levels of $GABA_A$ receptors after one and five electroshock-induced seizures. They found that a single seizure led to a rapid and transient increase in alpha4 mRNA in the dentate gyrus. A single shock led to an increase in alpha4 proteins in the dentate gyrus, and repeated electroshocks (48-h intervals) led to an enhanced response of the alpha4 subunit to the seizure. Esel et al. [48] compared the GABA system between 25 depressed patients who received a course of ECT and 23 healthy subjects. They found that one session of ECT produced a massive increase in the GABA levels. In addition, the effect of ECT may involve galanin, which is an important neuropeptide in the inhibition of classical neurotransmitter release [49]. Christiansen et al. [50] examined the effects of repeated electroconvulsive stimulation on the galanin system and found that repetitive electric shocks regulate the expression of both the GalR2 and GalR1 receptor subtypes and the receptor binding of galanin in the piriform cortex, in the hippocampal dentate gyrus, and in the amygdala.

7.2.5 Conclusion

ECT is the alternative treatment option when medications fail to treat RSE. It has also been used in recent years for RSE. In a variety of etiologies for RSE, ECT can lead to a termination of RSE or a reduction of the frequency of seizures. Cognitive impairment is the most common adverse effect in ECT.

7.3 Ketogenic Diet Treatment for Refractory Status Epilepticus

7.3.1 History Evolution

Hippocrates treated a patient with epilepsy by fasting and drink deprivation to control seizures, suggesting that fasting may be an important method for the treatment of epilepsy [51]. In 1921, Wilder [52] found that the high-fat, low-carbohydrate diet effectively controls the seizures, putting forward the notion of a ketogenic diet. Fatty acids produce beta-hydroxybutyrate (BHB), acetoacetic acid and acetone, and then ketosis; the body energy metabolism from glucose converts to ketone bodies. Seizures are controlled without calories limit, which is better than fasting and drink deprivation. This diet characteristically promotes the clinical application of the ketogenic diet (KD). In 1938, with the advent of phenytoin and the subsequent emergence of new AEDs, KD use is gradually reduced. In the mid-1990s, a TV show reported that a 2-year-old boy suffering from intractable epilepsy received KD treatment, whereupon the seizures were controlled after a few months. KD treatment thereby gained wider attention. During 2000–2007, the KD treatment of child patients with epilepsy in the UK increased to 50% [53]. In December 2006, 26 epileptic experts and nutrition experts from 9 countries developed an expert consensus on KD treatment, which is funded by Charlie Foundation and approved by the pediatric neurology practice committee. It describes in detail to whom it will apply the pretreatment evaluation, type of diet selection, subjects of follow-up and supervision, side effect monitoring, withdrawal indications, and so on [54]. In 2012, the National Institute for Health and Clinical Excellence in the United Kingdom developed guidelines for KD treatment in epilepsy, setting the level of clinical evidence and recommendation grading [55]. In 2015, as for the regions with limited resources, the diet treatment group of the International League Against Epilepsy (ILAE) developed KD treatment guidelines that were particularly cost-effective and readily available, thereby promoting the worldwide application of the KD [56].

7.3.2 The Types of KD and Derived Diets

7.3.2.1 Classic KD

The classic KD is the most widely used and is the easiest to accept. It is made up of long-chain fatty acids, moderate protein, and low carbohydrates; the ratio of fat and protein to carbohydrate (g) is 4:1. Eighty to ninety percent of calories are supplied by butter, vegetable oil, and other foods rich in fat, with the remaining calories provided by foods low in carbohydrates and with essential proteins, such as vegetables and fruits. After the first 1–2 days of fasting, the diet gradually transitions to a 4:1 ratio (fat: protein and carbohydrate), inducing the liver to produce ketone bodies. When ketosis occurs, blood glucose and urine ketone monitoring is required. Nutrition doctors need to adjust the dietary structure throughout the diet's administration.

7.3.2.2 Medium-Chain Triglycerides (MCTs)

MCTs are palatable and compliable, with 30% of the calories derived from medium-chain fatty acids (sunflower acid, caprylic acid, etc.) and 30% from long-chain fatty acids. One calorie of medium-chain fatty acids can produce more ketone bodies than long-chain fatty acids, resulting in the patient taking in more protein and carbohydrates when the total calories are limited.

7.3.2.3 Modified Atkins Diet (MAD)

The ratio of fat and protein to carbohydrates (g) is 1:1 in MAD. Unlike in the classical KD, only the amount of carbohydrate is limited, without fasting, hospitalization, or restriction of protein, calories, or fluid intake. Therefore, the patient is free to choose his food.

7.3.2.4 Low Glycemic Index Treatment (LGIT)

Only carbohydrates with glycemic indexes <50 can be ingested. Sixty percent of calories are from fat, and the amount of carbohydrates (40–60 g/day) is much higher than in the classic KD.

7.3.3 Clinical Application of KD in RSE

SE is a common neurological emergency. AEDs are effective for most SE, but some patients are not sensitive to AEDs, and their seizures are weakly controlled, leading to RSE. Recent reports suggest that the KD is also applied for treating adults and children with RSE, for ages ranging from 5 months to 49 years [57, 58]. Currently, approximately 50 children and ten adults with RSE under KD treatment have been reported [59]. These case reports indicate that the KD is effective and safe for RSE patients, but there is insufficient evidence to recommend the KD as an established treatment option.

7.3.3.1 KD Treatment for RSE Children

Caraballo et al. described two patients suffering from refractory myoclonic SE and treated with the KD. One patient was a 23-month-old boy who was admitted to the hospital because of myoclonic SE. The patient was refractory to different AEDs, such as midazolam, levetiracetam, ethosuximide, clobazam, topiramate, and corticosteroids. At 2 years and 6 months of age, the KD was started at a 4:1 ratio. After a 24 h fast, the patient was administered the KD via a nasogastric tube. During the first week on the KD, the patient slowly improved, achieving a 75–90% seizure reduction, with fewer electroencephalogram (EEG) abnormalities. Since then, his neuropsychological performance, but mainly his motor development, has significantly improved. After 1 year on the diet, the patient has isolated myoclonias. The number of AEDs has been reduced to one (valproic acid). The diet was switched to the classic oral diet at 3 years of age. Another patient was a 17-month-old boy. On the first day of life, he started with recurrent RSE requiring mechanical ventilation. At 1 year of age, the patient developed progressive encephalopathy and myoclonic epilepsy. The boy was admitted to the intensive care unit (ICU) because of refractory myoclonias, and intravenous levatiracetam, valproic acid, benzodiazepines, and corticosteroids were tried without response over 3 weeks before starting the KD. The KD was begun at a 4:1 ratio. After 24 h of fasting, the child was given the KD via a nasogastric tube. 1 week after KD initiation, the patient slowly improved, achieving a 50% seizure reduction. After a 6-month follow-up, in spite of the progressive encephalopathy, his quality of life improved, and the AEDs were reduced to levetiracetam and topiramate. The patient continues to receive the same formula orally [60].

In early 2014, Caraballo et al. assessed the efficacy and tolerability of the KD in patients with RSE who were followed for a minimum of 6 months. Two patients were seizure-free, and five patients had a 50–75% seizure frequency reduction after the onset of ketonuria in 2–5 days. Three patients had a < 50% seizure reduction and discontinued the diet because all had suffered severe side effects. Seven insisted on the diet for 6 months to 3 years, with seizures recurring in 4 months: two had weekly seizures, two had monthly seizures, two had occasional seizures, and one had one seizure. All of them established good tolerability of the KD, and their quality of life did not further worsen. The KD should be considered earlier in the treatment of focal SE, which is secondary to inflammation [61]. Lin et al. described a boy with super RSE who was administered an intravenous KD. Moderate ketosis appeared 24 h after admission, and thiamylal was successfully weaned 70 h after admission [62].

7.3.3.2 KD Treatment for RSE Adults

Thakur et al. [63] performed a retrospective case review of KD-treated adult patients with super RSE at four medical centers. Ten adult patients were enrolled. Four patients were male, and seven had encephalitis. The median age was 33 years. The median duration of SE before the KD was 21.5 days, and the median number of AEDs used before the KD was seven. Ninety percent of patients achieved ketosis, becoming SE-free in a median of 3 days. Three patients experienced transient acidosis and hypertriglyceridemia as side effects of the KD. Ninety percent of patients achieved resolution of SE. A major limitation of the current study was its retrospective nature. Many patients received adjunctive treatment with multiple AEDs, surgical intervention, steroids, plasmapheresis, and immunoglobulin while on the KD. The possibility that other interventions resulted in seizure relief cannot be excluded. An ongoing prospective multicenter trial using a standardized KD protocol will provide further data on the safety and efficacy of the KD in critically patients with RSE and/or super RSE.

Wusthoff et al. [64] describes two KD-treated adult patients with prolonged nonconvulsive status epilepticus (NCSE). A 29-year-old woman was diagnosed with Parry Romberg and Rasmussen's syndromes at 12 years of age after progressive left hemifacial atrophy. The first seizure appeared at age 14, and complex partial seizures appeared at age 21. Secondary generalization and recurrent SE occurred at age 24 after increased seizure frequency. After multiple AEDs (carbamazepine, lamotrigine, gabapentin, levetiracetam, topiramate, zonisamide, pregabalin, and clobazam) with poor seizure control, the KD was introduced via gastrostomy tube. Four days after initiation, seizure frequency was reduced to once every 3–4 days; seizures were controlled completely after 11 days. Another previously healthy 34-year-old man suffered from generalized tonic-clonic seizures (GTCS) progressing to SE as a result of viral encephalitis or postinfectious encephalitis. Because of the AEDs' (lorazepam, levetiracetam, phenytoin, topiramate, phenobarbital, pentobarbital, valproic acid, and midazolam) poor control of SE, fasting was introduced to initiate the KD via gastric tube. Within 6 days of KD initiation, the patient was weaned from AEDs without a return of seizures. He still suffered occasional self-limited breakthrough seizures for 1 year. Moreover, other clinical experts also have confirmed the effectiveness of the KD in RSE treatment [65–72].

7.3.3.3 Some Factors of the KD in RSE Treatment

Routes of administration can be divided into enteral and parenteral administration. Enteral administration is the most common, i.e., via a gastric tube; parenteral administration is less used, i.e., via an intravenous route. Whatever the method of administration, the proportion of fat and nonfat must be strictly maintained at 4:1, and glucose must be discontinued.

After starting a KD, ketosis can usually be accomplished within 2–3 days; the seizures will see improvement after 5–8 days.

If symptoms of SE patients are controlled, long-term adoption of the KD is applicable as an adjuvant therapy. If serious complications occur or the KD produces no effect, the diet can be terminated.

The KD is effective in the treatment of SE or RSE with various seizures types, such as viral encephalitis, autoimmune encephalitis, FIRES, and Dravet syndrome.

7.3.3.4 Precautions for Applying the KD in RSE Treatment

Before starting the KD, several steps are needed: (1) an assessment should be made as to whether any diseases are causing abnormal fatty acid metabolism, (2) a dietitian should design a 4:1 ketogenic allocation, (3) fasting should be initiated for 1–2 days, and intravenous infusion of carbohydrates should stop.

To initiate the KD, several factors should be monitored: (1) blood glucose every 4 h, (2) ketone or serum β-hydroxybutyric acid daily, (3) electrolytes daily, (4) triglycerides, (5) pH, and (6) blood routine and blood biochemistry.

7.3.3.5 Contraindications of the KD in RSE Treatment

The KD should not be implemented in certain contexts: metabolic disorder (continued hypernatremia, hyponatremia, hypoglycemia, acidosis, hypocalcemia), hemodynamic instability or cardiopulmonary dysfunction, coagulopathy, hepatic failure, pancreatitis, severe hyperlipidemia, enteral nutrition intolerance (including obstruction), pregnancy, receiving any propofol injection within 24 h, fatty acid oxidation disorder, or pyruvate carboxylase deficiency.

7.3.4 Adverse Reactions to the KD

7.3.4.1 Acidosis

Initially, the anticonvulsant property of the KD was hypothesized to be the reduction in cerebral pH. However, a change in cerebral pH has not been observed in rats receiving a KD, nor has blood pH changed in humans treated with KD [73]. Conversely, metabolic acidosis is a common side effect of KD therapy. Oral sodium bicarbonate is common to correct metabolic acidosis.

7.3.4.2 Dyslipidemia

Hyperlipidemia is the most common side effect in KD, with an incidence of up to 33–38% [74–76]. Zamani et al. [77] studied 33 children with refractory epilepsy after 6 months of KD treatment to detect adverse reactions to the KD on the serum lipid profile. Median triglyceride increased significantly (from 84 to 180 mg/dL), as well as median total cholesterol (from 180 to 285 mg/dL), median serum low-density lipoprotein (LDL) (from 91 to 175 mg/dL), and median serum high-density lipoprotein (HDL) (from 51 to 58 mg/dL). Kwiterovich et al. [78] conducted a 6-month prospective cohort study of 141 KD-treated children with refractory seizures. At 6 months, atherogenic apoB-containing lipoproteins increased significantly, and antiatherogenic HDL cholesterol decreased; the KD significantly increased mean total, LDL, VLDL, and non-HDL cholesterol, as well as triglycerides and total apoB. In addition, mean HDL cholesterol decreased significantly, although apoA-I increased. Coppola et al. [79] found that epilepsy patients treated with the KD developed higher arterial stiffness parameters, including AIx and beta-index. However, MCT may had less of an effect on lipids than did the classic KD. Lambrechts et al. [80] found that 7% of epilepsy patients with MTC had a relevant increase in total and LDL cholesterol values and triglyceride values during the KD.

7.3.4.3 Protein-Losing Enteropathy

Protein-losing enteropathy is a very rare side effect of the KD. Moriyama et al. [81] reported that a 9-year-old girl developed fever for 5 days, which then evolved into severe RSE. After multiple AEDs with poor control, the KD was introduced and her seizures stopped. However, she developed hypoproteinemia, and her abdominal dynamic scintigraphy and colonoscopy findings indicated protein-losing enteropathy with nonspecific mucosal inflammation. Because of the worsening nutritional status, the KD was discontinued. Her nutrition gradually improved, but her seizures increased.

7.3.4.4 Propofol Infusion Syndrome

Long-term (>48 h) infusion of propofol may result in rare but fatal propofol infusion syndrome with metabolic acidosis, rhabdomyolysis, lipemia, and myocardial failure. Baumeister et al. [82] reported that a 10-year-old boy with catastrophic epilepsy developed fatal propofol infusion syndrome after the KD was initiated. The KD aggravated the impaired fatty acid oxidation induced by propofol.

7.3.4.5 Others

Gastrointestinal reactions (i.e., abdominal pain, nausea, vomiting, constipation) are a common side effect [71, 74]. There have been reports that the KD for RSE treatment was discontinued because of gastroesophageal reflux [67]. Weight loss occurs in 19–60% of intractable epilepsy patients with KD [59, 74, 75, 83, 84], with an incidence as high as 60% in adolescents [85]. Forty-five percent of women are prone to menstrual disorders while on the KD [86]. Childhood and adolescence are critical periods for growth and development, with large nutritional demands; the side effect of the KD on growth rate and weight loss is an important reason for the KD to be discontinued. Sampath et al. [86] conducted a cohort study for the KD treatment of children with refractory epilepsy (n = 195): the incidence of kidney stones increased to 6.7% without regard to age or carbonic anhydrase inhibitors (such as zonisamide and topiramate). Oral potassium citrate improves kidney stones, and delays occurred.

7.3.5 Potential Mechanisms

In general, after a few hours on the KD, ketosis appears and continues for 2 weeks to achieve the best effect for controlling seizures. This time delay may be related to metabolic adaptation, mitochondrial proliferation, and other transport-related adjustments. However, once the low-carbohydrate diet is discontinued and ketosis is interrupted, the efficacy of seizure control will disappear in a few days [87].

No matter what type of KD, such as the long-chain fatty acid-based classic KD, the medium-chain fatty acid-based MCT, or the high-fat, high-protein, low-glucose MAD, significant inhibition of seizures via increasing ketone and/or restricting glucose and calories can occur. This conclusion is verified in acute or chronic epilepsy animal experiments as well as in clinical trials [87]. Compared with adults, children and young animals respond better to the KD. Melo et al. [88] also found that single-acid transporter MCT-1 expression is higher in younger patients, as well as ketone bodies (BHB and acetoacetate) transported from the blood-brain barrier and GABA in the cerebrospinal fluid (CSF). However, others have noted that the KD is not age dependent: its effect is similar on adults and children with epilepsy.

7.3.5.1 Ketones' Direct Antiepileptic Effects

In the 1930s, Keith showed that acetone or ethylacetoacetate protected rabbits from thujone-induced seizures [89]. In 2002, Likhodii et al. found that acetone appeared to have a broad spectrum of anticonvulsant effects by using four seizure rat models (maximal electroshock model, pentylenetetrazole (PTZ) model, amygdala kindling model, AY-9944 model) [90]. Gasior et al. found that acetone (1–32 mmol/kg, i.p.) showed a dose-dependent increase in the PTZ threshold and protects against 4-AP-induced seizures [91]. Rho et al. also found that acetoacetate, acetone, stereoisomers, and L-(+) of BHB were anticonvulsant in Frings audiogenic seizure-susceptible mice [92]. However, Nylen et al. found that the KD was unable to elevate amygdaloid after discharge thresholds in fully kindled rats [93].

7.3.5.2 The Increased GABAergic Hypothesis

It is popularly hypothesized that the KD influences the brain inhibitory neurotransmitter γ-aminobutyric acid, the main therapeutic target for epilepsy. In general, the KD is most effective against seizure models induced by GABAergic antagonists such as PTZ, bicuculline, picrotoxin, and γ-butyrolactone. Conversely, it shows little if any efficacy in seizure models activated by ionotropic glutamate receptors (such as kainic acid), voltage-dependent sodium channels (such as maximal electroshock), or glycine receptor inhibition (such as strychnine) [94].

Dahlin et al. examined the effect of the KD on the excitatory and inhibitory amino acids of CSF in 26 KD-treated children with refractory epilepsy. GABA levels were increased in responders (>50% seizure reduction) compared with in nonresponders. The GABA levels of very good responders (>90% seizure reduction) were dramatically higher either at baseline or during the diet [95]. Wang et al. also found increased GABA levels of 2 KD-treated patients through 2D MRI scans [96]. In animal studies, calorie restriction also increases brain glutamic acid decarboxylase (GAD) 65 and GAD67 expression in the superior colliculus, cerebellar cortex, and temporal cortex [97]. Ketotic mice showed an enhanced concentration of glutamine and GABA in the forebrain after the administration of acetate and nitrogen donor [98]. Astrocyte metabolism is found to be more active in the ketotic brain, with increased conversion of excitatory neurotransmitter glutamate to glutamine, which further converts to GABA [99].

7.3.5.3 Reduced Neuronal Excitability Via K_{ATP} Channels

In general, the mitochondrial metabolism of ketone bodies inhibits glycolysis, followed by an increase in mitochondrial ATP and a decrease in glycolytic ATP. Meanwhile, inhibition of glycolytic enzymes may activate a compartmentation of ATP at the plasma membrane. The submembrane consumption of glycolytic ATP by pumps—that is, for maintaining intracellular ionic concentrations—could activate nearby ATP-sensitive potassium (K_{ATP}) channels, producing a hyperpolarizing current that reduces neuron excitability [100].

Physiological levels of ketone bodies (β-hydroxybutyrate or acetoacetate) reduce the spontaneous firing in "seizure gate" substantia nigra pars reticulata of rats and mice. However, the anticonvulsant effect of ketone bodies is eliminated by sensitive K_{ATP} channel blockers or by gene knockout. It has been proposed that ketone bodies or glycolytic restriction enhances a natural activity-limiting action served by neuronal K_{ATP} channels [101].

7.3.5.4 Glycolytic Inhibition

Glycolytic inhibition is anticonvulsant [102, 103]. The decreased glucose levels produced by animals or human on the KD are consistent with a reduction of the glycolysis process. Stafstrom et al. found that glycolytic inhibitor 2-deoxy-D-glucose (2-DG) reduced interictal epileptiform bursts evoked by 4-AP and bicuculline in CA3 of the hippocampus, as well as by audiogenic stimulation in Frings mice. A potential mechanism may involve an increase of after-discharge thresholds in perforant path kindling and a twofold slowing in kindled seizure progression. However, 2-DG had no protection on maximal electroshock or Metrazol seizures [102]. Garriga-Canut et al. also showed that 2-DG potently blocks the progression of kindled seizures and decreases the expression of seizure-induced brain-derived neurotrophic factor (BDNF) and its receptor, TrkB. This reduced expression is proposed as the activation of transcription factor NRSF, which recruits the NADH-binding co-repressor CtBP around the BDNF promoter to suppress a transcription permissive chromatin environment [103]. Importantly, because 2-DG administered orally is fairly well tolerated, this compound may represent a novel and feasible treatment strategy for epilepsy.

7.3.5.5 Role of Fatty Acids

Chang et al. [104] confirmed that some specific medium-chain fatty acids serve to more effectively address seizure control and enhance neuroprotection with less sedation and cell toxicity, compared to the antiepileptic drug valproic acid. In 2016, Chang et al. [105] also found that decanoic acid, a medium-chain fatty acid, exhibits antiseizure activity in rat hippocampal slice models of epileptiform activity but that other medium-chain fatty acids, such as ketones (beta-hydroxybutyrate and acetone), do not. It has a strong direct inhibition on the α-amino-3-hydroxy-5-methyl-4-isoxazole-propionic acid (AMPA) receptor and excitatory neurotransmission in hippocampal neurons, which likely occurs via binding to the M3 helix of the AMPA-selective glutamate receptor 2 (GluA2) transmembrane domain, which ultimately contributes to the anticonvulsant effects of MCT.

Polyunsaturated fatty acids (PUFAs) such as arachidonic acid (AA, C20:4ω6), docosahexaenoic acid (DHA, C22:6ω3), arachidonic acid (AA, C20:4ω6), or eicosapentaenoic acid (EPA, C20:5ω3) have become popular foci of KD research. Specific PUFAs (i.e., AA and DHA) were found to be increased in both the sera and brains of KD-treated patients and animals [87]. Dietary supplementation with 5 g of n-3 PUFAs per day significantly reduced seizure frequency and intensity in epileptic patients [106]. EPA and DHA significantly raised the electrical-evoked threshold of action potentials and reduced the frequency of action potentials in CA1 neurons of hippocampal slices. EPA also restored PTZ- or glutamate-induced neuronal excitability [107]. It is likely that the Shaker K_V channel in open and closed states interacts with a PUFA-enriched lipid bilayer [108].

7.3.6 Conclusion

Due to its rapid onset, high efficiency, and mild side effects, the KD is a promising therapy for the treatment of intractable epilepsy and SE in children and adults. Importantly, it does not increase the seizure types of patients or exacerbate seizures. For neurological clinicians, a large number of randomized controlled multicenter clinical trials are needed for adult patients, especially regarding RSE treatment. At present, the mechanisms of the KD are still being explored because looking for key targets for the inhibition of seizures will provide a theoretical basis for improving the application of the KD among epilepsy patients—especially, adult patients with RSE. Dietitians also need to establish more consistent diet components for patients with different dietary habits. For patients, there exist websites and software for self-managing the daily diet for long-term treatment using the KD.

7.4 Neuromodulatory Treatment in Refractory Status Epilepticus

RSE cannot always be controlled by AEDs. When pharmacotherapy fails, neuromodulatory treatment becomes a possible option. At present, neuromodulatory technology that is applied to SE therapy includes vagus nerve stimulation (VNS), cortical responsive stimulation (CRS), and deep brain stimulation (DBS).

7.4.1 VNS

VNS was approved for the treatment of generalized or focal epilepsy in Europe in 1994 [109]. In 1997, it was also approved for the treatment of refractory focal epilepsy (age > 12) by the US FDA [110]. Thus far, more than 75,000 patients with drug-resistant epilepsy worldwide have received this surgery [111].

7.4.1.1 Surgical Procedures

The device is implanted below the patient's left clavicle (the left vagus nerve is usually used because stimulating the right vagus nerve may cause severe bradycardia); two continuous leads along the splitter inducer guide the electrode wires from the chest incision through the subcutaneous tunnel to the neck incision, and the electrode is entwined around the left vagus nerve and directly wrapped around the left vagus nerve, after which the short lead converges below and the long lead converges upward to make connect the wire and the stimulator. First, bradycardia and asystole tests caused by vagus nerve stimulation are conducted in the operation room; then, the implanted stimulator performs the function 2 weeks after surgery. The device program settings are installed on a command bar outside of the body; the command bar is connected to a magnet, and the magnet can directly activate the stimulator to transmit the set stimulation pulse. Patients can even use the command bar to induce the magnet to initiate stimulus pulses during seizures or auras to stop seizures or to reduce their severity. The entire device is usually programmed for 30 s in the powered-on state and 5 min in the powered-off state. The pulse width is usually set at 500 Hz, with the amplitude set from 0.25 to 3.5 mA. Most commonly, the most appropriate current is 1–2 mA. Parameters can be adjusted according to the degree of effect, and the speed of equipment cycle is directly related to the battery life of the pulse stimulator [112].

7.4.1.2 Clinical Application and Efficacy in Epilepsy

VNS is considered an effective treatment for intractable epilepsy. It is mainly suitable for patients with drug-resistant epilepsy who are not appropriate for focal excision, especially those with complex partial or secondary generalized epilepsy. For example, VNS has been shown to be effective in partial and secondary epilepsy therapy in children. It can also be used in other epilepsy syndromes, such as symptomatic and idiopathic generalized epilepsy [113], and Lennox-Gastaut syndrome, and it is better for young patients with primary generalized epilepsy and focal epilepsy [114]. A retrospective study also confirmed that the prognoses of younger patients or patients with unilateral interictal discharges and cortical dysplasia who had VNS surgery were superior [115].

Vonck et al. [116] used VNS to treat 118 patients with intractable epilepsy in 2004.

Seizures were significantly reduced by 55 and 7%; patients became seizure-free over the 6-month postoperative follow-up period. De Herdt et al. [117] found a significant reduction of seizures in 51% of 138 patients with refractory epilepsy and seizure cessation of 9% patients in the 44 months leading to follow-up. Kuba et al. [118] found seizure reduction in 55.9% patients with drug-resistant epilepsy approximately 6.6 years after VNS surgery. Although VNS is currently used as an adjunctive treatment for intractable epilepsy, it has been widely recognized for its efficacy.

7.4.1.3 Clinical Application and Efficacy in RSE

Patwardhan et al. [119] used VNS to treat a 30-year-old man with RSE. The patient received left vagus nerve stimulator implantation after nearly 9 days of pentobarbital anesthesia failed. As indicated by EEG monitoring, he became seizure-free for 19 consecutive days after surgery and was awakened from his coma. He only took levetiracetam and phenobarbital as antiepileptic drugs upon discharge from the hospital and became seizure-free. This was the first case in which it was reported that VNS completely controlled RSE [119]. In addition, VNS can completely terminate SE caused by other types of epilepsy, such as autosomal dominant nocturnal frontal lobe epilepsy [120]. O'Neill et al. [121] reported a 23-year-old male patient with primary generalized tonic-clonic epilepsy who received VNS after 3 weeks in SE when drug treatment had failed. On the second day, the patient's EEG showed that generalized epilepsy waves had decreased significantly, and 5 days after the placement of the VNS stimulator, the low-voltage theta electrical activity measured by the EEG had replaced general epileptic discharge. Nine days later, the patient regained consciousness. Although he still had myoclonic seizures at night, seizure frequency was reduced by 75% compared with the situation before VNS stimulation. Zeiler et al. [122] began systematically surveying VNS treatment for RSE cases, and they found that seizure was reduced in 19 patients and with complete freedom from seizure for some of 24 RSE cases with generalized tonic-clonic epilepsy; however, the onset times of termination differed, ranging from 3 days to 14 days. In addition, these patients needed to continue AEDs to maintain the curative effect after seizure termination. Thus far, at least 28 patients with RSE worldwide (7 months–82 years old) have been treated with VNS [123, 124] with good effects; such findings support the conclusion that VNS treatment of SE in adults and children has a known effect, especially in the treatment of RSE with GTCS. The effect of this intervention as an emergency treatment is positive (epilepsy reaction rate, 76%) [122], but for focal RSE, evidence is still lacking. Zeiler et al. [122] used VNS to treat 4 patients with partial RSE, and the average time of seizure termination was 37.5 days later. There were still three patients who experienced seizure recurrence during follow-up.

7.4.1.4 Potential Mechanisms and Existing Problems

The afferent connection of the vagus nerve is the main nucleus of the solitary tract; fibers start from this nucleus to the nuclei of the brain stem. These nuclei regulate the excitability of the cerebral cortex by releasing various neurotransmitters. Therefore, vagus nerve stimulation indirectly controls the excitability of the brain, thereby controlling epilepsy. So far, the improved VNS technique can also perceive tachycardia and heart rate variability by detecting changes in heart rate, and the latter can also be perceived by the VNS monitoring device when seizures or SE occurs. VNS implantation has no influence on MRI scans [125]. VNS treatment still leaves some questions, such as the reason for lagged onset times, the reason why it cannot completely prevent the recurrence of RSE despite effectively terminating it after acute treatment, and the reason why patients need to take AEDs for extended periods of time after seizure termination to prevent recurrence. Because VNS treatment for RSE is still in the clinical trial stage, the data provided are insufficient to persuade and guide clinicians to incorporate vagus nerve surgery into absolute indications for RSE.

7.4.2 CRS

The first instrument that used electrical stimulation to trace the function of the human brain was produced in 1884; brain stimulation used in clinical therapy began in the last century, first used by Heath and Delgado in the field of psychiatry [126]. Among the psychopaths treated, many patients also suffered from epilepsy, so when clinicians used the nerve stimulation system that was placed directly on the brain cortex to treat mental illness, they found that direct stimulation of epileptic lesions could terminate the seizure activity. Subsequent reports also suggested that electrical stimulation in animals and humans could interrupt laboratory and clinical seizures.

This cortical nerve stimulation system includes a pulse generator, epilepsy detection software, and an intracranial electrode which is used to record epileptic lesions and stimulate the brain [127, 128]. The closed-loop focal cortical stimulator was approved for adjuvant treatment of drug-resistant epilepsy in 2013 by the US FDA [128].

Initially, CRS was mainly used in 18-year-old patients with focal epilepsy and fewer than two epileptic foci. However, with advancements in technology, CRS can simultaneously stimulate two separate epileptic foci, even if these two lesions are located in different regions (including functional areas and areas that surgery cannot reach). Because CRS has wide stimulation parameters, the pulse width ranges from 40 to 1000 ms, the frequency ranges from 1 to 333 Hz, and the current ranges from 0.5 to 12 mA; clinicians can choose more stimulation sites and more individualized treatments of epileptic patients with different characteristics [129].

7.4.2.1 Surgical Procedures

At present, the technology works by implanting the instrument in the brain's cortical surface or deeper in patients, near the epileptic foci. The instrument consists of two electrodes with four contacts that are separately implanted subdurally or in the cortex by deep electrodes. When the deep electrodes are implanted and anchored around the epileptic foci, each electrode has four contacts connected to the lesion and uses two electrodes each time to record and stimulate the lesion. The device also has an epilepsy detection function by which it can directly detect seizures in patients. Continuous EEG can record and display epileptic activity over 24 h. When a seizure occurs, transient electrical stimulation will be delivered in a timely manner to the detected site to terminate the seizure. High frequencies (100–200 Hz) and shorter durations (100 ms) are usually used. Although frequent stimulation is delivered to the epileptic site, the overall current intensity remains low [130].

CRS is a personalized surgical treatment requiring that the subdural electrode stripes or deep brain electrodes are implanted near epileptic foci to detect seizures accurately and then turn on the stimulation mode. This means that epileptic foci must be identified prior to electrode implantation. Then, the system analyzes the epileptic signal according to the real-time EEG provided by the implanted electrode, automatically responding and sending the stimulus to the site to terminate the development and spread of epileptiform activity. The stimulating device is placed in the groove of the skull; the device is controlled by a type of electrode bar in the same way as VNS, and the electrode bar is linked to the computer, which sets up its programming. At the same time, due to the limited storage capacity of the device, patients must always connect the electrode bar to the computer to download the electricity needed by the cortical electrodes. Clinicians can also access the patient's cortical EEG records via a secure webpage and test or adjust the stimulus routine regularly based on each patient's specific condition.

7.4.2.2 Clinical Application and Efficacy in Refractory Epilepsy

The responsive neurostimulator system (RNS) is a closed-loop response brain stimulation treatment for epilepsy in CRS. This treatment is currently considered promising for intractable temporal lobe epilepsy. A large sample study of RNS treatment of refractory partial epilepsy confirmed that RNS significantly reduces seizure frequency in patients with refractory partial epilepsy and one or more lesions [128]. This study had achieved level I clinical evidence. However, more evidence is still needed to achieve level I clinical evidence about RNS for the treatment of RSE.

Among recent clinical trials, Bergey et al. [131] reported on the outcome of RNS treatment for 230 patients with refractory partial epilepsy with one or two lesions. The study found that 1 year after RNS, the average seizure percentage declined by 44%, which was 48–66% at the time of long-term follow-up. The seizures of 61% of patients with temporal epileptic foci decreased by 50% after 5 years, and 15% of patients with frontal epileptic foci experienced decreases in seizures of 50% after 5 years. A recent investigation of 795 cases with intractable epilepsy secondary to craniocerebral trauma during 1995–2014 found that the seizure rate declined by 4.5–79.8% after CRS stimulation, but seizure severity improved to a different degree [132].

7.4.2.3 Clinical Application and Efficacy in RSE

Animal experiments have found that CRS may be beneficial for RSE. In kainic acid-induced SE models, SE can be terminated in a timely manner for rats placed in RNS stimulation [133]. At present, CRS has not yet been widely applied to humans with RSE, but there are still some reports showing that CRS in the treatment of drug-resistant SE field has a positive effect. For example, Antonio Valentin et al. [134] reported on two patients with partial SE who received chronic cortical stimulation conducted by subdurally placed electrodes (continuous stimulation frequency 60–130 Hz, current 2–3 mA), resulting in seizures being reduced by 90% during the 22-month postoperative period. The study reported that this was a rare case of focal RSE, with frequent seizures usually affecting distal limb functions that ultimately caused long-lasting limb function damage. The above results suggest that CRS therapy may have a distinct advantage in patients with intractable epilepsy originating from functional cortical areas.

7.4.2.4 Potential Mechanisms

The mechanism of CRS has not yet been fully elucidated. Because cortical electrical stimulation leads to reversible changes of epileptic lesions, thus inhibiting the triggering and spreading of epileptic activity in lesions, this seems to be the mechanism of action [135]. Studies have shown that single-pulse stimulation of the cerebral cortex can cause prolonged cell discharge inhibition [136]. Repetitive stimulation in the correct conjectural frequency range can inhibit cortical electrical activity.

7.4.3 DBS

The history of deep brain stimulation can be traced back to 1940, when a study found that stimulation of the subthalamic nucleus, thalamus, striatum, globus pallidus, and cerebellum could influence seizures [136]. In 1985, deep brain stimulation of the anterior thalamic nucleus was first used in the treatment of comorbid epilepsy and psychiatric disorders [126, 137, 138]. DBS treatment of epilepsy was subsequently extended to Lennox-Gastaut syndrome and multifocal epilepsy, as demonstrated by the progress of a series of animal experiments on DBS treatment of epilepsy [139–141]. Such animal experiments have found that DBS can inhibit SE in animal models by selectively kindling the target of the anterior thalamic nucleus [130].

7.4.3.1 Surgical Indications

DBS is also suitable for intractable epilepsy that cannot be treated by lesion excision (i.e., unclear lesion, diffuse lesion distribution, lesions located in functional areas or in the deep cortex). DBS may be an effective alternative treatment to VNS. As new "unconventional" brain stereotactic targets are identified and used, the flexibility and expected results of DBS may be better than VNS [117].

7.4.3.2 Surgical Procedures

Positioning by MRI is needed before the DBS operation. Usually, four deep intracranial electrodes are implanted into the bilateral anterior thalamus under MRI location guidance (in the subthalamic nucleus or the posterior hypothalamus [pHyp] and caudal zona incerta [CZi] [136, 138]). Implanted electrodes link to an implantable pulse generator (IPG); this IPG is placed below the clavicle (and possibly implanted subcutaneously). The electrical stimulation program for setting up the IPG is similar to that for VNS: the stimulus frequency used in IPG is characterized by high-frequency stimulation (130–200 Hz), a pulse width of 90–450 Hz, and a voltage of 5–10 V. The set stimulus time is 1 min of stimulation followed by 1 min of intermittent stimulation and 5 min in a powered-off state. The stimulator is powered by the battery (a non-rechargeable battery with four typical settings that needs to be replaced every 6 years versus a rechargeable battery that needs to be replaced every 9–20 years) [142].

7.4.3.3 Clinical Application and Efficacy in Refractory Epilepsy

Deep brain stimulation, especially high-frequency stimulation (HFS), is another promising treatment modality for intractable epilepsy. In a randomized, placebo-controlled, multicenter trial of 110 patients with refractory partial epilepsy or secondarily generalized epilepsy, Fisher [142] and his colleagues found that after administering DBS on the anterior thalamic nucleus, the seizure frequency of patients was reduced to 40.5% of the average preoperative baseline level and to 58% 3 years after surgery.

Salanova et al. [143] followed up with patients aged 18–65 years with partial epilepsy or secondary generalized refractory epilepsy who had been treated with DBS. Their seizure frequencies decreased by 43% 1 year following surgery and by nearly 68% 5 years after DBS. The total seizure rate reduced to 50% 1 year after DBS in the 44% of patients who had temporal epileptic foci and to 76% 5 years later across all patients; the total seizure rate reduced to 50% 1 year after DBS in the 53% of patients who had frontal epileptic foci and to 59% 5 years later across all patients.

7.4.3.4 Clinical Application and Efficacy in RSE

DBS has a promising future in the treatment of RSE, and there are many successful cases in the clinical treatment of RSE. Angelo Franzini et al. [138] successfully controlled SE caused by Rasmussen encephalitis by DBS stimulation. In another case, after a clinician implanted a DBS electrode in the bilateral thalamic centromedial nucleus and applied stimulation, one patient with RSE secondary to encephalitis experienced the timely termination of GTCS and periodic epileptiform waves after 5 weeks. After the patient had no SE for at least 2 months, thalamic centromedial nuclear DBS treatment was confirmed to be an effective method for RSE [145]. Franzini A et al. also performed DBS operations for four epileptics (including two patients with SE secondary to refractory partial epilepsy), with surgical sites in the pHyp and the CZI; after deep brain stimulation, seizure frequency decreased by 70% in the patients with refractory focal epilepsy, whereas another patient with SE secondary to partial epilepsy achieved obvious relief [138].

7.4.3.5 Potential Mechanisms

The mechanism of DBS treatment of epilepsy may be related to the following factors: (1) The seizure threshold may be improved by affecting the epilepsy network. Considering the close connections between the ATN and the limbic structure, the ATN seems to be the ideal stimulus target in DBS. In animal models, stimulation of the ATN is actually a pre-convulsion stimulation [146]. This stimulation in epilepsy animal models can extend the interval before seizures develop into SE [130]. Therefore, it may play a particular role in the treatment of SE and RSE. In addition, in a hippocampal stimulation model, researchers found that high-frequency stimulation was more effective in suppressing seizures than low-frequency stimulation [147, 148]. (2) Stimulating brain structures cause interactions with the reticular-thalamic-cortical pathway (while considering how the reticular-thalamic-cortical system contains the diencephalon and mesencephalon, two structures that regularize the excitability of the cortex to varying degrees); therefore, DBS may play a role against SE through the stimulation of "interfering" brain cortical neuronal activity and synchronized discharge [149].

7.4.4 Adverse Reactions and Complications of the Neuromodulatory Treatment of Refractory Epilepsy

7.4.4.1 Infection

Infection is the common adverse complication of all surgeries: the postoperative infection rates are approximately 3.3% for VNS, 9.4% for CRS, and 0–15% for DBS [118, 150]. The infection incidence is related to the surgical wound area and surgical depth.

7.4.4.2 Nerve Injuries and Other Complications

VNS surgery may cause carotid artery or laryngeal nerve injury during the operation, unbearable chronic hoarseness, chronic vocal cord paralysis, simple hoarseness (especially upon stimulation), cough, different degrees of vagus nerve injury, throat discomfort, voice change, or transient vocal cord paralysis [151]. Studies of patients undergoing VNS surgery have found that in short-term post-VNS, there are positive effects on the reconstruction of cognitive and memory impairments induced by epilepsy; however, there are no data showing support for long-term memory recovery and reconstruction [152]. Moreover, patients still risk death (even sudden death) for a variety of reasons after surgery, thereby explaining the VNS mortality rate of 3.9% [153, 154].

CRS surgery may cause intracranial hemorrhage, skin erosion, depression, suicidal tendencies, and increased risk of seizures. Nerve stimulator implantation needs to accurately determine the localization of the seizure-onset zone. It is often necessary to carry out intracranial EEG recording early, and intracranial EEG recording and device implantation are also directly related to the need for postoperative skull reconstruction [155, 156]. RNS does not resolve all generalized epilepsy. MRI scans cannot be carried out after implanting this type of device. Some heat therapy for the brain is also contraindicated. RNS in CRS has shown no serious or unanticipated adverse events in clinical trials; nevertheless, in severe adverse reactions, the mortality of CRS is 4.3%, and the incidence of sudden unexpected death in epilepsy (SUDEP) is approximately 2.7% [156].

DBS surgery may cause intracranial hemorrhage, infection of the leads, superficial infection, or lead breakage. Different target stimulation sites cause different complications: for example, subthalamic nucleus (STN) stimulation may lead to behavior changes, verbal memory [157, 158] and executive dysfunction [159], depression [160], or abnormal feelings in the chest or other parts of the body. Some patients may develop SE, which may be mainly related to implantation procedures and hardware—for example, the stimulation site may experience paresthesia or infection, which may also be related to a high stimulating voltage [144]. The mortality of DBS in severe adverse reactions is 6.4%, and the incidence of SUDEP is approximately 3.6% [142, 161].

7.4.5 Other Emerging Therapies for Drug-Resistant Epilepsy and SE

In addition to the traditional surgeries and neuromodulatory surgeries listed above, emerging surgical treatments for drug-resistant epilepsy and SE currently include heart-reactive vagus nerve stimulation, trigeminal nerve stimulation, magnetic resonance-guided stereotactic laser ablation, and modified electroconvulsive therapy, among others. However, relevant evidence of the efficacy for these techniques is still lacking.

References

1. Hippocrates De Vetere Medicina. Harvard University Press, Loeb Classical Library:460–375 BC:461–432.
2. Gunn AJ, Laptook AR, Robertson NJ, Barks JD, Thoresen M, Wassink G, Bennet L. Therapeutic hypothermia translates from ancient history in to practice. Pediatr Res. 2017;81(1–2):202–9.
3. Westin B, Miller JA Jr, Nyberg R, Wedenberg E. Neonatal asphyxia pallida treated with hypothermia alone or with hypothermia and transfusion of oxygenated blood. Surgery. 1959;45(5):868–79.

4. Ommaya AK, Baldwin M. Extravascular local cooling of the brain in man. J Neurosurg. 1963;20:8–20.
5. Vastola EF, Homan R, Rosen A. Inhibition of focal seizures by moderate hypothermia. A clinical and experimental study. Arch Neurol. 1969;20(4):430–9.
6. Sourek K, Travnicek V. General and local hypothermia of the brain in the treatment of intractable epilepsy. J Neurosurg. 1970;33(3):253–9.
7. Orlowski JP, Erenberg G, Lueders H, Cruse RP. Hypothermia and barbiturate coma for refractory status epilepticus. Crit Care Med. 1984;12(4):367–72.
8. Corry JJ, Dhar R, Murphy T, Diringer MN. Hypothermia for refractory status epilepticus. Neurocrit Care. 2008;9(2):189–97.
9. Legriel S, Lemiale V, Schenck M, Chelly J, Laurent V, Daviaud F, Srairi M, Hamdi A, Geri G, Rossignol T, et al. Hypothermia for neuroprotection in convulsive status epilepticus. N Engl J Med. 2016;375(25):2457–67.
10. Elting JW, Naalt J, Fock JM. Mild hypothermia for refractory focal status epilepticus in an infant with hemimegalencephaly. Eur J Paediatr Neurol. 2010;14(5):452–5.
11. Guilliams K, Rosen M, Buttram S, Zempel J, Pineda J, Miller B, Shoykhet M. Hypothermia for pediatric refractory status epilepticus. Epilepsia. 2013;54(9):1586–94.
12. Lin JJ, Lin KL, Hsia SH, Wang HS, Group CS. Therapeutic hypothermia for febrile infection-related epilepsy syndrome in two patients. Pediatr Neurol. 2012;47(6):448–50.
13. Rossetti AO. What is the value of hypothermia in acute neurologic diseases and status epilepticus? Epilepsia. 2011;52(Suppl 8):64–6.
14. Holzer M. Targeted temperature management for comatose survivors of cardiac arrest. N Engl J Med. 2010;363(13):1256–64.
15. Cereda C, Berger MM, Rossetti AO. Bowel ischemia: a rare complication of thiopental treatment for status epilepticus. Neurocrit Care. 2009;10(3):355–8.
16. Rothman SM. The therapeutic potential of focal cooling for neocortical epilepsy. Neurotherapeutics. 2009;6(2):251–7.
17. Fujii M, Inoue T, Nomura S, Maruta Y, He Y, Koizumi H, Shirao S, Owada Y, Kunitsugu I, Yamakawa T, et al. Cooling of the epileptic focus suppresses seizures with minimal influence on neurologic functions. Epilepsia. 2012;53(3):485–93.
18. Volgushev M, Kudryashov I, Chistiakova M, Mukovski M, Niesmann J, Eysel UT. Probability of transmitter release at neocortical synapses at different temperatures. J Neurophysiol. 2004;92(1):212–20.
19. Wassink G, Gunn ER, Drury PP, Bennet L, Gunn AJ. The mechanisms and treatment of asphyxial encephalopathy. Front Neurosci. 2014;8:40.
20. Nakashima K, Todd MM, Warner DS. The relation between cerebral metabolic rate and ischemic depolarization. A comparison of the effects of hypothermia, pentobarbital, and isoflurane. Anesthesiology. 1995;82(5):1199–208.
21. Motamedi GK, Salazar P, Smith EL, Lesser RP, Webber WR, Ortinski PI, Vicini S, Rogawski MA. Termination of epileptiform activity by cooling in rat hippocampal slice epilepsy models. Epilepsy Res. 2006;70(2–3):200–10.
22. Hill MW, Wong M, Amarakone A, Rothman SM. Rapid cooling aborts seizure-like activity in rodent hippocampal-entorhinal slices. Epilepsia. 2000;41(10):1241–8.
23. Motamedi GK, Gonzalez-Sulser A, Dzakpasu R, Vicini S. Cellular mechanisms of desynchronizing effects of hypothermia in an in vitro epilepsy model. Neurotherapeutics. 2012;9(1):199–209.
24. Yu L, Zhou Y, Wang Y. Effect of mild hypothermia on glutamate receptor expression after status epilepticus. Epilepsy Res. 2012;101(1–2):56–69.
25. Aird RB, Tsubaki T. Common sources of error in the diagnosis and treatment of convulsive disorders: a review of 204 patients with temporal lobe epilepsy. J Nerv Ment Dis. 1958;127(5):400–6.
26. Capovilla G, Beccaria F, Beghi E, Minicucci F, Sartori S, Vecchi M. Treatment of convulsive status epilepticus in childhood: recommendations of the Italian League against epilepsy. Epilepsia. 2013;54(Suppl 7):23–34.
27. Viparelli U, Viparelli G. ECT and grand mal epilepsy. Convuls Ther. 1992;8(1):39–42.
28. Vigevano F, Cilio MR. Vigabatrin versus ACTH as first-line treatment for infantile spasms: a randomized, prospective study. Epilepsia. 1997;38(12):1270–4.
29. Zeiler FA, Matuszczak M, Teitelbaum J, Gillman LM, Kazina CJ. Electroconvulsive therapy for refractory status epilepticus: a systematic review. Seizure. 2016;35:23–32.
30. Lambrecq V, Villega F, Marchal C, Michel V, Guehl D, Rotge JY, Burbaud P. Refractory status epilepticus: electroconvulsive therapy as a possible therapeutic strategy. Seizure. 2012;21(9):661–4.
31. Regenold WT, Weintraub D, Taller A. Electroconvulsive therapy for epilepsy and major depression. Am J Geriatr Psychiatry. 1998;6(2):| 180–3.
32. Kucia KA, Stepanczak R, Tredzbor B. Electroconvulsive therapy for major depression in an elderly person with epilepsy. World J Biol Psychiatry. 2009;10(1):78–80.
33. Griesemer DA, Kellner CH, Beale MD, Smith GM. Electroconvulsive therapy for treatment of intractable seizures. Initial findings in two children. Neurology. 1997;49(5):1389–92.
34. Lisanby SH, Bazil CW, Resor SR, Nobler MS, Finck DA, Sackeim HA. ECT in the treatment of status epilepticus. J ECT. 2001;17(3):210–5.
35. Cline JS, Roos K. Treatment of status epilepticus with electroconvulsive therapy. J ECT. 2007;23(1):30–2.
36. Koong FJ, Chen WC. Maintaining electroconvulsive therapy for refractory epilepsy combined with psychotic symptoms. BMJ Case Rep. 2010;2010.
37. Kamel H, Cornes SB, Hegde M, Hall SE, Josephson SA. Electroconvulsive therapy for refractory

status epilepticus: a case series. Neurocrit Care. 2010;12(2):204–10.
38. Shin HW, O'Donovan CA, Boggs JG, Grefe A, Harper A, Bell WL, McCall WV, Rosenquist P. Successful ECT treatment for medically refractory nonconvulsive status epilepticus in pediatric patient. Seizure. 2011;20(5):433–6.
39. Carrasco Gonzalez MD, Palomar M, Rovira R. Electroconvulsive therapy for status epilepticus. Ann Intern Med. 1997;127(3):247–8.
40. Wusthoff CJ, Kranick SM, Morley JF, Christina Bergqvist AG. The ketogenic diet in treatment of two adults with prolonged nonconvulsive status epilepticus. Epilepsia. 2010;51(6):1083–5.
41. Trevino K, McClintock SM, Husain MM. A review of continuation electroconvulsive therapy: application, safety, and efficacy. J ECT. 2010;26(3):186–95.
42. Brodaty H, Berle D, Hickie I, Mason C. "Side effects" of ECT are mainly depressive phenomena and are independent of age. J Affect Disord. 2001;66(2–3):237–45.
43. Stoppe A, Louza M, Rosa M, Gil G, Rigonatti S. Fixed high-dose electroconvulsive therapy in the elderly with depression: a double-blind, randomized comparison of efficacy and tolerability between unilateral and bilateral electrode placement. J ECT. 2006;22(2):92–9.
44. Sackeim H, Decina P, Prohovnik I, Malitz S. Seizure threshold in electroconvulsive therapy. Effects of sex, age, electrode placement, and number of treatments. Arch Gen Psychiatry. 1987;44(4):355–60.
45. Khalilov I, Holmes GL, Ben-Ari Y. In vitro formation of a secondary epileptogenic mirror focus by interhippocampal propagation of seizures. Nat Neurosci. 2003;6(10):1079–85.
46. Sackeim HA, Decina P, Prohovnik I, Malitz S, Resor SR. Anticonvulsant and antidepressant properties of electroconvulsive therapy: a proposed mechanism of action. Biol Psychiatry. 1983;18(11):1301–10.
47. Clark M. Sensitivity of the rat hippocampal GABA(A) receptor alpha 4 subunit to electroshock seizures. Neurosci Lett. 1998;250(1):17–20.
48. Esel E, Kose K, Hacimusalar Y, Ozsoy S, Kula M, Candan Z, Turan T. The effects of electroconvulsive therapy on GABAergic function in major depressive patients. J ECT. 2008;24(3):224–8.
49. Yoshitake T, Reenila I, Ogren SO, Hokfelt T, Kehr J. Galanin attenuates basal and antidepressant drug-induced increase of extracellular serotonin and noradrenaline levels in the rat hippocampus. Neurosci Lett. 2003;339(3):239–42.
50. Christiansen SH, Woldbye DP. Regulation of the galanin system by repeated electroconvulsive seizures in mice. J Neurosci Res. 2010;88(16):3635–43.
51. Wheless JW. History of the ketogenic diet. Epilepsia. 2008;49(Suppl 8):3–5.
52. Wilder RM. The effect on ketonemia on the course of epilepsy. Mayo Clin Bull. 1921;2:307–8.
53. Lord K, Magrath G. Use of the ketogenic diet and dietary practices in the UK. J Hum Nutr Diet. 2010;23(2):126–32.
54. Kossoff EH, Zupec-Kania BA, Amark PE, et al. Optimal clinical management of children receiving the ketogenic diet: recommendations of the International Ketogenic Diet Study Group. Epilepsia. 2009;50(2):304–17.
55. National Clinical Guideline Centre, National Institute for Health and Clinical Excellence: Guidance. In: The epilepsies: the diagnosis and management of the epilepsies in adults and children in primary and secondary care: pharmacological update of Clinical Guideline 20. London: Royal College of Physicians; 2012.
56. Kossoff EH, Al-Macki N, Cervenka MC, et al. What are the minimum requirements for ketogenic diet services in resource-limited regions? Recommendations from the International League Against Epilepsy Task Force for Dietary Therapy. Epilepsia. 2015;56(9):1337–42.
57. Ferlisi M, Shorvon S. The outcome of therapies in refractory and super-refractory convulsive status epilepticus and recommendations for therapy. Brain. 2012;135(Pt 8):2314–28.
58. Shorvon S. Super-refractory status epilepticus: an approach to therapy in this difficult clinical situation. Epilepsia. 2011;52(Suppl 8):53–6.
59. Klein P, Tyrlikova I, Mathews GC, et al. Dietary treatment in adults with refractory epilepsy: a review. Neurology. 2014;83(21):1978–85.
60. Caraballo RH, Valenzuela GR, Armeno M, et al. The ketogenic diet in two paediatric patients with refractory myoclonic status epilepticus. Epileptic Disord. 2015;17(4):491–5.
61. Caraballo RH, Flesler S, Armeno M, et al. Ketogenic diet in pediatric patients with refractory focal status epilepticus. Epilepsy Res. 2014;108(10):1912–6.
62. Lin JJ, Lin KL, Chan OW, et al. Intravenous ketogenic diet therapy for treatment of the acute stage of super-refractory status epilepticus in a pediatric patient. Pediatr Neurol. 2015;52(4):442–5.
63. Thakur KT, Probasco JC, Hocker SE, et al. Ketogenic diet for adults in super-refractory status epilepticus. Neurology. 2014;82(8):665–70.
64. Wusthoff CJ, Kranick SM, Morley JF, et al. The ketogenic diet in treatment of two adults with prolonged nonconvulsive status epilepticus. Epilepsia. 2010;51(6):1083–5.
65. Strzelczyk A, Reif PS, Bauer S, et al. Intravenous initiation and maintenance of ketogenic diet: proof of concept in super-refractory status epilepticus. Seizure. 2013;22(7):581–3.
66. Nabbout R, Mazzuca M, Hubert P, et al. Efficacy of ketogenic diet in severe refractory status epilepticus initiating fever induced refractory epileptic encephalopathy in school age children (FIRES). Epilepsia. 2010;51(10):2033–7.
67. Nam SH, Lee BL, Lee CG, et al. The role of ketogenic diet in the treatment of refractory status epilepticus. Epilepsia. 2011;52(11):e181–4.

68. Cervenka MC, Hartman AL, Venkatesan A, et al. The ketogenic diet for medically and surgically refractory status epilepticus in the neurocritical care unit. Neurocrit Care. 2011;15(3):519–24.
69. Vaccarezza M, Silva W, Maxit C, et al. Super-refractory status epilepticus: treatment with ketogenic diet in pediatrics. Rev Neurol. 2012;55(1):20–5.
70. Bodenant M, Moreau C, Sejourné C, et al. Interest of the ketogenic diet in a refractory status epilepticus in adults. Rev Neurol (Paris). 2008;164(2):194–9.
71. Kossoff EH, Nabbout R. Use of dietary therapy for status epilepticus. J Child Neurol. 2013;28(8):1049–51.
72. Sort R, Born AP, Pedersen KN, et al. Ketogenic diet in 3 cases of childhood refractory status epilepticus. Eur J Paediatr Neurol. 2013;17(6):531–6.
73. Al-Mudallal AS, LaManna JC, Lust WD, et al. Diet-induced ketosis does not cause cerebral acidosis. Epilepsia. 1996;37(3):258–61.
74. Alberti MJ, Agustinho A, Argumedo L, et al. Recommendations for the clinical management of children with refractory epilepsy receiving the ketogenic diet. Arch Argent Pediatr. 2016;114(1):56–63.
75. Cervenka MC, Henry BJ, Felton EA, et al. Establishing an adult epilepsy diet center: experience, efficacy and challenges. Epilepsy Behav. 2016;58:61–8.
76. Ye F, Li XJ, Jiang WL, et al. Efficacy of and patient compliance with a ketogenic diet in adults with intractable epilepsy: a meta-analysis. J Clin Neurol. 2015;11(1):26–31.
77. Zamani GR, Mohammadi M, Ashrafi MR, et al. The effects of classic ketogenic diet on serum lipid profile in children with refractory seizures. Acta Neurol Belg. 2016;116(4):529–34.
78. Kwiterovich PO Jr, Vining EP, Pyzik P, et al. Effect of a high-fat ketogenic diet on plasma levels of lipids, lipoproteins, and apolipoproteins in children. JAMA. 2003;290(7):912–20.
79. Coppola G, Natale F, Torino A, et al. The impact of the ketogenic diet on arterial morphology and endothelial function in children and young adults with epilepsy: a case-control study. Seizure. 2014;23(4):260–5.
80. Lambrechts DA, de Kinderen RJ, Vles HS, et al. The MCT-ketogenic diet as a treatment option in refractory childhood epilepsy: a prospective study with 2-year follow-up. Epilepsy Behav. 2015;51:261–6.
81. Moriyama K, Watanabe M, Yamada Y, et al. Protein-losing enteropathy as a rare complication of the ketogenic diet. Pediatr Neurol. 2015;52:526–8.
82. Baumeister FA, Oberhoffer R, Liebhaber GM, et al. Fatal propofol infusion syndrome in association with ketogenic diet. Neuropediatrics. 2004;35:250–2.
83. Nei M, Ngo L, Sirven JI, et al. Ketogenic diet in adolescents and adults with epilepsy. Seizure. 2014;23:439–42.
84. Smith M, Politzer N, Macgarvie D, et al. Efficacy and tolerability of the modified Atkins diet in adults with pharmacoresistant epilepsy: a prospective observational study. Epilepsia. 2011;52:775–80.
85. Mady MA, Kossoff EH, McGregor AL, et al. The ketogenic diet: adolescents can do it, too. Epilepsia. 2003;44(6):847–51.
86. Sampath A, Kossoff EH, Furth SL, et al. Kidney stones and the ketogenic diet: risk factors and prevention. J Child Neurol. 2007;22(4):375–8.
87. Bough KJ, Rho JM. Anticonvulsant mechanisms of the ketogenic diet. Epilepsia. 2007;48(1):43–58.
88. Melo TM, Nehlig A, Sonnewald U. Neuronal-glial interactions in rats fed a ketogenic diet. Neurochem Int. 2006;48:498–507.
89. Keith HM. Factors influencing experimentally produced convulsions. Arch Neurol Psychiatr. 1933;29:148–54.
90. Likhodii SS, Serbanescu I, Cortez MA, et al. Anticonvulsant properties of acetone, a brain ketone elevated by the ketogenic diet. Ann Neurol. 2003;54(2):219–26.
91. Gasior M, French A, Joy MT, et al. The anticonvulsant activity of acetone, the major ketone body in the ketogenic diet, is not dependent on its metabolites acetol, 1,2-propanediol, methylglyoxal, or pyruvic acid. Epilepsia. 2007;48:793–800.
92. Rho JM, Anderson GD, Donevan SD, et al. Acetoacetate, acetone, and dibenzylamine (a contaminant in L-(+)-b-Hydroxybutyrate) exhibit direct anticonvulsant actions in vivo. Epilepsia. 2002;43(4):358–61.
93. Nylen K, Likhodii SS, Hum KM, et al. A ketogenic diet and diallyl sulfide do not elevate after discharge thresholds in adult kindled rats. Epilepsy Res. 2006;71:23–31.
94. Bough KJ, Gudi K, Han FT, et al. An anticonvulsant profile of the ketogenic diet in the rat. Epilepsy Res. 2002;50(3):313–25.
95. Dahlin M, Elfving A, Ungerstedt U, et al. The ketogenic diet influences the levels of excitatory and inhibitory amino acids in the CSF in children with refractory epilepsy. Epilepsy Res. 2005;64: 115–25.
96. Wang ZJ, Bergqvist C, Hunter JV, et al. In vivo measurement of brain metabolites using two-dimensional double-quantum MR spectroscopy--exploration of GABA levels in a ketogenic diet. Magn Reson Med. 2003;49:615–9.
97. Cheng CM, Hicks K, Wang J, et al. Caloric restriction augments brain glutamic acid decarboxylase-65 and -67 expression. J Neurosci Res. 2004;77:270–6.
98. Yudkoff M, Daikhin Y, Nissim I, et al. Response of brain amino acid metabolism to ketosis. Neurochem Int. 2005;47(1–2):119–28.
99. Yudkoff M, Daikhin Y, Horyn O, et al. Ketosis and brain handling of glutamate, glutamine, and GABA. Epilepsia. 2008;49(Suppl 8):73–5.
100. Lutas A, Yellen G. The ketogenic diet: metabolic influences on brain excitability and epilepsy. Trends Neurosci. 2013;36(1):32–40.
101. Ma W, Berg J, Yellen G. Ketogenic diet metabolites reduce firing in central neurons by opening K(ATP) channels. J Neurosci. 2007;27(14):3618–25.
102. Stafstrom CE, Ockuly JC, Murphree L, et al. Anticonvulsant and antiepileptic actions of 2-deoxy-D-glucose in epilepsy models. Ann Neurol. 2009;65(4):435–47.

103. Garriga-Canut M, Schoenike B, Qazi R, et al. 2-Deoxy-D-glucose reduces epilepsy progression by NRSF-CtBP-dependent metabolic regulation of chromatin structure. Nat Neurosci. 2006;9:1382–7.
104. Chang P, Terbach N, Plant N, et al. Seizure control by ketogenic diet-associated medium chain fatty acids. Neuropharmacology. 2013;69:105–14.
105. Chang P, Augustin K, Boddum K, et al. Seizure control by decanoic acid through direct AMPA receptor inhibition. Brain. 2016;139:431–43.
106. Schlanger S, Shinitzky M, Yam D. Diet enriched with omega-3 fatty acids alleviates convulsion symptoms in epilepsy patients. Epilepsia. 2002;43:103–4.
107. Xiao Y, Li X. Polyunsaturated fatty acids modify mouse hippocampal neuronal excitability during excitotoxic or convulsant stimulation. Brain Res. 1999;846:112–21.
108. Yazdi S, Stein M, Elinder F, et al. The molecular basis of polyunsaturated fatty acid interactions with the shaker voltage gated potassium channel. PLoS Comput Biol. 2016;12:e1004704.
109. Ben-Menachem E, Manon-Espaillat R, Ristanovic R, Wilder BJ, Stefan H, Mirza W, Tarver WB, Wernicke JF. Vagus nerve stimulation for treatment of partial seizures: 1. A controlled study of effect on seizures. First International Vagus Nerve Stimulation Study Group. Epilepsia. 1994;35:616–26.
110. Handforth A, DeGiorgio CM, Schachter SC, Uthman BM, Naritoku DK, Tecoma ES, Henry TR, Collins SD, Vaughn BV, Gilmartin RC, Labar DR, Morris GL III, Salinsky MC, Osorio I, Ristanovic RK, Labiner DM, Jones JC, Murphy JV, Ney GC, Wheless JW. Vagus nerve stimulation therapy for partial-onset seizures: a randomized active-control trial. Neurology. 1998;51:48–55.
111. Gooneratne IK, Green AL, Dugan P, Sen A, Franzini A, Aziz T, Cheeran B. Comparing neurostimulation technologies in refractory focal-onset epilepsy. J Neurol Neurosurg Psychiatry. 2016;87:1174–82.
112. Heck C, Helmers SL, DeGiorgio CM. Vagus nerve stimulation therapy, epilepsy, and device parameters: scientific basis and recommendations for use. Neurology. 2002;59:S31–7.
113. Amar AP, Apuzzo ML, Liu CY. Vagus nerve stimulation therapy after failed cranial surgery for intractable epilepsy: results from the vagus nerve stimulation therapy patient outcome registry. Neurosurgery. 2004;55:1086–93.
114. DeGiorgio CM, Schachter SC, Handforth A, Salinsky M, Thompson J, Uthman B, Reed R, Collins S, Tecoma E, Morris GL, Vaughn B, Naritoku DK, Henry T, Labar D, Gilmartin R, Labiner D, Osorio I, Ristanovic R, Jones J, Murphy J, Ney G, Wheless J, Lewis P, Heck C. Prospective long-term study of vagus nerve stimulation for the treatment of refractory seizures. Epilepsia. 2000;41:1195–200.
115. Ghaemi K, Elsharkawy AE, Schulz R, Hoppe M, Polster T, Pannek H, Ebner A. Vagus nerve stimulation: outcome and predictors of seizure freedom in long-term follow-up. Seizure. 2010;19:264–8.
116. Vonck K, Raedt R, Naulaerts J, De Vogelaere F, Thiery E, Van Roost D, Aldenkamp B, Miatton M, Boon P. Vagus nerve stimulation…25 years later! What do we know about the effects on cognition? Neurosci Biobehav Rev. 2014;45:63–71.
117. De Herdt V, Boon P, Ceulemans B, Hauman H, Lagae L, Legros B, Sadzot B, Van Bogaert P, van Rijckevorsel K, Verhelst H, Vonck K. Vagus nerve stimulation for refractory epilepsy: a Belgian multicenter study. Eur J Paediatr Neurol. 2007;11:261–9.
118. Kuba R, Brazdil M, Kalina M, Prochazka T, Hovorka J, Nezadal T, Hadac J, Brozova K, Sebronova V, Komarek V, Marusic P, Oslejskova H, Zarubova J, Rektor I. Vagus nerve stimulation: longitudinal follow-up of patients treated for 5 years. Seizure. 2009;18:269–74.
119. Patwardhan RV, Dellabadia J Jr, Rashidi M, Grier L, Nanda A. Control of refractory status epilepticus precipitated by anticonvulsant withdrawal using left vagal nerve stimulation: a case report. Surg Neurol. 2005;64:170–3.
120. Carreno M, Garcia-Alvarez D, Maestro I, Fernandez S, Donaire A, Boget T, Rumia J, Pintor L, Setoain X. Malignant autosomal dominant frontal lobe epilepsy with repeated episodes of status epilepticus: successful treatment with vagal nerve stimulation. Epileptic Disord. 2010;12:155–8.
121. O'Neill BR, Valeriano J, Synowiec A, Thielmann D, Lane C, Wilberger J. Refractory status epilepticus treated with vagal nerve stimulation: case report. Neurosurgery. 2011;69:E1172–5.
122. Zeiler FA, Zeiler KJ, Teitelbaum J, Gillman LM, West M. VNS for refractory status epilepticus. Epilepsy Res. 2015;112:100–13.
123. Winston KR, Levisohn P, Miller BR, Freeman J. Vagal nerve stimulation for status epilepticus. Pediatr Neurosurg. 2001;34:190–2.
124. Bayrlee A, Ganeshalingam N, Kurczewski L, Brophy GM. Treatment of super-refractory status epilepticus. Curr Neurol Neurosci Rep. 2015;15:66.
125. Boon P, Raedt R, de Herdt V, Wyckhuys T, Vonck K. Electrical stimulation for the treatment of epilepsy. Neurotherapeutics. 2009;6:218–27.
126. Delgado JM, Hamlin H, Chapman WP. Technique of intracranial electrode implacement for recording and stimulation and its possible therapeutic value in psychotic patients. Confin Neurol. 1952;12:315–9.
127. Skarpaas TL, Morrell MJ. Intracranial stimulation therapy for epilepsy. Neurotherapeutics. 2009;6:238–43.
128. Morrell MJ. Responsive cortical stimulation for the treatment of medically intractable partial epilepsy. Neurology. 2011;77:1295–304.
129. Ben-Menachem E. Neurostimulation-past, present, and beyond. Epilepsy Curr. 2012;12:188–91.
130. Hamani C, Hodaie M, Chiang J, del Campo M, Andrade DM, Sherman D, Mirski M, Mello LE, Lozano AM. Deep brain stimulation of the anterior nucleus of the thalamus: effects of electrical stimulation on pilocarpine-induced seizures and status epilepticus. Epilepsy Res. 2008;78:117–23.

131. Bergey GK, Morrell MJ, Mizrahi EM, Goldman A, King-Stephens D, Nair D, Srinivasan S, Jobst B, Gross RE, Shields DC, Barkley G, Salanova V, Olejniczak P, Cole A, Cash SS, Noe K, Wharen R, Worrell G, Murro AM, Edwards J, Duchowny M, Spencer D, Smith M, Geller E, Gwinn R, Skidmore C, Eisenschenk S, Berg M, Heck C, Van Ness P, Fountain N, Rutecki P, Massey A, O'Donovan C, Labar D, Duckrow RB, Hirsch LJ, Courtney T, Sun FT, Seale CG. Long-term treatment with responsive brain stimulation in adults with refractory partial seizures. Neurology. 2015;84:810–7.
132. Larkin M, Meyer RM, Szuflita NS, Severson MA, Levine ZT. Post-traumatic, drug-resistant epilepsy and review of seizure control outcomes from blinded, randomized controlled trials of brain stimulation treatments for drug-resistant epilepsy. Cureus. 2016;8:e744.
133. Huang L, van Luijtelaar G. The effects of responsive and scheduled subicular high frequency stimulation in the intra-hippocampal kainic acid seizure model. Epilepsy Res. 2013;106(3):326–37.
134. Valentin A, Ughratdar I, Cheserem B, Morris R, Selway R, Alarcon G. Epilepsia partialis continua responsive to neocortical electrical stimulation. Epilepsia. 2015;56:e104–9.
135. Alarcon G, Martinez J, Kerai SV, Lacruz ME, Quiroga RQ, Selway RP, Richardson MP, Garcia Seoane JJ, Valentin A. In vivo neuronal firing patterns during human epileptiform discharges replicated by electrical stimulation. Clin Neurophysiol. 2012;123:1736–44.
136. Chabardes S, Kahane P, Minotti L, Koudsie A, Hirsch E, Benabid AL. Deep brain stimulation in epilepsy with particular reference to the subthalamic nucleus. Epileptic Disord. 2002;4(Suppl 3):S83–93.
137. Cooper IS, Upton AR. Therapeutic implications of modulation of metabolism and functional activity of cerebral cortex by chronic stimulation of cerebellum and thalamus. Biol Psychiatry. 1985;20:811–3.
138. Franzini A, Messina G, Marras C, Villani F, Cordella R, Broggi G. Deep brain stimulation of two unconventional targets in refractory non-resectable epilepsy. Stereotact Funct Neurosurg. 2008;86:373–81.
139. Upton AR, Cooper IS, Springman M, Amin I. Suppression of seizures and psychosis of limbic system origin by chronic stimulation of anterior nucleus of the thalamus. Int J Neurol. 1985;19-20:223–30.
140. Velasco F, Velasco M, Ogarrio C, Fanghanel G. Electrical stimulation of the centromedian thalamic nucleus in the treatment of convulsive seizures: a preliminary report. Epilepsia. 1987;28:421–30.
141. Graber KD, Fisher RS. Deep brain stimulation for epilepsy: animal models. Bethesda, MD: National Center for Biotechnology Information; 2012.
142. Fisher R, Salanova V, Witt T, Worth R, Henry T, Gross R, Oommen K, Osorio I, Nazzaro J, Labar D, Kaplitt M, Sperling M, Sandok E, Neal J, Handforth A, Stern J, DeSalles A, Chung S, Shetter A, Bergen D, Bakay R, Henderson J, French J, Baltuch G, Rosenfeld W, Youkilis A, Marks W, Garcia P, Barbaro N, Fountain N, Bazil C, Goodman R, McKhann G, Babu Krishnamurthy K, Papavassiliou S, Epstein C, Pollard J, Tonder L, Grebin J, Coffey R, Graves N. Electrical stimulation of the anterior nucleus of thalamus for treatment of refractory epilepsy. Epilepsia. 2010;51:899–908.
143. Salanova V, Witt T, Worth R, Henry TR, Gross RE, Nazzaro JM, Labar D, Sperling MR, Sharan A, Sandok E, Handforth A, Stern JM, Chung S, Henderson JM, French J, Baltuch G. Long-term efficacy and safety of thalamic stimulation for drug-resistant partial epilepsy. Neurology. 2015;84(10):1017–25.
144. Fisher RS, Velasco AL. Electrical brain stimulation for epilepsy. Nat Rev Neurol. 2014;10:261–70.
145. Valentin A, Nguyen HQ, Skupenova AM, Agirre-Arrizubieta Z, Jewell S, Mullatti N, Moran NF, Richardson MP, Selway RP, Alarcon G. Centromedian thalamic nuclei deep brain stimulation in refractory status epilepticus. Brain Stimul. 2012;5:594–8.
146. Lado FA. Chronic bilateral stimulation of the anterior thalamus of kainate-treated rats increases seizure frequency. Epilepsia. 2006;47:27–32.
147. Wyckhuys T, Raedt R, Vonck K, Wadman W, Boon P. Comparison of hippocampal deep brain stimulation with high (130Hz) and low frequency (5Hz) on after discharges in kindled rats. Epilepsy Res. 2010;88:239–46.
148. Tyrand R, Seeck M, Spinelli L, Pralong E, Vulliemoz S, Foletti G, Rossetti AO, Allali G, Lantz G, Pollo C, Boex C. Effects of amygdala-hippocampal stimulation on interictal epileptic discharges. Epilepsy Res. 2012;99:87–93.
149. Velasco M, Velasco F, Velasco AL, Jimenez F, Brito F, Marquez I. Acute and chronic electrical stimulation of the centromedian thalamic nucleus: modulation of reticulo-cortical systems and predictor factors for generalized seizure control. Arch Med Res. 2000;31:304–15.
150. Bjerknes S, Skogseid IM, Saehle T, Dietrichs E, Toft M. Surgical site infections after deep brain stimulation surgery: frequency, characteristics and management in a 10-year period. PLoS One. 2014;9:e105288.
151. Ching J, Khan S, White P, Reed J, Ramnarine D, Sieradzan K, Sandeman D. Long-term effectiveness and tolerability of vagal nerve stimulation in adults with intractable epilepsy: a retrospective analysis of 100 patients. Br J Neurosurg. 2013;27:228–34.
152. Vonck K, Raedt R, Naulaerts J, De Vogelaere F, Thiery E, Van Roost D, Aldenkamp B, Miatton M, Boon P. Vagus nerve stimulation…25 years later! What do we know about the effects on cognition? Neurosci Biobehav Rev. 2014;45:63–71.
153. Elliott RE, Morsi A, Kalhorn SP, Marcus J, Sellin J, Kang M, Silverberg A, Rivera E, Geller E, Carlson C, Devinsky O, Doyle WK. Vagus nerve stimulation

in 436 consecutive patients with treatment-resistant epilepsy: long-term outcomes and predictors of response. Epilepsy Behav. 2011;20:57–63.
154. Granbichler CA, Nashef L, Selway R, Polkey CE. Mortality and SUDEP in epilepsy patients treated with vagus nerve stimulation. Epilepsia. 2015;56:291–6.
155. Loring DW, Kapur R, Meador KJ, Morrell MJ. Differential neuropsychological outcomes following targeted responsive neurostimulation for partial-onset epilepsy. Epilepsia. 2015;56: 1836–44.
156. Morrell M, Hirsch L, Bergey G, et al. Long-term safety and efficacy of the RNS™ system in adults with medically intractable partial onset seizures. Presented at the American Epilepsy Society 62nd Annual Meeting. Seattle, WA; December 8, 2008.
157. Daniele A, Albanese A, Contarino MF, Zinzi P, Barbier A, Gasparini F, Romito LM, Bentivoglio AR, Scerrati M. Cognitive and behavioural effects of chronic stimulation of the subthalamic nucleus in patients with Parkinson's disease. J Neurol Neurosurg Psychiatry. 2003;74:175–82.
158. Hershey T, Revilla FJ, Wernle A, Gibson PS, Dowling JL, Perlmutter JS. Stimulation of STN impairs aspects of cognitive control in PD. Neurology. 2004;62:1110–4.
159. Kleiner-Fisman G, Fisman DN, Sime E, Saint-Cyr JA, Lozano AM, Lang AE. Long-term follow up of bilateral deep brain stimulation of the subthalamic nucleus in patients with advanced Parkinson disease. J Neurosurg. 2003;99:489–95.
160. Doshi PK, Chhaya N, Bhatt MH. Depression leading to attempted suicide after bilateral subthalamic nucleus stimulation for Parkinson's disease. Mov Disord. 2002;17:1084–5.
161. Nagel SJ, Najm IM. Deep brain stimulation for epilepsy. Neuromodulation. 2009;12:270–80.

8 Treatment Strategies for Refractory Status Epilepticus

Xuefeng Wang

Abstract

Treatment strategies for refractory status epilepticus (RSE) consist of two phases, including the termination of RSE onset and addressing the secondary damage induced by status epilepticus (SE). In this chapter, we provide a detailed introduction regarding how therapies to treat RSE are chosen, how these treatments are administered, the precautions that should be taken, and the potential problems that can arise during their use. We also summarize the characteristics of the pathophysiological processes underlying SE, discuss how they affect the functions of different organs, and describe the corresponding countermeasures to these effects. The hope is that once the onset of RSE has been terminated, any secondary damage can simultaneously be reduced as much as possible. These efforts are aimed at achieving a state of stable vital signs in the patient, ensuring the presence of good perfusion and functioning in important organs, and, most importantly, decreasing the death rate and increasing the cure rate in patients with RSE.

8.1 Termination of the Onset of Refractory Status Epilepticus

The termination of the onset of RSE remains the primary focus of treatments for RSE.

X. Wang
Chongqing Key Laboratory of Neurology, Department of Neurology, The First Affiliated Hospital of Chongqing Medical University, 1 YouYi Road, Chongqing 400016, China
e-mail: xfyp@163.com

8.1.1 Treatment Objective

The clinical manifestations and electroencephalographic waveforms observed in patients with RSE are not fixed, and convulsive status epilepticus (CSE) can transform into nonconvulsive status epilepticus (NCSE) during treatment. Therefore, treatment for RSE should simultaneously terminate both clinical seizures and the epileptic discharges observed on electroencephalogram (EEG). Consequently, when using drugs to treat RSE, synchronous EEG monitoring is needed if a patient's medical condition allows. It may assist in determining the effects of drug treatment.

X. Wang, S. Li (eds.), *Refractory Status Epilepticus*, DOI 10.1007/978-981-10-5125-8_8

8.1.2 Treatment Options

The most prominent feature observed in RSE patients is drug resistance against the first-line antiepileptic drugs (AEDs) that are commonly used to treat SE. The occurrence of this resistance is often associated with a variety of neurotransmitter dysfunctions, especially GABA receptor deficiency. Therefore, the use of a variety of anesthetics, including midazolam, propofol, thiopental, and ketamine, is advocated to treat RSE. If this proves ineffective, mild hypothermia therapy, electroconvulsive therapy (ECT), a ketogenic diet (KD), and other non-drug therapies should be used. While this proposition is intended to provide a reference for a treatment option for RSE for clinical practitioners, we do not deny that other reasonable options exist.

8.1.3 Drug Selection

8.1.3.1 Midazolam

1. *Indications*: There is no evidence that the effect of midazolam is superior to that of diazepam or clonazepam. Its effects on respiratory depression and blood pressure are significantly stronger than those of diazepam, and the conditions under which it can be used are limited. Hence, the main indication for midazolam is RSE when treatment using diazepam or other benzodiazepines has failed.
2. *Administration routes*: Recommended intravenous medication.
3. *Dosage*: For adult SE patients, the intravenous administration of the midazolam can be performed using the following methods. Midazolam should be given via intravenous injection at a dosage of 0.1–0.2 mg/kg and at a slow rate (<4 mg/min). If administration is ineffective, it can be repeated once; if it still remains ineffective after a repeat, administration of midazolam must be stopped, and other recommended drugs should be provided. If the administration is effective, midazolam should be administered using an intravenous pump at a speed of 0.1–0.2 mg/kg/h for 12 h. It should then be gradually reduced because sudden withdrawal can trigger a rebound phenomenon. The intravenous injection can be repeated once if recurrence occurs during the maintenance period.

   The appropriate dosage of midazolam when administered intravenously in pediatric patients with RSE remains under exploration. Wilkes et al. [1] conducted a systematic review of 16 studies that involved 645 cases (521 of which were treated with midazolam) of children with RSE. The authors found that efficiency reached 76% when patients were treated using the following regiment: intravenous injection was applied at an initial dosage of 0.15–0.5 mg/kg at first, then a sustained intravenous infusion was administered at a speed of 1–2 μg/kg/min, and its maximum speed can reach 5–24 μg/kg/min. Another study that involved 27 pediatric patients with RSE (age: 5.1 ± 3.5 years old) showed that after an intravenous injection was administered at an initial dose of 0.2 mg/kg and followed by a sustained infusion at a speed of 1–5 μg/kg/min, seizures were controlled in 26 (96%) of the patients. Furthermore, none of these patients developed hypotension, bradycardia, respiratory depression, or other adverse events [2].
4. *Attention*: Midazolam has a significant inhibitory effect on respiration and a prominent antihypertensive effect. It is therefore best to administer it under close supervision in a neurological intensive care unit. If necessary, mechanical ventilation can be used to maintain respiratory function.
5. The clinical practice of using midazolam to treat RSE is discussed in Chap. 6.

8.1.3.2 Propofol

1. *Indications*: The preferred drugs to treat RSE are midazolam and propofol. Both are widely accepted. Propofol may increase the occurrence of SE, and it is therefore recommended only after treatment with midazolam has failed.
2. *Administration routes*: Recommended intravenous medication.
3. *Dosage*: For adult SE patients, propofol can be administered via slow intravenous injection

at a dosage of 1–2 mg/kg. If administration is ineffective, the injection can be repeated once; if it still remains ineffective after a repeat, administration must be stopped, and other recommended drugs should be provided. If administration is effective, propofol should be administered via intravenous pump at a speed of 1–2 mg/kg/h for 10–12 h and then gradually reduced. The injection can be repeated once if recurrence occurs during the maintenance period.

Most clinical professionals do not recommend using propofol to treat pediatric patients because it inhibits physiological functions in children and causes damage to immature brains.

4. *Attention*: (a) Similar to midazolam, it is better to use propofol under close supervision in a neurological intensive care unit. If necessary, mechanical ventilation can be provided to maintain normal respiratory function. (b) Small doses of propofol have been reported to cause SE. Therefore, intravenous applications should not be lower than the recommended dose except under exceptional circumstances. (c) The long-term use of propofol at high doses is of concern because propofol may cause rhabdomyolysis. If necessary, a periodic inspection of creatinine phosphokinase levels may be helpful to diagnose rhabdomyolysis.
5. The clinical practice of using propofol to treat RSE is discussed in Chap. 6.

8.1.3.3 Ketamine

1. *Indications*: Ketamine is mainly suitable for treating RSE that cannot be controlled by midazolam and propofol and as a combination therapy in patients in whom multiple drugs treatments have failed. Gaspard et al. [3] evaluated the statistical data regarding the ability of ketamine to successfully control RSE and reported that the median of drugs that were unsuccessfully used to treat RSE was six before ketamine was selected. Rosati et al. [4] reported similar results (the median of drugs was five). The effectiveness of adding ketamine after multiple drugs treatments have failed is reported to reach 66.7% (6/9), suggesting that ketamine is commonly used to treat RSE at an advanced stage and should be applied only when SE has not been controlled by five to six other types of drugs. Borris et al. [5] supported this conclusion with data from animal experiments. They found that when ketamine was administered 15 min after SE occurred, it remained uncontrolled in all animals (0/4). However, if ketamine was administered at 1 h after superrefractory status epilepticus (SRSE) occurred, its control rate for SE was 100% (4/4).
2. *Administration routes*: Recommended intravenous medication.
3. *Dosage*: For adult SE patients, the ketamine can be administered slowly via intravenous injection at a dosage of 1–2 mg/kg followed by administration via an intravenous pump at a speed of 0.5–2 mg/kg/h for 10–12 h to maintain the treatment after termination of the seizure.

   Synowiec et al. [6] reported that in RSE patients, an intravenous injection of ketamine at a dose of 1–2 mg/kg that was followed by a continuous intravenous drip at a speed of 0.45–2.1 mg/kg/h required an average duration of 9.8 days (4–28 days) to treat the disease. Eventually, the seizures were controlled in all of the patients (11/11), and no side effects were reported. Basha et al. [7] administered a continuous intravenous drip of ketamine to treat RSE at an initial rate of 1 mg/kg/h that was gradually increased to an average rate of 3.5 mg/kg/h (1–5 mg/kg/h) for 2–14 days to maintain the treatment. The RSE remission rate was 57% (4/7). One case experienced RSE relapse after ketamine was discontinued, and the case was resolved by surgery. And two patients died because one family ended treatment and one had cardiac arrest. Therefore, treatment with ketamine can be administered via two methods. One method is to first administer an intravenous injection and then to administer the drug via a continuous intravenous drip. Another method is to administer the drug via continuous intravenous drip only.
4. *Attention*: (a) The application of the anesthetic drug ketamine requires the guidance of an

anesthesiologist. It has a significant inhibitory effect on respiration. It is therefore best used in a neurological intensive care unit under close supervision. Mechanical ventilation may be required to maintain normal respiratory function. (b) Because of its significant effect on respiratory depression, the USFDA recommends beginning with a small dose of ketamine and increasing the amount slowly. (c) Ketamine may have excitatory effects in the central nervous system (CNS). Although such cases are rare, the FDA does not recommend ketamine for patients who have severe hypertension, a drug allergy to ketamine, coronary heart disease, cardiac dysfunction, glaucoma, arteriosclerosis, pulmonary hypertension, pulmonary heart disease, pregnancy, severe intracranial hypertension, a history of mental health issues, hyperthyroidism, tachyarrhythmia, or adrenal pheochromocytoma. A head CT scan must be performed to rule out intracranial lesions, which can induce intracranial hypertension, before ketamine is administered. (d) Ketamine should be administered cautiously in patients with SE that was caused by alcohol poisoning. (e) Ketamine causes increased skeletal muscle tension, and the diagnosis must therefore be differentiated from tonic-clonic seizures [8].

8.1.3.4 Combination Therapy

1. *Potential advantages*: SE is a multifactor and heterogeneous disease with many different causes and a complex underlying mechanism. Hence, a combined approach in which various AEDs that act via different mechanisms are applied may be more practical for treating SE than the use of drugs that act via a single mechanism. Researchers have also shown that SE is a continuous disease process, and its pathogenesis may not be identical among seizures with different lengths [9]. Wasterlain et al. [10] found that in recurrent and prolonged seizures, GABAA receptor activity decreased on postsynaptic membranes, while the number and activity of NMDA receptors increased, and these effects led to an increased incidence of benzodiazepine-resistant SE. Drug combination that affects a variety of neurotransmitters may provide more obvious advantages. In particular, a drug combination therapy that includes a selection of new AEDs as an additive was more beneficial in improving patient prognoses [9]. Sustained seizures can cause substantial brain damage, including cerebral edema and the loss of neurons. Thus, the early use of multi-mechanism AEDs for SE will help to achieve the early termination of seizures and thereby improve patient prognoses [11].
2. *Clinical application*: Currently, combined applications of AEDs to treat SE mainly include ketamine, levetiracetam, phenytoin, midazolam, stiripentol, barbiturates, and immunomodulatory drugs. Of these, levetiracetam, ketamine, and propofol are the most successful:

(a) *Levetiracetam*: Levetiracetam is a broad-spectrum AED that performs its antiepileptic effects by regulating calcium channels, glutamate receptors, and GABA transport [12–15]. Mazarati et al. [12] found that when treating SE, levetiracetam and diazepam had a strong synergistic effect in animal experiments. Uges et al. [13] used standard treatment regimens (e.g., benzodiazepines and phenytoin) in nine patients who were also simultaneously treated with 2500 mg of levetiracetam via intravenous injection (for more than 5 min) as an add-on therapy. With the exception of one patient who died 9 days later as a result of multiple organ failure (unrelated to levetiracetam), the remaining patients achieved complete control of their seizures within 24 h, and there were no significant side effects during this period. Gallentine et al. [14] retrospectively analyzed 11 cases of pediatric patients with RSE who were treated with the levetiracetam as an add-on therapy. The patients were treated with levetiracetam combined with other drugs (e.g., midazolam, pentobarbital, valproate, phenobarbital, phenytoin, or diazepam). In all, 45% (5/11) of the patients experienced obvious beneficial effects.

(b) *Ketamine*: Ketamine is a noncompetitive NMDA receptor antagonist that blocks NMDA transmission and exerts a neuroprotective effect. Ketamine also stabilizes hemodynamics, which reduces the chance of a patient developing hypotension [8]. In recurrent and prolonged seizures, there is a decrease in the number and activity of GABAA receptors on postsynaptic membranes and an increase in the number and activity of NMDA receptors, and these effects lead to the emergence of drug-resistant SE [10]. Wasterlain et al. [16] used animal experiments to demonstrate that a combination consisting of ketamine and benzodiazepines corrected both weakened GABA inhibition and enhanced glutamic acid excitation during the progression of SE. As a treatment for RSE, this synergistic effect provides more advantages when SE is in an advanced stage. Synowiec et al. [6] retrospectively analyzed 11 patients with RSE who were treated with ketamine as an add-on therapy. The patients were intravenously administered ketamine in combination with other drugs (e.g., lorazepam or phenytoin) after other AEDs were found to be ineffective. The duration of treatment with ketamine was 4–28 days. In all patients (11/11), RSE was fully controlled, and no significant side effects were reported.

3. *Indications*: When administrate a variety of drugs to treat RSE, the SE still cannot be terminated [8].
4. *Administration routes*: Recommended intravenous medication.
5. *Methods of administration*: (a) Simultaneous application: One drug is administered first, followed by the administration of another drug, regardless of how effective the first drug was. (b) Administer in order: once the current drug treatment has failed, the drug dose should be unchanged while another drug is added [8].
6. *Dosage*: Studies have reported that there are three different methods for dosing drug combination treatments, as follows: (a) for combinations consisting of two drugs, half of the dose of each of the two drugs is administered; (b) the full amount of the major drug and half the dosage of the another drug are administered; or (c) the full dose of both drugs is administered. Please refer to Chap. 6 for a description of combination treatments for SE.

8.1.3.5 Phenobarbital

1. *Indication*: Phenobarbital is mainly suitable for treating SE after treatment with diazepam and clonazepam has failed, and it is particularly effective in pediatric patients.
2. *Administration routes*: Administered intravenously.
3. *Dosage*: When treating adult SE patients, a slow intravenous injection of phenobarbital is first administered at a dosage of 10 mg/kg and at a speed of less than 100 mg/min. When effective, the phenobarbital should then be administered at a dose of 100–200 mg via intramuscular injection twice per day for 1–2 days to maintain the treatment effectiveness. If phenobarbital is not effective, its administration should be stopped, and other recommended drugs should be administered.

8.1.3.6 Valproic Acid

1. *Indication*: Valproic acid is mainly suitable for treating SE after treatment with benzodiazepines has failed. Valproic acid is particularly suitable for treating NCSE patients because the drug has no obvious effects on consciousness.
2. *Administration routes*: Administered intravenously.
3. *Dosage*: When treating adult SE patients, an initial intravenous injection of 800–1600 mg of valproic acid should be administered. Then, 800–1600 mg of valproic acid should be given via intravenous drip for a consecutive 2–3 days to maintain the treatment. If treatment is effective, valproic acid can be administered orally after seizures stop and the patient regains consciousness. If treatment is not effective, valproic acid administration should be stopped, and other recommended drugs should be provided.

4. *Attention*: (a) When using valproic acid to treat SE, the first dose should be doubled because a long-term intravenous drip of valproic acid at a small dose will not achieve the desired effect. (b) Caution should be exercised regarding the specific contraindications of valproic acid, which include seizures caused by mitochondrial encephalomyopathy. Generally, valproic acid is not recommended for treating SE caused by a genetic disease, seizures caused by hepatic encephalopathy, or other diseases that are otherwise contraindicated for treatment with valproic acid.

8.1.4 Non-drug Therapies for RSE

8.1.4.1 KD

The KD is a method for treating RSE that was developed in recent years. Caraballo et al. [17] summarized the results related to ten cases of pediatric RSE that occurred from 2010 to 2014 and found that when a KD was used as an adjuvant therapy, all of the patients reached a state of ketonuria within an average of 3 days, and after an average of 5 days, the following therapy-induced effect occurred: seizures stopped in two patients, and the frequency of seizures decreased by 50–75% in five patients. Moreover, the KD had been lasted for at least 6 months in these seven patients. However, in three of the patients, the frequency of seizures decreased by less than 50%, and in these patients, the KD therapy was stopped because of severe complications. Thakur et al. [18] evaluated ten adult RSE patients (seven with encephalitis and the remainder with cerebral cysticercosis, cortical dysplasia, or hypoxic-ischemic encephalopathy) who received classic KD therapy for a median time of 17.5 days. In nine of these patients (90%), the seizures were controlled after several days (the median time is 3 days) of KD therapy.

1. *Administration routes and dosage*: A KD can be administered in either an enteral or a parenteral way. Enteral administration is the most common and occurs through a stomach tube, whereas parenteral administration occurs through the venous system. Regardless of the administration route, the proportion of fat to nonfat components must be administered in strict 4:1 ratio, and glucose intake should be controlled. Generally, dietary intake and the infusion of glucose are forbidden for 24 h before beginning KD therapy because its treatment effect on SE disappears once glucose is infused.
2. *Onset time*: Generally, administration of KD therapy results in ketosis in 2–3 days and controls seizures after 5–8 days.
3. *Course of treatment*: If the condition of the SE patient improves, a KD can be used as a long-term adjuvant treatment. If it is not effective or if severe complications appear, the KD should be terminated.
4. *The type of SE that can be treated by KD*: A sufficient systematic analysis is lacking because there are few reports in which a KD was used to treat SE. According to previous data, a KD has been effective in improving RSE cases that arose from a variety of causes, such as viral encephalitis, autoimmune encephalitis, FIRES, and Dravet syndrome [19–21].
5. For matters that require attention when using a KD to treat RSE, please refer to Chap. 7 of this book.
6. *Contraindications*: Contraindications include metabolic disorders (such as persistent hyponatremia, hypoglycemia, hypocalcemia, hypernatremia, and acidosis), hemodynamic instability or cardiorespiratory dysfunction, blood coagulation disorders, pancreatitis, liver failure, severe hyperlipidemia, enteral nutrition intolerance (including intestinal obstruction), pregnancy, and the injection of any propofol within 24 h, previously known fatty acid oxidation disorder or pyruvate carboxylase deficiency [19–21].

8.1.4.2 Mild Hypothermia Therapy

Fifty years ago, research showed that mild hypothermia reduces electric activity in the cerebral cortex and that frozen brine terminated seizures in temporal lobe tumor patients. In 1984, Orlowski et al. [22] used physical cooling to control the complications of high fever in RSE patients and found that their seizures were controlled when the temperature was dropped. Thus, mild hypothermia had an adjuvant effect on RSE. In 2008, Corry et al. [24] reported the first study showing that mild hypothermia therapy is a physical method that can be used to treat RSE. The authors treated four patients with an endovascular cooling system to induce mild hypothermia while simultaneously administering antiepileptic therapy. Although the temperature of one patient should have been reduced more than it was, the seizures of the other patients were controlled. After the seizures were controlled and 24 h of burst-suppression in EEG, the administration of AEDs (e.g., midazolam) was stopped, and there was no recurrence during the next 41 h. After the patients were rewarmed, two of the patients improved and were discharged from the hospital with oral antiepileptic therapy. In 2013, Guilliams et al. [25] administered mild hypothermia therapy to five patients whose seizures were not controlled by the injection of drugs including phenobarbital and midazolam or whose seizures recurred after the drug was stopped. The authors found that mild hypothermia therapy provided a clear beneficial effect in epilepsy patients, and these results promoted the application of mild hypothermia therapy as a treatment for RSE.

1. *Indications*: Mild hypothermia therapy is mainly suitable for RSE that is not controlled by the drugs recommended above or in cases that recur after the cessation of the drugs recommended above.
2. *Methods of application*: When using sufficient AEDs to treat SE, an endovascular cooling system or hyperthermia therapy apparatus (e.g., an ice blanket and ice cap) should also be applied simultaneously to induce mild hypothermia or hypothermia, respectively. The target temperature is 31–35 °C. After seizures have been controlled or after 24–48 h of burst-suppression in EEG, the temperature should be increased to 36.5 °C, and the speed of rewarming should not be faster than 0.5–1 °C/day [22–25].
3. *Onset time*: Generally, within 3–48 h of reaching the target temperature, the therapy begins to work, and a state of suppression appears on EEG.
4. *Attention*: (a) EEG monitoring is necessary during the period in which mild hypothermia is induced and during treatment and rewarming. After rewarming, if the seizures do not recur, the AEDs that were used to treat SE should be withdrawn. However, if necessary, they should be administered orally. (b) If the patient experiences a chill while mild hypothermia is induced, the mild hypothermia treatment should be stopped, and the patient should be rewarmed. (c) The drugs used to treat SE (e.g., phenobarbital or midazolam) should be continually administered during mild hypothermia treatment [22–25]. (d) A temperature lower than 30 °C can result in side effects, including ventricular fibrillation, blood coagulation dysfunction, and venous thrombosis. Additionally, when mild hypothermia therapy is used to treat RSE, hypokalemia and acute intestinal ischemia and necrosis can occur because of the low temperature [22–25]. In 2013, Guilliams et al. [25] assessed five pediatric RSE patients who had undergone mild hypothermia treatment. During mild hypothermia and rewarming, electrolyte disturbances (hypokalemia, hypernatremia) occurred in some of the patients. Although these side effects can disappear after treatment has been terminated, it is still necessary to monitor blood gas, blood coagulation function, and electrolytes and to perform routine blood tests once every 6 h during mild hypothermia and rewarming. Additionally, if an endovascular cooling system is used, an ultrasound of the lower limb veins must be performed once per week [26].

8.1.4.3 ECT

Reports describing the use of ECT in patients with epilepsy date back to the 1930s. In 2005, the UK guidelines on ECT first introduced this type of therapy as the industry norms for treating RSE [27]. Similarly, in 2012, Ferlisi et al. [28] noted that ECT is an alternative method for treating

SE. These two events triggered an increase in the clinical use of ECT.

1. *Indication*: When SRSE cannot be controlled by the treatments described above.
2. *Parameters of ECT*: The two ways to determine the appropriate electric dosage for ECT are the fixed dose method and the dose titration method. The American Psychiatric Association recommends the dose titration method. The dose titration method means using the minimum electrical dosage that can induce a seizure as the initial dosage. This approach is advantageous because it implements the use of an individualized dosage, which means that the dosage matches the individual seizure threshold. Hence, the ECT will have a smaller effect on cognitive function while ensuring the therapeutic goal. In 2011, Shin et al. [30] successfully treated a pediatric RSE patient using ECT with the following parameters: ECT sessions, 12; pulse width, 0–2 s; pulse frequency, 37–120 HZ; and stimulus duration, 3–43 s. For different parameters that have been used in the clinical application of this treatment, please refer to the methods introduced by Yang et al. [23].
3. *Method*: (1) The electrodes are placed bilaterally, and (2) three consecutive single stimuli are used to form a group of consecutive stimuli. (3) The choice of anesthetics may influence the effect of ECT [28]. A combination of propofol and ECT is preferred because propofol reduces the hemodynamic response and cognitive impairment caused by ECT while allowing a quick recovery. Hence, in England, propofol is the most commonly used anesthetic in ECT [29].
4. *Attention*: ECT is relatively safe, and its primary complication is cognitive impairment. Thus, in ECT, the following precautions should be taken:

(a) Evaluate the condition of the patient and obtain informed consent.
(b) Ensure that the anesthesia is administered by professionals, because anesthesia can reduce tension in the patients and prevent the potential complications, including fractures and damage to teeth, tendons, and muscles, that can arise during ECT.
(c) Use the seizure threshold as the basis for determining the electrical dosage for ECT. While treating SRSE, the electrical dosage should match the patient's seizure threshold and be continuously regulated during the entire period. Adjustments to the electrical dosage or its timing and frequency can be made based on the reactions of the patient and the occurrence of possible complications.
(d) If the patient has other diseases, such as heart failure, severe valvular disease, or arrhythmia, the risks associated with the therapy are increased, and the treatment may induce cardiovascular complications. Thus, throughout the therapy, patient characteristics, including the duration of seizures, EEG, airway patency, vital signs, and side effects, must be closely monitored [23].
(e) It is also necessary to perform EEG monitoring after ECT because the therapy can induce seizures and NCSE.
(f) The clinical application of ECT is limited, and there is therefore no consensus regarding its protocol [23, 27–30].

8.1.4.4 Treatments That Are Under Exploration

1. *Neuromodulation therapy*: Neuromodulation therapy is a new method that was developed in recent years to treat RSE. Neuromodulation technologies that are under exploration for treating RSE include vagus nerve stimulation, cortical responsive stimulation, and deep brain stimulation. More details regarding this treatment are provided in Chap. 7.
2. *Levetiracetam*:

(a) Indications: Levetiracetam is mainly suitable for treating SE after treatment with diazepam and clonazepam has failed. It is also suitable for use in combined therapies aimed at treating seizures that cannot be controlled by many other drugs. Levetiracetam may have a treatment effect on pediatric electrical SE during sleep.

(b) Administration routes: Recommended intravenous medication.
(c) Dosage: When treating adult SE patients, the administration should be an intravenous injection of levetiracetam at an initial dose of 1000–1500 mg and a speed of 2–5 mg/(kg·min). This dosage can be increased if the seizures continue or if there is continuous epileptiform discharge on EEG. If the treatment is effective, levetiracetam can be administered via continuous infusion at a speed of 0.05–2 mg/(kg·h) at a recommended daily dose of 1500–3000 mg. If levetiracetam is ineffective, its administration should be stopped, and other recommended drugs should be administered.

The use of levetiracetam as a combination therapy is recommended in patients with SRSE. Levetiracetam is usually combined with benzodiazepines. When administering a combination therapy that includes levetiracetam and benzodiazepines, levetiracetam should be administered via a slow intravenous injection at a dose of 2500 mg over a period of more than 5 min. There are two methods for administering combination therapies including levetiracetam and benzodiazepines. Levetiracetam can be added when treatment with benzodiazepines fails, or levetiracetam and benzodiazepines can be simultaneously administered (for more details, please see Chap. 6).

8.2 Secondary Damage in Patients with Refractory Status Epilepticus and Countermeasures

Among the treatment strategies of RSE, in addition to the termination of RSE, addressing the secondary damage is also quite important. SE can influence the function of the entire body, especially the brain, which may be a direct cause of death in patients with epilepsy. A better understanding of the secondary damage may help to improve the prognosis of patients with RSE.

8.2.1 The Effect of RSE on Different Organs

8.2.1.1 The Effect of RSE on Cardiac Function and Cardiac Electrical Activity

During SE, skeletal muscle contraction can lead to excessive energy consumption and respiratory failure, causing hypoxia and anaerobic metabolism, which can result in lactic acidosis. Simultaneously, skeletal muscle contraction increases the peripheral resistance and cardiac load, which weakens cardiac ejection function, causing circulatory failure and further deepening hypoxia in the body. In SE, elevated plasma catecholamine levels release a large number of catecholamines, leading to abnormal myocardial excitability and producing pathological myocardial repolarization [31, 32]. In addition, SE attacks cause the acute and intense activation of the sympathetic nervous system, further resulting in myocardial damage, abnormal cardiac electrical activity, and increased susceptibility of ventricular arrhythmias, leading to arrhythmia, myocardial hemorrhage, subendocardial hemorrhage, acute myocardial ischemia and hypoxia, T wave variation, and bradycardia. These abnormalities are common in SE and can cause cardiac arrest when serious. Arrhythmia and acute heart failure are important causes of death in patients with epilepsy [33–42].

8.2.1.2 The Effect of RSE on Blood Pressure

Cerebral blood flow (CBF) is maintained by the elevation of its own blood pressure, and blood pressure is increased by regulating the concentration of catecholamine in the body. To protect the brain in the early stages of SE, CBF increases, and a large number of catecholamines are released, resulting in a sharp increase in blood pressure. In the late stages of SE, with the depletion of catecholamines and the desensitization of peripheral blood vessels on catecholamine, this compensation can only be maintained for 0.5–2 h. Consequently, CBF will decrease, and blood pressure likewise decreases. Hocker et al. [43] found that, in SE, blood pressure and heart rate can reach the peak in 1 min but may take 1 h to gradually return to baseline levels. With the progression of SE, blood pressure drops to baseline levels. Then, cerebral hypoperfusion may appear [44].

8.2.1.3 The Effect of RSE on Respiratory Function

In the tonic phase of CSE, sustained contraction of the diaphragm can cause airway obstruction and respiratory disorders, leading to pulmonary dysfunction and triggering a pulmonary vascular perfusion shunt. This can result in end-tidal carbon dioxide pressure and alveolar carbon dioxide (CO_2) pressure changes, causing asphyxia and hypoxia [45, 46].

Epilepsy seizures that last for a long period of time will cause extensive inhibition of the patient's EEG activity and acute CNS injury. The widespread inhibition of the brain affects the respiratory center of the brainstem, resulting in low central ventilation or apnea. Simultaneously, central respiratory depression can lead to sustained apnea, which can aggravate the rapid progress of respiratory failure. Respiratory failure, on the one hand, can aggravate seizures, forming a vicious circle; on the other hand, the brainstem may be inhibited for a long time, which may eventually lead to respiratory arrest. Some scholars believe that, after seizures, the synergy of the broad inhibition of brain and the dysfunction of the heart and lung is an important factor in sudden death of an unknown cause in epilepsy patients [47–49].

After experiencing tonic-clonic seizures, 2% of patients have neurogenic pulmonary edema (NPE), with a mortality rate reaching 60–100%. Intracranial pressure (ICP) increases suddenly in the onset of seizures, leading to arteriovenous vascular spasms, which then causes pulmonary vascular contraction and an increase in systemic peripheral vascular resistance, resulting in left ventricular failure and NPE. With the increasing numbers of seizures, pulmonary capillary pressure gradually increases. The synergy of the elevated pressure and the neurohumor causes the permeability of circulating endothelial cells in the lungs to increase, leading to the leakage of a large amount of protein-rich liquid, which is involved in the formation of NPE [50, 51].

8.2.1.4 The Effect of RSE on Renal Function

When SE occurs, myoclonus leads to excessive muscle contraction, shortage of muscle energy and oxygen supply, and cell membrane defects, which cause a large influx of calcium, while this influx of calcium strengthens the muscle contraction. In addition, SE may also activate a number of intracellular enzymes (such as phospholipase and protease), leading to cell lysis, muscle fiber necrosis, rhabdomyolysis, disseminated intravascular coagulation, and the production of a large amount of muscle cell contents, such as myoglobin, creatine kinase (CK), lactate dehydrogenase enzymes, and some other toxic ions and small molecules. In muscles, the hemoperfusion and the energy supply reorganization result in the release of cell contents into the extracellular fluid and the blood circulation. When the myoglobin concentration is greater than 15 mg/L, the body forms tube-type deposition, which may cause renal tubular obstruction and acute tubular necrosis, eventually producing acute renal failure. Simultaneously, a large amount of fluid flow into the tissue space after muscle injury induced by seizures, resulting in the shortage of effective circulating blood volume and eventually leading to acute renal failure. In the late stage of SE, catecholamine is depleted, blood pressure decreases, renal blood perfusion is insufficient, the glomerular filtration rate decreases significantly, and the damage of renal function occurs [52].

8.2.1.5 The Effect of RSE on Liver Function

Some anticonvulsants used to treat epilepsy have liver toxicity. Sustained seizures can lead to liver hypoxia and ischemia, and anticonvulsant drugs such as phenobarbital, phenytoin, and diazepam can cause the change of free radical metabolism, leading to liver cell membrane injury. Extensive hypoxia, ischemia, and the change of free radical metabolism promote liver failure together.

8.2.1.6 Cerebral Edema Induced by RSE

Cerebral edema is a quite common secondary damage of CNS. Current studies showed that both drugs (such as folic acid, kainic acid, lithium-pilocarpine, etc.), which are used to induce the SE animal model, and various types of SE (such as general, partial, convulsive, and nonconvulsive) can cause cerebral edema. Lee et al. [53] found that the cerebral edema may due to blood-brain barrier (BBB) damage. However, in an animal experiment, Seitelberger et al. [54] showed that in kainate-kindled rats, massive swelling of brain neurons and dysfunction of astrocyte microcirculation can induce cerebral edema. Relevant studies suggest that cerebral edema usually occurs 30 h to 20 days after SE [55, 56] and the degree of cerebral edema is different among different patients. In most cases, the patient's cerebral edema is mild to moderate and transient; however, a small number of patients can form malignant cerebral edema, leading to hernia and death.

8.2.2 Countermeasures

8.2.2.1 Maintenance of Vital Signs in Patients with RSE

In RSE, direct and indirect central and/or peripheral nerve injury can cause systemic hypoxia, aspiration pneumonia, lactic acidosis, CO_2 anesthesia, hyperkalemia, fever, leukocytosis, hypoglycemia, shock, arrhythmia, pulmonary edema, acute tubular necrosis, and high-output heart failure, which has become an important cause of sudden death in patients with epilepsy [57]. Therefore, the maintenance of vital signs in patients with epilepsy is particularly important.

1. General treatment: A vein channel must be established quickly, and electrocardiography (ECG), blood pressure, oxygen saturation, and EEG must be monitored.
2. Cardiovascular system function support:

(a) *ECG monitoring*: Conduct the ECG and myocardial enzyme spectrum examination as soon as possible to rule out arrhythmia, conduction abnormalities, acute myocardial ischemia, T wave variation, and other abnormal ECG activities. Early correction of arrhythmias can reduce the risk of heart attack. A survey found that heart rate variability was significantly lower in patients with RSE. A decrease in heart rate variability may increase the mortality of patients with epilepsy and is associated with an increased risk of fatal arrhythmia and sudden cardiac death. Thus, Mukherjee et al. [58] propose that high-risk patients may be given a cardiac pacemaker and defibrillator combined equipment in advance [59–61].

(b) *Maintenance of blood pressure*: To maintain blood pressure, establish a fluid infusion channel and monitor the blood pressure closely. In the early stages of SE, to ensure cerebral perfusion, there is massive catecholamine release, causing reflex hypertension, transient vasoconstriction, and organ hypoperfusion, which aggravates visceral ischemia, myocardial perfusion insufficiency, and arrhythmia. Because of its short duration, medication is generally not necessary for low blood pressure in the early stages of SE. However, when blood pressure is dramatically increased, such as systolic blood pressure (SBP) > 180 mmHg, diastolic blood pressure > 100 mmHg, or mean arterial pressure (MAP) > 90 mmHg, and lasts for 30–60 min, short-acting beta-blocker drugs or sodium nitroprusside can be used to reduce blood pressure. But, the inhibitory effects of beta-blockers in the myocardium must be monitored. Blood pressure in patients with SE increases sharply and is maintained at higher levels for approximately 0.5–2 h. With the depletion of catecholamines and the desensitization of peripheral blood vessels to catecholamines, CBF decreases, and blood pressure is gradually reduced, resulting in heart failure. This leads to insufficient effective blood volume, followed by more severe hypotension. When blood pressure drops below the baseline level, cerebral hypoperfusion may occur. At this stage, the patient should be given fluid infusion and hypertension drugs to ensure that the SBP is ≥100 mmHg or the MAP is >70 mmHg.

3. Respiratory function support:

   First, maintain airway patency and prevent aspiration. Emergency respiratory support treatment can prevent further cerebral ischemia and hypoxia.

   Second, epilepsy patients may receive tracheal intubation based on the following criteria: (a) cannot maintain or protect the airway, such as airway obstruction, etc., (b) ventilation or oxygenation dysfunction, and (c) expected clinical deterioration, such as seizure activity for more than 10 min, etc. [62, 63]. Establishment of an artificial airway and pulmonary management at the right time can significantly reduce the incidence of these respiratory complications and the mortality of the patients. The establishment of an artificial airway includes standard endotracheal intubation, rapid endotracheal intubation, and alternative airway devices and techniques [62–64].

   The last not the least, ensure that the body is being oxygenated and CO_2 is discharged, and NPE is actively corrected: reducing ICP based on treating the primary disease is central to reducing NPE. Simultaneously, ventilator-assisted breathing, the use of positive end-expiratory pressure, the application of glucocorticoids, the optimization of body oxygenation, reducing the before- and the afterload, and increasing the myocardial contractile force in heart failure patients are necessary measures [65].

4. Monitoring and support of renal function:

   Close monitoring is necessary to observe the change in renal function, urine routine, blood gas, blood and urine myoglobin, CK, creatinine, and urea nitrogen, and the ratio of these factors will be the routine examination. Dynamic changes must be noted and particularly be cautious about rhabdomyolysis and central diabetes insipidus. In the early stages of SE, we must pay attention to the protection of renal function; we must also reduce or control excessive contraction of the skeletal muscle, promote kidney blood circulation, strengthen the osmotic diuresis, correct acidosis, and supplement the effective circulating blood volume [40]. The key to the treatment of late-stage acute renal failure is to block the process of acute renal failure, including inadequate capacity, kidney tubule tubular formation, acidic urine, and oxygen-free radicals. In accordance with the diagnosis and treatment of acute renal failure, we should provide positive continuous blood filtration, correct electrolyte disorders, alkalize urine, give nutritional therapy, and care for follow-up on dynamic changes. The timely detection and treatment of these complications can improve the successful rate of rescue and prognosis of SE [66].

5. Monitoring and support of liver function:

   Liver function must be closely monitored, and drugs with liver toxicity should be used cautiously. In particular, be aware of the liver toxicity of anticonvulsant drugs for the treatment of SE. Patients with liver injury should eliminate causes of liver damage, reduce blood ammonia, correct plasma amino acid imbalances, promote normal neurotransmitter functions, eliminate toxic substances in the body, promote the recovery of liver function and liver regeneration, and provide nutritional support treatment. If liver failure occurs, it can be treated with plasma exchange or an artificial liver.

8.2.2.2 Treatment of Cerebral Edema

1. Commonly used dehydrating agent

   Dehydration is the most important method used to treat intracranial hypertension; it can protect many patients from the occurrence of herniation and reduce patient mortality.

(a) *Mannitol*: Mannitol is the most widely used clinical first-line drug to reduce ICP. The dosage of mannitol for the treatment of cerebral edema is decided by weight: 0.25–1 g/kg, formulated as a 20% concentration. It is provided via intravenous injection and usually takes effect immediately after medication; mannitol takes 1–2 h to reach a peak, which is maintained for 4–6 h. When the patient is weakened, the dose should be reduced to 0.5 g/kg, repeated once per 4–6 h if necessary. Mannitol has two primary effects: diuresis and dehydration. To dehydrate, its infusion rate cannot be less than 250 mL/30 min. Kumar et al. [67] believe that there is no difference between small doses (0.25–0.5 g/kg) of mannitol and high-dose (0.5–1.5 g/kg) mannitol treatment; however, small doses can reduce side effects, so small dose treatment is preferred. Notably, plasma osmolality must be monitored because when the plasma osmolality is high, side effects of mannitol can appear.

(b) *Hypertonic saline (HS)*: HS is an important osmotic agent. The literature reports that HS concentrations of 29.2% and 3% are used to treat cerebral edema caused by SE. Worthley et al. [68] analyzed five patients with severe hyponatremia and SE who received 50 mL of 29.2% HS (250 mmol) via a central venous catheter, and the time of injection was more than 10 min, followed by the continuous intravenous infusion of 80–150 mL of 29.2% HS (400–750 mmol) via a central venous catheter over a period of 8–12 h, with serum sodium increasing at 2–3 mmol/l/h until the serum sodium level reached 130–135 mmol/l. Serum sodium, potassium, blood urea, and blood sugar levels must be checked 30 min before and after the treatment and 2–4 h after the treatment to assess osmotic pressure. Sharf et al. [69] studied 56 infants with first-episode SE who were younger than 1 year of age. Fifteen of the infants had low-sodium seizures and were treated with 1.5 mL/kg (0.6–6.1 mL/kg) of 3% salt; their serum sodium increased at an average rate of 2.35 mmol/h (1–6 mmol/h) for an average duration of 6.63 h (2–11 h), effectively terminating the epileptic seizures. According to our experience (from a study that has not yet been published), the use of 3% HS (100 mL, 2–3 times a day) is safe and effective.

Although mannitol remains more widely used, HS therapy has become an alternative to mannitol in hyperosmolar therapy [70–76]. Because of the different osmotic reflection coefficients across the BBB, an intact BBB is less permeable to saline than to mannitol; therefore, HS may be more effective in decreasing cerebral edema than mannitol. In addition, HS provides patients with the benefit of increased intravascular volume while reducing ICP without exacerbating hypotension. HS has been increasingly used as a safe and effective osmotherapeutic agent for the treatment of cerebral edema. However, clinical experience with its use is limited compared to that with mannitol. The timing of the onset of therapy, the optimal dosage, the concentration of HS, the safest and most effective mode of administration, and the duration remain unknown. Further studies of carefully controlled experimental animal models and large-scale randomized clinical trials are needed to obtain high-quality data to elucidate the above problems.

2. Other treatments

In addition to the traditional dehydrating agents, corticosteroids, barbiturates, hyperventilation, low temperatures, decompressive craniectomy, and other methods can reduce ICP. Wang et al. [77] used kainic acid to establish an epilepsy and SE mouse model and found that immediately using low temperatures to treat a patient in an epileptic state can protect brain tissue, reduce the recurrence of epilepsy, and improve cognition. The low-temperature antiepileptic effect can primarily reduce cerebral edema caused by SE.

References

1. Wilkes R, Tasker RD. Intensive care treatment of uncontrolled status epilepticus in children: systematic literature search of midazolam and anesthetic therapies. Pediatr Crit Care Med. 2014;15(7):632–9.
2. Ozdemir D, Gulez P, Uran N, Yendur G, Kavakli T, Aydin A. Efficacy of continuous midazolam infusion and mortality in childhood refractory generalized convulsive status epilepticus. Seizure. 2005;14(2):129–32.

3. Gaspard N, Foreman B, Judd LM, et al. Intravenous ketamine for the treatment of refractory status epilepticus: a retrospective multicenter study. Epilepsia. 2013;54:1498–503.
4. Rosati A, Erario LM, Ilvento L, Cecchi C, Pisano T, Mirabile L, Guerrini R. Efficacy and safety of ketamine in refractory status epilepticus in children. Neurology. 2012;11(79):2355–8.
5. Borris DJ, Bertram EH, Kapur J. Ketamine controls prolonged status epilepticus. Epilepsy Res. 2000;42:117–22.
6. Synowiec AS, Singh DS, Yenugadhati V, Valereriano JP, Schramke CJ, Kelly KM. Ketamine use in the treatment of refractory status epilepticus. Epilepsy Res. 2013;105:183–8.
7. Basha MM, Alqallaf A, Shah AK. Drug-induced EEG pattern predicts effectiveness of ketamine in treating refractory status epilepticus. Epilepsia. 2015;56(4):e44–8.
8. Fang Y, Wang X. Ketamine for the treatment of refractory status epilepticus. Seizure. 2015;30:14–20.
9. Wang X, Jin J, Chen R. Combination drug therapy for the treatment of status epilepticus. Expert Rev Neurother. 2015;15(6):639–54.
10. Wasterlain CG, Chen JW. Mechanistic and pharmacologic aspects of status epilepticus and its treatment with new antiepileptic drugs. Epilepsia. 2008;49(Suppl 9):63–73.
11. Silbergleit R, Lowenstein D, Durkalski V, Conwit R. RAMPART (rapid anticonvulsant medication prior to arrival trial): a double-blind randomized clinical trial of the efficacy of intramuscular midazolam versus intravenous lorazepam in the prehospital treatment of status epilepticus by paramedics. Epilepsia. 2011;52(Suppl 8):45–7.
12. Mazarati AM, Baldwin R, Klitgaard H, Matagne A, Wasterlain CG. Anticonvulsant effects of levetiracetam and levetiracetam-diazepam combinations in experimental status epilepticus. Epilepsy Res. 2004;58(2–3):167–74.
13. Uges JW, van Huizen MD, Engelsman J, Wilms EB, Touw DJ, Peeters E, et al. Safety and pharmacokinetics of intravenous levetiracetam infusion as add-on in status epilepticus. Epilepsia. 2009;50(3):415–21.
14. Gallentine WB, Hunnicutt AS, Husain AM. Levetiracetam in children with refractory status epilepticus. Epilepsy Behav. 2009;14(1):215–8.
15. Zheng F, Du C, Wang X. Levetiracetam for the treatment of status epilepticus. Expert Rev Neurother. 2015;15(10):1113–21.
16. Wasterlain CG, Baldwin R, Naylor DE, Thompson KW, Suchomelova L, Niquet J. Rational polytherapy in the treatment of acute seizures and status epilepticus. Epilepsia. 2011;52(Suppl 8):70–1.
17. Caraballo RH, Flesler S, Armeno M, et al. Ketogenic diet in pediatric patients with refractory focal status epilepticus. Epilepsy Res. 2014;108(10):1912–6.
18. Thakur KT, Probasco JC, Hocker SE, et al. Ketogenic diet for adults in super-refractory status epilepticus. Neurology. 2014;82(8):665–70.
19. Chiusolo F, Diamanti A, Bianchi R, et al. From intravenous to enteral ketogenic diet in PICU: a potential treatment strategy for refractory status epilepticus. Eur J Paediatr Neurol. 2016;20(6):843–7.
20. Farias-Moeller R, Bartolini L, Pasupuleti A, et al. A practical approach to ketogenic diet in the pediatric intensive care unit for super-refractory status epilepticus. Neurocrit Care. 2016;26(2):267–72.
21. Appavu B, Vanatta L, Condie J, et al. Ketogenic diet treatment for pediatric super-refractory status epilepticus. Seizure. 2016;41:62–5.
22. Orlowski JP, Erenberg G, Lueders H, Cruse RP. Hypothermia and barbiturate coma for refractory status epilepticus. Crit Care Med. 1984;12(4):367–72.
23. Yang X, Wang X. Potential mechanisms and clinical applications of mild hypothermia and electroconvulsive therapy on refractory status epilepticus. Expert Rev Neurother. 2015;15(2):135–44.
24. Corry JJ, Dhar R, Murphy T, Diringer MN. Hypothermia for refractory status epilepticus. Neurocrit Care. 2008;9:189–97.
25. Guilliams K, Rosen M, Buttram S, et al. Hypothermia for pediatric refractory status epilepticus. Epilepsia. 2013;54(9):1586–94.
26. Lin JJ, Lin KL, Hsia SH, Wang HS. Therapeutic hypothermia for febrile infection-related epilepsy syndrome in two patients. Pediatr Neurol. 2012;47(6):448–50.
27. AIF S. College guidelines on electroconvulsive therapy: an update for prescribers. Adv Psychiatr Treat. 2005;11(2):150–6.
28. Ferlisi M, Shorvon S. The outcome of therapies in refractory and super-refractory convulsive status epilepticus and recommendations for therapy. Brain. 2012;135(Pt 8):2314–28.
29. Lomber SG, Payne BR, Horel JA. The cryoloop: an adaptable reversible cooling deactivation method for behavioral or electrophysiological assessment of neural function. J Neurosci Methods. 1999;86(2):179–94.
30. Shin HW, O'Donovan CA, Boggs JG, et al. Successful ECT treatment for medically refractory nonconvulsive status epilepticus in pediatric patient. Seizure. 2011;20(5):433–6.
31. Fountain NB. Status epilepticus: risk factors and complications. Epilepsia. 2000;41(Suppl 2):S23–30.
32. Legriel S, Mourvillier B, Bele N, et al. Outcomes in 140 critically ill patients with status epilepticus. Intensive Care Med. 2008;34:476–80.
33. Legriel S, Azoulay E, Resche-Rigon M, et al. Functional outcome after convulsive status epilepticus. Crit Care Med. 2010;38:2295–303.
34. Rossetti AO, Hurwitz S, Logroscino G, Bromfield EB. Prognosis of status epilepticus: role of aetiology, age, and consciousness impairment at presentation. J Neurol Neurosurg Psychiatry. 2006;77:611–5.
35. Scholtes FB, Renier WO, Meinardi H. Generalized convulsive status epilepticus: causes, therapy, and outcome in 346 patients. Epilepsia. 1994;35:1104–12.
36. Jehi L, Najm IM. Sudden unexpected death in epilepsy: impact, mechanisms, and prevention. Cleve Clin J Med. 2008;75(Suppl2):s66–70.

37. Téllez-Zenteno JF, et al. Sudden unexpected death in epilepsy: evidence-based analysis of incidence and risk factors. Epilepsy Res. 2005;65(1–2):101–15.
38. Ficker DM, et al. Population-based study of the incidence of sudden unexplained death in epilepsy. Neurology. 1998;51(5):1270–4.
39. Tellez-Zenteno JF, Ronquillo LH, Wiebe S. Sudden unexpected death in epilepsy: evidence-based analysis of incidence and risk factors. Epilepsy Res. 2005;65:101–15.
40. Wasterlain CG, Fujikawa DG, Penix L, et al. Pathophysiological mechanisms of brain damage from status epilepticus. Epilepsia. 1993;34(Suppl 1):S37–53.
41. Engrand N, Crespel A, et al. Pathophysiologic basis of status epilepticus. Rev Neurol (Paris). 2009;165(4):315–9.
42. Garzon E, Fernandes RM, Sakamoto AC. Analysis of clinical characteristics and risk factors for mortality in human status epilepticus. Seizure. 2003;12(6): 337–45.
43. Hocker S. Systemic complications of status epilepticus—an update. Epilepsy Behav. 2015;49:83–7.
44. Hampel KG, Jahanbekam A, Elger CE, et al. Seizure-related modulation of systemic arterial blood pressure in focal epilepsy. Epilepsia. 2016;57(10):1709–18.
45. Freeman R, Schachter SC. Autonomic epilepsy. Semin Neurol. 1995;15:158–66.
46. Oppenheimer SM, Gelb A, Girvin JP, et al. Cardiovascular effects of human insular cortex stimulation. Neurology. 1992;42:1727–32.
47. Manno EM, Pfeifer EA, Cascino GD, Noe KH, et al. Cardiac pathology in status epilepticus. Ann Neurol. 2005;58(6):954–7.
48. Surges R, Taggart P, Sander JW, et al. Too long or too short? New insights into abnormal cardiac repolarization in people with chronic epilepsy and its potential role in sudden unexpected death. Epilepsia. 2010;51(5):738–44.
49. Metcalf CS, Poelzing S, Little JG, et al. Status epilepticus induces cardiac myofilament damage and increased susceptibility to arrhythmias in rats. Am J Physiol Heart Circ Physiol. 2009;297(6):H2120–7.
50. Bealer SL, Little JG, Metcalf CS, et al. Autonomic and cellular mechanisms mediating detrimental cardiac effects of status epilepticus. Epilepsy Res. 2010;91(1):66–73.
51. Britton J, Gheating GR, Benarroch EE, et al. The ictal bradycardia syndrome: localization and lateralization. Epilepsia. 2006;47:737–44.
52. Zubair S, Arshad AB, Saeed B, et al. Ictal asystole-late manifestation of partial epilepsy and importance of cardiac pacemaker. Seizure. 2009;18:457–61.
53. Lee DJ, Amini M, Hamamura MJ, et al. Aquaporin-4-dependent edema clearance following status epilepticus. Epilepsy Res. 2012;98(2–3):264–8.
54. Seitelberger F, Lassmann H, Hornykiewicz O. Some mechanisms of brain edema studied in a kainic acid model. Acta Neurobiol Exp (Wars). 1990;50(4–5):263–7.
55. Lechner C, Auer D, Kümpfel T, et al. Prolonged non-convulsive status epilepticus as an early clinical manifestation of epilepsy in connection with HIV infection—case report with EEG and MRI follow-up. Fortschr Neurol Psychiatr. 1998;66(7):326–30.
56. Bailey B, Blais R, Letarte A. Status epilepticus after a massive intravenous N-acetylcysteine overdose leading to intracranial hypertension and death. Ann Emerg Med. 2004;44(4):401–6.
57. Schuele SU. Effects of seizures on cardiac function. J Clin Neurophysiol. 2009;26:302–8.
58. Mukherjee S, Tripathi M, Chandra PS, et al. Cardiovascular autonomic functions in well-controlled and intractable partial epilepsies. Epilepsy Res. 2009;85(2–3):261–9.
59. Brambrink AM, Dick WF. Neurogenic pulmonary edema. Pathogenesis, clinical picture and therapy. Anaesthesist. 1997;46(11):953–63.
60. Johnston SC, Horn JK, Valente J, Simon RP. The role of hypoventilation in a sheep model of epileptic sudden death. Ann Neurol. 1995;37(4):531–7.
61. Heled Y, Zarian A, Moran D, et al. Exercise induced rhabdomyolysis-characteristics,mechanisms and treatment. Harefuah. 2005;144(1):34–38, 7O.
62. Seyal M, Bateman LM, Albertson TE, et al. Respiratory changes with seizures in localization-related epilepsy: analysis of periictal hypercapnia and airflow patterns. Epilepsia. 2010;51(8):1359–64.
63. Nguyen TT, Hussain E, Grimason M, et al. Neurogenic pulmonary edema and acute respiratory distress syndrome in a healthy child with febrile status epilepticus. J Child Neurol. 2013;28(10):1287–91.
64. Surges R, Thijs RD, Tan HL, et al. Sudden unexpected death in epilepsy: risk factors and potential pathomechanisms. Nat Rev Neurol. 2009;5(9):492–504.
65. So EL, Sam MC, Lagerlund TL. Postictal central apnea as a cause of SUDEP: evidence from near-SUDEP incident. Epilepsia. 2000;41(11):1494–7.
66. Walczak T, et al. Do antiepileptic drugs play a role in sudden unexpected death in epilepsy? Drug Saf. 2003;26(10):673–83.
67. Kumar G, Kalita J, Misra UK. Raised intracranial pressure in acute viral encephalitis. Clin Neurol Neurosurg. 2009;111(5):399–406.
68. Worthley LI, Thomas PD. Treatment of hyponatraemic seizures with intravenous 29.2% saline. Br Med J (Clin Res Ed). 1986;292(6514):168–70.
69. Sharf RE. Seizure from hyponatremia in infants. Early recognition and treatment. Arch Fam Med. 1993;2(6):647–52.
70. Sakellaridis N, Pavlou E, Karatzas S, et al. Comparison of mannitol and hypertonic saline in the treatment of severe brain injuries. J Neurosurg. 2011;114:545–8.
71. Francony G, Fauvage B, Falcon D, et al. Equimolar doses of mannitol and hypertonic saline in the treatment of increased intracranial pressure. Crit Care Med. 2008;36:795–800.
72. Harutjunyan L, Holz C, Rieger A, et al. Efficiency of 7.2% hypertonic saline hydroxyethyl. Starch 200/0.5 versus mannitol 15% in the treatment of increased

intracranial pressure in neurosurgical patients—a randomized clinical trial [ISRCTN62699180]. Crit Care. 2005;9:R530–40.
73. Ichai C, Armando G, Orban JC, et al. Sodium lactate versus mannitol in the treatment of intracranial hypertensive episodes in severe traumatic brain-injured patients. Intensive Care Med. 2009;35:471–9.
74. Kamel H, Navi BB, Nakagawa K, et al. Hypertonic saline versus mannitol for the treatment of elevated intracranial pressure: a meta-analysis of randomized clinical trials. Crit Care Med. 2011;39:554–9.
75. Kerwin AJ, Schinco MA, Tepas JJ III, et al. The use of 23.4% hypertonic saline for the management of elevated intracranial pressure in patients with severe traumatic brain injury: a pilot study. J Trauma. 2009;67:277–82.
76. Bennett TD, Statler KD, Korgenski EK, et al. Osmolar therapy in pediatric traumatic brain injury. Crit Care Med. 2012;40:208–15.
77. Wang Y, Liu PP, Li LY, et al. Hypothermia reduces brain edema, spontaneous recurrent seizure attack, and learning memory deficits in the kainic acid treated rats. CNS Neurosci Ther. 2011;17(5):271–80.

9 Complications and Other Conditions in Refractory Status Epilepticus That Require Attention

Shengnian Zhou and Xinshi Wang

Abstract

Refractory status epilepticus (RSE) is one of the most common diseases seen in neurological intensive care and is associated with a high mortality rate. Complications in epilepsy, including fever, acidosis, blood pressure disorders, and brain edema, are often directly implicated in the death of affected patients. They are therefore key factors that contribute to the failure of antiepileptic treatments. In this chapter, we focus on rare complications in RSE. These include hyponatremia and rhabdomyolysis as well as other conditions that require attention, such as malnutrition, in patients with status epilepticus (SE), status epilepticus caused by alcohol withdrawal syndrome (AWS), and sudden unexpected death in epilepsy (SUDEP). We explore the underlying pathogenesis and treatments for these conditions and describe the measures used to control their relevant complications with the aim of reducing mortality and greatly improving the survival rate and quality of life of affected patients.

9.1 Hyponatremia in Patients with Status Epilepticus

9.1.1 Introduction

Hyponatremia in patients with SE attracts less attention in the clinic. A severe and acute drop in sodium levels has been reported as a metabolic cause of status epilepticus. With numerous physiologic changes occurring in the background of SE, hyponatremia induced by cerebral salt-wasting syndrome (CSWS) within the first 24 h of SE onset is also common in SE patients. Carbamazepine (CBZ) or oxcarbazepine (OXC) for the treatment of epilepsy also increases the

S. Zhou (✉)
Department of Neurology, Qilu Hospital of Shandong University and Brain Science Research Institute, Shandong University, 107 Wenhuaxi Road, Jinan, Shandong 250012, China
e-mail: zhoushengnian126@126.com

X. Wang, Ph.D.
Department of Neurology, The First Affiliated Hospital of Wenzhou Medical University, Nanbaixiang Street, Ouhai District, Wenzhou City, Zhejiang Province 325015, China

X. Wang, S. Li (eds.), *Refractory Status Epilepticus*, DOI 10.1007/978-981-10-5125-8_9

possibility of hyponatremia in SE patients. Oxcarbazepine is the most common antiepileptic drugs (AEDs) used to induce the syndrome of inappropriate antidiuretic hormone (SIADH) and hyponatremia. The differentiation between CSWS- and SIADH-induced hyponatremia is important because each condition is treated differently.

9.1.2 Definition

Sodium is one of the most important cations in the human body. The normal concentration of serum sodium is 135–145 mmol/L. Hyponatremia is defined as sodium levels less than 135 mmol/L [1]. Acute hyponatremia (<48 h) is more serious and recognizable than chronic hyponatremia (>48 h) [2]. The main clinical symptoms of hyponatremia are nervous and muscle system disturbances. Falling sodium levels lead to a decrease in extracellular osmolality and cell swelling. If the latter occurs in a cavity with a fixed volume, such as the brain, the resultant increase in intracranial pressure causes a series of central nervous system symptoms, such as headache, nausea, vomiting, fatigue, restlessness, disorientation, and seizures. Severe acute hyponatremia may lead to cerebral herniation, followed by convulsions, coma, permanent brain damage, apnea, or even death. Falling sodium levels cause reductions in extracellular sodium concentrations and subsequent decreases in action potential amplitude. If these changes occur in skeletal muscle cells, patients may suffer from fatigue. If these changes occur in gastrointestinal smooth muscle cells, patients may develop nausea and vomiting [3].

9.1.3 Historical Evolution and Epidemiology

In 1986, Tilelli et al. [4] identified cases of girls suffering from hypoglycemia with SE. These patients who reported drinking large quantities of water were diagnosed with water poisoning hyponatremia and secondary SE. In the 1995, Farrar et al. [5] reported that the incidences of hyponatremic SE in infants and young children were 56% and 27%, respectively, which represented the first clinical trial data supporting hyponatremic SE. Since then, there have been reported cases of mental illness in elderly patients with secondary hyponatremic SE due to polydipsia, and these cases were primarily categorized as complex partial SE [6–8]. Although hyponatremia is one of the most common metabolic disorders after SE, it was not until 2005 that clinical trial data were available, revealing that the risk of hyponatremia was 34.5% within 24 h after RSE [9].

9.1.4 Etiology Classification of Hyponatremia

In patients with central nervous system disorders, the three main etiologies of hyponatremia are osmotic diuresis, SIADH, and CSWS. The differentiation between CSWS and SIADH is important because each condition is treated differently.

SIADH is due to inappropriately elevated antidiuretic hormone levels caused by an expanded effective arterial blood volume. CSWS is caused by the renal loss of sodium, resulting in a decrease in the effective arterial blood volume and thus providing a baroreceptor stimulus for vasopressin release. Distinguishing CSWS from SIADH relies primarily on the presence of hypovolemia and a negative salt balance.

SIADH is characterized by a low serum sodium level, a high urinary sodium level, inappropriately concentrated urine compared to serum osmolality, and the absence of peripheral edema or dehydration with no adrenal, thyroid, or renal dysfunction.

CSWS clinically manifests as polyuria, excessive urinary sodium loss resulting in extracellular fluid loss, dehydration, and hyponatremia. CSWS is defined by the following criteria: hyponatremia (serum sodium <130 mmol/L), increased urinary sodium (>120 mmol/L), increased urine osmolarity (>300 mOsm/kgH_2O), increased urine volume (>3 mL/kg/h), and negative fluid balance during the last 24 h. The most important element of treatment is to replace the volume and sodium loss.

9.1.5 Hyponatremia-Induced SE

Hyponatremia is a well-known etiology and/or aggravating factor for generalized tonic-clonic seizures. Notably, the severity of hyponatremic SE depends primarily on both the severity and the acuity of the decline in sodium levels rather than the degree of the drop. Zelano et al. [10] artificially established acute hyponatremia in C57/BL6 mice via intraperitoneal injection of 1-deamino-8-D-arginine vasopressin and water loading, resulting in a serum sodium level of 125–130 mmol/L. EEG (electroencephalogram) showed an enhanced frequency of epileptiform spikes in the hyponatremic mice, and electrographic seizures were found in 5/9 hyponatremic mice. Kainic acid injection in hyponatremic mice significantly increased the duration of electrographic seizure activity, which was also observed after diazepam treatment.

9.1.5.1 Hyponatremic SE in Infants

In infants with SE, hyponatremia is an important etiological factor. In early 1995, Farrar et al. [5] reviewed 59 infants (<2 years old) and reported that the incidence of hyponatremic seizures in infants without other causes of seizures was 56%. Hyponatremic seizures are usually shown as generalized seizures. Seizure duration was approximately 30 min in patients with hyponatremic seizures and 17 min in normonatremic patients. The incidence of SE was 73% in hyponatremic patients and 36% in normonatremic patients.

Sharf et al. [11] also found that in 56 infants (<1 year old) with first-time seizures, 15 (27%) had hyponatremic seizures. Risk factors for hyponatremic seizure include age less than 6 months, recent febrile illness, status epilepticus, hypothermia, hyperglycemia, the absence of evidence of trauma, and formula with solute-poor fluid.

Hyponatremic SE is also induced by the intentional ingestion of water by a child as a form of punishment. A 5-year-old girl was forced to drink a significant amount of water as a punishment measure by her mother. She has severe failure to thrive; her weight, height, and bone age were similar to that of 2.5-year-old girl. She was unconscious and only responsive to deep pain; she had hypertonic extensor posturing. Her serum sodium level had dropped to 107 mmol/L, indicating severe hyponatremic SE and acute water intoxication. After 3% saline was administrated, her sodium levels returned to normal. She regained consciousness and the seizure activity stopped [4].

9.1.5.2 Hyponatremic SE in Polydipsia

Generalized nonconvulsive SE has also been attributed to hyponatremia in elderly patients, particularly in those with a polydipsia background. Polydipsia and polyuria are prevalent in psychiatric patients. Some polydipsic patients develop water intoxication and brain swelling. Primavera et al. [6] reported that a 53-year-old woman had three episodes of absence SE as a result of polydipsia-hyponatremia. She suffered confusion with slowing of mentation and automatism after episodes of compulsive water drinking and abuse of diuretics. Her serum sodium levels dropped to 90–98 mmol/L. During her hospitalization, repeated EEGs showed continuous or paroxysmal generalized 3 Hz sharp waves intermixed with irregular spikes, indicating recurrent absence SE. Electrolyte infusion and water restriction increased her serum sodium levels to 136–138 mmol/L, and her EEG and symptoms improved. Another 57-year-old man who had the habit of drinking large amounts of water suffered two absence status episodes and recovered after sodium infusion treatment. His EEG showed continuous spiking and slow wave complexes bilaterally over the frontal area in both episodes, and some spikes appeared in the left frontal area after recovery from absence status. Polydipsia-hyponatremia is believed to be involved in epileptogenicity in the left frontal lobe, when followed by generalized focal activity and absence status [8].

Barolomei et al. [7] described a patient with complex partial SE who recovered fully when unexplained hyponatremia was corrected. A 68-year-old man experienced two syncopal attacks before admission. He was admitted for recent-onset fatigue with muscle cramps and weakness. Two days later, he suffered confused and unresponsive to simple instructions. Laboratory tests demonstrated hyponatremia at a concentration of 117 mmol/L. His EEG showed continuous and irregular spikes and slow waves in the left hemisphere. Complex partial SE provoked by hyponatremia was considered after excluding other seizure causes. Saline was administered to correct the hyponatremic SE. His EEG gradually returned to normal, accompanied by increasing sodium levels. On the fourth day, his serum sodium levels rose to 138 mmol/L. The patient fully regained consciousness, and his EEG was completely normal.

9.1.6 SE-Induced Hyponatremia

Considering the numerous physiologic changes in blood pressure, electrolytes, glucose, hypophysis function, etc., the appearance of hyponatremia is not surprising during status epilepticus. The potential mechanism may involve seizures evoking ANP (atrial natriuretic peptide) and BNP (brain natriuretic peptide) secretions, which increase urinary sodium excretion and aldosterone, resulting in CSWS [12].

Tolunay et al. [13] reported two children with SE who developed CSWS. One patient was a 12-year-old boy with epilepsy and cognitive and motor retardation; he was admitted and received intravenous midazolam because of SE. He had serum sodium levels of 122 mmol/L, urine sodium levels of 100 mmol/L, a urine output of 7 mL/kg/h, a blood osmolarity of 270 mOsmol/kg, and a urine specific gravity of 1030; based on these values, he was diagnosed with CSWS caused by SE after excluding other possible causes of hyponatremia. Intravenous fluid and 3% hypertonic saline solution were administered, but he showed little improvement; thus, fludrocortisone (0.1 mg/12 h) was added. His laboratory tests showed recovery (sodium, 138 mmol/L; urine output, 2 mL/kg/h; urine sodium, 25 mmol/L) after 13 days of administration. Another 10-year-old boy with refractory epilepsy and severe mental retardation developed resistant hyponatremia (sodium, 120 mmol/L). He had a high urine output of 6 mL/kg/h, high urine sodium levels of 150 mmol/L, and a high urine specific gravity of 1025. When other possible causes of hyponatremia were excluded, SE-induced CSWS was considered. A 3% hypertonic saline solution was administered intravenously, and appropriate volume replacement was initiated. CSWS was resolved on the eighth day of follow-up with normal serum sodium, urine output, and sodium levels.

Holtkamp et al. [9] found that hyponatremia within the first 24 h of SE onset occurred significantly more often in refractory SE patients (10/29, 34.5%) than in non-refractory SE patients (6/44, 13.6%). These patients did not receive CBZ, OXC, or other drugs possibly inducing hyponatremia. The authors indicated that hyponatremia occurring early in SE progression may promote the development of refractoriness.

9.1.7 AED-Induced Hyponatremia Induces Increasing Seizures

9.1.7.1 Carbamazepine

CBZ is one of the most common AEDs that causes hyponatremia in patients with epilepsy at a rate of 1.8–40% depending primarily on the studied epileptic patient population. An increase in seizure frequency, which is one clinical manifestation of CBZ-induced symptomatic hyponatremia, may develop into SE in epileptic patients [15, 16].

Kuz et al. [15] reported a 44-year-old woman who developed acute hyponatremia and experienced subsequent generalized tonic-clonic seizures after mistakenly taking 600 mg of CBZ, which is twice of her usual evening dosage. On admission, her CBZ concentration was 8.6 mg/mL, and her serum sodium level was 122 mmol/L. An infusion of 0.9% saline was administrated, and her serum sodium levels increased to 136 mmol/L within 24 h. Holtschmidt et al. also reported a 54-year-old woman taking

CBZ (600 mg, then 200 mg) for 6 weeks who suddenly suffered from a generalized seizure. Laboratory tests showed that she had a serum sodium level of 125 mmol/L. EEG revealed a left temporal focus with slow waves. The patient quickly recovered to a sodium level of 137 mmol/L after 63 days of treatment. Unfortunately, her EEG was no longer normal after hyponatremia recovery.

9.1.7.2 Oxcarbazepine

Clinical trials have shown that OXC causes hyponatremia at a rate of 23–73.3% [16]. Importantly, OXC treatment for refractory SE increases the risk of hyponatremia. Kellinghaus et al. [17] identified 13 patients (median age 79 years) who were treated with OXC for refractory SE. Relevant hyponatremia was observed in three of the patients, in whom the minimum sodium serum levels were 112, 121, and 125 mmol/L.

As early as 1987, Johannessen et al. [18] reported that a 4-year-old OXC-treated (46 mg/kg) patient with epilepsy experienced increases in seizure frequency due to hyponatremia (sodium values not described). In 2014, Kim et al. [14] observed that 6.8% ($n = 69$) of patients in a larger sample of 1009 OXC-treated patients with epilepsy developed symptomatic hyponatremia, including increasing seizures ($n = 26$).

9.1.7.3 Possible Mechanisms Underlying CBZ-/OXC-Induced Hyponatremia

The mechanisms underlying CBZ-/OXC-induced hyponatremia have not been fully elucidated. SIADH is believed to be an important factor in the development of CBZ-/OXC-induced hyponatremia [19]. Kloster et al. [19] reported two CBZ-/OXC-treated epileptic patients who experienced sudden death. A 45-year-old man with epilepsy was treated with 1800 mg/d of OXC 5 days before his death. An autopsy revealed that his sodium level was 117 mmol/L, his blood osmolality was 240 mOsmol/kg, his urine sodium was normal, and his urine osmolality had increased (406 mOsmol/kg). Another 30-year-old epileptic man was treated with OXC (1500 mg/d) for 2 years before his death. An autopsy showed a serum sodium level of 124 mmol/L, a urine osmolality of 911 mOsmol/kg, a urine sodium level of 63 mmol/L, and an OXC concentration of 112 μmol/L.

9.1.8 Treatment

9.1.8.1 Treatment of Hyponatremic SE

Hyponatremic seizures are more difficult to treat. A 3% bolus of saline is effective and safe for treating hyponatremic seizures among infants; early use decreases morbidity from antiseizure therapy. Three of seven hyponatremic infants given a 3% bolus of saline required intubation [11]. Worthley et al. [20] gave five patients with severe hyponatremic epileptiform seizures 50 mL of 29.2% saline (250 mmol) by central venous catheter. Ten minutes later, their seizures were completely controlled, and the mean serum sodium level increased by 7.4 mmol/L. Further saline was then administered over 10 h, increasing the serum sodium level by 2–14 mmol/L/h until it reached 133 mmol/L.

9.1.8.2 Treatment of CBZ-/OXC-Induced Hyponatremia

Checking baseline serum sodium levels and regularly performing sodium tests during the first 3 months after initiating CBZ/OXC treatment is recommended. Treatment is focused on the removal of risk factors, fluid restriction, dosage reduction, or drug discontinuation [21]. Risk factors that increase the rate of CBZ-/OXC-induced hyponatremia include old age, high dosages, low-baseline serum sodium concentrations, the concomitant use of medications associated with hyponatremia, and female gender [21].

9.1.9 Conclusion

SE and hyponatremia comorbidity is not uncommon in clinical settings, indicating that the causal relationship is the prerequisite regarding the development of treatment programs. First, a systematic laboratory check is necessary, including serum sodium, urinary sodium, plasma osmolality, urinary excretion, and urine specific gravity analyses. Second, these parameters should be combined with the patient's age, history of water consumption, and intake of drugs known to cause hyponatremia, especially OXC, CBZ, and so on.

Clinicians should recommend the appropriate treatment based on individual causes. In some cases, symptoms can disappear in the short term after appropriate treatment is administered, but serious cases can lead to death or irreversible neurological disease.

9.2 Rhabdomyolysis Induced by Refractory Status Epilepticus

9.2.1 Introduction

RSE is one of the most serious neurological illnesses; currently, it is primarily treated using drugs. Anti-status epilepticus drugs and seizures can both cause rhabdomyolysis. This paper summarizes the related factors of rhabdomyolysis that are caused by commonly used antiepileptic drugs and status epilepticus itself to understand and learn the laws of its occurrence and the effects of the prevention and treatment of status epilepticus.

9.2.2 Definition and Historical Evolution

Necrosis of various causes in the skeletal muscle leads directly to the release of muscle cell contents into the blood, including myoglobin, creatine kinase (CK), and lactate dehydrogenase; this phenomenon is known as rhabdomyolysis [22]. In 1965, Diamond et al. [23] first reported on the relationship between status epilepticus and rhabdomyolysis. In 1979, MacDonald et al. [24] reported the relationship between rhabdomyolysis and renal dysfunction. In 1987, Rasmussen et al. [25] reported a case of rhabdomyolysis after grand mal epilepsy. In 1988, Murray et al. [26] systematically summarized the characteristics of rhabdomyolysis caused by status epilepticus, emphasizing the role of myoglobin in causing acute renal failure after seizures. Since then, status epilepticus and anti-status epilepticus drug-induced rhabdomyolyses have received extensive attention.

9.2.3 Epidemiology

Clinical data and statistics are relatively rare because the diagnostic criteria for rhabdomyolysis syndrome are not universally unified. Some patients with mild rhabdomyolysis may not be diagnosed. Therefore, prospective studies related to the incidence of rhabdomyolysis syndrome are rare and unreliable [27]. Approximately 26,000 individuals are suspected to have rhabdomyolysis every year in the United States [28, 29]. Chamberlain et al. [30] found that four out of 1500 pediatric patients who came for consultations were diagnosed with rhabdomyolysis syndrome. A retrospective study on pediatrics reported a rhabdomyolysis syndrome recurrence rate of 5% over 6 years [31]. A study of 475 patients who were diagnosed with rhabdomyolysis suggested that 11% of patients with rhabdomyolysis will relapse [32]. Mackay et al. [33] reported a similar recurrence rate. Currently, although many cases of rhabdomyolysis caused by status epilepticus and antiepileptic status drugs have been reported, the incidence of rhabdomyolysis associated with status epilepticus remains unknown because of the small number of patients and the lack of systematic analyses and prospective investigations.

9.2.4 Etiology Classification of Rhabdomyolysis

9.2.4.1 Rhabdomyolysis Caused by Status Epilepticus

Seizures that lead to rhabdomyolysis are common in status epilepticus [34, 35]. Status epilepticus can cause excessive muscle fiber stretch, leading to striated muscle damage. Simultaneously, the body produces a large amount of heat, degrading enzyme activity increases, and skeletal muscle integrity is destroyed, which affects Na^+-K^+ ATPase and Na^+-Ca^{2+} exchange. This causes extracellular sodium, calcium influx, cell content leakage (enzymes, potassium ions, phosphate ions, lactate, myoglobin, etc.), and increased intracellular free calcium; moreover, calcium-dependent protease and phospholipase are activated, leading to muscle cell damage and consequent rhabdomyolysis.

In 2015, Yamazaki et al. [36] reported a patient with status epilepticus-induced rhabdomyolysis. Within 3 h of recurrent seizures, the 24-year-old male epilepsy patient experienced a loss of consciousness, glazed eyes, twitching limbs, tongue biting, and no incontinence. Each episode lasted 5–10 min for a total of five episodes with intermittent disturbance of consciousness. The patient was diagnosed with status epilepticus and immediately received 2 mg of midazolam via intravenous injection; the patient no longer had convulsions, and consciousness was gradually restored. After discharge, the patient had aggravated lower back pain and oliguria, was diagnosed with "acute kidney injury," and was hospitalized. His CK increased to 4807 IU/L after admission, and his urine volume increased gradually after hemodialysis and fluid therapy. In 2008, Kreft et al. [37] reported on two children with fatal rhabdomyolysis syndrome following refractory status epilepticus. The two children were admitted to the hospital after seizures; they received tracheal intubation and midazolam administration, according to the guidelines for antiepileptic drug management by the Danish Paediatric Society. One day after the termination of their seizures, both children had a sharp increase in CK values, manifested as limb pain and weakness, which later developed into rhabdomyolysis, followed by the emergence of acute renal failure. Despite active hemodialysis, the patients finally developed disseminated intravascular coagulation (DIC) and died. Guven, Navarrete, Navarro, and Sato have also reported similar cases.

9.2.4.2 Related Antiepileptic Drugs

The main drugs that can induce rhabdomyolysis syndromes include statins, other lipid-lowering drugs, and psychotropic substances [38]. Rhabdomyolysis syndromes caused by anti-status epilepticus drugs have recently become an issue [39].

Phenytoin

Phenytoin has been used for antiepileptic treatment since 1938. The main side effects include hypersensitivity, gingival hyperplasia, nystagmus, and hematopoietic dysfunction [40]. The first case of rhabdomyolysis caused by phenytoin was reported in 1986 [41]. This case involved a 22-year-old male patient who was taking 300 mg of phenytoin every day. Three months after phenytoin administration, myalgia, fever, and rash appeared. His creatine kinase level was 85,000 IU/L at admission and then increased to 242,000 IU/L, and his urine color appeared brown. He was diagnosed with phenytoin-induced rhabdomyolysis. Phenytoin was discontinued after complications occurred. The patient received 30 mg of methylprednisolone bolus and intravenous pulse therapy with 30 mg of methylprednisolone for 3 days, which was then changed to 100 mg of oral prednisone every day; hormone therapy was gradually stopped beginning on the seventh day after admission. The patient's condition improved gradually. Santos-Calle et al. [42] reported a 46-year-old patient with the sudden onset of generalized tonic-clonic seizures at home. An intravenous infusion of 250 mg of phenytoin was administered after emergency endotracheal intubation and mechanical ventilation, and the serum drug concentration was within the valid range. The CK value reached 54,000 IU/L 5 days later (presumably because of the phenytoin). After the withdrawal of phenytoin, the CK value decreased to 14,229 IU/L and gradually returned to normal, followed by the disappearance of symptoms. The laboratory examination and clinical symptoms supported the diagnosis of phenytoin-induced rhabdomyolysis syndrome. In 2016, Hyunjin Kim et al. [43] reported a case of status epilepticus with phenytoin treatment that caused rhabdomyolysis. A 37-year-old man visited the emergency center after three events of generalized tonic-clonic seizures without recovery of consciousness between the seizures. Upon admittance to the emergency center, his blood pressure was 125/55 mmHg, his heart rate was 112/min, and his body temperature was 37.2 °C. The patient was intubated, and lorazepam 4 mg was injected twice. Next, 20 mg/kg phenytoin was given, while 24-h EEE was simultaneously monitored. The patient regained consciousness, and no additional clinical seizures were observed after phenytoin treatment. In initial laboratory tests, his creatine kinase was elevated to 727 IU/L, but his estimated glomerular filtration rate (eGFR), blood urea nitrogen (BUN), and creatinine (CRE) levels were within normal ranges (eGFR, 70 mL/min/1.73 m^2; BUN, 13 mg/dL; creatinine, 1.31 mg/dL). Because the levels of CK and creatinine increased to 1823 IU/L and 2.93 mg/dL, respectively, on the second day of hospitalization, massive hydration with bicarbonate therapy was initiated to treat acute kidney injury. Serum CK decreased to 824 IU/L transiently after starting hydration, but it increased again on the sixth day of hospitalization, and his serum CK levels peaked at 3825 IU/L on the seventh day of hospitalization. Because phenytoin might be the cause of rhabdomyolysis, phenytoin was substituted with levetiracetam on the seventh day of hospitalization. Subsequently, serum CK levels promptly decreased and normalized by day 13. In the present case, the second increase in CK levels on the seventh day after the last seizure could not be explained by the seizure itself. CK levels were normalized after phenytoin discontinuation; thus, we diagnosed the cause of the second rise in CK levels as rhabdomyolysis by phenytoin.

Propofol

Propofol was approved by the Food and Drug Administration (FDA) in 1989, and it is currently used to treat a growing number of patients with status epilepticus [44]. During use, propofol infusion-related syndrome (PRIS) may appear. The symptoms include hyperkalemia, heart failure, metabolic acidosis, rhabdomyolysis, and related signs and symptoms that cannot be explained by other causes but occur in response to long-term use or high doses of propofol. In 1992, Parke et al. [45] reported on a pediatric patient who presented with PRIS after being administered propofol at 7.5–10 mg/kg/h for 66–115 h. Zaccheo et al. [46] found that propofol infusion-related syndrome will occur when high doses of propofol (more than 4 mg/kg/h) are administered for long periods (greater than 48 h) of time. Diaz et al. [47] revealed the incidence, risk factors, and biomarkers of propofol infusion-related syndrome in a 1-year retrospective investigation. The incidence of PRIS was 4.1%, and the mortality rate was 33%. Propofol infusion syndrome appears over time, and triglyceride levels are correlated positively with these measures. In 1998, Hanna et al. [48] found that the administration of propofol for refractory status epilepticus could induce progressive hypoxia, metabolic acidosis, and rhabdomyolysis in adolescents and children. One of the patients was a 17-year-old male who was first administered 80 mg of propofol at a rate of 167 μg/kg/min in the first hour, which was then increased to 147 mg/kg/min and again increased to 292 mg/kg/min. The patient presented with severe low oxygen, dark brown urine, and CK levels of 83,000 IU/L after 44 h. Propofol was disabled when a total dose of 19,275 mg (482 mg/kg) had been administered. The patient died 84 h later, and an autopsy showed rhabdomyolysis syndrome. In another case, a 7-year-old male was first administered propofol at 33.3 mg/kg/min, which was then increased to 449 mg/kg/min. The patient presented with brown urine, and his CK levels were 49,992 IU/L after 38 h of propofol administration. Then, 63 h later, propofol was discontinued and after a total dose of 35,330 mg (1275 mg/kg) had been administered. The autopsy revealed the presence of rhabdomyolysis syndrome. Some experts believe that the propofol dosage should be limited to 67 μg/kg/min in children with a severe illness [49]. Zarovnaya et al. [50] reported an adult patient with epilepsy who presented with PRIS after propofol treatment. In 2015, Zhou et al. [39] described the most recent case of propofol-induced rhabdomyolysis syndrome. In this case, a 54-year-old female patient was scheduled for a hysterectomy, but shortly after the induction of anesthesia with propofol, the patient began exhibiting rhabdomyolysis. The patient experienced extensive skeletal and cardiac dissolution; although active treatment was provided, she eventually died. When propofol infusion-related syndrome occurs, propofol should be immediately discontinued, and cardiopulmonary support, the application of hemodialysis, and plasmapheresis should be initiated immediately [51].

Levetiracetam

Levetiracetam (an acetyl pyrrolidine compound) is a novel, comparatively recent, clinical antiepileptic drug. In December 1999, the FDA of the United States formally approved levetiracetam as an adjunctive therapy in adults (over 16 years of age) with partial seizures. This indication was expanded to children over 4 years old in June 2005 [52]. Akiyama et al. [53] reported a 29-year-old female patient with a previous history of epilepsy. The patient was stably treated with oral valproic acid (1000 mg/d) and Clobazam (20 mg/d). After an epilepsy relapse, the patient was treated with levetiracetam (1000 mg/d) and valproic acid (800 mg/d) on the third day post-admission. On the fourth day post-admission, the patient presented with back muscle pain and lower extremity weakness, and the symptoms gradually worsened. A laboratory examination revealed that the CK values were greater than 2410 IU/L. Levetiracetam was discontinued immediately, and the use of sodium valproate (800 mg/d) was continued. Muscle pain and weakness immediately improved after levetiracetam discontinuation, and serum CK quickly returned to normal levels. Based on these clinical and laboratory data, the rhabdomyolysis in this patient was attributed to levetiracetam.

Valproate

Valproate was first applied clinically in 1963. Because of its high blood-brain barrier permeability and low toxicity, this drug is often prescribed to children. The side effects mostly include a gut reaction, pancreatitis, liver damage, headache, nystagmus, ataxia, and dizziness [54].

Roodhooft et al. [55] first reported a case of valproic acid overdose in a child in 1990. The child presented with progressive unconsciousness, no urine, rhabdomyolysis, and renal failure. In 1997, Pinkston et al. [56] reported that one patient appeared drowsy and complained of a headache after a 500 mg dose of valproic acid. Within 24 h, the patient had no urine output, and the laboratory CK value was 1242 IU/L. The authors believed that the rhabdomyolysis was related to valproate toxicity. Kottlors et al. [57] reported a case of one patient with Carnitine palmitoyltransferase type II (CPTII) defect who presented with rhabdomyolysis after treatment with valproic acid. Deficiencies in patients with CPTII can include intermittent myoglobinuria and even rhabdomyolysis. The patient's use of valproate resulted in the appearance of rhabdomyolysis and acute renal failure. We believe that patients with CPTII deficiencies (which are typically the result of a serine to leucine mutation at position 113) should use valproate with caution. Wieser et al. [58] also support this view and suggest that when using valproic acid therapy in high-risk rhabdomyolysis patients, carnitine treatment should be included. In addition to adults, newborns can present with rhabdomyolysis caused by valproic acid. Valproic acid is also used to treat bipolar disorder or prevent migraines and may result in rhabdomyolysis. Thus, CK levels should be closely monitored to facilitate early rhabdomyolysis treatment.

9.2.5 Clinical Manifestations

Rhabdomyolysis has many types of clinical manifestations, from a single asymptomatic elevation in serum CK to severe electrolyte imbalance, cardiac arrhythmia, acute renal failure, DIC, and other symptoms [59]. Symptoms are related to the extent and area of muscle damage.

9.2.5.1 Main Symptoms

1. Acute or subacute myalgia
2. Urinary pigmentation
3. Muscle weakness

However, the probability of presenting with a simultaneous triad in one person is less than 10% [60]. In addition, many nonspecific symptoms are associated with rhabdomyolysis, including muscle pain, swelling, nausea, vomiting, weakness, fever, and delirium.

9.2.5.2 Complications

Acute Renal Failure

Acute renal failure is the most serious complication of rhabdomyolysis and has an incidence rate of 14–46%. Tubular necrosis can occur as a result of the accumulation of myosin. Pediatric patients with rhabdomyolysis have a higher rate of acute renal failure, ranging from 42 to 50%. When the serum CK level reaches 5000–15,000 IU/L, the occurrence rate of acute renal failure is 35%. When the serum CK is >15,000 IU/L, the rate is 70% [61]. The main mechanisms of acute renal failure are (1) renal vasoconstriction and renal ischemia, (2) myoglobin tube formation, and (3) myoglobin cytotoxicity [62].

Compartment Syndrome

Compartment syndrome is not uncommon when there is rhabdomyolysis. Most skeletal muscle tissue is enclosed in an inelastic space composed of bones, fascia, and other structures. Compartment syndrome is usually more likely to occur in the limb muscle gap, such as the upper limb biceps muscle gap and triceps gap, forearm dorsal wrist and extensor digitorum gap, hip muscle gap, front and rear thigh gap, etc [27]. Cells are damaged when rhabdomyolysis occurs, followed by an influx of calcium and sodium and a large amount of extracellular fluid into the cells, leading to local edema and an increase in intramuscular pressure. The increase in internal muscle pressure not only hinders the blood supply for local muscle tissue, but it also hinders venous blood reflux, which further increases tissue edema. In addition, local ischemia can increase the permeability of the capillaries, further aggravate edema, and form a vicious circle. Clinical manifestations of compartment syndrome include local limb pain, pale color, and weakened or undetectable pulse. Sensory and motor dysfunction may occur following severe limb ischemia [63].

Electrolyte Imbalance

Other complications include hypercalcemia (late), hypocalcemia, hyperphosphatemia, hyperkalemia, etc. Hyperkalemia (serum potassium levels >5.0 mmol/L) can lead to fatal arrhythmias. Nearly all (98%) of potassium in the body is stored in cells, and skeletal muscle cells accounted for 60–70% of human cells. Therefore, even if there is 100 g of skeletal muscle necrosis in the short term, serum potassium levels can also increase by 1 mmol/L. Organic acid-induced metabolic acidosis will further aggravate hyperkalemia. Hypocalcemia often occurs in the early stages of rhabdomyolysis and may aggravate the cardiotoxic effects of hyperkalemia. Patients with serum potassium levels less than 6.0 mmol/L are often asymptomatic, whereas serum potassium levels greater than 6.0 mmol/L require urgent treatment. High blood potassium electrocardiogram may have the following changes: high, sharp acute T wave and shortening of the Q-T interval. Some of the more serious cases can display a flat P wave, widened QRS, ventricular arrhythmias, etc. Broken skeletal muscle cells can also release inorganic phosphorus and lead to hyperphosphatemia, causing the formation of calcium phosphate deposition in the damaged muscle cells and other tissues, which further increases hypocalcemia. However, the calcium in the cytoplasm of myocytes can be released into the plasma in the process of RM, which may cause high blood calcium later [64–66].

9.2.6 Diagnostic Criteria

9.2.6.1 Clinical Manifestations

The possibility that anti-status epilepticus drugs can cause rhabdomyolysis is the most important consideration for the early diagnosis of rhabdomyolysis syndrome. Only 10% of patients present with all symptoms of the triad. Thus, physicians should be more concerned about the presence of other nonspecific symptoms. A detailed neuromuscular examination, blood pressure, sensory disturbances, and muscle strength and muscle volume abnormalities can all provide an important diagnostic basis.

9.2.6.2 Laboratory Examination

The serum CK level is an important consideration for diagnosis. It is generally accepted that levels more than five times higher than normal are problematic although there is no consensus on the diagnostic criteria [67]. CK values can also predict the occurrence rate of acute renal failure. The kidneys can be easily damaged when CK >5000 IU/L. CK levels should be detected using a urine dipstick regardless of whether myoglobinuria is positive. Myoglobinuria is also important evidence supporting a diagnosis of rhabdomyolysis syndrome, but rhabdomyolysis cannot be excluded when urine is negative for myoglobin. Myoglobin concentrations will return to normal levels within 6–8 h because the half-life of myoglobin is shorter than that of serum CK during muscle injury. Therefore, the serum myoglobin levels are not as sensitive as the serum CK levels. In some patients with rhabdomyolysis syndrome, electrolyte levels and renal function are abnormal when muscle destruction releases large quantities of creatine, which is converted into creatinine in the blood, leading to a greater rise in creatinine than urea nitrogen. Thus, a decrease in the BUN/creatinine ratio can help differentiate rhabdomyolysis from other causes of renal failure [68].

9.2.6.3 Pathology

A muscle biopsy can identify the interstitial infiltration of inflammatory cells and the disappearance of striated muscle tissue [69]. A renal biopsy may show myoglobin casts within the distal nephron, epithelial cell shedding, and proximal tubular necrosis when the disease is associated with acute renal failure. Monoclonal antibodies will also be positive [68].

9.2.6.4 Imaging

B-mode ultrasound or magnetic resonance imaging can show local tissue swelling, which is used to detect muscle necrosis. These imaging modalities can also detect the degree of muscle damage, range, and liquefaction situation. Imaging is a noninvasive method that can diagnose muscle necrosis [70].

9.2.7 Treatment

9.2.7.1 General Treatment

Patients should undergo electrocardiography (ECG) and EEG monitoring [71], close observation of vital signs and changes in state of consciousness, and regular measurement of body temperature every day; these data should be recorded.

9.2.7.2 Treated with Convulsions

Patients with status epilepticus should be closely observed for changes in their condition and should be given drug treatment; a detailed record of the number and duration of seizures in patients should be maintained. The safety of the patients should be closely monitored through the placement of guard rails and protective belts to prevent falling off the bed and the self-removal of intravenous tubes and other tubes in the stomach, catheters, etc. The airway must be kept open to prevent tongue bites. Convulsions will increase secretions; thus, it is necessary to aspirate in a timely manner and turn the head to one side [72, 73].

9.2.7.3 Rehydration Therapy

Patients with rhabdomyolysis require rehydration to maintain blood volume, improve renal ischemia, prevent kidney damage, increase the glomerular filtration rate, and dilute myoglobinuria to prevent tube formation [74]. Therefore, rehydration is one of the most important treatment measures; it is also key to the prevention and treatment of renal failure. In the process of rehydration, patients should be closely observed for the appearance of chest tightness, suffocation, palpitations, and other symptoms. In particular, during the first 30 min when drugs are administered, the infusion rate should be controlled, and the patient should be closely observed. Timely symptomatic treatment can prevent the occurrence of adverse consequences if an exception occurs [75, 76].

9.2.7.4 Prevention of Acute Renal Failure

The urine and electrolyte balance must be monitored. Close observation of the patient's urine color and urine output can be conducted through storing urine samples and comparing them to previous samples. We can identify changes in renal function based on urine volume and color. A change in urine color from light to dark or even to a soy sauce color suggests that the condition is deteriorating. The timely detection of blood BUN, blood electrolytes, creatinine, and the endogenous creatinine clearance rate is necessary for the early detection of renal failure and early treatment [23, 24, 77].

9.2.7.5 Alkaline Urine

Urine and plasma pH levels should be maintained at <6.5 and <7.5, respectively, to avoid the blockage of renal tubules [76].

9.2.8 Prognosis

The prognosis of rhabdomyolysis primarily depends on the complications presented and their underlying causes. The patient's prognosis is good when the syndrome is treated promptly and properly, whereas the patient's prognosis is poor if the syndrome further develops into acute renal failure. The mortality rate of rhabdomyolysis is 8–10% [48]. However, the mortality rate can reach up to 42% when associated with acute renal failure. The mortality rate of rhabdomyolysis in children is 7–10% [31].

9.2.9 Conclusion

SE and AEDs both can induce rhabdomyolysis. Understanding their association will facilitate a rational approach for the clinical use of these drugs. Rhabdomyolysis is characterized by the emergence of unpredictable adverse reactions. The early detection, diagnosis, and treatment of rhabdomyolysis are key to avoiding mortality.

9.3 Nutritional Assessments in Refractory Status Epilepticus Patients

9.3.1 Introduction

Malnutrition is an independent risk factor for clinical adverse outcomes in patients with RSE. On the one hand, it is difficult for patients with acute stage RSE to intake food because of dysphagia or disturbance of consciousness; on the other hand, many antiepileptic drugs can suppress appetite, interfere with the absorption of nutrients, and even cause nausea, vomiting, constipation, and other side effects, leading to problems regarding nutrient and energy intake and metabolism; thus, malnutrition is more obvious in RSE patients. Nutritional problems directly affect the prognosis of RSE patients. Thus, they are important clinical problems requiring attention.

9.3.2 Historical Evolution and Epidemiology

The investigation of Guigoz et al. [78, 79] found that in common neurological disease inpatients, the incidence rate of malnutrition risk was 46.5%, the rate of malnutrition was 15.8%, and the incidence rate of malnutrition in refractory status epilepticus patients was as high as 40% [80]. On the one hand, during a sustained state of refractory seizures, patients cannot eat; they may have difficulty swallowing or experience vomiting, resulting in reduced dietary intake. On the other hand, the long-term use of antiepileptic drugs will also affect energy or nutrient intake and metabolism; therefore, the risk of malnutrition in patients can increase significantly because antiepileptic drugs may suppress appetite and interfere with the absorption of nutrients, resulting in the decreased uptake of foods or nutrients such as iron and zinc [81]. Simultaneously, many antiepileptic drugs have side effects such as drowsiness, nausea, vomiting, and constipation, which interfere with the intake of nutrients. Anticonvulsants also interfere with the metabolism of certain vitamins such as calcium and folic acid. Carbamazepine, ethosuximide, phenobarbital, phenytoin, valproate, and other drugs can inhibit intestinal calcium transport and can interfere in the synthesis of vitamin D [82]. Lipid oxidation as an independent predictor of seizure frequency was significantly increased in patients with refractory seizures [83]. A study found that patients with epilepsy were underweight and had a smaller upper arm circumference than normal [84]. Therefore, it is difficult for patients with refractory status epilepticus to avoid nutritional deficiencies.

Leibovitz et al. [85] found that serum albumin levels directly affect the prognosis of patients and are closely related to neonatal intensive care unit (NICU) hospitalization time, the total length of hospital stay, increased hospital consumption, etc. An increased risk of undernutrition was associated with increased mortality in hospitalized patients [86]. Reasonable clinical nutrition support can reduce mortality and complications in the treatment of refractory status epilepticus in patients with nutritional deficiencies, thus improving the success rate and quality of life of the patient [87]. Consequently, it is imperative to increase focus on the nutritional conditions of refractory epilepsy patients and improve nutritional risk screening and nutrition management. Emphasis should also be placed on using effective assessment methods and tools for "fast, objective, comprehensive, and accurate" assessments to achieve early detection.

9.3.3 Nutritional Assessment Tools and Methods

Currently, the application of nutrition assessment tools in clinical work includes a single index and a composite index. The single index has certain limitations: it can only reflect the nutritional status of a patient from the past or at a certain period of time in the present. Thus, in recent years, research has primarily focused on the composite index screening tool to improve the sensitivity and specificity of screening.

9.3.3.1 Human Body Measurement Index

Anthropometric measurements are suitable for the assessment of short-term and long-term nutritional status. They are convenient, inexpensive, and noninvasive [88]. Existing ergonomic indicators include weight, body mass index (BMI), arm and calf fat measurements, and body composition measurements:

1. Body weight assessment is the earliest used ergonomic evaluation index [89]. Short-term weight change is a benign index of fluid balance changes, whereas long-term changes in body weight (such as 5% weight loss within 1 month of admission or 10% weight loss within 6 months of admission) can infer a general nutritional status change, suggesting the need for a further nutritional assessment [88].
2. BMI is an indicator of weight and height that is closely related to total body fat. The advantages of BMI include ease of use, no need for in-depth procedures, and good specificity and sensitivity [90, 91].
3. Upper arm circumference and calf circumference are important indicators of nutritional status [92]. The upper arm measurements include triceps skinfold (TSF) thickness, arm circumference (AC), and arm muscle circumference (AMC) measurements. TSF is used to measure subcutaneous fat thickness and reflects body fat storage, whereas upper arm AC and AMC reflect changes in protein content and storage of skeletal muscle in vivo. Notably, people of different races and regions have certain differences in their diagnostic values of upper arm circumference. Researchers of different countries use different cutoff values of the upper arm and calf in the diagnosis of patients with malnutrition. For example, the Canadian researcher Campillo [93] used an upper arm circumference cutoff of 26.9 cm, whereas the Swiss researcher Guigoz [94] believed that the cutoff was 22 cm. The body composition analysis method is generally applied in the clinic because it is noninvasive and simple, provides abundant information, and is easily accepted by doctors and patients; however, it requires some technical equipment that can increase the economic burden on patients.

9.3.3.2 Laboratory Biochemical Indexes

Clinical laboratory biochemical parameters include plasma protein, metabolite determination, and immune function evaluation. Plasma proteins commonly used include albumin, prealbumin, transferrin, and retinol-binding protein. Prealbumin and retinol-binding protein are sensitive markers of the early diagnosis of acute malnutrition:

1. Albumin: currently, the most commonly used clinical determination for the prognosis of patients (such as mortality, complication rate, etc.) is the serum albumin level. Risk evaluation is very important, but because of the long half-life (20 days) of serum albumin [95], it is not specific for the diagnosis of malnutrition; thus, its clinical application is limited. Seres [96] noted that all visceral proteins should be questioned for their reliability. Therefore, no single visceral protein measurement can be used as a nutritional assessment for patients.
2. Metabolite indexes: creatinine height index (CHI), nitrogen balance, 3-methyl histidine, urinary hydroxyproline, and blood and urine creatinine.
3. CHI is an indicator to observe muscle protein consumption and a sensitive index to measure protein levels. However, CHI is susceptible to a variety of factors, such as advanced age, muscular dystrophy, renal insufficiency, being long-term bedridden, catabolic state, high animal protein diet, and other factors [95].
4. Nitrogen balance: reflects whether the protein intake meets the needs of the body for protein synthesis and catabolism; it is the most common indicator of protein nutritional status evaluation. For hospitalized patients, the goal is to maintain a positive nitrogen balance (2–4 g/d); if the patient is in an acute catabolic state, the goal is to reduce the occurrence of a negative nitrogen balance [95].
5. Immunologic function test: usually evaluated by total lymphocyte count and the intensity of delayed skin hypersensitivity [95], but the application is limited, and the results are easily influenced by many factors [97]. This test is not applicable in liver cirrhosis patients and patients undergoing chemotherapy, so the clinical application value of immune function is small.

Laboratory biochemical examination is mainly used to identify early malnutrition, distinguish malnutrition types, and provide objective indicators. For all anthropometric measurements, laboratory biochemical examinations of patients with nutritional deficiencies provide a nonspecific diagnosis; thus, a nutritional status assessment should be combined with patient history and clinical data [88].

9.3.4 Composite Nutritional Assessment Tools and Methods

9.3.4.1 Nutritional Risk Screening (NRS)-2000

The nutritional risk screening (NRS)-2002 is summarized from 128 randomized controlled trials by Espen that used evidence-based medical methods; it was published in 2003. This table is recommended by most researchers as a new nutritional assessment tool for hospitalized patients [98]. There are more studies confirming that, combined with the Chinese BMI normal value, the NRS-2002 applies to more than 99% of Chinese inpatients [99]. Compared to other screening tools, the NRS-2002 has a high sensitivity to critically ill patients with nutritional risk screening [100]. It includes four aspects: anthropometric measurement, recent weight change, dietary intake, and severity of disease. The NRS-2002 has simple, noninvasive, strong operability characteristics; it can detect whether the current patient has nutritional deficiencies as well as assess whether the patient has a nutritional risk and decide whether to provide nutritional support. Notably, the NRS-2002 method is not suitable for the elderly (>90 years old), those with delirium (refractory status epilepticus), or those who are unable to stand up or have serious chest ascites. Furthermore, reductions in dietary intake and the degree of weight loss are affected by subjective factors, which may reduce the accuracy of the screening results.

9.3.4.2 Malnutrition Universal Screening Tool (MUST)

The malnutrition universal screening tool (MUST) is developed based on a community population [101] and is used to assess the nutritional status of all inpatients. MUST includes three aspects: BMI, weight loss, and disease impact score. Advantages of this tool are that it can be easily and rapidly used, and procedures can generally be completed within 5 min [102]. The results showed that MUST and other tools (mini nutritional assessment, NRS, SGA, etc.) have a good consistency [103] (kappa value range 0.551–0.893). Stratton [102] also noted that MUST is effective in predicting prognosis (mortality and length of stay) in elderly hospitalized patients.

9.3.4.3 Mini Nutritional Assessment (MNA)

The mini nutritional assessment (MNA) is a special method used to evaluate the nutritional status of the elderly [97]. The MNA is suitable not only for nutritional screening but also for nutritional assessment. It is often used in the community, inpatient and elderly outpatients, chronic disease patients, and surgical patients [104]. It includes anthropometric measurements, an overall assessment, a dietary questionnaire, and a subjective assessment of four dimensions of the 18 elements. One study found that the MNA and traditional nutritional assessment methods (BMI, upper arm midpoint circumference, calf circumference, etc.) have good consistency [105]. However, because the MNA includes subjective and objective evaluations, the measurement results may be affected by human error; therefore, operators must receive professional training before conducting the MNA. In 2001, a simpler mini nutritional evaluation method was proposed based on the MNA. The short form of the mini nutritional assessment (MNA-SF) has been validated in various communities in Switzerland and in hospitalized elderly patients [106]. A recent systematic evaluation of the study also noted that for nutritional assessment in elderly patients, the MNA-SF is the most appropriate tool [107]. The method is rapid (within 3 min), noninvasive, and simple, can be repeatedly measured, and can be used to dynamically evaluate the nutritional status of patients. The MNA-SF is effective and practicable; for refractory epilepsy patients and bedridden patients in whom BMI cannot be obtained, small leg or arm circumference can replace the BMI value.

9.3.4.4 Patient-Generated Subjective Global Assessment (PG-SGA)

The patient-generated subjective global assessment (PG-SGA) has good applicability, validity, reliability, specificity, and sensitivity [97]. It includes history of weight change, diet, gastrointestinal symptoms, stress reactivity, etc.; its ergonomic parameters include subcutaneous fat thickness, muscle, and edema measurements [108]. However, the tool focuses on nutrient intake and body composition assessment; it does not consider the intrinsic protein levels, resulting in PG-SGA results with a low correlation to serum ALB levels [108]. To improve its accuracy and reliability and to enhance its ability to predict clinical adverse outcomes of patients, Mariana Raslan [109] noted that the PG-SGA can be combined with NRS-2002 requirements; furthermore, the NRS-2002 should be completed within 48 h of admission. After screening patients for nutritional risk, the PG-SGA is then performed, resulting in an excellent complementary effect of the two assessments.

9.3.5 Conclusion

Refractory status epilepticus is accompanied by malnutrition, leading to adverse outcomes; thus, early detection of nutritional risk and malnutrition has a positive effect on the prevention of complications and outcomes. However, the current general nutritional risk screening and assessment tools have their own advantages. Thus, how to properly use clinical assessment tools, develop a treatment for the early detection of malnutrition risk, and create a nutritional management strategy are worthy of further research.

9.4 A Phenomenon Requiring Attention in the Intensive Care Unit: Acute Alcohol Withdrawal Syndrome

9.4.1 Introduction

Drinking alcohol has become increasingly prevalent worldwide. Alcohol abuse or dependence can cause psychological and physiological dependence. A series of adverse reactions may occur after discontinuing drinking. Severe cases can progress to alcohol withdrawal syndrome, producing delirium tremens (DTs), generalized tonic-clonic seizures, and potentially endangering the patient's life. Intensive care unit (ICU) patients generally must stop drinking passively, which can cause acute withdrawal syndrome, leading to problems for the diagnosis and treatment of the primary disease. Understanding the specific phenomenon in the neuroscience ICU will help us better manage our patients.

9.4.2 Definition

AWS includes a series of adverse reactions that are likely to occur when alcohol is consumed in large quantities for a prolonged period and then abruptly discontinued [110]. The long-term or excessive use of alcohol can increase the body's tolerance and nerve dependence. Without alcohol stimulation, the central nervous system will produce autonomic nerve dysfunction and nerve symptoms, namely, withdrawal symptoms. Mild cases include symptoms of anorexia, nausea, vomiting, palpitations, high blood pressure, anxiety, depression, and bad mood changes. It may become life-threatening in severe cases with delirium tremens, seizures, and other symptoms. Alcohol withdrawal symptoms depend on the last alcohol intake amount rather than the blood alcohol concentration [111]. The metabolic rate of alcohol is 15 mg/dL per hour, independent of the initial concentration. Thus, withdrawal symptoms usually appear 6–72 h after discontinuing drinking, and generalized tonic-clonic seizures usually appear within 24–48 h. However, there are also reports that seizures can occur in the early stage (2 h after discontinuing drinking). Delirium tremens usually occur 48–72 h after discontinuing drinking, but they can be delayed up to 5 days [112].

9.4.3 Historical Evolution and Epidemiology

Early in the dawn of human civilization, the ancient art of wine culture had already sprouted. For thousands of years, as the most influential drink, wine permeated daily life and social, economic, and cultural activities. Moreover, alcohol is a common choice for people to ease the pressure of social life. Consequently, alcohol is the most addictive substance in the world. Drinking induces brain function, cognitive function, and emotional and behavioral changes. There are two billion global drinkers, of whom approximately 140 million are classified as alcohol-dependent individuals [113]. According to the World Health Organization (WHO) "2014 alcohol and health global status report," in 2012, the harmful use of alcohol caused 3.3 million deaths worldwide, accounting for 5.9% of global deaths [114]. In the United States, alcohol dependence occurs at twice the rate of other drugs of abuse, and there were more than 80 million people with alcohol dependence [115].

Alcohol dependence refers to the frequency and amount of alcohol consumed; to a certain extent, the drinkers cannot control their drinking behavior and often experience somatization and alcohol withdrawal symptoms. As a result of alcohol dependence, alcohol withdrawal syndrome occurs in approximately 50% of abstainers [116, 117]. Most patients experience mild withdrawal symptoms such as anxiety and trembling, which can be effectively controlled. However, approximately 5% of patients will experience severe seizures and delirium tremens [117]. Bayard and others [112] noted that, in the United States alone, more than two million people each year are treated for seizures as a result of acute alcohol withdrawal. The possibility of seizures during the period of alcohol withdrawal is approximately 10% [118, 119]. In addition, approximately 3–5% of patients who are treated for alcohol withdrawal symptoms meet the clinical criteria for the diagnosis of delirium tremens [117, 120]. Untreated delirium tremens can reach a mortality of 5–15% [118, 121]. A timely and clear identification of withdrawal symptoms will help patients to navigate the risk period during alcohol withdrawal.

9.4.4 Clinical Features

Alcohol withdrawal syndrome displays a wide variety of symptoms. The severity of the symptoms is related to the alcohol intake, the length between the last time of drinking and the number of previous instances of drinking [111].

9.4.4.1 Simple Withdrawal Symptoms

Simple withdrawal symptoms usually occur 6–36 h after discontinuing drinking [122]. The patient will exhibit a series of autonomic dysfunction symptoms, such as sleep disorders (sleep difficulties, nightmares, shallow sleep), trembling, mild anxiety, gastrointestinal discomfort, headache, sweating, palpitations, anorexia, and other symptoms. These symptoms will gradually disappear in a few days.

9.4.4.2 Withdrawal Seizures

Withdrawal epilepsy refers to the appearance of seizures in chronic alcoholics after absolute or relative drinking prohibition. LaRoche and others [123] believe that withdrawal seizures usually occur 48–72 h after discontinuing drinking. The patients who have a history of long-term high concentrations of drinking or previous withdrawal seizures are more likely to develop status epilepticus, and status epilepticus can also occur 6–48 h after the first drink [124]. The severity of alcohol withdrawal symptoms, EEG abnormalities, and changes in the same type of semi-amino acids will have a certain effect on the prediction of alcohol withdrawal after discontinuing drinking. In 2011, Eyer et al. [125] conducted a study in a large cohort of patients treated for AWS; they found that a significant predictor of withdrawal seizures during AWS therapy was the severity of withdrawal symptoms after admission. EEG plays an important role in the diagnosis of epilepsy. Bleich et al. [126] analyzed 191 patients with withdrawal seizures; 91.4% of those patients found EEG had different degrees of abnormality in their results, which indicates that high homocysteine levels are associated with alcohol withdrawal seizures. Homocysteine levels may be helpful to predict which patients are at risk for first-onset alcohol withdrawal seizures.

9.4.4.3 Delirium Tremens

Delirium is an acute brain syndrome that occurs once individuals with alcohol dependence stop drinking. Delirium tremens is the most severe alcohol withdrawal symptom, and it can be fatal. Delirium patients not only exhibit disturbance of consciousness and increased action and thinking disorders, but they also cannot correctly identify the surrounding environment [127]. Patients with alcohol withdrawal first exhibit tremors; when they occur in the morning, they are called morning tremors. Severe hallucinations with photism and tactile elements may also occur. In 1996, Ferguson et al. [128] analyzed 200 patients with alcohol withdrawal and found that 24% of patients exhibited delirium during hospitalization. A multivariate logistic regression analysis shows that those whose last drinking episode was longer are more prone to delirium tremens. If not accompanied by other influencing factors, the delirium incidence rate was 9%. If there was a precipitating factor, the incidence rate was 25%, and with two types of precipitating factors, it was 54%. Lee et al. [129] showed that a previous history of delirium tremens and a higher pulse rate (more than 100 bpm) were important predictive factors of delirium tremens. In 2011, Eyer et al. [125] conducted a study in a large cohort of patients treated for AWS. Significant predictors at admission for the occurrence of DTs were lower serum potassium, a lower platelet count, and the presence of structural brain lesions. A recent prospective study about the severity of alcohol withdrawal symptom scale prediction of alcohol withdrawal severity scale (PAWSS) showed that the PAWSS includes useful psychological characteristics and has a good predictability, which can help clinicians identify complex alcohol withdrawal symptoms for the timely prevention and treatment of AWS [130].

9.4.5 Pathogenesis

9.4.5.1 Central Neurotransmitter Mechanism

Alcohol is a fat-soluble neurotrophic substance that can penetrate the blood-brain barrier, inhibiting the central nervous system. Large amounts of alcohol can cause acute alcohol poisoning, and long-term drinking can result in alcohol abuse and dependence. In the central nervous system, related transmitters such as γ-aminobutyric acid (GABA), glutamate, and dopamine participate in the formation of this process.

Neurotransmitter Mechanisms Related to Withdrawal Seizures

When a small dose of ethanol reaches the blood, it can inhibit the inhibitory effect of GABA on the brain and show exciting benefits. However, high doses directly inhibit the central nervous system, causing lethargy and coma. Long-term exposure to alcohol can increase the effect of GABA on the GABA receptor and reduce the binding of glutamate and the *N*-methyl-D-aspartic acid (NMDA) receptor. Thus, a reduced excitatory stimulus response occurs with later episodes of alcohol drinking. Brain GABA-A receptors decrease compensatively, and the number of NMDA receptors increases, thus increasing the tolerance to alcohol; likewise, blood alcohol levels must increase to maintain the same effect [131, 132]. The occurrence of seizures is closely related to the excitatory neurotransmitter glutamate and its receptor. Long-term drinking can inhibit the combination of glutamate and its receptor. Conversely, upon discontinuing drinking, the inhibitory effect of alcohol diminishes, and the excitatory effect of glutamate becomes hyperactive, leading to ion changes in Na^+, Ca^{2+} flow, and K^+ efflux, producing depolarization. The ion imbalance causes seizures [133].

The Neurotransmitter Associated with Delirium Tremens

Under normal physiological conditions, the function of two neurotransmitter systems, GABA and dopamine, is antagonistic in the nigrostriatal system. The dopamine system in the brain is the most important euphoric area and includes the midbrain ventral tegmental area (VTA) and the nucleus accumbens (NAC). Addictive drugs can increase the level of the dopamine in the two regions, producing a euphoric feeling [134]. Long-term alcohol consumption exposes dopamine neurons to long-term stimulation with alcohol; thus, their reactivity and sensitivity decrease. Upon discontinuing drinking, the function of dopamine neurons will rebound. Heinz et al. [135] noted that increasing dopamine activity can lead to more severe withdrawal symptoms. Clements [136] also stressed that the high concentrations of dopamine in the synapse during the process of neural signal transmission can cause severe withdrawal symptoms. In addition, delirium tremens of alcohol withdrawal is closely related to the polymorphism of dopamine-related genes. In 2010, Munster et al. [137] found that dopamine transporter gene SLC6A3 can reduce the risk of delirium and dopamine receptor DRD2 genes are related to the occurrence of delirium [138].

9.4.5.2 Neuroendocrine Mechanism

Tremors are the most common symptom of comprehensive abstinence syndrome. Discontinuing drinking makes the central and peripheral nervous beta-adrenergic receptors hyperactive, blood catecholamines increase, and the skeletal muscle contraction rate increases, interfering with the transmission of nerve-muscle, or muscle spindle activity, resulting in an increase of tremor strength. A series of autonomic dysfunctions appear after discontinuing drinking because of sympathetic nerve activity, which weakens the inhibition of the central nervous system.

9.4.6 Treatment

The primary method of treatment is to relieve symptoms. The clinical symptoms in patients with alcohol withdrawal differ, and the risk of withdrawal seizures and delirium tremens must be properly assessed in each patient. The early treatment and prevention of severe symptoms and maintaining normal vital signs are important.

9.4.6.1 Benzodiazepines

Benzodiazepines have strong inhibitory effects on the central nervous system and can enhance the inhibitory effect of GABA neurotransmission and synapses, which promotes its receptor-binding function, improves the symptoms of alcohol withdrawal and duration, and delays progress to withdrawal seizures and delirium tremors. As early as 1969, a study about benzodiazepines in the management of alcohol withdrawal syndrome identified its role as a first-line therapy in the treatment of alcohol withdrawal [139]. A long-term benzodiazepine such as diazepam has the advantages of a fast-acting time and a long half-life. It does not need to be combined with other drugs [140]. Muzyk et al. [140] showed that compared to traditional treatment, diazepam can effectively improve alcohol withdrawal symptoms, including delirium tremens. However, absorption by intramuscular injection is not stable. Because it is metabolized in the liver, diazepam can damage the liver function. Compared to diazepam, lorazepam does not undergo the same degree of metabolism in the liver, but its onset time is slow. Stehman et al. [141] compared the effects of diazepam, lorazepam, and alprazolam on alcohol withdrawal syndrome. The results showed that lorazepam was the weakest and alprazolam had the strongest effect.

9.4.6.2 Barbiturates

Barbiturates work by enhancing the function of central GABA (extending Cl^- channel opening time, increasing Cl^- flow); the excitatory responses after depolarization can be reduced or blocked in the corresponding receptor of glutamate, causing central inhibition [142]. Thus, it can be used for alcohol withdrawal, but supporting evidence is limited [143, 144]. When barbiturates are used simultaneously with any type of benzodiazepine, they can enhance the inhibitory effect of the latter. Gold et al. [145] selected 54 patients in clinical trials; the results showed that for delirium tremens in patients, the combination of the two drugs can reduce the time of mechanical ventilation and hospitalization of patients. Recently, Askgaard et al. [146] compared 1063 patients receiving long-term benzodiazepine chlorodyne treatment with 1365 patients receiving phenobarbital treatment and found that phenobarbital did not reduce the risk of alcohol relapse, but it reduced the mortality rate.

9.4.6.3 Propofol

Propofol is a nonbarbiturate anesthetic that has antiepileptic effects. It has stable, obvious, and rapid effects in the induction of anesthesia, a short half-life, rapid recovery of consciousness, and few respiratory and cardiac side effects, and it can reduce the metabolism of brain tissue and intracranial pressure. Because propofol can enhance GABA-mediated presynaptic or postsynaptic inhibition and reduce excitatory neurotransmitter (such as glutamate and aspartate) release, it plays a role in antiepileptic mechanisms [131]. In view of the above reasons, propofol can control the symptoms of alcohol withdrawal [147]. There have been some cohort analyses and retrospective studies demonstrating that propofol can be used to treat refractory tremor delirium in patients [148–152]. However, the side effects of propofol cannot be ignored. Compared to the use of benzodiazepines alone, propofol increases the use of benzodiazepines, resulting in increased mechanical ventilation and hospital complications [153].

9.4.6.4 Dexmedetomidine

Patients with alcohol withdrawal syndrome use gamma amino acid agonists, such as benzodiazepines, even if the symptoms are still not completely alleviated after increasing the dose of the drug. At this time, dexmedetomidine may be beneficial to some patients. As an alpha-2 adrenergic receptor agonist, dexmedetomidine should be considered the adjuvant treatment for severe alcohol withdrawal symptoms. Dexmedetomidine can reduce the short-term demand for benzodiazepines and improve the epinephrine-driven hemodynamic parameters of alcohol withdrawal [154].

9.4.6.5 Other Treatment Measures

During the alcohol withdrawal period, the patient must be provided with adequate nutritional support. Thiamine in alcohol withdrawal patients is usually lacking, which leads to the development of Wernicke's encephalopathy, mental abnormalities, ophthalmoplegia, and ataxia. The recommended daily thiamine intake is 1–2 mg [155]. However, with the occurrence of Wernicke's encephalopathy, acute treatment requires initial doses up to 1500 mg [156]. Because chronic alcohol consumption is associated with hyperhomocysteinemia, which is generally considered to be caused by a lack of folic acid, folic acid must be added to the diet [157]. The use of a variety of vitamins can supplement the nutritional deficiencies caused by chronic alcohol consumption. In the process of alcohol withdrawal, patients often encounter a water-electrolyte imbalance. Hypokalemia appears at this time; thus, the timely supplementation of potassium is very important to maintain normal renal function. Hypophosphatemia is common in alcohol withdrawal and should be promptly identified. When the patient is experiencing severe seizures and delirium tremens, mechanical ventilation and monitoring of normal vital signs are necessary to maintain airway patency.

9.4.7 Conclusion

The management of patients with alcohol withdrawal syndrome is also a challenge, particularly in critically ill patients. A correct understanding of the mechanisms of alcohol withdrawal, clinical manifestations, and risk factors is the key for the treatment of patients.

9.5 Refractory Status Epilepticus and SUDEP

9.5.1 Introduction

SUDEP is dissimilar to death caused by status epilepticus. Because of this, the diagnostic criteria for SUDEP need to exclude status epilepticus; however, given that refractory epilepsy is one of the independent risk factors of SUDEP, refractory status epilepticus is one of the most serious outcomes of refractory epilepsy. Therefore, refractory epilepsy may produce SUDEP in the progression of the disease from refractory epilepsy to refractory status epilepticus. At the same time, people with refractory status epilepticus have a higher mortality from SUDEP than other epileptics. Therefore, realizing SUDEP and its relationship to both epilepsy and refractory epilepsy will help us to understand refractory status epilepticus from a different perspective.

9.5.2 Definition

SUDEP refers to deaths that are sudden, unfounded, and nontraumatic or uncomplicated drownings that occur in patients with epilepsy. These deaths do not present with evidence of epileptic seizure and are not caused by status epilepticus. In addition, these deaths are not caused by poisoning or by any anatomical structural abnormalities found on the autopsy after death. Both refractory epilepsy and refractory status epilepticus are independent risk factors for SUDEP.

9.5.3 Historical Evolution and Epidemiology

The concept of SUDEP was first distinguished by the American President George Washington, because of the sudden death of his stepdaughter who had developed refractory epilepsy after a seizure [158]. Although at that time it was controversial that epilepsy could lead to death, the sudden death phenomenon of epilepsy was further confirmed by Bacon [159] in 1868 and was then increasingly valued and standardized.

First proffered by Nashef [160] in 1997, the notion of SUDEP as a criteria-based diagnosis is still in use today as the sudden death of the epileptic, that is, with or without cause, without warning, nontraumatic in nature, and without occult causes. Regarding the actual death, there is neither evidence of a real-time epileptic event nor is it preceded by status epilepticus. In addition, the autopsy results after the death find a lack of evidence to support poisonings or any anatomical structural defect as the cause. It is worth noting that SUDEP has been called as a special cause of death for epileptics that is associated with epilepsy.

The number of people with epilepsy accounts for 0.5–1% of the world's total population. The mortality of patients with epilepsy is 24–28 times higher than that of people who do not suffer from epilepsy. In addition, the mortality of children with epilepsy is 90 times greater than those who are never diagnosed with epilepsy [161, 162]. Approximately 0.4–1 per 1000 of epileptic patients die from SUDEP [163], with a mortality that increases to 9.3% when referring only to patients who have refractory epilepsy (about a third of people with epilepsy develop refractory epilepsy due to various reasons) [164, 165]. SUDEP is also one of the most common causes of death from chronic refractory epilepsy and is the leading cause of death of refractory status epilepticus and drug-resistant epilepsy [166]. The incidence of SUDEP in children with epilepsy is 24–28 times higher than that of other age groups [167–170] and most frequently occurs in persons aged 21–40, of which 31–40-year-olds have the highest incidence. In people with epilepsy in the 15- to 44-year-old age group, the highest incidence of SUDEP was close to 9%, and the reported rate of SUDEP in patients who underwent surgery for refractory epilepsy and still had a recurrence of epilepsy was nearly 50% [171]. In a 10-year follow-up, approximately 1012 children with epilepsy found that in 42 deaths, 11 of those children died from SUDEP. Therefore, SUDEP has become one of the specific causes of death in epileptic children [172].

9.5.4 Pathogenesis

9.5.4.1 Fatal Arrhythmias

Research on the pathogenesis of SUDEP has mostly focused on the complication of the cardiovascular system [173]. In a retrospective study of SUDEP in patients with epilepsy, 11 patients had generalized tonic-clonic seizures (GTCS), and during the process of the seizure, the heart and respiratory rates increased, which then developed into a central apnea and significant bradycardia. One clinic found that during a seizure episode, nearly every type of arrhythmia can appear [174–176]. The insula controls the autonomic nervous system, which is composed of the visceral sensory cortex, the cingulate gyrus, and the prefrontal cortex. The hypothalamus is the secondary center of neuroendocrine function and the autonomic nervous response. The connection of the amygdala to the prefrontal cortex in addition to the subcortical part of the limbic system is responsible for the integration of the autonomic nervous system's response to emotion. These structures are part of a common cause of sexual epilepsy. Therefore, a series of changes in the autonomic nervous system can be observed when epileptic seizures (especially partial seizures) occur [177, 178]. For example, patients whose seizure activity is monitored can present with an accompanying arrhythmia, and generalized tonic-clonic seizures have a higher probability of serious arrhythmia than complex partial seizures [179, 180]. The sensitivity of baroreceptors may also be associated with SUDEP, despite the acute reactivity of common pressure sensors, but SUDEP occurs because of heart rate variations that result from the chronic response of the vagus nerve. In addition, all the factors that resulted in cardiac death, such as inflammation, fever, and high levels of C-reactive protein, may increase the risk for SUDEP [181].

In addition, certain genetic defects can cause arrhythmias and include short or long QT syndrome, Brugada syndrome, or catecholamine-induced polymorphic ventricular tachycardia. The KCNQ1 and KCNH2, RyR2, and SCN1A genes have a dual effect on the heart and brain, and some of those genes are associated with sodium-calcium ion channels [181]. Seizures with excitatory responses in the sympathetic division are simultaneously accompanied by aggregation of the solute of the muscle and excessive parasympathetic tone, which are all likely causes of SUDEP. In experimental epileptic animal models, it was observed that the brain released signals that directly connected to the cardiac autonomic nervous system, which would induce arrhythmias. For example, the stimulation of the parasympathetic nervous system can induce a sensation of euphoria after seizures that can cause cardiac arrest, excessive activation of baroreceptors, etc. Increased levels of cardiac catecholamines can be one of the main causes of cardiac damage after a seizure. This idea is unique as the cause of myocardial ischemia in patients with atherosclerosis but can also increase the risk for SUDEP in people with epilepsy. Other possible mechanisms for SUDEP include arrhythmia, ion channel disease, nerve conduction block, or specific exogenous factors or all of the above caused by or during the use and withdrawal of epileptic drugs [181].

Ryvlin [182] conducted a systematic retrospective survey on SUDEP patients over a 2-year period across 160 epilepsy centers in Europe, Israel, Australia, and New Zealand. The results showed that, out of 147 epilepsy centers that responded to the survey, 29 epileptic patients died from cardiopulmonary arrest, and 16 patients died from SUDEP with cardiopulmonary arrest. The survey also showed that, in epileptic patients who suffered a cardiopulmonary arrest, at least ten of those patients' arrests were due to secondary GTCS that caused an increase in respiratory frequency (18–25 breaths per min) and a short period (within 3 min) of cardiopulmonary dysfunction. Although this was a short period of dysfunction, that cardiopulmonary dysfunction recurred within 11 min after the seizures, which eventually lead to suffocation and cardiac arrest [182].

9.5.4.2 Lethal Respiratory Arrest

SUDEP is associated with the respiratory system mainly in terms of the resultant respiratory arrest, and laboratory studies have shown that 5-hydroxytryptamine (5-HT) serotonin receptors are associated with breathing in patients with epilepsy. 5-HT receptors can increase the respiratory dynamics and the body's sensitivity to hypercapnia, while simultaneously reducing the incidence of apnea.

Central and obstructive apnea, acute neurogenic pulmonary edema, hypoxia, and laryngospasm are causes of SUDEP that occur in people with epilepsy. Central apnea is particularly important since clinical observations have suggested that a period of central apnea that lasts for just 10 s may induce 40% of the seizures in people with epilepsy [183]. Similarly, central apnea is regulated by large amounts of substances including adenosine, which is an anesthetic neurotransmitter that affects calcium efflux and is produced after the occurrence of epilepsy and, after the onset of epilepsy, may appear "close" to the brain and may also include the cessation of respiratory function [184]. A specific explanation may be that the function of monoamine neurons includes these 5-HT serotonin neurons which are lost after an epileptic seizure, and the failure of these single amine neurons is simultaneous when central apnea is associated with a lower arousal level in the postictal state. These two kinds of clinical symptoms appear in SUDEP [181]. In addition, the clinical pathological changes in neurogenic pulmonary edema can be found in a large number of patients with SUDEP; the mechanism is likely to produce continuous seizures with systemic vasoconstriction, while simultaneously causing excessive stimulation of the sympathetic nervous system associated with the actual epileptic seizure, which causes increased pulmonary vascular resistance and finally progressed into pulmonary edema [185]. In addition to epileptic seizures, concurrent subarachnoid hemorrhage, brain damage, and hypoventilation can also lead to acute pulmonary edema [186].

9.5.4.3 The Endocrine and Microenvironmental Disorders

Studies have found that in the process of status epilepticus, the endocrine system secretes multiple hormones that can lead to microenvironmental changes. These changes may promote the mechanism for the occurrence of SUDEP. For example, adrenocorticotropic hormone, prolactin, oxytocin, vasopressin, cortisol, and adrenaline are all secreted in patients with tonic-clonic seizure activity (especially status epilepticus) [171, 187, 188]. The secretion of hormones lowers the body's pH, and there is a characteristic hyperkalemia and acidosis that is caused by status epilepticus [189, 190]. The acid environment in vivo can induce cardiac excitability and can produce changes in the heart rate, myocardial infarction, and even bradyarrhythmia or tachyarrhythmia, which promote the occurrence of SUDEP [191, 192]. In addition, the latest research has also confirmed that the onset of autonomic dysfunction is associated with episodes of hypoxemia after a seizure. Long-term damage of parasympathetic tone will increase the likelihood that patients will experience SUDEP [193].

9.5.4.4 SUDEP-Related Genes

Research has shown that some genes may be associated with SUDEP and may be biological risk assessment indicators for the clinical presentation of SUDEP in epileptic patients. Most of these genes are commonly related genes of either the brain and cardiac or the brain and respiratory systems. For example, the KCNA1 gene is responsible for encoding one part of a voltage-gated potassium channel called the Kv1.1 alpha subunit, and laboratory studies have found that when they knocked out the KCNA1 gene in rats, they not only seized, but 75% of the rats died within 10 weeks. The experimental rats also presented with atrioventricular blocks and cardiac abnormalities, such as paroxysmal bradycardia [194]. The SCN1A gene is responsible for encoding one part of a voltage-gated sodium channel called the Nav1.1 gene, whose mutation has been confirmed to be one of the main causes for SUDEP in Dravet syndrome (infant severe myoclonic epilepsy) and in generalized epilepsy in patients with febrile seizures [195, 196]. The SCN5A [197, 198] and SCN8A (encoding the Nav1.6 alpha subunit of nerve cells through voltage-gated sodium channels) [199], the HCN2 (encoding hyperpolarization-activated nucleotide-gated potassium channel) [200], the KCNQ1 gene (encodes voltage-gated potassium channels, the Kv7.1 alpha subunit,which can activate the slow delayed potassium rectifier current and may be associated with congenital long QT syndrome) [201, 202], and the KCNH2 gene (encoding proteins that are associated with congenital long QT syndrome) [203], the PRRT2 gene (encodes genes that regulate the release of neurotransmitter protein genes) [204, 205], and the RYR2 (encoding ryanodine receptor-mediated Ca^{2+} release in cardiac cells) [206], have been confirmed in reports to be associated with SUDEP in laboratory animal models or in clinical epilepsy patients. Recently, researchers used second-generation sequencing technology to conduct gene analysis to screen potential genes that may be associated with SUDEP, which included FBN1, HCN1, SCN4A, EFHC1, CACNA1A, SCN11A, and SCN10A [207].

9.5.5 Clinical Manifestations

SUDEP patients usually have the following clinical characteristics: (1) patients with definitive epilepsy who have died and who have a history of recurrent seizure activity; (2) patients who have died without warning with a relatively stable health status prior to death; (3) patients whose death occurs suddenly, and before the occurrence of a terminal event (death), patients have presented as completely lucid or suffering from other diseases that were controlled or were in remission; (4) patients whose death can be witnessed or not; (5) patients that have seizures prior to the death but this criteria is not required; (6) patients whose surrounding environments are considered safe at the time of death; (7) patients whose deaths are not due to status epilepticus, drowning, or traumatic causes; and (8) patients whose autopsy results are not definitive as to the cause of death [208].

9.5.6 Diagnostic Criteria

Over the past 20 years, both in clinical and scientific research, researchers have studied epilepsy on the basis of the definition of sudden death. Recently, Nashef [209] and other scholars have redefined SUDEP by collecting large amounts of clinical data. Consequently, they have created the unified standards for the identification of SUDEP.

9.5.6.1 Definitive SUDEP

Sudden death, that is, with or without cause, without warning, nontraumatic in nature, and without occult causes that occur in epileptic patients. Death that occurred when the surroundings were safe, death that occurs in epileptic patients without evidence of an epileptic seizure, or death that is not caused by status epilepticus (seizure activity that lasts more than 30 min or multiple seizures of greater than 5-min duration without periods of lucidity) and autopsy results without a clear cause of death.

9.5.6.2 Definitive SUDEP Additional

Meets the diagnostic criteria for definitive SUDEP, but whose death was accompanied by other symptoms of proven non-epileptic seizures before and after death, or the symptoms and the death occurred at the same time, or the autopsy, direct observation, or medical records found the accompanying symptoms of a terminal illness that was not the direct cause of death.

9.5.6.3 Probable SUDEP

Conforms to definitive SUDEP but without confirmation on the autopsy and the accidental death of the epileptic patient whose body is in a stable state, was performing regular activities, and was in safe environment and that the patient has no obvious structural damage to the body that could have led to death.

9.5.6.4 Possible SUDEP

Cannot be ruled out, but there is insufficient evidence to support a diagnosis of SUDEP.

9.5.6.5 Near-SUDEP

The epileptic patient recovered from a cardiopulmonary arrest that occurred for a period of more than 1 h and was confirmed by inspection. The event does not constitute a structural damage that caused the arrest.

9.5.6.6 Non-SUDEP

There is a clear cause that leads to the patient's death.

9.5.6.7 Unclassified

Cannot completely access the information regarding a confirmed diagnosis of SUDEP.

9.5.7 Differential Diagnosis

Epileptic mortality is two to three times that of the general population, and the death of patients with epilepsy can be divided into epilepsy-related death, pathological changes after epilepsy that caused death, and cause of death unrelated to seizures. Among these, SUDEP, status epilepticus, and suicide all belong to accidental deaths in epilepsy [210].

9.5.7.1 Deaths Caused by Status Epilepticus

SUDEP needs to be differentiated from deaths that are caused by status epilepticus. Although status epilepticus is caused by epilepsy, the direct cause of death is status epilepticus, and the morbidity is approximately 10–60 per 100,000, which constitutes approximately 0.5–10% of epilepsy-related mortality [211–213]. There are no significant gender differences, and SE often occurs in older patients (approximately 40% of the SE death rate), and there is a positive correlation between mortality and status epilepticus duration [214, 215]. Short-term mortality (SE attacks within 30 days) is correlated to the severity of the symptoms of SE and other combined causes. Long-term mortality (30 days after the onset of SE and in the subsequent 10 years) is related to the severity of the acute symptoms of SE, the myoclonic seizure activity, and the duration of SE (if more than 24 h). The clinical diagnosis of SE before death can show characteristics of status epilepticus on EEG, which have been clearly shown [216].The main risk factors that cause death include cerebrovascular accident, ischemia anoxic encephalopathy, brain tumors, metabolic disorders, and systemic infection. Secondary risk factors include the decrement of antiepileptic drugs, alcohol, or other organ diseases. Regarding the secondary risk factors, the clinical characteristics of SUDEP include death without a clear etiology, and patients are often found dead in their beds, even if there was evidence that epileptic patients may have had a recent seizure, but before the death without status epilepticus occurred. The incidence of SUDEP is higher in men than in women, and the incidence of SUDEP in patients with symptomatic epilepsy is relatively higher than for patients with cryptogenic epilepsy.

9.5.7.2 Suicide

Suicide is also a common cause of death associated with epileptic patients, and the incidence of suicide accounts for 5–14% of the mortality in epileptic patients. These patients are more easily identified if they have a history of mental illness, especially depression, and use psychotropic drugs [217, 218].

9.5.7.3 Accidental Death

Correlations between epilepsy and larger accidental death include trauma, traffic collisions, high-altitude falls, burns, and submersions. These are fatal events that occur more often in epileptic patients than in ordinary patients [219, 220]. Accidental death in the majority of patients can be because of accidental death after a seizure that occurs at the same time. There may be a clear cause of death, a specific environment and structural damage to the body that is easy to find, making these events easy to distinguish from SUDEP.

9.5.7.4 Death After Surgery for Epilepsy

It is worth mentioning that death associated before and after surgery for the epileptic condition may be directly related to whether the epilepsy was cured or the seizures recurred after the procedure [221]. A large number of investigations on mortality that were based on race, disease characteristics, and different surgical methods concluded that postoperative patients with epilepsy could still experience SUDEP; however, the mortality of SUDEP after surgery in patients with epilepsy has been shown to be less than in nonsurgical patients with epilepsy. Therefore, we can speculate that death after surgery for epilepsy may be due to a variety of other causes.

9.5.8 The Prevention of SUDEP

9.5.8.1 Prevention of SUDEP by Controlling Epilepsy, Refractory Epilepsy, and Refractory Status Epilepticus

A recent survey showed that the incidence of SUDEP in ordinary people is 0.7–1.3 per 1000 and in patients with severe epilepsy (refractory epilepsy or refractory status epilepticus) the risk of SUDEP increases by at least tenfold. Because at least 30% of epileptic patients may develop refractory epilepsy and the independent risk factors of SUDEP are refractory epilepsy, the effect of antiepileptic drugs to reduce the incidence of SUDEP is mainly utilized to reduce the seizure frequency and the drug side effects [222]. Consequently, controlling epilepsy is the primary endpoint in the prevention of SUDEP [223, 224]. Before the combination we could identify patients with epilepsy earlier who may develop refractory epilepsy and adopt other measures as early as possible, such as an early surgical intervention, etc., that may reduce the incidence of SUDEP. Clinical studies have found that in patients with refractory epilepsy, the incidence of SUDEP can be reduced sevenfold when patients use the appropriate doses of their AEDs to treat refractory epilepsy relative to the inappropriate use of AED treatments in patients [225].

9.5.8.2 Adjusting the Cardiovascular System to Prevent SUDEP

The cardiac autonomic nervous response caused by epilepsy may include arrhythmias, such as bradycardia, tachyarrhythmias, cardiac arrest, and heart failure [226, 227]. Therefore, monitoring and evaluating epileptic patients using an ECG is particularly important so as to distinguish long QT syndrome that can be easily misdiagnosed as epilepsy, although some patients may also suffer from long QT syndrome concomitant with epilepsy. These patients have a higher incidence of SUDEP. Therefore, the treatment for long QT syndrome can reduce the incidence of SUDEP. For example, implanting the patient with a cardiac pacemaker to prevent cardiac arrest is one option, but clinical evidence still lacks that epilepsy patients will have a reduced incidence of SUDEP after cardiac pacemaker implantation. Currently, we cannot be certain that in this group of patients with implanted pacemakers, the treatment is helpful for improving the prognosis of patients with epilepsy [173, 174, 177].

9.5.8.3 Adjusting the Respiratory System to Prevent SUDEP

Preventing or reducing the respiratory distress, the hypoventilation, and the hypoxia caused by epilepsy is useful to prevent or reduce reflexes of the secondary autonomic nervous system, cardiovascular abnormalities, and death. In a laboratory study, Bateman [228, 229] found that drugs similar to fluoxetine, a type of selective serotonin reuptake inhibitor (SSRI), could reverse the occurrence of respiratory failure in epileptic animal models. However, there is no direct or current evidence that these drugs can reduce the incidence of SUDEP. Regulation of sleep at night has obvious effects on the reduction of SUDEP [230]. Adjusting the sleeping posture of patients can awaken the patients' consciousness, which stimulates breathing. In one study of 105 patients with generalized tonic-clonic seizures, there were 39 patients who obtained a benefit from sleep regulation, and breathing disorders and postictal generalized electroencephalography suppression (PGES) were significantly reduced [231].

In addition, a portable oxygen saturation monitor can remind the patient and the surrounding family members to improve the patient's ventilation in a timely manner. Positive pressure ventilation equipment for the treatment of patients with obstructive sleep apnea can also help reduce the incidence of SUDEP. Diaphragm pacemakers [231, 232] may also be an effective way to improve hypoventilation after epilepsy [227].

9.5.8.4 Prevention of SUDEP Through Surgical Intervention

Patients with complex partial seizures can treat their epilepsy and prevent SUDEP by electing to have the epileptic foci and part of their frontal or temporal lobe resected, if necessary. There is evidence in multiple clinical case reports to suggest that surgical intervention is positive. In 70 patients with epilepsy, 39 epileptic patients underwent a frontal lobe resection and only two experienced SUDEP. Another study showed that, because of the curative surgery for epilepsy, 31 patients were followed up for 10 years and none experienced SUDEP. In addition, of 371 epileptic patients who had the epileptogenic zone of their temporal lobe resected, 141 of them had recurrent seizure activity, but only two experienced SUDEP. Lastly, because of this curative surgery, 230 patients with epilepsy received follow-up for 5.5 years, and none of those patients experienced SUDEP [233, 234]. However, even though there is a surgery that can decrease epilepsy-related mortality, the stimulation of the vagus nerve does not decrease the incidence of SUDEP in epilepsy [235, 236]. However, a recent study that used a vagus nerve stimulation surgery in epileptic patients with drug resistance has shown that vagus nerve stimulation is helpful to stabilize cardiac electrophysiology and reduce the risk of arrhythmias in drug-resistant epilepsy and in drug-resistant status epilepticus [237].

Although not all surgeries can achieve complete control of seizures, surgical intervention may serve the neural circuit that has formed in the brain to help interrupt the pathological connection that nerve has to the cardiovascular and respiratory systems to reduce the occurrence of SUDEP. Future studies will need to evaluate what kinds of surgical intervention can reduce the risk of SUDEP. This research not only can reduce the incidence of SUDEP but can also provide further understanding of the pathogenesis of SUDEP. However, just because epileptic patients passed the preoperative screening does not mean that they will elect to have the surgery to treat epilepsy, so these patients also face a risk for SUDEP. Therefore, auxiliary antiepileptic drugs and palliative surgeries can also be adequately considered.

9.5.9 Conclusion

Refractory status epilepticus is the most serious outcome of refractory epilepsy, although for a diagnosis of SUDEP, we must first exclude that the patient experienced status epilepticus before death or for at least 24 h prior to death, and the differential diagnosis of death caused by status epilepticus is different from SUDEP. However, patients with refractory status epilepticus may experience any of the above two causes of death in various circumstances. Thus, patients with refractory status epilepticus have a higher risk for death than any other type of epilepsy.

References

1. Goh KP. Management of hyponatremia. Am Fam Physician. 2004;69(10):2387–94.
2. Schrier RW, Sharma S, Shchekochikhin D. Hyponatraemia: more than just a marker of disease severity? Nat Rev Nephrol. 2013;9(1):37–50.
3. Ortenzi A, Paggi A, Foschi N, Sabbatini D, Pistoli E. Oxcarbazepine and adverse events: impact of age, dosage, metabolite serum concentrations and concomitant antiepileptic therapy. Funct Neurol. 2008;23(2):97–100.
4. Tilelli JA, Ophoven JP. Hyponatremic seizures as a presenting symptom of child abuse. Forensic Sci Int. 1986;30(2–3):213–7.
5. Farrar HC, Chande VT, Fitzpatrick DF, Shema SJ. Hyponatremia as the cause of seizures in infants: a retrospective analysis of incidence, severity, and clinical predictors. Ann Emerg Med. 1995;26(1):42–8.
6. Primavera A, Fonti A, Giberti L, Cocito L. Recurrent absence status epilepticus and hyponatremia in a patient with polydipsia. Biol Psychiatry. 1995;38(3):189–91.
7. Barolomei F, Gastaut JL. Complex partial status epilepticus provoked by hyponatremia. Eur Neurol. 1998;40(1):53–4.
8. Azuma H, Akechi T, Furukawa TA. Absence status associated with focal activity and polydipsia-induced hyponatremia. Neuropsychiatr Dis Treat. 2008;4(2):495–8.
9. Holtkamp M, Othman J, Buchheim K, Meierkord H. Predictors and prognosis of refractory status epilepticus treated in a neurological intensive care unit. J Neurol Neurosurg Psychiatry. 2005;76(4):534–9.
10. Zelano J, Halawa I, Clausen F, Kumlien E. Hyponatremia augments kainic-acid induced status epilepticus in the mouse: a model for dysmetabolic status epilepticus. Epilepsy Res. 2013;106(1–2):29–34.
11. Sharf RE. Seizure from hyponatremia in infants. Early recognition and treatment. Arch Fam Med. 1993;2(6):647–52.
12. Celik T, Tolunay O, Tolunay I, Celik U. Cerebral salt wasting in status epilepticus: two cases and review of the literature. Pediatr Neurol. 2014;50(4):397–9.
13. Tolunay O, Celik T, Celik U, et al. Cerebral salt wasting in pediatric critical care; not just a neurosurgical disorder anymore. Neuro Endocrinol Lett. 2015;36(6):578–82.
14. Kim YS, Kim DW, Jung KH, et al. Frequency of and risk factors for oxcarbazepine-induced severe and symptomatic hyponatremia. Seizure. 2014;23(3):208–12.
15. Kuz GM, Manssourian A. Carbamazepine-induced hyponatremia: assessment of risk factors. Ann Pharmacother. 2005;39(11):1943–6.
16. Van Amelsvoort T, Bakshi R, Devaux CB, Schwabe S. Hyponatremia associated with carbamazepine and oxcarbazepine therapy: a review. Epilepsia. 1994;35(1):181–8.
17. Kellinghaus C, Berning S, Stogbauer F. Use of oxcarbazepine for treatment of refractory status epilepticus. Seizure. 2014;23(2):151–4.
18. Johannessen AC, Nielsen OA. Hyponatremia induced by oxcarbazepine. Epilepsy Res. 1987;1(2):155–6.
19. Kloster R, Borresen HC, Hoff-Olsen P. Sudden death in two patients with epilepsy and the syndrome of inappropriate antidiuretic hormone secretion (SIADH). Seizure. 1998;7(5):419–20.
20. Worthley LI, Thomas PD. Treatment of hyponatraemic seizures with intravenous 29.2% saline. Br Med J (Clin Res Ed). 1986;292(6514):168–170.
21. Asconape JJ. Some common issues in the use of antiepileptic drugs. Semin Neurol. 2002;22(1):27–39.
22. Dawley C. Myalgias and myopathies: rhabdomyolysis. FP Essent. 2016;440:28–36.
23. Diamond I, Aquino TI. Myoglobinuria following unilateral status epilepticus and ipsilateral rhabdomyolysis: a clinicopathological report. N Engl J Med. 1965;272:834–7.
24. MacDonald I, Benaroya S, Zidulka J. Acute renal failure, rhabdomyolysis and hemolytic anemia. Can Med Assoc J. 1979;120(6):640.
25. Rasmussen KT, Garsdal P. Rhabdomyolysis with acute renal failure after a grand mal seizure. Ugeskr Laeger. 1987;149(14):917.
26. Murray AN, Riordan G, Swanepoel CR, Eastman RW. Myoglobinuric renal failure after generalised tonic-clonic seizures. A case report. S Afr Med J. 1988;74(5):236–7.
27. Zutt R, van der Kooi AJ, Linthorst GE, Wanders RJ, de Visser M. Rhabdomyolysis: review of the literature. Neuromuscul Disord. 2014;24(8):651–9.
28. Sauret JM, Marinides G, Wang GK. Rhabdomyolysis. Am Fam Physician. 2002;65(5):907–12.
29. Brown CV, Rhee P, Chan L, Evans K, Demetriades D, Velmahos GC. Preventing renal failure in patients with rhabdomyolysis: do bicarbonate and mannitol make a difference? J Trauma. 2004;56(6):1191–6.
30. Chamberlain MC. Rhabdomyolysis in children: a 3-year retrospective study. Pediatr Neurol. 1991;7(3):226–8.
31. Perreault S, Birca A, Piper D, Nadeau A, Gauvin F, Vanasse M. Transient creatine phosphokinase elevations in children: a single-center experience. J Pediatr. 2011;159(4):682–5.
32. Alpers JP, Jones LK Jr. Natural history of exertional rhabdomyolysis: a population-based analysis. Muscle Nerve. 2010;42(4):487–91.
33. Mackay MT, Kornberg AJ, Shield LK, Dennett X. Benign acute childhood myositis: laboratory and clinical features. Neurology. 1999;53(9):2127–31.
34. Zhou J, Luo B, Peng G. A single seizure attack induced rhabdomyolysis. Neurol India. 2017;65(Supplement):S93-94.
35. Mishra A, Dave N. Acute renal failure due to rhabdomyolysis following a seizure. J Family Med Prim Care. 2013;2(1):86–7.

36. Yamazaki H, Tajima S, Takeuchi T. Refractory status epilepticus, serious rhabdomyolysis, acute liver injury, and pancytopenia after a massive intake of ethyl methanesulfonate: a case report. Int J Clin Exp Med. 2015;8(9):16863–7.
37. Kreft A, Rasmussen N, Hansen LK. Refractory status epilepticus in two children with lethal rhabdomyolysis. Ugeskr Laeger. 2008;170(42):3339.
38. Torres PA, Helmstetter JA, Kaye AM, Kaye AD. Rhabdomyolysis: pathogenesis, diagnosis, and treatment. Ochsner J. 2015;15(1):58–69.
39. Zhou ZB, Yang XY, Zhou X, et al. Propofol-induced rhabdomyolysis: a case report. Int J Clin Pharmacol Ther. 2015;53(10):890–4.
40. Haruda F. Phenytoin hypersensitivity: 38 cases. Neurology. 1979;29(11):1480–5.
41. Engel JN, Mellul VG, Goodman DB. Phenytoin hypersensitivity: a case of severe acute rhabdomyolysis. Am J Med. 1986;81(5):928–30.
42. Santos-Calle FJ, Borras-Blasco J, Navarro-Ruiz A, Plaza MI. Unsuspected rhabdomyolysis associated with phenytoin. Int J Clin Pharmacol Ther. 2005;43(9):436–40.
43. Kim H, Jo S, Park KW, Han SH, Lee SA. A case of phenytoin-induced rhabdomyolysis in status epilepticus. J Epilepsy Res. 2016;6(1):36–8.
44. Rossetti AO, Logroscino G, Bromfield EB. Refractory status epilepticus: effect of treatment aggressiveness on prognosis. Arch Neurol. 2005;62(11):1698–702.
45. Parke TJ, Stevens JE, Rice AS, et al. Metabolic acidosis and fatal myocardial failure after propofol infusion in children: five case reports. BMJ. 1992;305(6854):613–6.
46. Zaccheo MM, Bucher DH. Propofol infusion syndrome: a rare complication with potentially fatal results. Crit Care Nurse. 2008;28(3):18–26. quiz 27.
47. Diaz JH, Prabhakar A, Urman RD, Kaye AD. Propofol infusion syndrome: a retrospective analysis at a level 1 trauma center. Crit Care Res Pract. 2014;2014:346968.
48. Hanna JP, Ramundo ML. Rhabdomyolysis and hypoxia associated with prolonged propofol infusion in children. Neurology. 1998;50(1):301–3.
49. Cornfield DN, Tegtmeyer K, Nelson MD, Milla CE, Sweeney M. Continuous propofol infusion in 142 critically ill children. Pediatrics. 2002;110(6):1177–81.
50. Zarovnaya EL, Jobst BC, Harris BT. Propofol-associated fatal myocardial failure and rhabdomyolysis in an adult with status epilepticus. Epilepsia. 2007;48(5):1002–6.
51. Levin PD, Levin V, Weissman C, Sprung CL, Rund D. Therapeutic plasma exchange as treatment for propofol infusion syndrome. J Clin Apher. 2015;30(5):311–3.
52. Crepeau AZ, Treiman DM. Levetiracetam: a comprehensive review. Expert Rev Neurother. 2010;10(2):159–71.
53. Akiyama H, Haga Y, Sasaki N, Yanagisawa T, Hasegawa Y. A case of rhabdomyolysis in which levetiracetam was suspected as the cause. Epilepsy Behav Case Rep. 2014;2:152–5.
54. Ponchaut S, Van Hoof F, Veitch K. Valproate and cytochrome c oxidase deficiency. Eur J Pediatr. 1995;154(1):79.
55. Roodhooft AM, Van Dam K, Haentjens D, Verpooten GA, Van Acker KJ. Acute sodium valproate intoxication: occurrence of renal failure and treatment with haemoperfusion-haemodialysis. Eur J Pediatr. 1990;149(5):363–4.
56. Pinkston R, Walker LA. Multiorgan system failure caused by valproic acid toxicity. Am J Emerg Med. 1997;15(5):504–6.
57. Kottlors M, Jaksch M, Ketelsen UP, Weiner S, Glocker FX, Lucking CH. Valproic acid triggers acute rhabdomyolysis in a patient with carnitine palmitoyltransferase type II deficiency. Neuromuscul Disord. 2001;11(8):757–9.
58. Wieser T. Carnitine palmitoyltransferase II deficiency. Seattle: University of Washington; 1993.
59. Huerta-Alardin AL, Varon J, Marik PE. Bench-to-bedside review: rhabdomyolysis—an overview for clinicians. Crit Care. 2005;9(2):158–69.
60. Bosch X, Poch E, Grau JM. Rhabdomyolysis and acute kidney injury. N Engl J Med. 2009;361(1):62–72.
61. Veenstra J, Smit WM, Krediet RT, Arisz L. Relationship between elevated creatine phosphokinase and the clinical spectrum of rhabdomyolysis. Nephrol Dial Transplant. 1994;9(6):637–41.
62. Kalim S, Rhee EP. An overview of renal metabolomics. Kidney Int. 2017;91(1):61–9.
63. Zimmerman J, Granatir R, Mummert K, Cioffi R. Sickle crisis precipitated by exercise rhabdomyolysis in a patient with sickle cell trait: case report. Mil Med. 1974;139(4):313–5.
64. Ferraz C, Reis ME, Lopes MM, Cardoso ML, Barbosa CR. Hypoglycaemia without ketosis. A case report. Rev Neurol. 2005;41(6):349–53.
65. Chatzizisis YS, Misirli G, Hatzitolios AI, Giannoglou GD. The syndrome of rhabdomyolysis: complications and treatment. Eur J Intern Med. 2008;19(8):568–74.
66. Better OS, Abassi ZA. Early fluid resuscitation in patients with rhabdomyolysis. Nat Rev Nephrol. 2011;7(7):416–22.
67. Cervellin G, Comelli I, Lippi G. Rhabdomyolysis: historical background, clinical, diagnostic and therapeutic features. Clin Chem Lab Med. 2010;48(6):749–56.
68. Al-Ismaili Z, Piccioni M, Zappitelli M. Rhabdomyolysis: pathogenesis of renal injury and management. Pediatr Nephrol. 2011;26(10):1781–8.
69. Fernandez WG, Hung O, Bruno GR, Galea S, Chiang WK. Factors predictive of acute renal failure and need for hemodialysis among ED patients with rhabdomyolysis. Am J Emerg Med. 2005;23(1):1–7.

70. Yeon EK, Ryu KN, Kang HJ, et al. Characteristic MR image finding of squatting exercise-induced rhabdomyolysis of the thigh muscles. Br J Radiol. 2017;90(1072):20160740.
71. Park A, Chapman M, McCredie VA, et al. EEG utilization in Canadian intensive care units: a multicentre prospective observational study. Seizure. 2016;43:42–7.
72. Dubey D, Kalita J, Misra UK. Status epilepticus: refractory and super-refractory. Neurol India. 2017;65(Supplement):S12–17.
73. Bayrlee A, Ganeshalingam N, Kurczewski L, Brophy GM. Treatment of super-refractory status epilepticus. Curr Neurol Neurosci Rep. 2015;15(10):66.
74. Gunal AI, Celiker H, Dogukan A, et al. Early and vigorous fluid resuscitation prevents acute renal failure in the crush victims of catastrophic earthquakes. J Am Soc Nephrol. 2004;15(7):1862–7.
75. Zager RA. Rhabdomyolysis and myohemoglobinuric acute renal failure. Kidney Int. 1996;49(2):314–26.
76. Altintepe L, Guney I, Tonbul Z, et al. Early and intensive fluid replacement prevents acute renal failure in the crush cases associated with spontaneous collapse of an apartment in Konya. Ren Fail. 2007;29(6):737–41.
77. Ward MM. Factors predictive of acute renal failure in rhabdomyolysis. Arch Intern Med. 1988;148(7):1553–7.
78. Kyle UG, Pirlich M, Lochs H, et al. Increased length of hospital stay in underweight and overweight patients at hospital admission: a controlled population study. Clin Nutr. 2005;24:133–42.
79. Guigoz Y. The mini nutritional assessment (MNA) review of the literature—what does it tell us. J Nutr Health Aging. 2006;10(6):466–87.
80. Cardinali S, Veggiotti P, et al. Evaluation of nutritional status in children with refractory epilepsy. Nutr J. 2006;5:14.
81. Volpe SL, Schall JI, Gallagher PR, et al. Nutrient intake of children with intractable epilepsy compared with healthy children. J Am Diet Assoc. 2007;107:1014–8.
82. Neala EG, Zupec-Kaniab B, Pfeifer HH. Carnitine, nutritional supplementation and discontinuation of ketogenic diet therapies. Epilepsy Res. 2012;100:267–71.
83. Tagliabue A, Bertoli S, Trentani C, et al. Effects of the ketogenic diet on nutritional status, resting energy expenditure, and substrate oxidation in patients with medically refractory epilepsy: a 6-month prospective observational study. Clin Nutr. 2012;31(2):246–9.
84. Vaid N, Fekadu S, Alemu S, et al. Epilepsy, poverty and early under-nutrition in rural Ethiopia. Seizure. 2012;21(9):734–9.
85. Leibovitz E, Giryes S, Makhline R, et al. Malnutrition risk in newly hospitalized overweight and obese individuals: Mr NOI. Eur J Clin Nutr. 2013;67(6):620–4.
86. Lim SL, Ong KCB, Chan YH, et al. Malnutrition and its impact on cost of hospitalization, length of stay, readmission and 3-year mortality. Clin Nutr. 2012;31:345–50.
87. Tappenden KA, Quatrara B, Parkhurst ML, et al. Critical role of nutrition in improving quality of care: an interdisciplinary call to action to address adult hospital malnutrition. J Acad Nutr Diet. 2013;113(9):1219–37.
88. Habek M, Hojsak I, Brinar VV. Nutrition in multiple sclerosis. Clin Neurol Neurosurg. 2010;112:616–20.
89. DeLegge MH, Drake LM. Nutritional assessment. Gastroenterol Clin N Am. 2007;36(1):1–22.
90. Sheard JM, Ash S, Mellick GD, et al. Nutrition screening and assessment in Parkinson's disease: a comparison of methods. e-SPEN J. 2013;8:e187–92.
91. Shen H-C, Chen H-F, Peng L-N, et al. Impact of nutritional status on long-term functional outcomes of post-acute stroke patients in Taiwan. Arch Gerontol Geriatr. 2011;53:149–52.
92. Allard JP, Aghdassi E, McArthur M, et al. Nutrition risk factors for survival in the elderly living in Canadian Long-term care facilities. J Am Geriatr Soc. 2004;52(1):59–65.
93. Campillo B, Paillaud E, Uzan I, et al. Value of body mass index in the detection of severe malnutrition: influence of the pathology and changes in anthropometric parameters. Clin Nutr. 2004;23(4):551–9.
94. Guigoz Y, Vellas B, Garry PJ. Assessing the nutritional status of the elderly: the mini nutritional assessment as part of the geriatric evaluation. Nutr Rev. 1996;54(2):59–65.
95. Alberda C, Graf A, McCargar L. Malnutrition: etiology, consequences, and assessment of a patient at risk. Best Pract Res Clin Gastroenterol. 2006;20(3):419–39.
96. Seres DS. Surrogate nutrition markers, malnutrition, and adequacy of nutrition support. NCP. 2005;20(3):308–13.
97. Kubrak C, Jensen L. Malnutrition in acute care patients: a narrative review. Int J Nurs Stud. 2007;44:1036–54.
98. Velasco C, García E, Rodríguez V, et al. Comparison of four nutritional screening tools to detect nutritional risk in hospitalized patients: a multicentre study. Eur J Clin Nutr. 2011;65(2):269–74.
99. Jiang ZM, Chen W, Zhan WH, et al. Parenteral and enteral nutrition application in West, Middle and East of China: a multi-centre investigation for 15098 patients in 13 metropolitans using NRS tool. Clin Nutr. 2007;2(Suppl):133–4.
100. Sheean PM, Peterson SJ, Chen Y, et al. Utilizing multiple methods to classify malnutrition among elderly patients admitted to the medical and surgical intensive care units (ICU). Clin Nutr. 2013;32:752–7.
101. Tsai AC, Chang TL, Chen JT, et al. Population-specific modifications of the short-form mini nutritional assessment and malnutrition universal

screening tool for elderly Taiwanese. Int J Nurs Stud. 2009;46(11):1431–8.

102. Stratton RJ, King CL, Stroud MA, et al. 'Malnutrition universal screening tool' predicts mortality and length of hospital stay in acutely ill elderly. Br J Nutr. 2006;95:325–30.

103. Stratton RJ, Hackston A, Longmore D, et al. Malnutrition in hospital outpatients and inpatients: prevalence, concurrent validity and ease of use of the "malnutrition universal screening tool"("MUST") for adults. Br J Nutr. 2004;92(5):799–808.

104. Benedik B, Farkas J, Kosnik M, et al. Mini nutritional assessment, body composition, and hospitalisations in patients with chronic obstructive pulmonary disease. Respir Med. 2011;105(Suppl 1):38–43.

105. Pereira Machado RS, Santa Cruz Coelho MA. Risk of malnutrition among brazilian institutionalized elderly: a study with the mini nutritional assessment (MNA) questionnaire. J Nutr Health Aging. 2011;15(7):532–5.

106. Guigoz Y. The mini nutritional assessment (MNA) review of the literature-what does it tell us? J Nutr Health Aging. 2006;10(6):466–87.

107. Phillips MB, Foley AL, Barnard R, et al. Nutritional screening in community-dwelling older adults: a systematic literature review. Asia Pac J Clin Nutr. 2010;19(3):440–9.

108. Bauer J, Egan E, Clavarino A. The scored patient-generated subjective global assessment is an effectivenutrition assessment tool in subjects with chronic obstructivepulmonary disease. e-SPEN J. 2011;6:e27–30.

109. Raslan M, Gonzalez MC, Torrinhas RS, et al. Complementarity of Subjective Global Assessment (SGA) and Nutritional Risk Screening 2002 (NRS 2002) for predicting poor clinical outcomes in hospitalized patients. Clin Nutr. 2011;30:49–53.

110. Perry EC. Inpatient management of acute alcohol withdrawal syndrome. CNS Drugs. 2014;28(5):401–10. doi:10.1007/s40263-014-0163-5.

111. Liskow BI, Rinck C, Campbell J, DeSouza C. Alcohol withdrawal in the elderly. J Stud Alcohol. 1989;50:414–42.

112. Bayard M, McIntyre J, Hill KR, Woodside J Jr. Alcohol withdrawal syndrome. Am Fam Physician. 2004;69:1443–50.

113. Mann K, Hermann D. Individualised treatment in alcohol-dependent patients. Eur Arch Psychiatry Clin Neurosci. 2010;260(Suppl 2): S116–20. doi:10.1007/s00406-010-0153-7. Epub 2010 Oct 16.

114. Gowing LR, Ali RL, Allsop S, et al. Global statistics on addictive behaviours: 2014 status report. Addiction. 2015;110(6):904–19.

115. Carlson RW, Kumar NN, Wong-Mckinstry E, Ayyagari S, Puri N, Jackson FK, et al. Alcohol withdrawal syndrome. Crit Care Clin. 2012;28(4):549–85.

116. Kosten TR, O'Connor PG. Management of drug and alcohol withdrawal. N Engl J Med. 2003;348:1786–95.

117. Schuckit MA. Recognition and management of withdrawal delirium (delirium tremens). N Engl J Med. 2014;371:2109–13.

118. Zilker T. Alkoholentzugssyndrom und Delirium tremens. MMW. 1999;141:26–30. [PubMed].

119. Hillbom M, Pieninkeroinen I, Leone M. Seizures in alcohol-dependent patients: epidemiology, pathophysiology and management. CNS Drugs. 2003;171:013–30. [PubMed].

120. American Psychiatric Association. Diagnostic and statistical manual of mental disorders. 5th ed. Washington, DC: American Psychiatric Association; 2013.

121. Erwin WE, Williams DB, Speir WA. Delirium tremens. South Med J. 1998;91:425–32. [PubMed].

122. Eastes LE, Alcohol withdrawal syndrome in trauma patients: a review. J Emerg Nurs. 2010;36(5): 507–9.

123. LaRoche SM, Shivdat-Nanhoe R. Subacute encephalopathy and seizures in alcoholics (SESA) presenting with non-convulsive status epilepticus. Seizure. 2011;20(6):505–8.

124. Hughes JR. Alcohol withdrawal seizures. Epilepsy Behav. 2009;15(2):92–7. doi:10.1016/j.yebeh.2009.02.037. Epub 2009 Feb 26.

125. Eyer F, Schuster T, Felgenhauer N, Pfab R, Strubel T, Saugel B, Zilker T. Risk assessment of moderate to severe alcohol withdrawal--predictors for seizures and delirium tremens in the course of withdrawal. Alcohol Alcohol. 2011;46(4):427–33. doi:10.1093/alcalc/agr053. Epub 2011 May 18.

126. Bleich S, Bayerlein K, Hillemacher T, Degner D, Kornhuber J, Frieling H. An assessment of the potential value of elevated homocysteine in predicting alcohol-withdrawal seizures. Epilepsia. 2006;47(5):934–8.

127. Schmidt KJ, Doshi MR. Treatment of severe alcohol withdrawal. Ann Pharmacother. 2016;50(5): 389–401.

128. Ferguson JA, Suelzer CJ, Eckert GJ, Zhou XH, Dittus RS. Risk factors for delirium tremens development. J Gen Intern Med. 1996;11(7):410–4.

129. Lee JH, Jang MK, Lee JY, Kim SM, Kim KH, Park JY, Lee JH, Kim HY, Yoo JY. Clinical predictors for delirium tremens in alcohol dependence. J Gastroenterol Hepatol. 2005;20(12):1833–7.

130. Maldonado JR, Sher Y, Das S, Hills-Evans K, Frenklach A, Lolak S, Talley R, Neri E. Prospective Validation Study of the Prediction of Alcohol Withdrawal Severity Scale (PAWSS) in medically ill inpatients: a new scale for the prediction of complicated alcohol withdrawal syndrome. Alcohol Alcohol. 2015;50(5):509–18. doi: 10.1093/alcalc/agv043. Epub 2015 May 21.

131. Brunton L, Chabner B, Knollmann B, editors. Goodman and Gilman's the pharmacological basis of therapeutics. 12th ed. New York, NY: McGraw-Hill; 2011.
132. Yip L. Ethanol. In: Nelson L, Lewin N, Howland M, Hoffman R, Goldfrank L, Fomenbaum N, eds. Goldfrank's Toxicologic emergencies. 9th. New York, NY: McGraw-Hill; 2011. http://0-accesspharmacy.mhmedical.com.libcat.ferris.edu/content.aspx?. Accessed 18 Dec 2014.
133. Mizielinska SM. Ion channels in epilepsy. Biochem Soc Trans. 2007;35:1077–9.
134. Enoch MA. The role of GABA (a) receptors in the development of alcoholism. Pharmacol Biochem Behav. 2008;90(1):95–104. doi:10.1016/j.pbb.2008.03.007. Epub 2008 Mar 15.
135. Heinz A, Schmidt K, Baum SS, Kuhn S, Dufeu P, Schmidt LG, Rommelspacher H. Influence of dopaminergic transmission on severity of withdrawal syndrome in alcoholism. J Stud Alcohol. 1996;57(5):471–4.
136. Clements JD. Transmitter time course in the synaptic cleft: its role in central synaptic function. Trends Neurosci. 1996;19(5):163–71.
137. van Munster BC, de Rooij SE, Yazdanpanah M. The association of the dopamine transporter gene and the dopamine receptor 2 gene with delirium, a meta-analysis. Am J Med Genet B Neuropsychiatr Genet. 2010;153B(2):648–55. doi:10.1002/ajmg.b.31034.
138. van Munster BC, Yazdanpanah M, Tanck MW, de Rooij SE, van de Giessen E, Sijbrands EJ, Zwinderman AH, Korevaar JC. Genetic polymorphisms in the DRD2, DRD3, and SLC6A3 gene in elderly patients with delirium. Am J Med Genet B Neuropsychiatr Genet. 2010;153B(1):38–45. doi:10.1002/ajmg.b.30943.
139. Kaim SC, Klett CJ, Rothfeld B. Treatment of the acute alcohol withdrawal state: a comparison of four drugs. Am J Psychiatry. 1969;125(12):1640–6.
140. Muzyk AJ, Leung JG, Nelson S, Embury ER, Jones SR. The role of diazepam loading for the treatment of alcohol withdrawal syndrome in hospitalized patients. Am J Addict. 2013;22(2):113–8. doi: 10.1111/j.1521-0391.2013.00307.x. Epub 2013 Feb 1.
141. Stehman CR, Mycyk MB. A rational approach to the treatment of alcohol withdrawal in the ED. Am J Emerg Med. 2013;31(4):734–42. doi:10.1016/j.aj.
142. Kim SJ, Lee DY, Kim JS. Neurologic outcomes of pediatric epileptic patients with pentobarbital coma. Pediatr Neurol. 2001;25(3):217–220. em.2012.12.029. Epub 2013 Feb 8.
143. Young GP, Rores C, Murphy C, Dailey RH. Intravenous phenobarbital for alcohol withdrawal and convulsions. Ann Emerg Med. 1987;16(8): 847–50.
144. Matz R. Barbiturates and alcohol withdrawal. J Gen Intern Med. 1990;5(2):182.
145. Gold JA, Rimal B, Nolan A, Nelson LS. A strategy of escalating doses of benzodiazepines and phenobarbital administration reduces the need for mechanical ventilation in delirium tremens. Crit Care Med. 2007;35(3):724–30.
146. Askgaard G, Hallas J, Fink-Jensen A, Molander AC, Madsen KG, Pottegård A. Phenobarbital compared to benzodiazepines in alcohol withdrawal treatment: a register-based cohort study of subsequent benzodiazepine use, alcohol recidivism and mortality. Drug Alcohol Depend. 2016;161:258–64.
147. Orser BA, Bertlik M, Wang LY, MacDonald JF. Inhibition by propofol (2,6 di-isopropylphenol) of the N-methyl-D-aspartate subtype of glutamate receptor in cultured hippocampal neurons. Br J Pharmacol. 1995;116:1761–8.
148. Coomes TR, Smith SW. Successful use of propofol in refractory delirium tremens. Ann Emerg Med. 1997;30:825–8.
149. McCowan C, Marik P. Refractory delirium tremens treated with propofol: a case series. Crit Care Med. 2000;28:1781–4.
150. Mahajan R, Singh R, Bansal P, Bala R. Use of propofol as adjuvant therapy in refractory delirium tremens. Ind Psychiatry J. 2010;19:58–9.
151. Hughes DW, Vanwert E, Lepori L, Adams BD. Propofolfor benzodiazepine-refractory alcohol withdrawal in a non-mechanically ventilated patient. Am J Emerg Med. 2014;32:112.e3–112.e4.
152. Lorentzen K, Lauritsen AO, Bendtsen AO. Use of propofol infusion in alcohol withdrawal-induced refractory delirium tremens. Dan Med J. 2014;61:A4807.
153. Sohraby R, Attridge RL, Hughes DW. Use of propofol-containing versus benzodiazepine regimens for alcohol withdrawal requiring mechanical ventilation. Ann Pharmacother. 2014;48:456–61.
154. Wong A, Smithburger PL, Kane-Gill SL. Review ofadjunctive dexmedetomidine in the management of severe acute alcohol withdrawal syndrome. Am J Drug Alcohol Abuse. 2015;41(5):382–91. doi:10.3109/00952990.2015.1058390.
155. Latt N, Dore G. Thiamine in the treatment of Wernicke encephalopathy in patients with alcohol use disorders. Intern Med J. 2014;44:911–5.
156. Lexi-Comp, Inc. (Lexi-Drugs). Lexi-Comp, Inc.; May 11, 2015.
157. Cravo ML, Selhub J, et al. Hyperhomocysteinemia in chronic alcoholism: correlation with folate, vitamin B-12, and vitamin B-6 status. Am J Clin Nutr. 1996;63:220–4.
158. Tomson T, Nashef L, Ryvlin P. Sudden unexpected death in epilepsy: current knowledge and future directions. Lancet Neurol. 2008;7(11):1021–31.
159. Bacon GM. On the modes of death in epilepsy. Lancet. 1868;91:555–6.
160. Nashef L. Sudden unexpected death in epilepsy: terminology and definitions. Epilepsia. 1997;38(11 Suppl):S6–8.

161. Nickels KC, Grossardt BR, Wirrell EC. Epilepsy-related mortality is low in children: a 30-year population-based study in Olmsted County, MN. Epilepsia. 2012;53(12):2164–71.
162. Ficker DM, So EL, Shen WK, et al. Population-based study of the incidence of sudden unexplained death in epilepsy. Neurology. 1998;51(5):1270–4.
163. Weber P, Bubl R, Blauenstein U, Tillmann BU, Lutschg J. Sudden unexplained death in children with epilepsy: a cohort study with an eighteen-year follow-up. Acta Paediatr. 2005;94(5):564–7.
164. Ficker DM. Sudden unexplained death and injury in epilepsy. Epilepsia. 2000;41(Suppl 2):S7–12.
165. Pedley TA, Hauser WA. Sudden death in epilepsy: a wake-up call for management. Lancet. 2002;359(9320):1790–1.
166. Ryvlin P, Tomson T, Montavont A. Excess mortality and sudden unexpected death in epilepsy. Presse Med. 2009;38(6):905–10.
167. Annegers JF. United States perspective on definitions and classifications. Epilepsia. 1997;38(11 Suppl):S9–12.
168. Forsgren L, Hauser WA, Olafsson E, Sander JW, Sillanpaa M, Tomson T. Mortality of epilepsy in developed countries: a review. Epilepsia. 2005;46(Suppl 11):18–27.
169. Nashef L, Hindocha N, Makoff A. Risk factors in sudden death in epilepsy (SUDEP): the quest for mechanisms. Epilepsia. 2007;48(5):859–71.
170. Asadi-Pooya AA, Sperling MR. Clinical features of sudden unexpected death in epilepsy. J Clin Neurophysiol. 2009;26(5):297–301.
171. Sperling MR, Feldman H, Kinman J, Liporace JD, O'Connor MJ. Seizure control and mortality in epilepsy. Ann Neurol. 1999;46(1):45–50.
172. Terra VC, Scorza FA, Arida RM, et al. Mortality in children with severe epilepsy: 10 years of follow-up. Arq Neuropsiquiatr. 2011;69(5):766–9.
173. Ryvlin P, Nashef L, Lhatoo SD, et al. Incidence and mechanisms of cardiorespiratory arrests in epilepsy monitoring units (MORTEMUS): a retrospective study. Lancet Neurol. 2013;12(10):966–77.
174. Keilson MJ, Hauser WA, Magrill JP, Goldman M. ECG abnormalities in patients with epilepsy. Neurology. 1987;37(10):1624–6.
175. Galimberti CA, Marchioni E, Barzizza F, Manni R, Sartori I, Tartara A. Partial epileptic seizures of different origin variably affect cardiac rhythm. Epilepsia. 1996;37(8):742–7.
176. Duplyakov D, Golovina G, Lyukshina N, Surkova E, Elger CE, Surges R. Syncope, seizure-induced bradycardia and asystole: two cases and review of clinical and pathophysiological features. Seizure. 2014;23(7):506–11.
177. Jehi L, Najm IM. Sudden unexpected death in epilepsy: impact, mechanisms, and prevention. Cleve Clin J Med. 2008;75(Suppl 2):S66–70.
178. Leung H, Schindler K, Kwan P, Elger C. Asystole induced by electrical stimulation of the left cingulate gyrus. Epileptic Disord. 2007;9(1):77–81.
179. Nei M, Ho RT, Sperling MR. EKG abnormalities during partial seizures in refractory epilepsy. Epilepsia. 2000;41(5):542–8.
180. Opherk C, Coromilas J, Hirsch LJ. Heart rate and EKG changes in 102 seizures: analysis of influencing factors. Epilepsy Res. 2002;52(2):117–27.
181. Hirsch LJ, Donner EJ, So EL, et al. Abbreviated report of the NIH/NINDS workshop on sudden unexpected death in epilepsy. Neurology. 2011;76(22):1932–8.
182. Goldman AM. Mechanisms of sudden unexplained death in epilepsy. Curr Opin Neurol. 2015;28(2):166–74.
183. Claes L, Del-Favero J, Ceulemans B, Lagae L, Van Broeckhoven C, De Jonghe P. De novo mutations in the sodium-channel gene SCN1A cause severe myoclonic epilepsy of infancy. Am J Hum Genet. 2001;68(6):1327–32.
184. So EL, Sam MC, Lagerlund TL. Postictal central apnea as a cause of SUDEP: evidence from near-SUDEP incident. Epilepsia. 2000;41(11):1494–7.
185. Terrence CF, Rao GR, Perper JA. Neurogenic pulmonary edema in unexpected, unexplained death of epileptic patients. Ann Neurol. 1981;9(5):458–64.
186. Johnston SC, Horn JK, Valente J, Simon RP. The role of hypoventilation in a sheep model of epileptic sudden death. Ann Neurol. 1995;37(4):531–7.
187. Meierkord H, Shorvon S, Lightman SL. Plasma concentrations of prolactin, noradrenaline, vasopressin and oxytocin during and after a prolonged epileptic seizure. Acta Neurol Scand. 1994;90(2):73–7.
188. Aminoff MJ, Simon RP, Wiedemann E. The hormonal responses to generalized tonic-clonic seizures. Brain. 1984;107(Pt 2):569–78.
189. Lipka K, Bulow HH. Lactic acidosis following convulsions. Acta Anaesthesiol Scand. 2003;47(5):616–8.
190. Mameli O, Caria MA, Pintus A, Padua G, Mameli S. Sudden death in epilepsy: an experimental animal model. Seizure. 2006;15(5):275–87.
191. Lee S, Harris ND, Robinson RT, Yeoh L, Macdonald IA, Heller SR. Effects of adrenaline and potassium on QTc interval and QT dispersion in man. Eur J Clin Investig. 2003;33(2):93–8.
192. Holbrook M, Malik M, Shah RR, Valentin JP. Drug induced shortening of the QT/QTc interval: an emerging safety issue warranting further modelling and evaluation in drug research and development? J Pharmacol Toxicol Methods. 2009;59(1):21–8.
193. Szurhaj W, Troussiere AC, Logier R, et al. Ictal changes in parasympathetic tone: Prediction of postictal oxygen desaturation. Neurology. 2015;85(14):1233–9.
194. Glasscock E, Qian J, Yoo JW, Noebels JL. Masking epilepsy by combining two epilepsy genes. Nat Neurosci. 2007;10(12):1554–8.
195. Escayg A, MacDonald BT, Meisler MH, et al. Mutations of SCN1A, encoding a neuronal sodium channel, in two families with GEFS+2. Nat Genet. 2000;24(4):343–5.

196. Meisler MH, O'Brien JE, Sharkey LM. Sodium channel gene family: epilepsy mutations, gene interactions and modifier effects. J Physiol. 2010;588(Pt 11):1841–8.
197. Parisi P, Oliva A, Coll Vidal M, et al. Coexistence of epilepsy and Brugada syndrome in a family with SCN5A mutation. Epilepsy Res. 2013;105(3):415–8.
198. Aurlien D, Leren TP, Tauboll E, Gjerstad L. New SCN5A mutation in a SUDEP victim with idiopathic epilepsy. Seizure. 2009;18(2):158–60.
199. Papale LA, Beyer B, Jones JM, et al. Heterozygous mutations of the voltage-gated sodium channel SCN8A are associated with spike-wave discharges and absence epilepsy in mice. Hum Mol Genet. 2009;18(9):1633–41.
200. Tu E, Waterhouse L, Duflou J, Bagnall RD, Semsarian C. Genetic analysis of hyperpolarization-activated cyclic nucleotide-gated cation channels in sudden unexpected death in epilepsy cases. Brain Pathol. 2011;21(6):692–8.
201. Goldman AM, Glasscock E, Yoo J, Chen TT, Klassen TL, Noebels JL. Arrhythmia in heart and brain: KCNQ1 mutations link epilepsy and sudden unexplained death. Sci Transl Med. 2009; 1(2):2ra6.
202. McLean BN, Wimalaratna S. Sudden death in epilepsy recorded in ambulatory EEG. J Neurol Neurosurg Psychiatry. 2007;78(12):1395–7.
203. Iannotti LL, Zavaleta N, Huasaquiche C, Leon Z, Caulfield LE. Early growth velocities and weight gain plasticity improve linear growth in Peruvian infants. Matern Child Nutr. 2015;11(1):127–37.
204. Heron SE, Grinton BE, Kivity S, et al. PRRT2 mutations cause benign familial infantile epilepsy and infantile convulsions with choreoathetosis syndrome. Am J Hum Genet. 2012;90(1):152–160.
205. Labate A, Tarantino P, Palamara G, et al. Mutations in PRRT2 result in familial infantile seizures with heterogeneous phenotypes including febrile convulsions and probable SUDEP. Epilepsy Res. 2013;104(3):280–4.
206. Johnson JN, Tester DJ, Bass NE, Ackerman MJ. Cardiac channel molecular autopsy for sudden unexpected death in epilepsy. J Child Neurol. 2010;25(7):916–21.
207. Coll M, Allegue C, Partemi S, et al. Genetic investigation of sudden unexpected death in epilepsy cohort by panel target resequencing. Int J Legal Med. 2016;130(2):331–9.
208. Donner EJ. Explaining the unexplained; expecting the unexpected: where are we with sudden unexpected death in epilepsy? Epilepsy Curr. 2011;11(2):45–9.
209. Nashef L, So EL, Ryvlin P, Tomson T. Unifying the definitions of sudden unexpected death in epilepsy. Epilepsia. 2012;53(2):227–33.
210. Hitiris N, Mohanraj R, Norrie J, Brodie MJ. Mortality in epilepsy. Epilepsy Behav. 2007;10(3):363–76.
211. DeLorenzo RJ, Hauser WA, Towne AR, et al. A prospective, population-based epidemiologic study of status epilepticus in Richmond, Virginia. Neurology. 1996;46(4):1029–35.
212. Hesdorffer DC, Logroscino G, Cascino G, Annegers JF, Hauser WA. Incidence of status epilepticus in Rochester, Minnesota, 1965-1984. Neurology. 1998;50(3):735–41.
213. Wu YW, Shek DW, Garcia PA, Zhao S, Johnston SC. Incidence and mortality of generalized convulsive status epilepticus in California. Neurology. 2002;58(7):1070–6.
214. Sagduyu A, Tarlaci S, Sirin H. Generalized tonic-clonic status epilepticus: causes, treatment, complications and predictors of case fatality. J Neurol. 1998;245(10):640–6.
215. Garzon E, Fernandes RM, Sakamoto AC. Serial EEG during human status epilepticus: evidence for PLED as an ictal pattern. Neurology. 2001;57(7):1175–83.
216. Nei M, Lee JM, Shanker VL, Sperling MR. The EEG and prognosis in status epilepticus. Epilepsia. 1999;40(2):157–63.
217. Pompili M, Girardi P, Ruberto A, Tatarelli R. Suicide in the epilepsies: a meta-analytic investigation of 29 cohorts. Epilepsy Behav. 2005;7(2):305–10.
218. Swinkels WA, Kuyk J, van Dyck R, Spinhoven P. Psychiatric comorbidity in epilepsy. Epilepsy Behav. 2005;7(1):37–50.
219. Beghi E, Cornaggia C, RESt-1 Group. Morbidity and accidents in patients with epilepsy: results of a European cohort study. Epilepsia. 2002;43(9):1076–83.
220. Hauser WA, Annegers JF, Elveback LR. Mortality in patients with epilepsy. Epilepsia. 1980;21(4):399–412.
221. McIntosh AM, Wilson SJ, Berkovic SF. Seizure outcome after temporal lobectomy: current research practice and findings. Epilepsia. 2001;42(10):1288–307.
222. Tebo CC, Evins AI, Christos PJ, Kwon J, Schwartz TH. Evolution of cranial epilepsy surgery complication rates: a 32-year systematic review and meta-analysis. J Neurosurg. 2014;120(6):1415–27.
223. Engel J Jr, McDermott MP, Wiebe S, et al. Early surgical therapy for drug-resistant temporal lobe epilepsy: a randomized trial. JAMA. 2012;307(9):922–30.
224. Wiebe S, Blume WT, Girvin JP, Eliasziw M, Effectiveness, Efficiency of Surgery for Temporal Lobe Epilepsy Study Group. A randomized, controlled trial of surgery for temporal-lobe epilepsy. N Engl J Med. 2001;345(5):311–8.
225. Ryvlin P, Cucherat M, Rheims S. Risk of sudden unexpected death in epilepsy in patients given adjunctive antiepileptic treatment for refractory seizures: a meta-analysis of placebo-controlled randomised trials. Lancet Neurol. 2011;10(11): 961–8.
226. Nishimura Y, Saito Y, Kondo N, et al. Ictal central apnea and bradycardia in temporal lobe epilepsy complicated by obstructive sleep apnea syndrome. Epilepsy Behav Case Rep. 2015;4:41–4.

227. Strollo PJ Jr, Soose RJ, Maurer JT, et al. Upper-airway stimulation for obstructive sleep apnea. N Engl J Med. 2014;370(2):139–49.
228. Faingold CL, Tupal S, Randall M. Prevention of seizure-induced sudden death in a chronic SUDEP model by semichronic administration of a selective serotonin reuptake inhibitor. Epilepsy Behav. 2011;22(2):186–90.
229. Faingold CL, Kommajosyula SP, Long X, Plath K, Randall M. Serotonin and sudden death: differential effects of serotonergic drugs on seizure-induced respiratory arrest in DBA/1 mice. Epilepsy Behav. 2014;37:198–203.
230. Langan Y, Nashef L, Sander JW. Case-control study of SUDEP. Neurology. 2005;64(7):1131–3.
231. Seyal M. Frontal hemodynamic changes precede EEG onset of temporal lobe seizures. Clin Neurophysiol. 2014;125(3):442–8.
232. Bialasiewicz P, Nowak D. Obstructive sleep apnea syndrome and nocturnal epilepsy with tonic seizures. Epileptic Disord. 2009;11(4):320–3.
233. Jeha LE, Najm I, Bingaman W, Dinner D, Widdess-Walsh P, Luders H. Surgical outcome and prognostic factors of frontal lobe epilepsy surgery. Brain. 2007;130(Pt 2):574–84.
234. Wieshmann UC, Larkin D, Varma T, Eldridge P. Predictors of outcome after temporal lobectomy for refractory temporal lobe epilepsy. Acta Neurol Scand. 2008;118(5):306–12.
235. Granbichler CA, Nashef L, Selway R, Polkey CE. Mortality and SUDEP in epilepsy patients treated with vagus nerve stimulation. Epilepsia. 2015;56(2):291–6.
236. Annegers JF, Coan SP, Hauser WA, Leestma J. Epilepsy, vagal nerve stimulation by the NCP system, all-cause mortality, and sudden, unexpected, unexplained death. Epilepsia. 2000;41(5):549–53.
237. Schomer AC, Nearing BD, Schachter SC, Verrier RL. Vagus nerve stimulation reduces cardiac electrical instability assessed by quantitative T-wave alternans analysis in patients with drug-resistant focal epilepsy. Epilepsia. 2014;55(12):1996–2002.

Special Cases of Refractory Status Epilepticus

10

Xuefeng Wang

10.1 Case 1: Anesthetics and Status Epilepticus

Abstract
Anesthetic-induced refractory status epilepticus (RSE) has been shown to be resistant to five anticonvulsants. However, it can be resolved using a combined therapy consisting of diazepam and propofol. In this chapter, we discuss the incidence, rate, and timing of the onset of anesthetic-induced RSE with a particular focus on its characteristics. We also describe the relevant anesthesia protocols and their appropriate use in patients with epilepsy. In addition, when and how to initiate polytherapy to treat RSE is also discussed in this chapter.

10.1.1 Case Summary

The patient was a 28-year-old parturient with a 20-year history of epilepsy. Seizures were characterized by loss of consciousness, twitching of the right limbs and angulus oris, blank stares, teeth clenching, and foaming at the mouth. The seizures could last approximately 1 min, but the patient could not recall the details during seizures. Her epilepsy relapsed many times during the course of the disease, and the symptoms were similar each time. Fortunately, no seizure attacks had occurred in recent 4 years after she began treatment with carbamazepine (0.1 g tid).

Five days before admission, the patient was admitted to the local hospital due to parturition and received epidural anesthesia with lidocaine (0.1 g) and ropivacaine (0.9 g) prior to a cesarean delivery. However, seizures began after 5 min of anesthesia and recurred twice during the following operation, and these attacks were not addressed by doctors. After the patient gave birth to a boy, her seizures frequently relapsed every 2–5 min, lasting for 20–60 s each time, and she was unconscious between attacks. As a result, she was admitted to the neurology intensive care unit (NICU) in our hospital.

Upon admission, the patient was unconscious and had persistent clonic twitches of her right limbs. An electroencephalogram (EEG) showed a long-range outbreak of spike and wave discharges in both hemispheres. A head CT scan revealed decreased density of the left parietal lobe, right temporal lobe, and right cerebellum. First, she was injected with 20 mg of diazepam (DZP), which failed; then, we increased the bolus dose to 30 mg, followed by an infusion of 80–100 mg for 10 h, but her seizure frequency decreased only slightly. Therefore, we used valproic acid (VAP) treatment (a bolus of 1200 mg,

X. Wang
Department of Neurology, The First Affiliated Hospital of Chongqing Medical University, Chongqing Key Laboratory of Neurology, 1 YouYi Road, Chongqing 400016, China
e-mail: xfyp@163.com

X. Wang, S. Li (eds.), *Refractory Status Epilepticus*, DOI 10.1007/978-981-10-5125-8_10

followed by an infusion of 1200 mg/day), but the results were not satisfactory. On the second day, midazolam was used with a bolus of 10 mg, followed by 5–10 mg/h infusion. However, status epilepticus (SE) continued, and the patient presented dyspnea and decreased oxygen saturation. As a result, propofol anesthesia (a bolus of 100 mg) was added soon after intubation and mechanical ventilation. This time her SE was controlled for 40 min; therefore, infusion was maintained at a rate of 100 mg/h, and the seizure interval was reduced to 2–5 h during propofol infusion. Unfortunately, she began twitching frequently again on the morning of day 3; thus, propofol was stopped and was substituted by two boluses of clonazepam (2 mg/bolus), which was also ineffective. Thus, DZP combined with propofol was selected. We first injected 40 mg of DZP followed by a continuous infusion of 100 mg. An injection of propofol (100 mg) was also simultaneously administered. Five minutes later, we obtained immediate, complete clinical and EEG control. On day 4, the patient's condition and EEG remained stable, and she gradually regained consciousness. She was successfully extubated 5 days later and was uneventfully discharged from the NICU on day 11.

10.1.2 Case Analysis

1. In this case, an established epilepsy patient exhibited seizures during cesarean delivery, which developed into SE that was resistant to five anticonvulsants for 3 days, consistent with the definition of RSE.
2. The woman had no seizures for 4 years before the operation, but seizures relapsed after use of anesthetics; therefore, anesthetic-induced epilepsy should be considered in this patient.

10.1.2.1 Epileptic Seizures During the Perioperative Period

It is known that seizures often occur without warming, and no method exists to predict seizure occurrence. However, the risk of seizures is increased when patients are subjected to certain conditions such as during the perioperative period, which should be noted. By investigating patients with or without epilepsy, researchers have found that the incidence of anesthetic-induced seizures is 0.031% in typical patients [1]; however, in epileptic patients, the seizure incidence could be as high as 3.4%, and if the patients have suffered from seizures within 1 month of the preoperative period, the seizure incidence could be up to 18.7% [2]. In addition, for preoperative patients who experience seizures more than once per week, the anesthetic-induced seizure rate is 26.3% [2]. All data indicate that the risk of anesthetic-induced seizures is much higher in epilepsy patients than in patients without this disease.

10.1.2.2 Lidocaine and Ropivacaine Can Induce Epileptic Seizures

Satsumae [3] reported a patient with a history of febrile convulsions who suffered from a generalized seizure after he received a brachial plexus block with ropivacaine (300 mg). Tsai [4] et al. also reported a young man who immediately experienced seizures after local anesthesia using lidocaine. These results are supported by other studies including a report by Rezvani [5]. In this case, the patient received both lidocaine and ropivacaine, which produces a higher risk of anesthetic-induced seizures.

10.1.2.3 Reasons for Epileptic Seizures During the Perioperative Period

The reasons for epileptic seizures during the perioperative period are not clear; they may be related to several factors. First, the serum concentrations of antiepileptic drugs (AEDs) are decreased in cases of jejunitis before surgery, and poor gastrointestinal function could result in slow drug absorption, both of which could induce epileptic seizures [2]. Second, anesthetics can induce epileptic seizures by inhibiting ion channels or exciting N-methyl-D-aspartic acid (NMDA) receptors [6].

10.1.2.4 Treatment of Anesthesia-Induced SE

Anesthesia-induced SE often occurs during the perioperative period while under monitoring by medical professionals, and these patients have the opportunity to receive timely and effective treatment. However, if treatment fails, the seizures could develop into RSE, as reported by Kim [7].

Most anesthesia-induced SE is multidrug resistant and exhibits no response to initial treatment; thus, polytherapy should be considered when initial treatment fails. For the treatment of the patient described here, we previously initiated DZP and propofol monotherapy separately, but her seizures were not resolved. However, the seizures were terminated after combined DZP and propofol administration, indicating that polytherapy may be a rational protocol for anesthesia-induced SE.

10.1.2.5 Prophylaxis of Anesthesia-Induced SE

Not all anesthetics induce seizures, but when anesthesia is necessary for epilepsy patients, anesthetics that exert the strongest seizure-promoting effects, such as sevoflurane, desflurane, enflurane, etomidate, and methohexital, should be avoided. It is better to choose anesthetics that have a lower risk of inducing epileptic seizures, such as midazolam combined with propofol. Additionally, it has been found that anesthesia-induced seizures are often related to the concentrations of anesthetics. When the concentration of sevoflurane is below 1MAC, the incidence of anesthesia-induced seizures is markedly decreased, and similar results are observed when the concentration of lidocaine is below 15 mg/ml [6].

10.2 Case 2: The Misdiagnosis and Mistreatment of Status Epilepticus and Epilepsy

Abstract

Non-epileptic seizures that occur following a head injury are often misdiagnosed as post-traumatic epilepsy, which is treated using long-term administration of AEDs. During the course of this treatment regimen, AEDs can cause seizures and drug-induced systemic lupus erythematosus (SLE), which are generally not detected in affected patients in a timely manner. The subsequent use of high-dose methylprednisolone treatment induces status epilepticus, and low-dose propofol aggravates the onset of epilepsy, which leads to the emergence of adverse consequences. In this report, we discuss the key factors that are targeted during the identification of epileptic and non-epileptic seizures following a head injury, the methods used to diagnose hyperventilation syndrome, the characteristics and differential diagnosis of drug-induced SLE, and precautions that should be taken when using both methylprednisolone and propofol.

10.2.1 Case Summary

The patient was a 24-year-old female. In June 2009, the patient was riding a motorcycle on her way home and was injured after being struck head-on by a vehicle. The patient was unresponsive on the ground, and bystanders immediately sent her to the local hospital for treatment. A physical examination indicated a left-sided occipital hematoma that was 2 × 3 cm; a physical examination of the patient's cranial nerves and limbic nervous system indicated no obvious abnormalities. A CT scan of the patient did not indicate a skull fracture or an intracranial hematoma. After 22 days of hospitalization, the patient's condition improved, and she was discharged. After discharge, the patient experienced intermittent dizziness and headaches. After 6 months, the patient presented with numbness of the left hand, which lasted for approximately 10 min, self-improved, and was not accompanied by a loss of consciousness, chest tightness, or respiratory difficulty. These symptoms were recurrent, with a duration from 2 to 30 min. The family's description of the events indicated that the patient had three episodes that included limb twitching, a fall, and an unknown level of consciousness. In July 2010, as a result of the frequent occurrence of the patient's limb twitching, the patient was emergently transferred to the local hospital, where a physical examination indicated that the patient was unable to answer questions and had shallow breathing and positive bilateral pathological reflexes; the patient was ultimately diagnosed with SE. An intravenous injection of 20 mg diazepam was administered, and the episode was terminated. The routine blood work indicated that the patient's white blood cell count was 8.2×10^9/L, her electrolytes were normal, and the partial pressure of carbon dioxide was 37 mmHg (normal 35–45 mmHg). An EEG examination revealed paroxysmal slow waves (another EEG examination indicated a similar episode), and an MRI of the brain suggested no abnormal findings. The patient was hospitalized for 6 days and did not exhibit further seizure activity; a repeat blood panel indicated normal results. The partial pressure of carbon dioxide was 42 mmHg, which had improved; thus, the patient was discharged from the hospital. The patient was discharged with a prescription for carbamazepine 0.1 g tid. The patient continued to have occasional episodes; thus, the carbamazepine dose was adjusted to 0.1 g in the morning and at noon and 0.2 g in the evening. The patient gradually stopped taking her medications over a 4-month period. Family members subsequently reported that the patient had an episode of unresponsiveness, which was described as a sudden, unexplained "daze" that was, in some cases, accompanied by a slight twitch at the left side of the patient's mouth, during which the patient was unresponsive to verbal commands. Afterwards, the patient could not recall the event, and she had repeated episodes with similar symptomatology. The duration of each episode was very short. Family members claimed that the duration of each episode was not more than 1 min, and the episodes occurred once every 3 months. The patient was readmitted, and her prescription for carbamazepine was changed to 0.2 g tid. In March 2011, the patient was admitted to the hospital for general surgery as a result of abdominal pain, and a routine preoperative examination indicated that the patient had a white blood cell count of 1.2×10^9/L. She was positive for antinuclear antibodies and lupus cells. A routine scalp EEG examination was without exception, and an immediate request was made for a neurology consultation. Considering the patient had SLE-induced seizures, hormone therapy was recommended. The subsequent day, the patient was started on 1000 mg of methylprednisolone via intravenous infusion. More frequent seizures occurred 4 days later. The patient was transferred to the intensive care unit (ICU), where 20 mg of intravenous DZP was administered with no effect. The treatment protocol was repeated 10 min later, once again with no effect. Sodium valproate was administered without an effect. On the ninth day after admission, 200 mg of continuous intravenous propofol (2 h) was initiated, and blood tests indicated that the patient's serum sodium level was 128 mmol/L. On the tenth day after admission, the patient died, which resulted in a doctor-patient dispute.

Autopsy report: The patient had a normal appearance of the skull, with no skull fracture. Extensive swelling in the brain tissue, shrunken ventricles, an obvious cerebellum, and a cerebellar tonsil embedded in the foramen magnum were noted. The morphologies of both sides of the hippocampus were normal, symmetrical, and displayed no hardening or atrophy. A microscopic examination showed that the number of neurons was normal, glial hyperplasia was not identified, and silver staining of the slices indicated no obvious mossy fiber buds. An examination of the other body organs did not indicate pathological changes consistent with SLE.

10.2.2 Case Analysis

10.2.2.1 Seizures After a Head Injury

Head injuries may cause seizures; however, more often than not, these seizures are non-epileptic. It must be determined whether the onset of seizures after a head injury is epilepsy, in addition to identifying the diagnostic criteria for epilepsy according to the common presentation (i.e., sexual, transient, stereotyped, and repetitive) and personality changes (which are characteristic of this type of seizure) that determine epilepsy. The relationship between a head injury and epilepsy should be determined by the following factors:

1. The time of epilepsy: in general, the onset of seizures after headache occurs within 1 week after a head injury or 1 week to 2 years after the head injury. The former is referred to as early-onset epilepsy, which is rarely recurrent and does not require special treatment. The latter is referred to as delayed epilepsy, and the possibility of recurrence is high.
2. Accompanying factors: these factors include whether the onset of seizures after a head injury is also related to the head injury severity. An epidemiological survey indicated that head injuries with concomitant skull fracture, cerebral contusion, intracranial hematoma, or a duration of >24 h of amnesia in patients produce a greater risk for seizures. If none of these four factors are present, then there is a limited chance of a seizure because there is no basis for an epileptic seizure to occur.
3. Types of seizures: SE and generalized tonic-clonic seizures may occur after a head injury; however, the more common seizure types are partial seizures, whereas other types of seizures are rare. If the patient presents with other types of seizures, the relationship of the seizure to the head injury is not significant.
4. Non-epileptic seizures after head injury are diverse and, in general, do not have a stereotypical seizure presentation pattern.
5. Epilepsy after a head injury is often refractory, and traditional drug treatments are not ideal. If various drug treatments have no effect, the clinician must consider the presence of epilepsy after a head injury. In this case, despite the time of onset and seizure type, the drug treatment effects were similar to epilepsy that presents after a head injury; however, the patient's head injury was mild, and there was no basis for a lesion that was induced by a traumatic brain injury. These findings do not support the presence of epilepsy after this patient's head injury, and it was more likely that the patient had non-epileptic seizures after her head injury [8–10].

10.2.2.2 Hyperventilation Syndrome

Hyperventilation syndrome (HVS) is one of the most common onsets of the disease, and its variable presentation may be easily misdiagnosed as epileptic seizures. In general, it is thought that the occurrence of HVS is related to psychological factors; however, the prevalence of HVS in patients with neurological disorders is often not the result of psychological trauma. In addition, the mere presence of the disease may be its predisposing factor, particularly when the ineffectiveness of chronic disease treatment is more likely to be an incentive. In the present case, the patient with non-epileptic seizures secondary to a head injury was both misdiagnosed and treated for epilepsy, which produced an ineffective treatment course. The patient was prone to develop HVS under long-term stress [11, 12].

According to the literature, HVS does not necessarily occur when the respiratory rate is accelerated; increasing the volume of the breaths may also induce clinical seizures. The general diagnosis of clinical HVS is based on the following characteristics: (1) The reproducibility of symptoms. When HVS is considered, the patient may be given excessive ventilation and, this may induce the same or similar performance at the time of onset. (2) Blood gas analysis results in the normal-to-low range: the partial pressure of CO_2 would be decreased or in the normal-to-low range based on blood gas measurements obtained during the seizure period compared to those obtained during the intermittent period, which corresponds to the initial onset of the seizure compared to 4 h after the onset, respectively. (3) Excessive ventilation may lead to respiratory alkalosis, and when it reaches a specific level, there may be diffuse or focal neurological damage; seizures are not uncommon in these situations. At this point, there may be a transition from the original non-epileptic seizures to real SE. Therefore, the existence of excessive HVS in a patient's history should not be overlooked because of the existence of organ damage. (4) HVS is complex: limb twitching in patients is very common and is a presentation that requires special attention.

For the patient in this case, the episode in July 2010 was accompanied by significant difficulty in breathing and a normal-to-low partial pressure of CO_2. This was a completely different presentation from the apnea of epileptic seizures; in addition, the duration of the episode was longer than the duration of a typical seizure. Therefore, HVS cannot be ruled out in this case.

10.2.2.3 Side Effects of Carbamazepine

The serious adverse effects caused by carbamazepine include rash and arrhythmia. In addition to these common side effects, carbamazepine may cause epilepsy and pseudo "SLE" and drug-induced hyponatremia. Patients with long-term use of carbamazepine may have blood that appears anti-nuclear antibody positive, and the presence of lupus cells is possible. Once identified, the patient cannot simply be diagnosed with SLE; the clinician must consider the adverse effects caused by the drugs. Identification may be considered from the following aspects: (1) In general, carbamazepine-induced lupus appears in the long-term medication administration process. Toepfer [13] reported a case of a patient with medication-induced SLE that occurred after 8 years of treatment with carbamazepine. Therefore, if the use of short-term carbamazepine may produce "lupus," the possibility of primary disease must be considered. (2) If the patient with drug-induced SLE stops using their prescribed AEDs, clinical manifestations may self-correct, and the amount of anti-nuclear antibodies will be significantly reduced, whereas real SLE is rarely self-limiting. (3) Compared with nonpharmacological SLE, drug-induced SLE produces anti-double-stranded DNA and anti-SSA antibodies that are not obvious, and the amount of complement reduction is less than the former.

This patient had been taking carbamazepine; however, the patient also had clinical manifestations of a transient "absence" of clinicopathologic symptoms and blood tests with lupus cells, and in addition to considering the presence of SLE, the clinician must also consider the presence of drug-induced SLE. If the drug could have been stopped at this time, a series of iatrogenic lesions may have been subsequently avoided. In addition, the hyponatremia in this patient might be related to carbamazepine because diluted hyponatremia was observed, and treatment should have consisted of limited water intake. Death resulting from increased salt and water intake is not a rarity in clinical practice.

10.2.2.4 Methylprednisolone

The current treatment regimen of SLE advocates large doses of methylprednisolone; however, the most serious side effect of methylprednisolone is that it causes SE. In the presence of epilepsy, the use of methylprednisolone should be monitored with particular vigilance. Once the original episodes are aggravated or there is an emergence of new types of seizures, the consideration of the possibility of drug-induced injury or a reduction or withdrawal is a reasonable choice; moreover, continuing the medication is not conducive to patient health.

10.2.2.5 Treatment of SE with Propofol

When two or more first-line AEDs fail in the treatment of SE, the seizure activity may be subsequently diagnosed as RSE. RSE is advocated by the use of treatment with propofol; however, low doses of propofol may induce SE, and only high doses of propofol play an antiepileptic role in SE. Therefore, in clinical applications, high-dose intravenous infusions should be advocated for rather than a low-dose method. In this case, the use of low doses of intravenous infusions to treat SE was clearly unreasonable.

The diagnosis and treatment of epilepsy are an art. Not only are the diagnosis and treatment very complex, but comorbidities with epilepsy are also very common, which make it easy to misjudge. In the general epilepsy center, the typical misdiagnosis rate is approximately 20% [12, 14, 15]. In the initial treatment of this patient, the non-epileptic seizures after the patient's head injury were misdiagnosed as epilepsy, which led to the long-term use of AEDs. As a result of this misdiagnosis, the standard medications will not be effective. In addition, long-term episodes as a negative factor that causes psychogenic disorders are common in the clinical practice of epilepsy. As a result of the rare side effects of common drugs that are seldom understood, the clinicians in this case did not make timely and correct clinical decisions, which ultimately contributed to the occurrence of a poor prognosis in this patient.

References

1. Akavipat P, Rungreungvanich M, Lekprasert V, et al. The Thai Anesthesia Incidents Study (THAI Study) of perioperative convulsion. J Med Assoc Thai. 2005;88(Suppl 7):S106–12.
2. Niesen AD, Jacob AK, Aho LE, et al. Perioperative seizures in patients with a history of a seizure disorder. Anesth Analg. 2010;111(3):729–35.
3. Satsumae T, Tanaka M, Saito S, et al. Convulsions after ropivacaine 300 mg for brachial plexus block. Br J Anaesth. 2008;101(6):860–2.
4. Tsai CJ, Wang HM, Lu IC, et al. Seizure after local anesthesia for nasopharyngeal angiofibroma. Kaohsiung J Med Sci. 2007;23(2):97–100.
5. Rezvani M, Finkelstein Y, Veriee Z, et al. Generalized seizures following topical lidocaine administration during circumcision: establishing causation. Paediatr Drugs. 2007;9(2):125–7.
6. Zhao X, Wang X. Anesthesia-induced epilepsy: causes and treatment. Expert Rev Neurother. 2014;14(9):1099–113.
7. Kim MJ, Lim DG, Yeo JS. Refractory status epilepticus occurred at the end of sevoflurane anesthesia in patient with epilepsy. Korean J Anesthesiol. 2013;65(1):93–4.
8. Ritter AC, Wagner AK, Fabio A, Pugh MJ, Walker WC, et al. Incidence and risk factors of posttraumatic seizures following traumatic brain injury: A Traumatic Brain Injury Model Systems Study. Epilepsia. 2016;57:1968–77.
9. Bennett KS, DeWitt PE, Harlaar N, Bennett TD. Seizures in children with severe traumatic brain injury. Pediatr Crit Care Med. 2017;18:54–63.
10. Dautovic E, de Roos C, van Rood Y, Dommerholt A, Rodenburg R. Pediatric seizure-related posttraumatic stress and anxiety symptoms treated with EMDR: a case series. Eur J Psychotraumatol. 2016;7:30123.
11. Rapin A, Deslee G, Percebois-Macadre L, Jonvel AC, Demangeon S, et al. Which treatments for the hyperventilation syndrome in adults? Rev Mal Respir. 2017;34:93–101.
12. Doss RC, LaFrance WC Jr. Psychogenic non-epileptic seizures. Epileptic Disord. 2016;18:337–43.
13. Toepfer M, Sitter T, Lochmuller H, Pongratz D, Muller-Felber W. Drug-induced systemic lupus erythematosus after 8 years of treatment with carbamazepine. Eur J Clin Pharmacol. 1998;54:193–4.
14. Oto MM. The misdiagnosis of epilepsy: appraising risks and managing uncertainty. Seizure. 2017;44:143–6.
15. Tinuper P, Bisulli F, Cross JH, Hesdorffer D, Kahane P, et al. Definition and diagnostic criteria of sleep-related hypermotor epilepsy. Neurology. 2016;86:1834–42.

MIX
Papier aus verantwortungsvollen Quellen
Paper from responsible sources
FSC® C105338

If you have any concerns about our products,
you can contact us on
ProductSafety@springernature.com

In case Publisher is established outside the EU,
the EU authorized representative is:
Springer Nature Customer Service Center GmbH
Europaplatz 3, 69115 Heidelberg, Germany

Printed by Libri Plureos GmbH
in Hamburg, Germany